Scientific Basis of Medical Imaging

Scientific Basis of Medical Imaging

Edited by
P. N. T. Wells

Department of Medical Physics,
Bristol General Hospital, Bristol

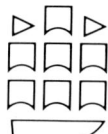

CHURCHILL LIVINGSTONE
EDINBURGH LONDON MELBOURNE AND NEW YORK 1982

CHURCHILL LIVINGSTONE
Medical Division of Longman Group Limited

Distributed in the United States of America by Churchill Livingstone Inc., 19 West 44th Street, New York, N.Y. 10036, and by associated companies, branches and representatives throughout the world.

© Longman Group Limited 1982

All rights reserved. No part of this publication may be reproduced, stored in a retrieval system, or transmitted in any form or by any means, electronic, mechanical, photocopying, recording or otherwise, without the prior permission of the publishers (Churchill Livingstone, Robert Stevenson House, 1–3 Baxter's Place, Leith Walk, Edinburgh, EH1 3AF).

First published 1982

ISBN 0 443 01986 X

British Library Cataloguing in Publication Data
Wells, P.N.T.
   Scientific basis of medical imaging
   1. Imaging systems in medicine
   I. Title
   616.07′5   R857.06

Library of Congress Catalog Card Number 81–68397

Printed and bound in Great Britain by
William Clowes (Beccles) Limited, Beccles and London

Preface

A new medical specialty is rapidly evolving, and there is little time for those who are involved to build the necessary foundations. The horizons of radiology are expanding beyond traditional X-ray imaging to embrace computed tomography, radionuclide and ultrasonic imaging, thermography and nuclear magnetic resonance imaging. In parallel with this, there is fresh insight into the processes of image perception, and there are now quantitative methods of image evaluation.

This new specialty is known as *medical imaging*. The rapidity of its evolution, and the importance of its impact on clinical medicine, make it vital for everyone concerned to have a grasp of its scientific basis.

This book aims to meet the needs of doctors, radiographers, technicians, engineers and physicists involved in medical imaging. The contributors have chosen a level similar to that of articles published in, for example, *Scientific American*. The fundamental principles are described in easily understood physical terms, with the use of mathematics restricted to the minimum necessary to convey essential concepts without recourse to wordy and unsatisfactory descriptions.

Oliver Heaviside, a great scientist, once asked: 'Shall I refuse my dinner because I do not fully understand the process of digestion?' Likewise, readers who find that some of this book is hard to grasp should not be discouraged; it is inevitable, with such a vast and complex subject, that the contributors have had to cite references to key publications where lack of space has made this necessary.

I make no apology for this. The new specialty of medical imaging is one which will depend, to an increasing extent, on collaboration between experts. This book establishes its foundation in physics, engineering, technology and medicine; each expert needs a thorough knowledge of matters for which he is responsible, and a working familiarity with others' problems. If there is something which you don't understand, *ask your expert colleague to explain it!*

Our objective is to inform those involved in medical imaging about the scientific basis of the techniques which they use every day, so that they will use them better. I believe that the contributors have been remarkably successful in achieving this, and I am grateful to them all.

Bristol   P. N. T. Wells
1982

Contributors

E. R. Andrew
Department of Physics, University of Nottingham, University Park, Nottingham NG7 2RD, UK

M. Susan Chesters
Department of Medical Physics, University of Leeds, The General Infirmary, Leeds LS1 3EX, UK

Malcolm Davison
Department of Clinical Physics and Bioengineering, Greater Glasgow Health Board, 11 West Graham Street, Glasgow G4 9LF, UK

G. A. Hay
Department of Medical Physics, University of Leeds, The General Infirmary, Leeds LS1 3EX, UK

C. H. Jones
Physics Department, The Royal Marsden Hospital, Fulham Road, London SW3 6JJ, UK

R. E. O'Mara
Division of Nuclear Medicine, University of Rochester Medical Center, 601 Elmwood Avenue, Rochester, NY 14642, USA

D. A. Weber
Division of Nuclear Medicine, University of Rochester Medical Center, 601 Elmwood Avenue, Rochester, NY 14642, USA

P. N. T. Wells
Department of Medical Physics, Bristol General Hospital, Bristol BS1 6SY, UK

Contents

1. **Traditional X-ray imaging** — 1
   G. A. Hay

2. **X-ray computed tomography** — 54
   Malcolm Davison

3. **Radionuclide imaging** — 93
   D. A. Weber and R. E. O'Mara

4. **Ultrasonic imaging** — 138
   P. N. T. Wells

5. **Thermographic imaging** — 194
   C. H. Jones

6. **Nuclear magnetic resonance imaging** — 212
   E. R. Andrew

7. **Perception and evaluation of images** — 237
   M. Susan Chesters

Index — 281

1

Traditional X-ray imaging

G. A. Hay

THE HISTORY AND NATURE OF X-RAYS

The discovery and nature of X-rays

X-rays were discovered by Wilhelm Konrad Röntgen in 1895.[32] They are often called 'roentgen rays' (particularly in the USA). They are emitted from the positive electrode in an electrical discharge tube through which a current is passing. One of their first applications was in the 'medical' field: Röntgen made a radiograph of his wife's hand showing the soft tissue and bone structure and the great radiopacity of the wedding ring. The properties of X-rays that are of significance in medical radiology are: (1) they penetrate matter to a greater or lesser degree; (2) they produce ionisation and excitation in the atoms of matter; (3) they produce fluorescence and hence visible light from certain materials; (4) they affect photographic emulsions; and (5) they produce biological effects in living tissues.

During the next two decades it was shown that X-rays were a form of electromagnetic radiation. They therefore share that strange duality peculiar to such radiation: that is they behave as a wave motion in space and are emitted and absorbed in the form of discrete particles of energy, known as quanta or photons.

The particulate nature of X-rays

The wavelengths of the X-rays used in medical diagnostic radiology range from about 100–5 pm, corresponding to a range of quantum energies from about 10–200 keV. Such quantum energies are relatively so large (visible light has a quantum energy of about 3 eV), however, and the devices used to detect X-ray images are so sensitive, that the particulate nature of X-rays is clearly evident in clinical practice. Therefore it is more useful to refer to the quantum energy of the radiation rather than to its wavelength, and this we shall do in the remainder of this chapter.

X-RAY IMAGE FORMATION AND DETECTION

When a beam of X-rays from an X-ray tube falls on a patient, interactions take place between energy and matter, and part of the energy is removed from the beam either by absorption or by scattering. The energy remaining in the beam that emerges unmodified from the patient carries information about the internal structures of the body in the form of a distribution of intensity perpendicular to the beam axis. This distribution in any given plane may be called the *X-ray image*, and the process may be called *X-ray image formation* (Fig. 1.1).

X-ray energy is not directly visible; therefore the X-ray image is allowed to fall on an X-ray image transducer. This converts the X-ray image into visible form in which it is detected and perceived by the visual system of the radiologist. Transduction may occur almost instantaneously, as in fluoroscopy, or there may be a time delay between transduction and perception, as in radiography.

It is common practice to consider the whole process from the X-ray tube to the radiologist's brain as one, yet considerable simplification in treatment is possible by dividing the process into three, as shown in Figure 1.1. The divisions occur naturally at the X-ray image and at the visible light image, as shown.

Most X-ray imaging processes produce a two-dimensional representation of a three-dimensional

2 SCIENTIFIC BASIS OF MEDICAL IMAGING

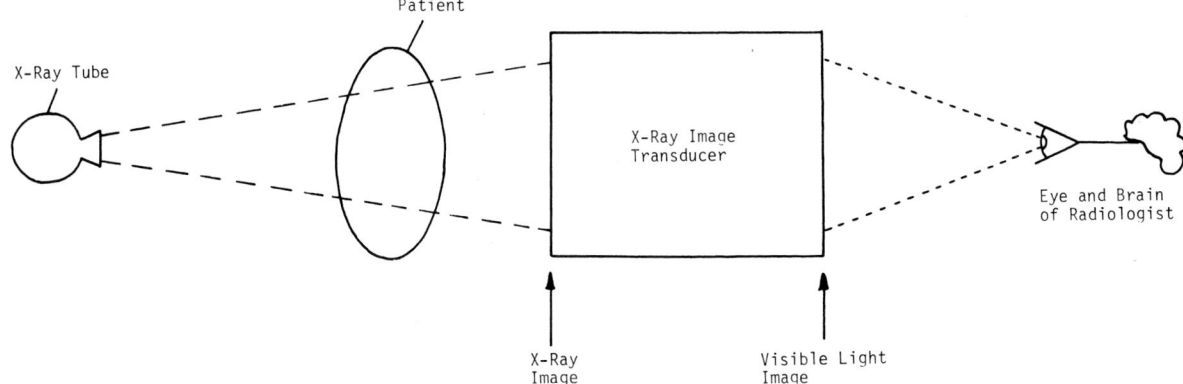

Fig. 1.1 A typical X-ray diagnostic system, showing the formation of the X-ray image, its transduction into a visible light image, and the detection and perception of the latter by the radiologist.

object. The relative intensities (contrasts) in this representation convey information about the radiological thicknesses (attenuations) of various structures in the body parallel to the beam axis, whereas the spatial distribution of the intensities conveys information about the shapes and fine structures of the organs of the body perpendicular to the beam axis. Because the X-ray image is a *shadowgraph*, no unequivocal interpretation in terms of body structure is possible (except in the case of tomographic techniques (p. 11). It is sometimes said whimsically of the medical radiologist that often he can diagnose a pathological condition only when he already knows what it is! Nevertheless, medical radiology is an invaluable and essential adjunct to other clinical methods of diagnosis.

THE PRODUCTION OF X-RAYS: X-RAY SPECTRA

X-ray tubes

In a modern X-ray tube for diagnostic use (Fig. 1.2a) electrons from a heated filament *in vacuo* are attracted to an anode or *target* by a potential difference ranging from 30 kVp (kV peak) to 200 kVp (most usually from 60–120 kVp). There they interact with the atoms of the target to produce X-rays, which are then emitted through the walls of the tube, in particular through the tube *window*. The production of X-rays is accompanied also by very large amounts of heat, less than 1 per cent of the electron energy being converted into X-rays.

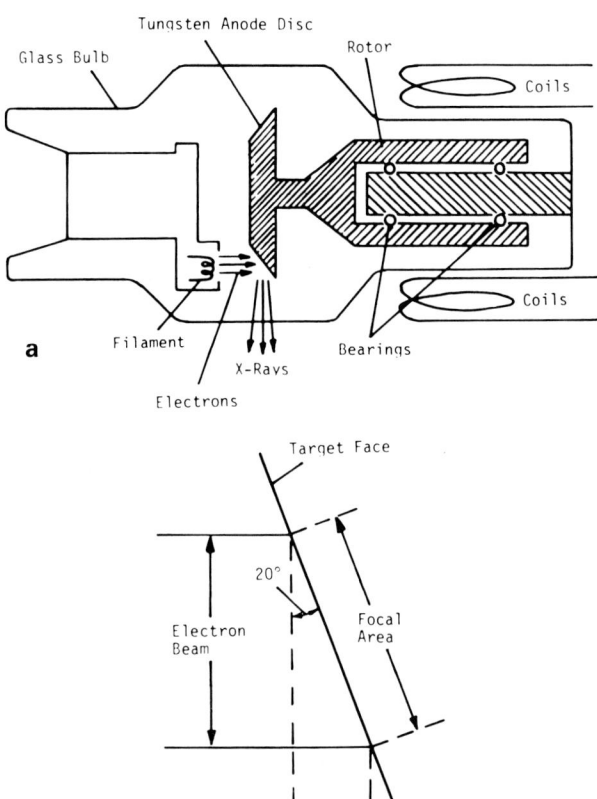

Fig. 1.2 (a) A modern rotating-anode diagnostic X-ray tube in diagrammatic form. The rotor is part of an induction motor; its bearings are dry-lubricated for the life of the tube. (b) Showing how a relatively large area of electron bombardment (focal area) can be made to appear as a small effective source size by steep angulation of the target face.

This creates a crucial difficulty for the X-ray tube designer, who must ensure that the heat is removed from the bombarded area (the *focal area*) of the target sufficiently fast to ensure that the focal area does not become excessively hot and therefore deteriorate or even melt. This is done in several ways, of which two are important in diagnostic radiology and are shown in Figure 1.2. First, the target is made in the form of a disc (with a bevelled edge) which is caused to rotate whenever X-ray emission is required; thus the heat is spread out over the periphery of the disc from which it is mainly radiated but partially conducted away. Nevertheless, the X-rays appear to emerge only from that small area of target opposite to the filament. Second, the angulation of the target periphery, combined with the long narrow shape of the filament, as shown in Figure 1.2b, ensures that the electrons are spread out over a long narrow rectangle (known as *line focus*) although the X-rays appear from the direction of the patient to emanate from a roughly square area (the *effective focal spot*). Focal spot sizes in diagnostic radiology range from about 0·1–2 mm square, though because of difficulties in electron focusing the X-ray intensity is far from uniform over this area. Clearly, the smaller the effective focal spot size, the sharper is the X-ray image (see p. 11), and in practice a compromise must be sought between size and heat dissipation.

The nature of the target material is important. For clinical work tungsten is in almost universal use because it has a high melting point, reasonable thermal conductivity, desirable mechanical properties and a high atomic number which increases the efficiency of X-ray production.

X-ray tube spectra and outputs

The fundamental physical processes at the target of an X-ray tube[16] lead to three products: (1) heat (> 99 per cent); (2) a continuous spectrum of X-rays (Bremsstrahlung); and (3) a spectrum of X-rays that is characteristic of the electron energy levels of the target material (characteristic radiation). The latter appears only when the incident electron energy is sufficient to displace electrons from the inner shells of the tungsten atoms (about 70 keV). The two X-ray spectra are superimposed on each other but the continuous spectrum represents the greater proportion of energy and hence is the more important.

Figure 1.3 shows typical X-ray spectra produced in a variety of conditions. Each spectrum has an upper energy limit that is determined by the maximum kVp across the X-ray tube; in such a case the whole energy of the maximum-energy electron is converted into Bremsstrahlung. The remainder

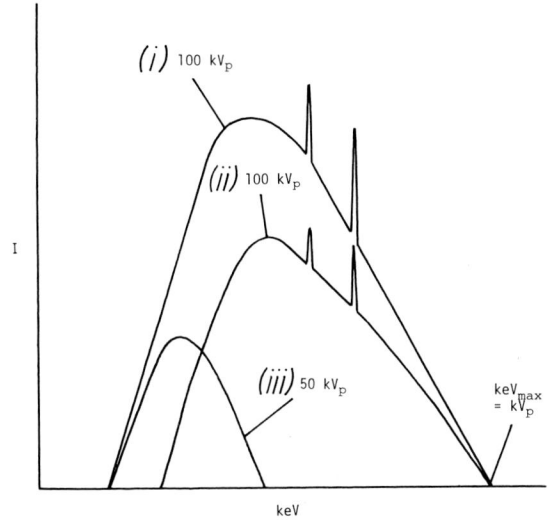

Fig. 1.3 Typical X-ray spectra: (i) 100 kV$_p$ showing both continuous and characteristic X-radiation; (ii) same kV$_p$ but heavier filtration showing decreased proportion of low-energy (soft) radiation and decreased total radiation intensity (exposure rate); and (iii) 50 kV$_p$ showing decreased peak keV, absence of characteristic radiation and decreased total radiation intensity (exposure rate).

of the continuous spectrum is composed of quanta that have been produced by electrons, only part of whose energy has been converted into X-rays. This mixture comprises the continuous spectrum. The characteristic lines of the tungsten atom are evident in spectra (i) and (ii), but not in (iii) because the maximum electron energy lies below 70 keV.

X-rays of high quantum energy (*hard* X-rays) are more penetrating than those of low quantum energy (*soft* X-rays) (Fig. 1.3). Hence if a *filter* of aluminium or copper is placed in the beam, the soft X-rays are attenuated to a greater extent than are the hard X-rays; the whole beam becomes more penetrating and is said to be *harder*. This technique is of importance in clinical radiology because the softer components in a spectrum are preferentially absorbed in the superficial layers of patient tissue nearest to the X-ray tube, with unwanted biological effects. Therefore it is customary partially to remove the soft components by means of an aluminium filter, though a more radical solution is to ensure that the potential difference across the X-ray tube is always at its maximum, i.e. is *constant potential* and not *pulsating*. Constant-potential generators, or their equivalent, are rapidly displacing the older pulsating voltage generators from the modern X-ray department. They have the outstanding advantage that not only is less soft X-radiation produced but that the heat that would have accompanied its production is absent also, thus rendering the X-ray tube design easier.

If the X-ray tube current (colloquially called the 'mA') is changed, the intensity of the X-ray output changes in proportion.[16] If the potential difference across the tube (colloquially called the 'kV') is increased, two things happen. First, the X-ray output intensity increases in proportion approximately to the square of the kV change, and second, the beam as a whole becomes more penetrating (harder), because all the components of the continuous spectrum become harder and also because the characteristic radiation (if any) increases in intensity.

The quality of an X-ray beam

It is often desirable to specify the *quality* or penetrating power of a beam of X-rays. As this consists of a complex spectrum, it cannot be done unequivocally in terms of quantum energy. In such a case recourse is had to a concept known as the *equivalent energy* of the beam. The latter is passed through various thicknesses of matter, and the thickness of a given material (for example, aluminium) that reduces the beam to one-half of its intensity is noted. This is called the *half-value layer* of the beam in that particular material. The measurement is then repeated using monoenergetic sources of X-rays and the quantum energy of the monoenergetic X-ray beam that has the same half-value layer as the beam in question is known as its equivalent energy. For example, the equivalent energy of a spectrum produced by 100 kVp across the X-ray tube is about 60 keV. (For other equivalents see Fig. 1.7).

THE INTERACTION OF X-RAYS WITH MATTER

The exponential law of absorption

In the absence of matter, X-rays obey the same laws of propagation as does all electromagnetic radiation. In particular, their intensity (energy per unit area per unit time) varies inversely as the square of the distance from a point source of the radiation. A small increase in the source size makes hardly any difference to this *inverse-square law*. Hence it is valid for the average diagnostic X-ray tube. Moreover, in the useful clinical range of quantum energies the attenuation caused by air can be neglected.

When X-rays traverse matter, interactions take place between the energy (in quantum steps) and the matter, and part of the energy in the incident beam is removed from the beam, partly by absorption and partly by scattering, both by the atoms of the matter. An explanation of those aspects of the phenomenon relevant to the diagnostic range of quantum energies follows.[16]

Assume that a monoenergetic beam of X-rays falls upon matter. If the intensity of the incident radiation is I_o, that of the transmitted intensity I, and the thickness of the matter is x cm, then

$$I = I_o \exp(-\mu x) \qquad (1.1)$$

μ is called the *total linear attenuation coefficient* of that particular kind of matter for that particular monoenergetic radiation. It is clearly the fractional decrease per centimetre for that radiation in that substance. This law may be recognised as the ubiquitous *exponential* law; equal incremental thicknesses of matter produce equal fractional decrements in intensity. Note that this law is not followed exactly in the case of heterogeneous radiation, i.e. for the radiation from an X-ray tube. Nevertheless it is a useful approximation, particularly in the case of heavily filtered beams, and is used here to demonstrate some of the basic phenomena of X-ray image formation.

The mechanisms of X-ray interaction with matter

The exponential law of attenuation describes the gross phenomenon, and does not differentiate between the various interactions that cause it. These, in the diagnostic range of quantum energies, are as follows:

1. If X-ray energy interacts with a tightly-bound electron in one of the inner shells of an atom of the matter, the electron may be ejected completely from the atom, forming a so-called *secondary electron*. This, having low energy, is soon absorbed by excitation or ionisation giving rise to heat in the material. The vacant place in the inner shell of the atom is filled by an electron from a shell farther out, the energy change giving rise to the emission of a quantum of radiation characteristic of the atom. The process is analogous to that which results in the production of characteristic radiation from the target of an X-ray tube (see p. 3). In this case, however, the quantum energy of the characteristic radiation is very low because of the generally low atomic number of the materials concerned, and therefore the low binding energy of the electron shells. Hence this characteristic radiation is very soon absorbed, and thus the whole of the energy of the original interacting quantum is absorbed and appears as heat. This process is called *photoelectric absorption*. The contribution it makes to μ, the total linear attenuation coefficient, is usually called τ. Figure 1.4 shows the variation of τ with quantum energy.[9] It is seen to be inversely proportional to the cube of the keV. It is also proportional to the fourth power of the atomic number of the material. These are facts of the utmost importance in diagnostic radiology.

2. If X-ray energy interacts with a less tightly-bound electron in an atom of the matter, the electron behaves as though it were free, and recoils in a direction at an angle to the path of the incident energy. This is called a *Compton interaction* or *Compton scatter*. The energy of this electron is soon absorbed by ionisation and excitation processes and appears as heat. It represents energy that is truly absorbed, and the contribution it makes to μ is usually called σ_a. The quantum of X-ray energy, on the other hand, is scattered away in another direction, and, though it loses energy in the collision, it may still have sufficient to escape from the material completely. It is energy that, though not truly absorbed, may nevertheless be removed from the beam; the contribution it makes to μ is usually called σ_s. It is called *Compton scattered radiation*.

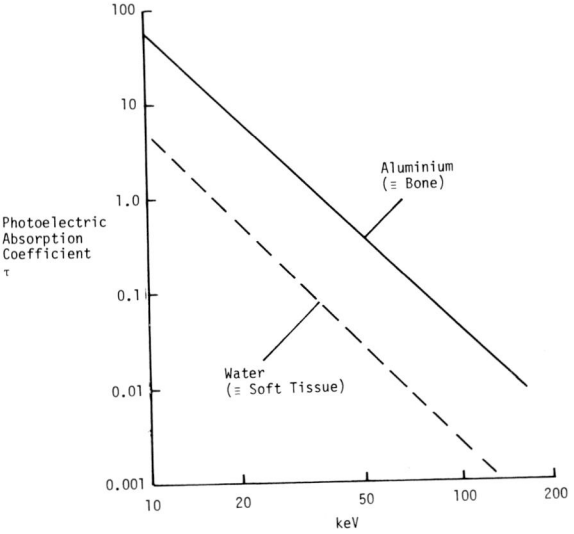

Fig. 1.4 The variation of the linear photoelectric absorption coefficient τ with keV for water (representing soft tissue) and for aluminium (representing bone).

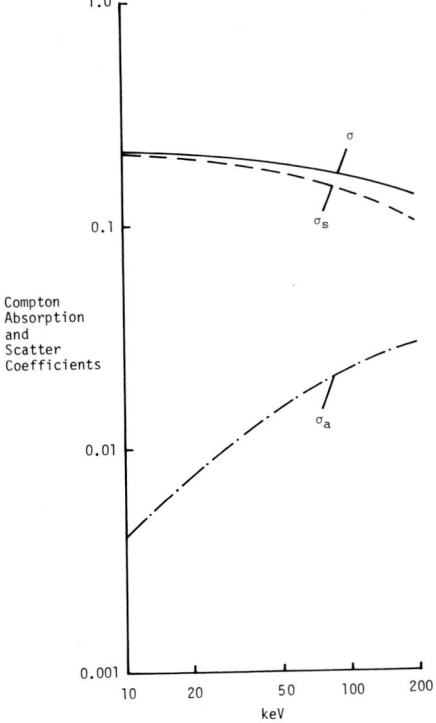

Fig. 1.5 The variation of Compton absorption and scatter coefficients (σ_a, σ_s) and their sum (σ) with keV. Note that (contrary to popular belief) the scatter component does not increase with kV.

Figure 1.5 shows the variation of σ_a and σ_s, and also that of their total ($\sigma_a + \sigma_s = \sigma$), with quantum energy.[9] Scattered radiation is of the utmost importance in diagnostic radiology. It helps to produce contrast (p. 6) it may destroy contrast (p. 8) and it can irradiate radiological personnel with undesirable biological consequences.

GENERAL RELATIONSHIPS IN THE CLINICAL PROCESS

Information in continuous and intermittent exposures

X-ray beam intensity may be expressed in the form of X-ray exposure rate, measured in roentgens per unit time ($R\,s^{-1}$) or some related units. The roentgen is a measure of the ionisation produced in air by the X-rays under carefully specified conditions.[33] (Exposure rate may also be measured in SI units, viz in $C\,kg^{-1}\,s^{-1}$.) X-ray energy, however, is absorbed in the transducer in the form of discrete quanta. Intuitively, the information available to the transducer and hence to the ultimate detector is an increasing function of the quanta absorbed (p. 18). In other words, each quantum can be loosely regarded as a *unit* of information. Hence, for a given X-ray spectrum, the amount of information carried by the X-ray beam is an increasing function of the X-ray exposure to the transducer.

For exposures of finite duration, e.g. in radiography, this concept presents no difficulty. In a typical case an X-ray exposure of about 1 mR ($2.5 \times 10^{-7}\,C\,kg^{-1}$) produces a photographic density of 1.0. It is indicated on page 36 how this exposure may in general be related to information. In continuous examinations such as fluoroscopy, however, it is highly unlikely that the information conveyed to the observer accumulates without limit as time progresses. In this case the information is determined by the system *storage time*, which is usually determined by a little-understood temporal parameter of the human brain, normally assigned a value of about 100 ms. Thus for a typical exposure rate of 50 $\mu R\,s^{-1}$ ($1.29 \times 10^{-8}\,C\,kg^{-1}\,s^{-1}$), the perceived information is associated with an exposure of $50 \times 0.1 = 5\,\mu R$ ($1.29 \times 10^{-9}\,C\,kg^{-1}$). (From the present point of view, this value compares unfavourably with 1 mR for a radiograph; this partially explains the great difference in information content and hence in quality of image between the two techniques.) If artificial means are used to increase the system storage time, information *can* be accumulated, theoretically without limit. To a certain extent this is what the time-integrating property of the photographic emulsion achieves.

Typical attenuation of X-rays in the clinical situation

The medical X-ray image-forming process is unfavourable to the problem of instrumentation design. The mean exposure in the beam emerging from an average chest is only one-tenth of the incident exposure, from an antero-posterior abdomen only one-hundredth, and from a lateral abdomen only one-thousandth. Yet the incident exposure to the patient must be kept within limits set by the maximum permissible exposure to the individual (for somatic effects) or to the population (for genetic effects). Thus the transducer must always be a highly sensitive device. This is achieved in radiography by photographic sensitivity and time integration, and in modern fluoroscopy by energy gain in a form of image intensifier.

CONTRAST

Contrast represents the relationship between two exposures or intensities or luminances, usually adjacent. It is the contrast between adjacent areas that enables the interface between two radiopacities to be detected. Therefore contrast is a factor of outstanding importance to the radiologist.

Mechanisms of contrast formation

Contrast has many definitions; the one we shall use at present is in the form of the natural logarithm of a ratio. For an area of intensity I, against a background I_o, the X-ray contrast $C_r = \ln(I_1/I_o)$.

What are the processes by which contrast is formed in the X-ray image? When an X-ray beam, within the diagnostic range of quantum energy, is incident on a patient, three different types of behaviour can be envisaged: (1) Energy can proceed directly in a straight line through the patient to be absorbed in the transducer. *This is the only energy that conveys direct information about the structures of the patient.* (2) Energy can be truly absorbed from the beam by a photoelectric interaction (τ). (3) Last, but not least important, energy can take part in a Compton interaction, part being truly absorbed (σ_a) and part scattered (σ_s). In both parts energy is removed from the beam; the Compton scatter process is thus wholly beneficial in contrast formation. If the scattered part of the energy proceeds in such a direction that it falls on the transducer surface, however, it *reduces* contrast, because it represents energy that has not travelled in a straight line from the X-ray source to the transducer and that therefore is not directly related to the patient structures. It is a common fallacy that the process of Compton scatter is wholly deleterious to contrast. It is only its by-product, however, *scattered radiation*, that may reduce contrast. In many practical situations, if it were not for the contrast-forming action of the Compton scatter process, there would be no contrast at all! For example, Table 1.1 shows the fraction of the total linear attenuation coefficient (μ) that is due to Compton scatter ($\sigma = \sigma_a + \sigma_s$), for water (representing soft tissue) and for aluminium (representing bone), at various quantum energies. For soft

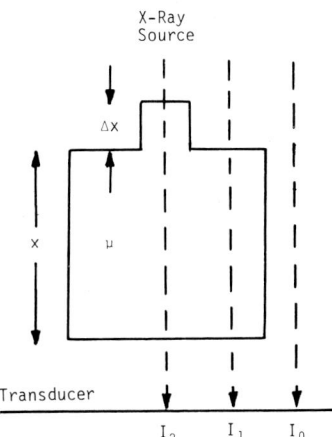

Fig. 1.6 A simulated 'patient' of thickness x and total linear attenuation coefficient μ with a 'tumour' of thickness Δx.

Calculation of primary contrast

The primary X-ray contrast, i.e. the contrast in the beam whose rays travel in a straight line from the X-ray focus to the transducer, can be calculated making certain approximations, and the result reveals a number of important principles of X-ray image formation. Imagine a 'patient' of linear attenuation coefficient μ cm^{-1} and thickness x cm as represented in Figure 1.6, having a 'tumour' of thickness Δx cm which it is desired to detect by X-ray examination. With the notation of Figure 1.6, and assuming monoenergetic X rays

$$I_1 = I_0 \exp(-\mu x), \text{ and } I_2 = I_0 \exp -\mu(x + \Delta x)$$

hence the contrast produced by the tumour is expressed as:

$$C_r = \ln(I_2/I_1) = -\mu \Delta x \qquad (1.2)$$

Several interesting conclusions can be drawn from Equation 1.2:

1. The contrast is the negative of the structure; for example, the presence of an increment of matter in the beam results in a decrement in X-ray exposure.

2. The contrast is proportional to the linear attenuation coefficient of the material.

3. The contrast is proportional only to the tumour thickness, and does not depend at all on the patient thickness. This conclusion is at first sight remarkable, as practical experience shows that contrast decreases rapidly with increase of total patient thickness x. The conclusion is indeed true for the

Table 1.1 The fraction of the total linear attenuation coefficient μ that is due to the Compton scattered radiation σ_s.

keV	kVp	Water (= soft tissue)	Aluminium (=bone)
20	32	0·31	0·053
30	50	0·44	0·16
40	65	0·72	0·31
60	100	0·84	0·58
80	120	0·86	0·72
100	150	0·85	0·78
150	200	0·80	0·81

tissue, especially at high quantum energy, by far the greater part of μ results from Compton scatter (σ). There is a technique known as *high-kV radiography* (see p. 8) which is used to examine (among other things) lung fields for evidence of pathology. If it were not for the Compton scatter process no detail at all would be visible in the lungs. *Scattered radiation*, however, if it falls on the transducer, very significantly reduces contrast (see p. 8).

primary X-ray beam, however, the practical situation being influenced by the presence in large amounts of secondary or scattered radiation, causing a marked reduction in contrast (see next Section).

4. For a cavity of thickness Δx, $C_r = + \mu \Delta x$.

5. For an inclusion of attenuation coefficient μ_2 in a material of μ_1, a similar calculation shows that $C_r = - |\mu_2 - \mu_1| \Delta x$. This result is of especial significance for inclusions of bone and other highly absorbing materials in soft tissue.

Factors affecting primary contrast in practice

Important practical consequences of these conclusions are as follows:

1. Figure 1.7 shows that the linear attenuation coefficient of bone is greater than that of soft tissue; hence the contrast for detail *within* bone is greater than that for detail *within* soft tissue (for equal thickness differences).

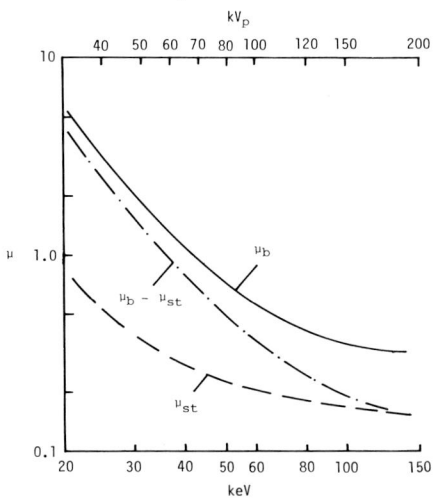

Fig. 1.7 The variation of total linear attenuation coefficient μ with keV and with kVp for bone and soft tissue. Their difference also is shown.

2. The linear attenuation coefficients of both soft tissue and of bone, and hence the contrasts *within* these body materials, decrease with increasing kVp (see Fig. 1.7).[9]

3. The difference in linear attenuation coefficient *between* soft tissue and bone, and hence the contrast *between* these body materials, decreases with increase of kVp (see Fig. 1.7). This effect is sometimes used in so-called *high-kV radiography*, from 150–200 kVp, when it is desired to preserve both bone and soft-tissue detail on the same radiograph.[30]

4. When it is desired to increase contrast above the normal, for example in the case of the digestive tract or of blood vessels that would normally be invisible because of inadequate contrast against their surroundings, a *contrast medium* may be used. This may consist of a material either of high μ, for example barium compounds ingested into the digestive tract or iodine compounds injected into the blood stream, or of a material of low μ, such as air injected into the ventricles of the brain. The introduction of contrast media is often accompanied by clinical risk, and alternative procedures are always to be preferred where available.

Calculation of the effect of scattered radiation on primary contrast

The reduction of primary contrast by scattered or secondary radiation is not so easily calculated. Secondary radiation is the scattered by-product of the Compton process that falls on the X-ray transducer. A rigorous treatment of its effect is complex, but the magnitude of these effects can be simply deduced by regarding the scattered X-rays as a uniform *flood* of radiation at the transducer surface. The effect is analogous to the loss of contrast in the image from an optical slide projector when the room lights are switched on. (This simple treatment is less true for large X-ray-opaque objects.[19])

Suppose I_p is the mean primary intensity and I_s the mean secondary intensity ($I_s/I_p = s$); then the modified contrast

$$C'_r = \ln \left(\frac{I_2 + I_s}{I_1 + I_s} \right).$$

At low contrasts (common in radiology) $I_1 \sim I_2 \sim I_p$, and $C_r = \ln (I_2/I_1)$, so it is easily shown that $C'_r = C_r/(1 + s)$.
Therefore

$$C'_r = S\, C_r = -S\, \mu\, \Delta x \qquad (1.3)$$

where $S = 1/(1 + s)$ is the factor by which the primary contrast (Equation 1.2) is reduced by the presence of scattered radiation at the transducer surface.

Figure 1.8 shows the magnitude of this effect at

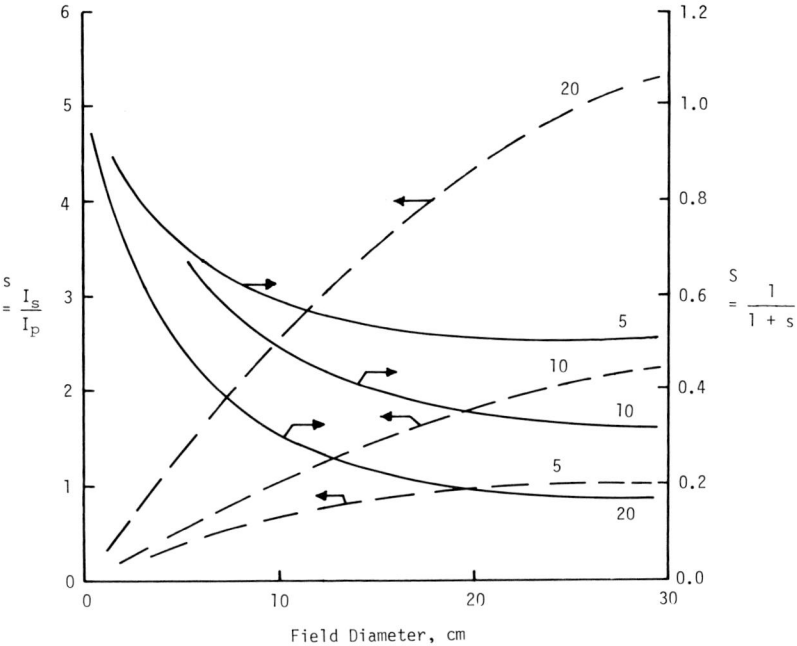

Fig. 1.8 The variation of scattered radiation expressed as a multiple of primary radiation (s), and the consequent fractional decrease of contrast (S), with field diameter and with patient (water) thickness in cm.

100 kVp for different patient thicknesses and X-ray field diameters. The ratio s has been both calculated and experimentally determined.[27] It increases both with patient thickness and with field diameter to values greater than five; in other words, in certain situations the greater part of the X-ray image consists of secondary or scattered radiation. The value of s increases also with kVp. σ_s and hence the absolute amount of scattered radiation actually decrease somewhat with increase of kV (see Fig. 1.5), but μ decreases rapidly with increase of kV (see Fig. 1.7), hence the amount of scattered radiation that actually emerges from the patient increases with kV.

This very large amount of scattered radiation must have a profound influence on contrast. The effect it has is shown by the factor S (see Fig. 1.8) which is calculated from s, as already explained. The contrast is seen to decrease to as little as one-fifth of the original value of the primary contrast. Another important source of image deterioration due to scattered radiation that is not often recognised is its effect in producing a background of X-ray quantum noise (see p. 18) that adds to the noise inherent in the signal and further reduces its detectability (see p. 39).

These deleterious effects cannot be tolerated in clinical radiology, and several methods are available to reduce the effects of scattered radiation. These are as follows:

1. The X-ray field size is reduced by adjustable lead diaphragms or by fixed conical field limiting devices to the minimum practicable for the particular examination. This is known as *coning down*.

2. The patient thickness may be reduced where possible by compression; it is obviously necessary to displace the patient tissues rather than merely air, however, and the application of the technique is limited.

3. An air space (or *exit gap*) may be left between the patient and the transducer surface. This ensures that scattered radiation emerging at an oblique angle has a greater probability of missing the transducer.

4. The kVp is reduced as far as practicable. It must be high enough, however, to ensure adequate penetration of the patient by the primary radiation.

5. The most important and effective method is

to use a device that provides greater absorption for the oblique secondary radiation than for the primary radiation. A flat metal foil can be used, but by far the most effective device is a *secondary-radiation grid* or *diaphragm* which consists of lead slats (separated by low-atomic-number material) orientated in the direction of the primary radiation. This is illustrated in Figure 1.9. The first grids consisted of parallel strips of lead, but later grids (so-called *focused grids*) have their slats orientated in the direction of the X-ray source. This avoids the selective attenuation of the primary radiation towards the edges of the parallel grid where the primary rays are no longer parallel to the slats. The grid ratio is the ratio of the depth of the lead slats to the distance between them; grids are also characterised by the number of slats per inch or per centimetre. Of course, grids absorb a considerable portion of the primary radiation as well as a large part of the scattered radiation; the ratio of primary transmission to secondary transmission is known as the *selectivity* of the grid.[25] A high value of selectivity is clearly desirable.

A disadvantage of the technique is that the slats may produce a striped pattern in the X-ray image, but this is often prevented by moving the grid during exposure, as in the so-called *Potter-Bucky* diaphragm.

SHAPES AND FINE STRUCTURE; FOURIER TECHNIQUES

Radiological magnification and distortion

The X-ray image is a two-dimensional projection of a three-dimensional object. Hence no unique interpretation of the image in terms of patient structure is possible, partly because many layers of the patient are superimposed in the image. Moreover, because the image is formed by a divergent beam, both geometrical magnification and distortion occur and must be allowed for by the radiologist when making his diagnosis.

Figure 1.10 shows the imaging of an object of infinitesimal thickness x_0 mm wide by an X-ray tube with an infinitesimal effective focal spot. From similar triangles, the magnification is given by:

$$\frac{x_i}{x_0} = \frac{ST}{SO} \qquad (1.4)$$

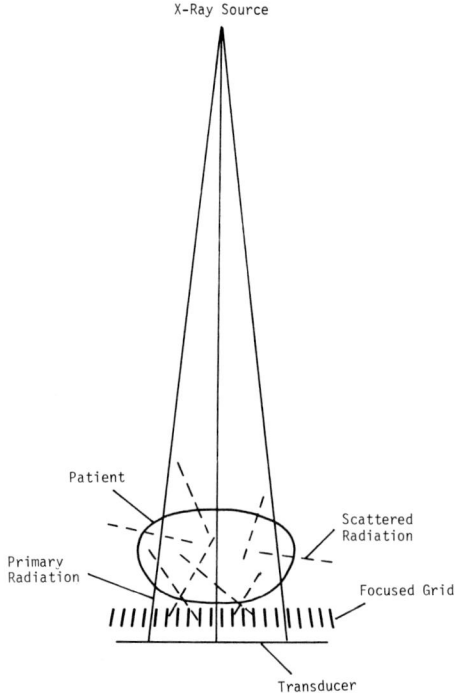

Fig. 1.9 Showing the action of a 'focused' secondary radiation grid in transmitting a large fraction of the primary radiation but absorbing a large fraction of the secondary or scattered radiation, thus improving contrast.

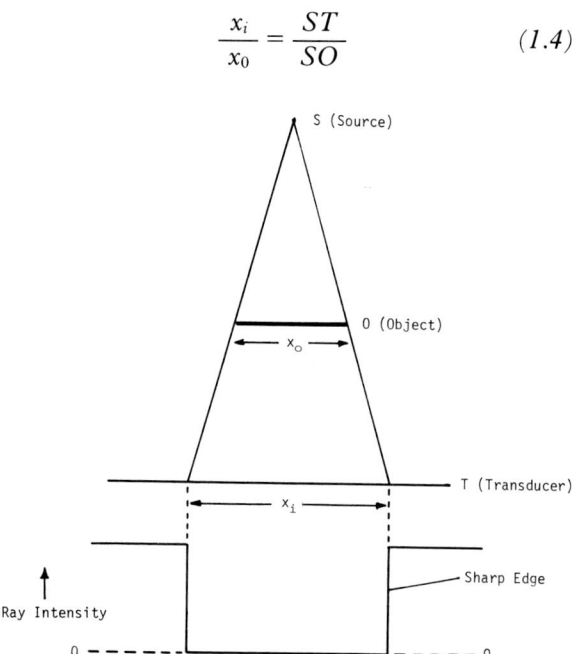

Fig. 1.10 The image of an object of infinitesimal thickness produced by an X-ray source of infinitesimal size. Note the magnification of the image and its 'sharp' edges.

Patients are not infinitesimal in thickness, however, and therefore the magnification varies for structures at different depths in the patient. This is called differential magnification. Equation 1.4 shows that the closer to the transducer is the structure of interest, the less is the magnification. If an infinitesimally thick object is in intimate contact with the input plane of the transducer, the magnification is unity. This situation is often approximated in chest radiography, when the X-ray tube is placed several metres from the patient and the latter is placed in contact with the transducer. This technique is especially valuable when it is desired to obtain an accurate estimate of heart size. Similarly, planar test objects are often placed as near to the transducer surface as possible to avoid undue magnification. In other radiographic techniques, it is often important to decide whether to make the exposure from front to back of the patient (antero–posterior, A–P) or vice versa (postero–anterior, P–A). In other situations, radiological magnification is deliberately encouraged (see p. 13), in which case it is called *macroradiography*. The technique of macroradiography affords an excellent example of the type of compromise that enters into every radiological technique, but before describing it unsharpness must be discussed.

Figure 1.11 shows the imaging of a three-dimensional object (a sphere) in two positions in the X-ray field. Intuition suggests that when the sphere lies on the perpendicular from the focal spot to the centre of the field, the image is nearly circular. On the other hand, when the sphere is near the periphery of the field, the image is an ellipse. This effect is called differential distortion. It is important because the dimensions of the patient are appreciable compared with the geometry of the image-forming system. These effects must be taken into account by the radiologist when interpreting the image.

Unsharpness or blurring: tomography

The ideal X-ray source is infinitesimal in size; also the ideal X-ray transducer would form a light image that reproduced the X-ray image without any degradation of sharpness. In practice, such ideals are unattainable. The finite size of the focal spot and the imperfections of the transducer, as well as possible movement of the object, combine to produce *unsharpness* or *blurring* in the image. There are two possible types of analytical treatment of this effect: the first, the classical treatment, deals with the spatial domain, and the second, Fourier analysis, operates in the spatial-frequency domain. The basic phenomena in the spatial domain are described here first.

Figure 1.12 shows the effect on image sharpness of the finite size of the X-ray tube focal spot, assumed to produce an effectively square distribution of X-ray intensity. Its effect is to destroy the sharpness of the edge of the image and to produce a *penumbra* that in this simple example has a unique extent U_g, known as the *geometrical unsharpness*. If u_g mm is the extent of the effective focal spot size, then similar triangles show that

$$\frac{U_g}{u_g} = \frac{OT}{SO} \qquad (1.5)$$

If the object is in contact with the transducer, $OT/SO = 0$, and the geometrical unsharpness is zero. If, however, the object is taken closer to the X-ray source (as it is in macroradiography), the extent of U_g increases as indicated in Equation 1.5. This is one facet of the compromise mentioned previously. Geometrical unsharpness is two-dimensional but not necessarily isotropic, as X-ray focal spot distributions are rarely centrally symmetrical.

The above discussion applies to a stationary object. When patient structures are moving at all rapidly, for example the heart, or the intestine in irritable colon, a type of unsharpness known as

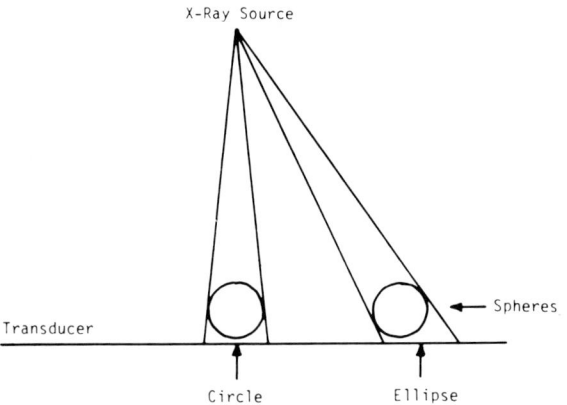

Fig. 1.11 Showing how the X-ray image is a two-dimensional representation of a three-dimensional object, also how distortion can occur in the image.

12 SCIENTIFIC BASIS OF MEDICAL IMAGING

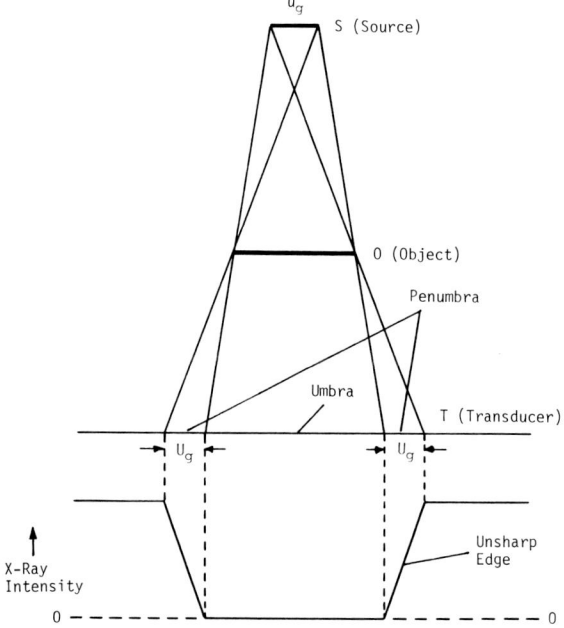

Fig. 1.12 Geometrical unsharpness: the effect of an X-ray source of finite dimensions in producing an unsharp image of an object.

movement unsharpness (U_m) is produced. Figure 1.13 shows a moving object in two extreme positions (separated by a distance u_m mm) imaged by an X-ray source of infinitesimal size. Again, similar triangles reveal that

$$\frac{U_m}{u_m} = \frac{ST}{SO} \quad (1.6)$$

Movement unsharpness obviously blurs the image of the desired structure and thus renders it less perceptible. For this reason the trend in radiography today is towards X-ray generators and tubes that can produce exposures with higher and higher tube currents (mA), amounting to as much as 2000 mA, thus enabling time exposures of the order of 10 ms to produce adequate density in the radiograph. Similarly, television camera tubes of exceedingly rapid response are now available (p. 32) which enable the image-intensifier-television image to be relatively free from movement unsharpness. In extremely high-speed cine-fluorography (200 frames s^{-1}) the movement unsharpness is set by the response time of the image intensifier itself (see p. 35). Movement unsharpness differs from geometrical unsharpness in that it is usually approximately unidimensional.

Movement unsharpness is usually a disadvantage. There is one radiographic technique, however, called tomography, in which it is used to great advantage. It was previously pointed out that the conventional X-ray image represents an infinity of planes in the patient, all superimposed on each other. In tomography, selective movement unsharpness is deliberately used to render more or less unsharp all planes but the one that it is desired to image. For example, studies of the middle ear are rendered possible which otherwise would be

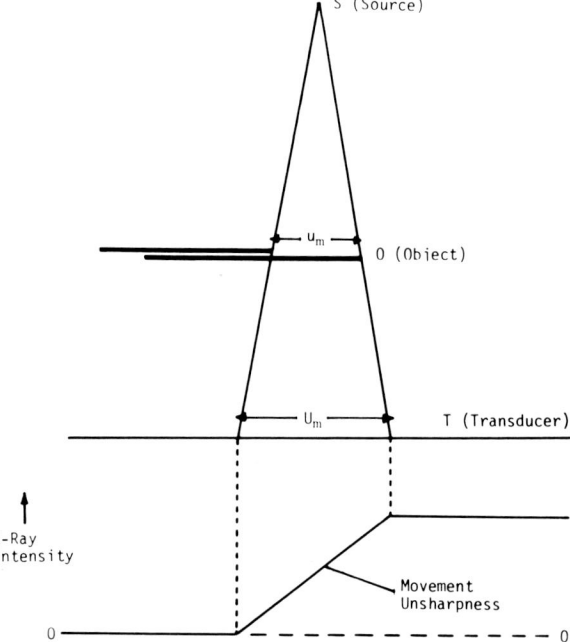

Fig. 1.13 Movement unsharpness: this shows how a moving object can produce an unsharp image of an otherwise sharp edge.

quite impracticable. Figure 1.14 shows how this is done. During the exposure, the X-ray source is moved through a certain distance, from position 1 to position 2. This results in the displacement of the image of the edge of the object from 1' to 2' on the transducer, which would normally result in gross movement unsharpness. Simultaneously with the source movement, however, the transducer is moved in the opposite direction by a corresponding distance so that the two positions 1' and 2' remain stationary on the transducer. Hence all details in the object plane A remain unaffected by movement

TRADITIONAL X-RAY IMAGING

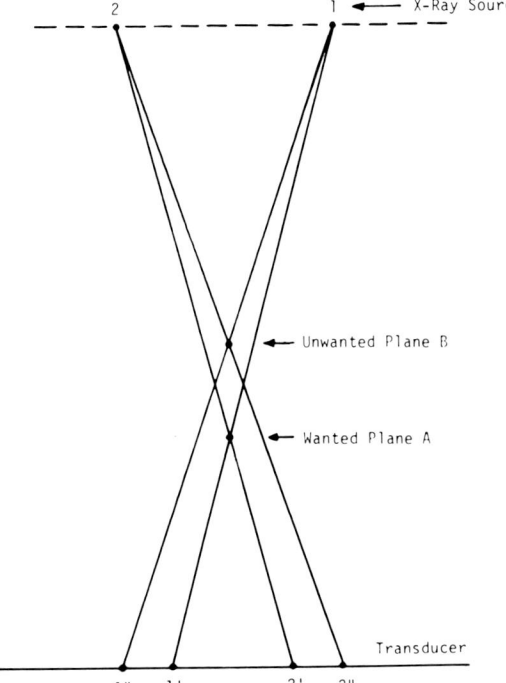

Fig. 1.14 The principles of tomography: as the X-ray source is moved from 1 to 2, the transducer is given a contrary motion of distance 1'2', thus retaining the sharpness of the wanted plane A. Because the images of structures in the unwanted plane B move through a different distance 1" 2", their images are subject to gross movement unsharpness, and therefore are less readily detectable.

unsharpness. The converse is true for details in all other planes, however, for example plane B. Figure 1.14 shows that the distance moved by the image of the object edge moves a distance 1" 2" that is different from 1' 2'. Hence all other planes suffer gross movement unsharpness which renders them less perceptible. Figure 1.14 implies a linear movement for ease of representation, but advantages are claimed for many other types of movement, e.g. circular and elliptical. Traditional tomography, though clinically invaluable, is not to be confused with the relatively new and powerful technique of computed tomography (*CT scanning*), which operates on an entirely different principle, and shares only a common etymology with the former (Greek τομος, a section; see Ch. 2).

Practical X-ray transducers introduce unsharpness into the light image they produce. Because most transducers in clinical use incorporate a fluorescent screen as a vital part of their functioning, this unsharpness is usually called *screen unsharpness* (U_s), though it can arise in many other components of a complex system, for example in electron optical devices and in electronic amplifiers. Screen unsharpness is approximately isotropic and is fully discussed later.

The three preceding types of unsharpness are all undesirable. There is a type of unsharpness, however, that is useful; it is usually called *absorption unsharpness* (U_a). Figure 1.15 shows the imaging of an object with a tapered edge. It is clear how the presence of the taper in the object introduces a type of unsharpness in the image intensity distribution. This unsharpness, however, is diagnostic of a characteristic of the object, and as such must be preserved and revealed at all costs. For example, its presence could reveal the difference between normal bone and bone whose cortex has been eroded for one reason or another.

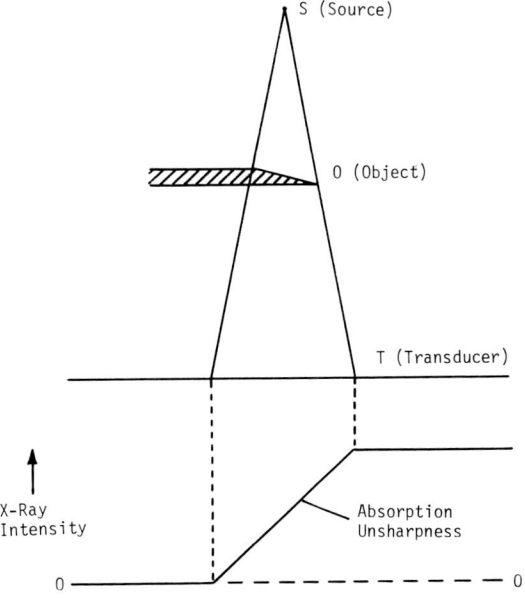

Fig. 1.15 Absorption or structure unsharpness: this shows how image unsharpness can often be diagnostic of structural details in the object.

The addition and effects of unsharpness

Unsharpness is difficult to analyse rigorously in the spatial domain. The examples of unsharpness so far considered are idealised, but in practice unsharpness is more complex. For example, the unsharpness profile of a fluorescent screen is roughly bell-shaped as in Figure 1.16. Two difficulties then arise: first, how is it possible to assign a unique value to its spatial extent, and second, how can the various unsharpnesses in a complex system be compounded? The rigorous answer to both difficulties

with the unsharpness, the only effect of the latter is to blur the edges of the resulting light image. As the slit becomes narrower, i.e. as the object becomes smaller, the edges of the slit approximate to each other, and the light image has a distribution midway between that of the X-ray image and the

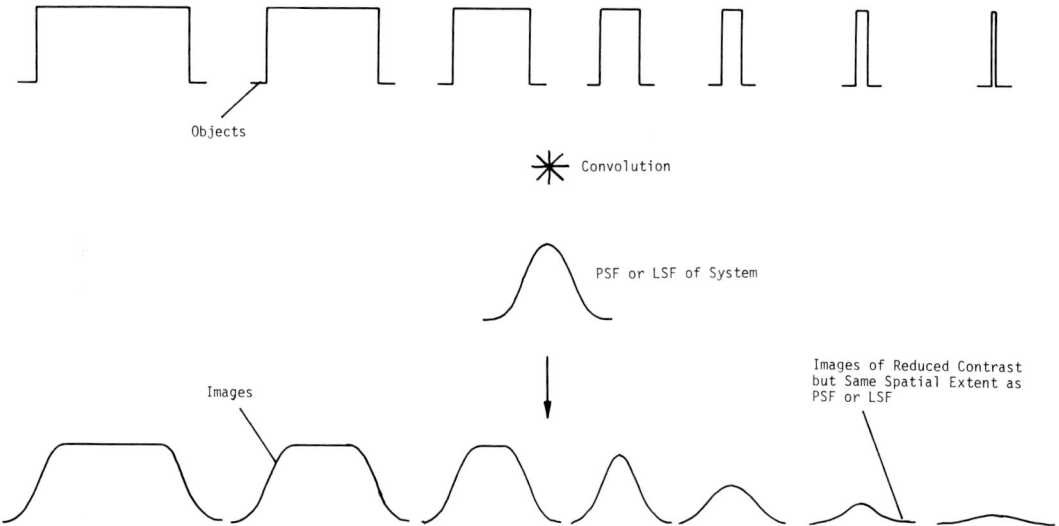

Fig. 1.16 The effects of unsharpness on isolated sharp details in an object: for large objects the image contrast is unaltered but the edges are rendered unsharp; for small objects the image contrast progressively decreases with decrease of object size but the image retains the extent of the point or line spread-function of the system.

lies either in a process called *convolution*, or by Fourier techniques in the spatial frequency domain (see p. 15), but for rough practical purposes approximations can be made. For example, the width of an unsharpness profile can be taken between, say, the 10 per cent levels in the distribution, and unsharpness can be compounded by a quadratic law: the total unsharpness U_t in a system is given roughly by

$$U_t = (U^2_g + U^2_m + U^2_s + U^2_a)^{1/2} \quad (1.7)$$

This equation, moreover, is exactly true if all the unsharpnesses are Gaussian in shape.

Unsharpness is an exceedingly important factor in radiological systems, hence before discussing Fourier analysis a brief resume of its most important effects is given. Figure 1.16 shows the effect of screen unsharpness on the X-ray image distributions produced by a number of slits cut in lead. When the incident X-ray image is wide compared

unsharpness profile. When the slit becomes narrower than the unsharpness, two things happen. First, the shape of the light image distribution loses the character of the original X-ray image and progressively takes on the form of the unsharpness profile. Second, the amplitude (contrast) of the light image decreases, being inversely proportional to the slit width (for unidimensional object distributions) but in the case of two-dimensional object distributions such as would be produced by circular apertures in the lead, the amplitude is inversely proportional to the square of the object diameter. This is one very important reason why small objects such as small stones (two-dimensional) and thin blood vessels (unidimensional) are difficult to see in radiology: their contrast has been markedly reduced by the overall unsharpness of the system.

The technique of *macroradiography*, or radiological magnification, was previously described as a typical example of a radiological compromise. The reason for this is as follows. When imaging an object with an X-ray source of finite size, as the object is separated from the transducer and approximated to the source, not only does the size of its image increase (Equation 1.4), but so also does the geometrical unsharpness (Equation 1.5). This may at first sight appear to be deleterious to image quality, especially as it can be shown from Equations 1.4 and 1.5 that

$$\frac{U_g}{x_i} = \frac{x_0}{u_g} \cdot \frac{OT}{ST} = \text{constant} \cdot \frac{OT}{ST} = \text{constant} \cdot OT$$

Hence as magnification is increased the geometrical unsharpness becomes an increasing proportion of the total image size.

The focal spot size, however, is not the only source of unsharpness in the system. The geometrical unsharpness U_g is added, roughly quadratically, to the transducer unsharpness U_s, and so long as the former is small compared with the latter, progressively increasing magnification results in the transducer unsharpness (which is constant) becoming an ever-decreasing fraction of the image size x_i, with a consequent improvement in image quality. When the degree of magnification is such that U_g becomes approximately equal to U_s further magnification results in a deterioration of image quality because of the dominance of the progressively increasing U_g. There is thus a break-even point of optimum image quality for each particular set of conditions. This break-even point is not sharply defined, and as the patient structures of interest are not often approximately in contact with the transducer, it is likely that many clinical procedures already automatically make partial use of this effect. Another facet of this compromise is that if the patient as a whole, as distinct from the structures of interest only, is separated from the transducer there is a welcome reduction in scattered radiation falling on the transducer, because of the *air-gap* effect (p. 8).

There are radiological techniques, however, where a deliberate use of macroradiography is found of value, for example in skeletal radiography and in the diagnosis of lung pathology. For these purposes it is obviously desirable to decrease U_g to a minimum by the use of an 0·3 mm or even an 0·1 mm focal spot.

Fourier techniques: modulation transfer function

We shall now discuss the application of Fourier techniques to the treatment of unsharpness. The ultimate constituent element of an image is a point. An ideal system would image a point object as a point image. Practical deficiencies lead to a spread of energy around the point, however, known as the *point spread-function (PSF)* (Fig. 1.17a). The PSF is variant in two dimensions, and thus is unnecessarily complex for analysis. Instead, we may consider a line object (e.g. a slit of infinite length and infinitesimal width in a lead plate), whose image is similarly spread in one dimension, forming the *line spread-function* (LSF) (Fig. 1.17b). (In both cases illustrated, some energy from the original point or line is shown scattered to quite large distances from its origin, giving the appearance of *skirts* to the PSF or LSF and resulting in a large-area contrast loss that is reminiscent of that resulting from scattered X-rays, see p. 8). This type of behaviour is particularly characteristic of image intensifiers (see p. 35).

How can we compound two LSFs? In the spatial domain, the process known as 'convolution' must be used as shown in Figure 1.18.[4, 26] By resolving the LSF into sinusoidal spatial-frequency components by the process known as Fourier transformation (FT), however, the two functions can be compounded by simple multiplication. The compounded LSF can then be recovered by inverse Fourier transformation. Fourier transformation essentially resolves the original function into sinusoidal components of infinite spatial extent that do not alter in waveform when processed by a linear system. In general, short, rapid spatial changes correspond to high spatial-frequency components and vice versa. Thus the reproduction of small, sharp detail demands a system that can transmit high spatial frequencies; on the other hand, the presence of large-area detail (e.g. the scattered energy in Fig. 1.17a) corresponds to very low spatial frequencies.[4, 26, 36]

Figure 1.17 shows also how the unsharpness of a system or process can be represented in the spatial-frequency domain by simple division; the result is called the *modulation transfer function* (MTF); it is a property of systems that is widely

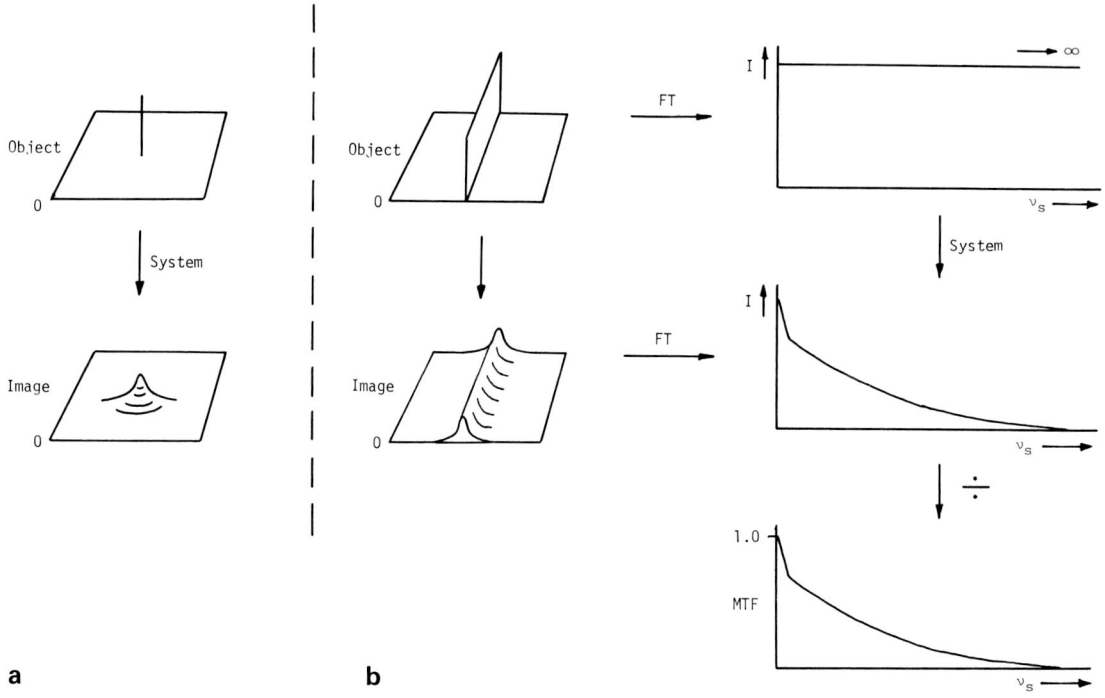

Fig. 1.17 (a) Point spread function (PSF). A point object can result in an unsharp image, energy being scattered in two dimensions, some to relatively large distances resulting in a large-area contrast loss. (b) The one-dimensional component of (a), the line spread-function (LSF), is an important property of an imaging system. By analysis of the LSF into sinusoidal components by Fourier analysis (FT: Fourier transform) the 'modulation transfer function' (MTF) of the system can be derived. ν_s represents spatial frequency in cycles mm^{-1}. The rapid drop in MTF near zero frequency represents the large-area contrast loss.

quoted. Figure 1.19 shows modulation transfer functions of typical radiological imaging systems. Any image can be resolved into a series of sinusoidal components of different spatial frequencies, amplitudes, phases and azimuths; by comparison of the frequency content of the signal with the MTF of the system it can be ascertained if that system can reproduce the signal without loss. It is generally accepted that most medical X-ray images contain little relevant information above a frequency of about 2 cycles mm^{-1}.

The use of the spatial frequency domain has both advantages and disadvantages. On the one hand, functions can readily be compounded by multiplication of their transforms (Fig. 1.18). On the other hand, Fourier transformation applies to linear systems, and no clinical radiological system even approaches linearity. Moreover, while a computer is required for convolution, so it is also for Fourier transformation.

X-ray tube intensity distributions

The ideal X-ray source is a point. In practice, the effective source area is the projection, in the direction of the patient, of the image of the X-ray tube filament on the target. Conventional tubes have long, narrow filaments; the effective source is then an approximately square distribution containing two adjacent peaks, as shown in Figure 1.18. In addition, much radiation is produced from other parts of the tube anode and by scatter from external parts of the tube housing. This is called *extra-focal radiation* and results in contrast loss similar to that caused by X-ray energy scattered in the patient.

It can be shown that the best finite source distribution is Gaussian,[38] and much effort is now being devoted to the production of tubes with Gaussian focal spots and with a minimum of extra-focal radiation.

The X-ray source distribution cannot be con-

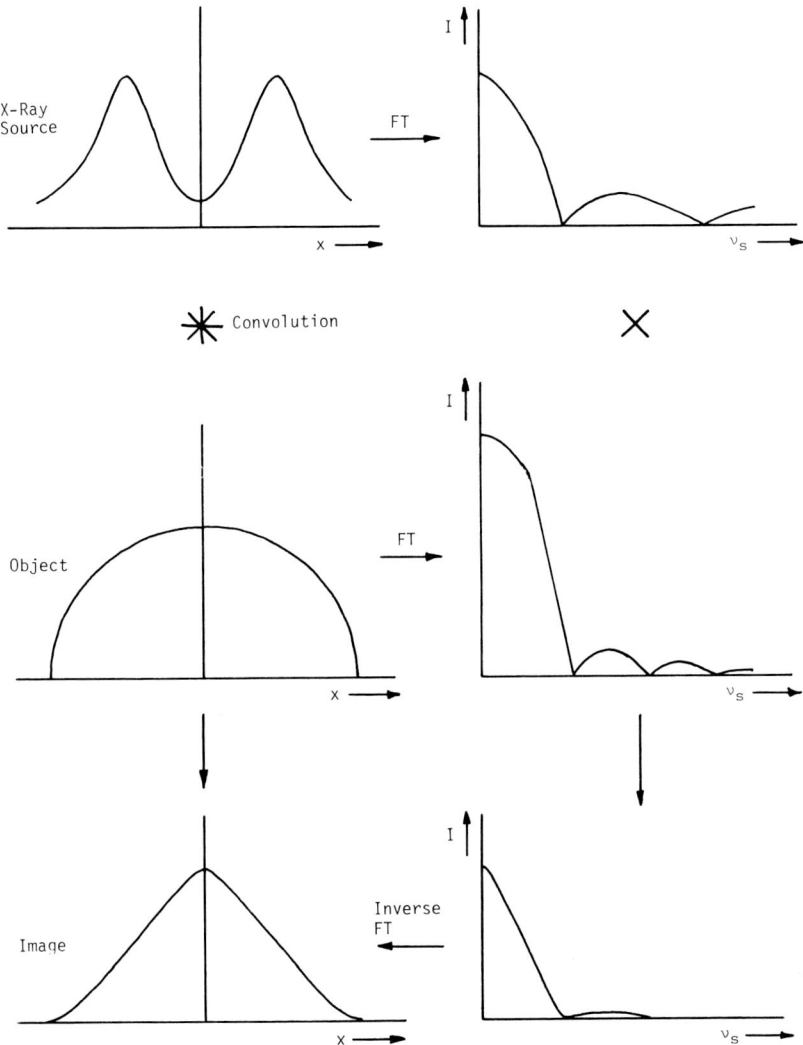

Fig. 1.18 Source and object distributions may be compounded by convolution to yield the resultant image distribution. An alternative method is simply to multiply the Fourier transforms (FT) and then to take the inverse Fourier transform. The X-ray source distribution is typical of a medical X-ray tube perpendicular to its long axis. The object distribution represents the X-ray image of a cylindrical object (such as a blood vessel with contrast medium) produced by a point X-ray source. The functions are to a certain extent idealised for ease of representation. I is intensity and ν_s spatial frequency.

sidered without reference to the heat produced at the X-ray tube target. The process of X-ray production is highly inefficient, less than 1 per cent of the electron energy appearing as X-ray energy. The size and distribution of the X-ray source are thus inextricably linked with the ability of the tube to dissipate heat from the electron-bombarded area. A well-known device to assist this process is the rotating-anode X-ray tube (see p. 2) and improvements in the direction of increased anode thermal capacity are currently being made.

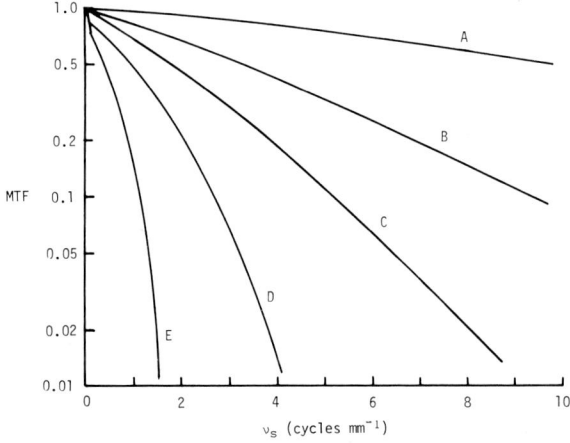

Fig. 1.19 Modulation transfer functions of typical X-ray imaging systems: A, 'non-screen' film; B, film with high-definition intensifying screens; C, film with medium-speed screens; D, a 150 mm CsI: Na image intensifier; and E, the same intensifier with television display. The intensifier-television system, and to a lesser extent the intensifier alone, exhibit the 'zero-frequency drop' which is characteristic of systems exhibiting large-area contrast loss, and which is absent in the screen-film systems. For comparison, many authorities believe that there is little important diagnostic information in the average medical X-ray image above about 2 cycles mm^{-1}.

X-RAY IMAGE TRANSDUCERS: FLUORESCENT SCREENS

Fluorescent screens: the quantum limit: noise

It is a remarkable fact that most X-ray image transducers in routine clinical use today commence with a simple fluorescent screen, which converts absorbed X-ray energy into light. The screen consists of a layer of powdered, crystalline, fluorescent material such as zinc-cadmium sulphide laid on a plastic or other substrate with a white reflective layer such as titanium oxide intervening. The fluorescent crystals most often include impurity atoms which have the effect of introducing free electrons into the crystal lattice (for example, caesium iodide with sodium impurity). X-ray energy is absorbed in the crystals in the form of quanta of energy; each quantum raises the energies of many free electrons to higher levels. When electrons return to the original energy levels, visible light is emitted whose colour is characteristic not of the particular atoms involved but of the crystalline substance itself. Part of the light emerges in a forward direction and is usefully emitted; that which is directed towards the substrate is partially reflected by the titanium oxide layer and some emerges in a forward direction.

The light that is emitted from the absorption of a single quantum of X-ray energy consists of a large number of photons whose emission is correlated in space and in time. Moreover, the absorption of the X-ray energy, which takes place predominantly by photoelectric interactions (as explained on p. 4), occurs within a very small volume of the fluorescent material (of the order of several μm in extent). Hence the absorption of a quantum of X-ray energy in an ideal fluorescent screen should be signalled by a flash of light of very small dimensions. The whole image is then made up of apparently infinitesimal flashes of light, and as the absorption of X-rays is a stochastic process, that is, random in space and time, the image is composed of flashes of light appearing randomly, the mean distribution of which composes the details of the light image. Thus the image does not have a smooth, continuous appearance, but appears rough and granular, the amount of information in the image, or in other words the quality of the image, depending on the average number of quantum absorptions per unit area per unit time, and hence on the exposure rate to the fluorescent screen (p. 6). This limitation to image quality that results from the limited number of absorbed X-ray quantum interactions is an exceedingly important concept in medical radiology and is known as the *X-ray quantum limit*. The random fluctuation about the mean intensity that is produced by the random X-ray quantum absorptions is called *noise*.

The preceding discussion depends on the ability of the observer to see every separate flash, and to compose the image in his brain from the aggregate of all the flashes. Whether or not this can occur is not at this point clear, but it is discussed later on page 28. Moreover, a less vital but still important fact is that it is assumed above that each flash (if it is seen at all) is seen as an infinitesimal point. Unfortunately, light scattering within the phosphor crystals, combined with the light that is directed back from the titanium oxide layer, causes each minute flash to degenerate into a blur of light. This process is the basis of *screen unsharpness* (U_s) (p. 11) or point spread-function (p. 15).

Characteristics of fluorescent screens

Important characteristics of screens are: (1) the fraction of X-ray energy absorbed; (2) the fraction of absorbed X-ray energy converted into light; (3) the fraction of such light usefully emitted; and (4) the PSF of the composite layer. To absorb a large part of the incident X-ray energy (an obviously desirable feature), a screen should be thick. A thick screen absorbs its own light radiation excessively, however, and also exhibits a large PSF due to light scatter. In practice, a suitable compromise must be sought between X-ray absorption efficiency (or *speed*) and unsharpness.

The simplest use of the fluorescent screen, common in clinical practice until the mid-1960s, was in traditional *fluoroscopy* or *screening*. The emergent beam from the patient (the X-ray image) fell on the fluorescent screen; the resulting light image was observed by the radiologist with the unaided eye. A sheet of lead glass between the screen and the radiologist protected the latter from transmitted X-rays. Although this technique permitted the observation of moving organs (for example, its use in oesophageal and stomach investigations) it is now obsolescent for reasons given later. The two main applications of the fluorescent screen are in radiography (in conjunction with a photographic emulsion) and in the image intensifier (in conjunction with a television camera for fluoroscopy or a small-format film camera for fluorography). In all uses of the fluorescent screen it is necessary to match its colour output to the colour sensitivity curve of the light detector. This is done by choice of a suitable material. Table 1.2 shows examples of screen materials in current use together with their important properties.[40, 46]

The fluorescent screen considered as an imaging device has many advantages: (1) it is linear (light output against X-ray input); (2) it has no background (except a small degree of spatial fluctuation due to its crystalline structure); (3) it has a high *quantum efficiency*, e.g. one absorbed X-ray quantum in zinc-cadmium sulphide gives rise to about 2000 photons usefully emitted in the forward direction. This property ensures that the information inherent in the original X-ray quantum has a high probability of being transmitted forward. On the other hand, the fluorescent screen exhibits un-

Table 1.2 Typical fluorescent screens used in clinical practice. The values shown for absorption and efficiency are approximate only. CsI:Na has an anisotropic structure that enables the conflicting requirements of thickness and unsharpness to be overcome (p. 35). $Gd_2O_2S:Tb$ is representative of a new class of phosphor and enhanced efficiency and X-ray absorption; these phosphors are being advocated for use in radiography, with dose reduction as their main advantage.

Substance and main application	Colour	Typical fraction of X-rays absorbed (η_a)	Fraction of absorbed X-ray energy emitted as light (η_e)	Figure of merit ($\eta_a\eta_e$)
(Zn, CdS): Ag Traditional fluoroscopy, image intensifiers	Green	0·25	0·15	0·04
$CaWO_4$ Radiography	Blue	0·45	0·03	0·015
CsI:Na (evaporated) Image intensifiers	Blue	0·6	0·10	0·06
$Gd_2O_2S:Tb$ Radiography	Green	0·6	0·15	0·09

sharpness; it is shown on page 35, however, how the use of evaporated CsI:Na can to a certain extent circumvent this disadvantage.

The light image produced by the fluorescent screen is detected in two ways in current clinical practice. This is either by a photographic emulsion in radiography, or by the human eye (directly or indirectly) in fluoroscopy.

X-RAY IMAGE TRANSDUCERS: RADIOGRAPHY

The photographic emulsion

The full-size radiograph is still the method of choice for the permanent recording of the X-ray image. The world shortage of silver, however, combined with the high cost of the large films and their associated storage difficulties, have led to a search for alternative techniques, which are described later.

Radiography makes use of the remarkable properties of the ordinary photographic emulsion.[18, 25] Figure 1.20 shows a cross-section of a typical radiographic cassette. In the centre is the photographic film. This consists of a substrate of cellulose acetate with a coating of sensitive *emulsion* on each side. The emulsion consists of a layer of gelatine in which is suspended minute crystals of silver bromide. The crystals have a range of sizes, but a typical X-ray emulsion contains crystals with an average linear dimension of 1 µm. The emulsion in turn is protected on each side by a layer of clear gelatine. On each side of the film is a fluorescent screen known as an *intensifying screen*, with the fluorescent material facing the film, and the whole is enclosed in an aluminium cassette with pressure plates to hold the film and screens together in intimate contact. If the components were not held in close contact, an additional source of unsharpness would be introduced, due to lateral diffusion of light. This is a common fault in old cassettes.

In use, X-rays are absorbed in the intensifying screens and produce visible and ultra-violet light. The light is absorbed by the photographic emulsion, in which it produces a *latent image*. This, as its name implies, is an invisible *record* of the incident light pattern, which can be rendered visible by the action of a liquid known as a photographic *developer*. The mechanism of the photographic emulsion is exceedingly complex, and is still not fully understood; for example, the gelatine that carries the silver bromide is not merely a passive carrier but acts as a *sensitiser* whose action is still somewhat obscure.[18] In broad terms, however, the following is the mode of action of the emulsion. A silver bromide grain absorbs an amount of light energy equivalent to many quanta; the energy thus absorbed ionises one AgBr molecule to produce a silver ion, Ag^+, which acts as a latent-image centre in the crystal. The crystals that have not absorbed the requisite amount of light energy remain unaltered. When the film is placed in the developer, the latter, which is a chemical reducing agent, penetrates and permeates the emulsion and its gelatine protective layer; it is so composed chemically that it completes the reduction to black silver of all the grains that carry latent-imaging centres, while leaving the other grains almost unaffected. The image is now visible because of the blackening so produced. Blackening occurs where light originally

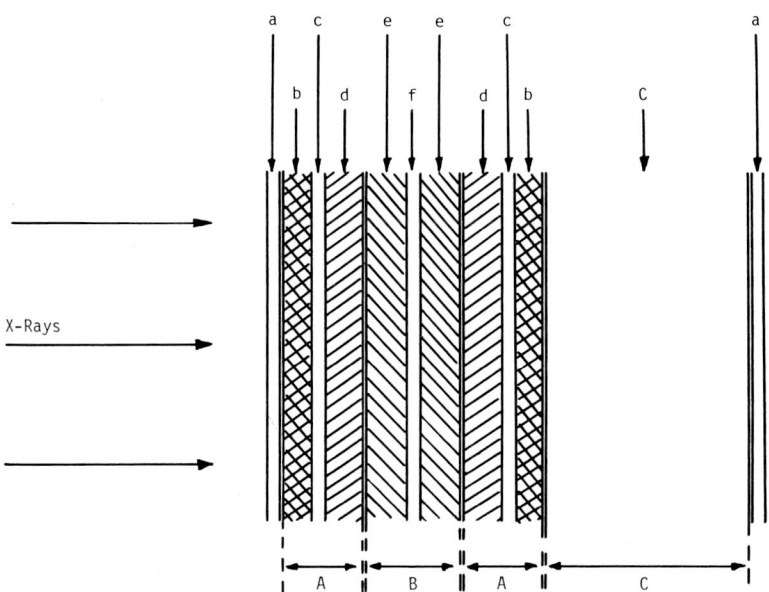

Fig. 1.20 A cross-section of part of a typical radiographic cassette. A, the intensifying screens; b, their substrate (card or plastic); c, reflecting layer of TiO_2; d, fluorescent layer; B, the film; e, sensitive emulsion; f, the substrate (cellulose acetate); C, a plastic foam pressure pad; a, aluminium sides of cassette.

fell, so the image is a so-called *negative*. The film, after washing, is then placed in a fixing and hardening solution, consisting of an acidified mixture of sodium thiosulphate (*hypo*) solution with a solution of a salt such as chrome alum. The former dissolves out the unaffected silver bromide, thus rendering the emulsion no longer sensitive to light, while the latter tans and therefore hardens the gelatine, rendering it less susceptible to scratching. The chemical processing is completed by a period of washing, and then drying by a current of warm air. Formerly, processing was carried out by hand in a dark room in solutions at room temperature, the whole process lasting about 25 min to produce a visible wet film, but about 1½ h to the final dry state. Automatic processors have now been developed that function at higher temperatures around 35°C; the films are led through the various solutions by rollers; the whole process takes about 90 s and can proceed in daylight after the initial loading. (The unused silver bromide in solution in the fixing agent is valuable and steps are often taken to recover it.) The first radiographs were made without intensifying screens, the X-ray energy being absorbed directly in the film, where it produced a latent image. Subsequently it was found that sensitivity could be greatly increased, by a factor of 10 to 40, by the use of fluorescent screens. The name *intensifying screens* is ill-chosen because it implies that the screens somehow merely intensify the image that is directly produced in the film by the X-rays. Instead, most of the blackening of the film is produced by the light from the screens, only about 3–10 per cent of the X-ray energy being directly absorbed in the film emulsions. This fact is of profound importance in determining the characteristics of the radiographic cassette.

The film is viewed by placing on a *viewing box* consisting of a sheet of opal plastic uniformly illuminated from behind, usually by fluorescent lamps. A small area of illumination of much higher intensity may be provided against which especially dark parts of the film may be viewed. Most modern viewing boxes are deficient in that they have no provision for masking off the illuminated area around the film; this peripheral region of high intensity results in intense glare and hence light scatter and related effects in the eye which seriously reduce the perceptibility of the desired details in the radiograph. In many cases, for example a film of a barium meal, where contrasts are high, this effect is not important. When the desired detail is near visual threshold, however, a concept discussed on page 36, for example in calcification in heart valves, the effect may make the difference between seeing and not seeing.

Table 1.3 shows that the transitions that take place in the exposure, development and viewing of the photographic emulsion comprise three powerful stages of *amplification*, as well as the property of time integration; these are the reasons for its great sensitivity.

Table 1.3 Stages in the photographic process: those features that make it a detector of outstanding sensitivity are shown by★.

Light (small energy)
★ ↓ Absorption and integration
Latent image
★ ↓ Chemical
↓ development
Silver image (blackening)
★ ↓ Viewing
light source
Light image (large energy)

The characteristic curve of the photographic emulsion: density

The blackening of the photographic emulsion is described quantitatively by the concept *density*. In the viewing process, if L_i is the light intensity incident on the film and L_t the light intensity transmitted by the film, then the density D is given by

$$D = \log (L_t/L_i) \quad (1.8)$$

For example, if the transmitted intensity is one-tenth of that incident on the film, the density is $D = \log 10 = 1$. A density of 1 represents a medium gray area; the range of densities in an average radiograph is from 0·2–3·0, with most of the diagnostic information lying between values of 0·5 and 2·0. The difference (ΔD) between the densities of two regions, usually adjacent, is called *radiographic contrast*, to distinguish it from X-ray contrast (see p. 6). It is also called *objective contrast*, to distinguish it from its appearance to the eye, which is known correspondingly as *subjective contrast*. Note that both radiographic contrast and X-ray contrast are in the form of the logarithm of a ratio, though the one makes use of base 10 and the other base e (some authorities use base 10 also for X-ray contrast, though this introduces certain disadvantages, see p. 36). It is the radiographic contrast that enables the radiologist to distinguish between regions of differing radiopacities; it is thus a very important property of the radiograph, and the mechanisms by which it results from X-ray contrast are of profound importance. They are described quantitatively in the form of the *characteristic curve*, *sensitometric curve* or *H and D curve*, of the emulsion. (H and D refers to Hurter and Driffield, the two photographic workers who originated the concept in the 19th century.)

It may be wondered why a logarithmic measure such as density is used to represent blackening. There seem to be three possible reasons: (1) to encompass a large range of light transmission without using very large or very small numbers; (2) in the belief that the response of the human eye is logarithmic, an assumption that is dubious to say the least; and (3) perhaps the best reason: from Equation 1.8, $L_t = L_i 10^{-D}$. This is an exponential law of absorption similar to Equation 1.1; D is proportional to the mass of developed metallic silver per unit area of the emulsion and hence is of great importance to those who design emulsions.

Density is measured by means of an instrument called a *densitometer* which measures the transmitted light but is calibrated directly in density. A microdensitometer is an instrument that measures the density of exceedingly small areas of film; most microdensitometers scan the film continuously, and automatically plot the density on linear graph paper.

Density is not a unique measure of blackening, because light is not only absorbed by the metallic silver but is also scattered by it (compare the attenuation of X-rays in matter, discussed on p. 4). Hence the value of density obtained from a densitometer depends on the angle of illumination of the film and the angle of collection of the light detector. In radiography, the film is diffusely illuminated (over a large angle) by the viewing box, and the light is *specularly* collected by a small aperture (the pupil of the eye) at a distance of about 300 mm.

The standard method of measuring density makes use of specular illumination and diffuse collection, a method that can be shown to be equivalent to the radiographic condition.

Figure 1.21 shows the characteristic curve of a typical X-ray film exposed to light. On the ordinate is plotted density D, while on the abscissa is the logarithm to the base 10 of the exposure, log E. *Exposure* is a word that has many connotations, of which four are important in radiology. It can mean exposure in roentgens (p. 6), exposure time in radiography, exposure in kVp and mA × s in radiography, but photographically it has a less precise meaning, having the dimensions of intensity × time in units that are not often specified. For the present purpose it can be regarded as being proportional to the exposure to the cassette in roentgens. Note that the characteristic curve is plotted on effectively double logarithmic coordinates, because D is already a logarithmic measure of blackening.

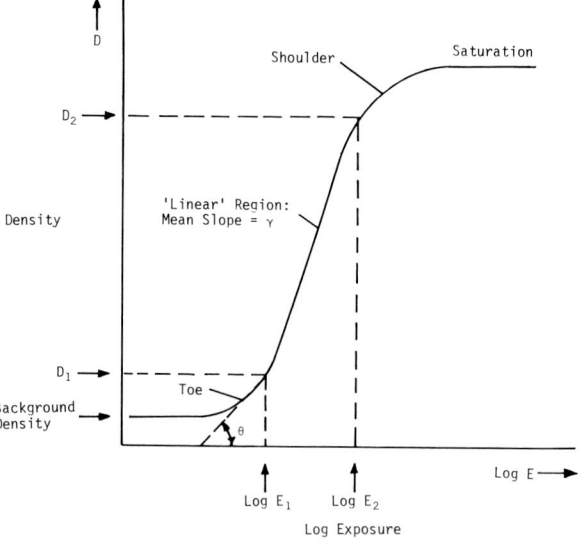

Fig. 1.21 The characteristic curve of a photographic emulsion exposed to visible light showing the variation of density D with exposure E. The quasi-linear region of mean slope γ represents a power-law relationship between input exposure and output viewed light. The γ at any point on the curve (the 'point-γ') is equal to tan θ. In an X-ray film used with intensifying screens, γ has typical values of 2–5, thus acting as an 'amplification factor' for contrast (Equation 1.11).

For zero exposure (not shown, of course, on a logarithmic scale) the density is not zero but varies from 0·15–0·3. This represents light absorbed in the film substrate and also in the few grains of AgBr that are converted to silver without being exposed, the so-called *chemical fog* that increases with the age of emulsions; it is always best to use fresh films.

With gradually increasing exposure, the density increases, first slowly, then with ever-increasing speed. This is known as the *toe* of the curve, and represents the light parts of the film up to a density of about 0·7. Then there follows a region that is often called *linear* but which in fact is sigmoid in shape; then the increase of density becomes progressively slower at the *shoulder* of the curve. The density at which this occurs depends on the total amount of AgBr in the emulsion; ultimately a state is reached, known as *saturation*, in which all the AgBr has been reduced to metallic silver. This occurs at densities around 3·5–4·0 for typical X-ray films, but emulsions can be designed that saturate at $D = 5$ or 6.

From Figure 1.21 the radiographic contrast $D_2 - D_1 = \gamma (\log E_2 - \log E_1)$. Hence

$$\Delta D = \gamma \log (E_2/E_1) \quad (1.9)$$

(γ, often written gamma, is the slope of the characteristic curve at any given point, in this case the average slope of the 'linear' part of the characteristic. Figure 1.21 shows that it is identical to the tangent of the angle with the abscissa made by the tangent to the curve at that particular point ($\gamma = \tan \theta$).)

Now the light exposures to the film are proportional to the X-ray exposures to the radiographic cassette (see p. 19); therefore

$$\Delta D = \frac{\gamma}{2 \cdot 303} \ln \left(\frac{I_2 + I_s}{I_1 + I_s} \right) = \frac{\gamma}{2 \cdot 303} C'_r \quad (1.10)$$

Hence from Equation 1.3

$$\Delta D = - \frac{\gamma \mu S \Delta x}{2 \cdot 303} \quad (1.11)$$

This Equation enables the radiographic contrast (i.e. the factor that enables the radiologist to distinguish between areas of differing radiopacities) to be calculated from the basic factors such as attenuation coefficient, thickness of structure and amount of scattered radiation.

Equation 1.11 shows that the gamma of the emulsion acts as a further *amplification factor* for contrast; X-ray emulsions have high maximum values of gamma of 2 to 4 so that the low values of contrast common in radiology are the more readily detected.

The 'linear' part of the characteristic curve is not linear in the sense that the fluorescent screen is linear, i.e. the light transmitted through the film is not proportional to the exposure to the film. In the first place, the radiograph is a negative image of the X-rays falling on the cassette, because light produces blackening in the emulsion. Hence the radiograph is a positive image of the structures in the patient (p. 7); a bone produces an increment of light from the film! In the second place, the so-called 'linear' part is quasilinear only on logarithmic co-ordinates, hence the relation between exposure and transmitted light is a negative power law whose exponent is equal to the gamma of the emulsion.

The radiographer is often recommended to expose the film so that the structures of interest lie within the 'linear' part of the characteristic. This is not because the characteristic is linear *per se*, however, but because the gamma and therefore the radiographic contrast is a maximum at the centre of the 'linear' part. At all points above and below this centre, the gamma is less. For example, if a chest radiograph is exposed so that the detail of the lung fields receives maximum contrast amplification, the detail in the ribs lies on the toe of the curve and the contrast is much reduced. Alternatively, the exposure (mA × s) to the film can be increased so that the images of the ribs lie in the linear region, then the lung fields are overexposed and not only is their contrast less but their density is greater, thus necessitating the use of a higher intensity viewing illuminator.

Non-screen films: emulsion design

Most, but not all, clinical radiographic techniques use a conventional cassette. Some use plain film without intensifying screens, and thus the mechanism of the direct response of the emulsion to X-rays, as well as the effect of different emulsion designs, are discussed here.

Radiography of the extremities, for example hair-line wrist fractures, demands a transducer with an exceedingly small unsharpness (or a correspondingly good MTF; see p. 15), otherwise the fracture will not be detectable (p. 13). Formerly, this was achieved by omitting the intensifying screens and making use of the direct action of X-rays on the film (which itself has a very small unsharpness indeed). This was called *non-screen radiography*. In recent years, however, intensifying screens with sufficiently small unsharpness have been produced; they result in a welcome reduction in patient dose. Another area in which the direct action of X-rays on film is used is that of radiation protection; the blackening of the film is used as a measure of the radiation received by the *film badge* worn by a radiation worker.

The response of the photographic emulsion to direct X-ray exposure is quite different from that due to visible light. This is because each X-ray quantum interaction dissipates so much energy (via its secondary electron) within a small region of the emulsion that many AgBr grains are rendered developable. Figure 1.22 shows the variation of density with exposure; the relationship is approximately linear until saturation is approached.

On the other hand, because of the small energy (3 eV) of the light quantum, many such absorptions are needed to render a grain developable, the average number depending on the quantum energy of the light and particularly on the size of the grain. The relation between absorbed quanta and developable grains is stochastic, so it is possible to speak only of average values (n); some grains require more quanta, some less. Figure 1.23 shows a highly idealised form of three film emulsions exposed to visible light. The first, with a large average grain size, requires an average of only two quantum absorptions per grain to render the grains developable. This number of grains, however, has approximately a Poisson distribution, and because of the small average number, its relative standard deviation is large. The second, with a medium average-grain-size, requires a larger average number of quantum absorptions per grain, with a correspondingly smaller relative standard deviation, while the third, with its small grain size, requires the largest number quantum absorptions per grain, with a very small relative standard deviation. The idealised characteristic curves of Figure 1.23 are obtained from the Poisson distributions of n by integration over n. The characteristic curve is clearly a sigmoid, and the figure shows how large-grain emulsions have high sensitivity (*speed*), low gamma, relatively large unsharpness (though not approaching that of screens), and large *latitude*, whereas small-grain emulsions have low sensitivity (speed), high gamma, very small unsharpness and small latitude. The term *latitude* simply refers to the range of exposures that can be accommodated within a reasonable range of density of the film. It is possible, by including a wide variety of AgBr grain sizes, to produce almost any desired shape of characteristic curve; special films with high gamma in one region yet wide overall latitude are now being offered by some of the film manufacturers and provide an alternative technique to high-kV radiography (p. 7). This account of emulsion design is highly idealised and simplified yet gives an impression of the mechanisms involved.

The preceding discussion shows how gamma can be varied by design of film emulsion. Gamma depends also on processing; for example, the longer

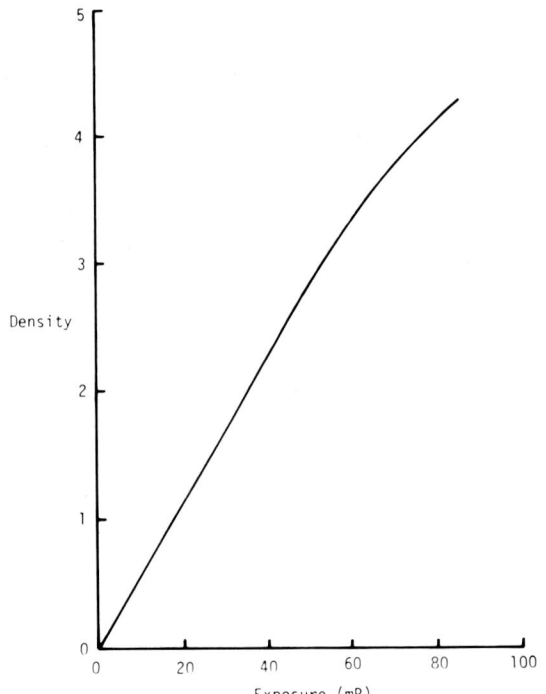

Fig. 1.22 The characteristic curve of a photographic emulsion exposed to X-rays. Because of the high energy of the secondary electrons, each electron produces several developable grains. Hence the relationship between density and exposure is linear until saturation is approached.

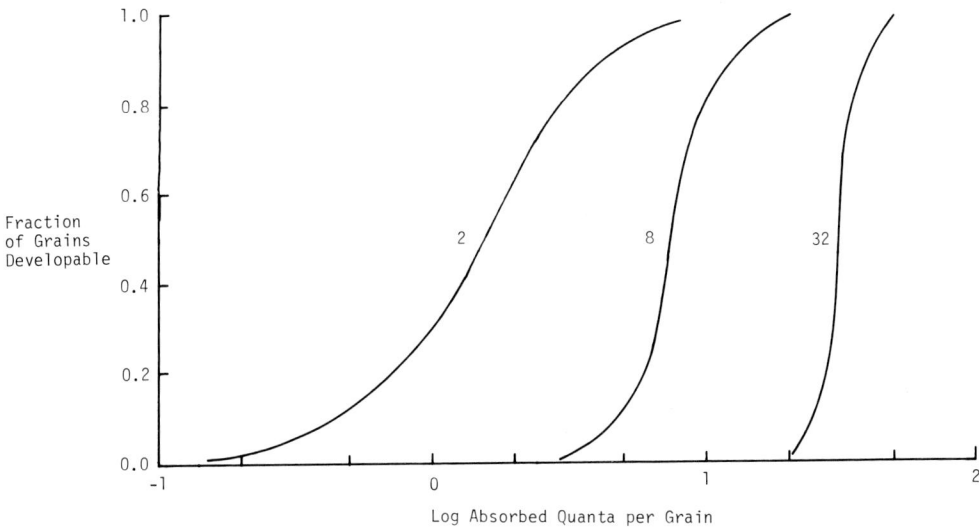

Fig. 1.23 Showing the fraction of grains made developable in a photographic emulsion as a function of the logarithm of the number of absorbed quanta per grain. The parameter is the mean number of quanta required to make a grain developable. The curves are the integrals of Poisson distributions and are related in general form to the characteristic curve of the emulsion. This presentation is highly simplified and idealised (see text).

the development time or the higher the development temperature, the higher is the gamma. Attempts to increase gamma beyond the capabilities of the emulsion merely lead to increase the chemical fog (p. 21), and the use of automatic processors has led to a general loss of interest in the changes that can be achieved in this way.

Radiography as an imaging system

Radiography as an imaging method shows many of the common defects of imaging systems: (1) it is nonlinear (this may not necessarily be a disadvantage); (2) it has a background of both density and noise (discussed later); (3) it is unsharp, mainly due to the PSF of the screens; and (4) it exhibits the common property of imaging systems that results in spatial and sometimes temporal random fluctuations of luminance, commonly called *noise*. In radiography the significant noise sources are: (a) the silver grains themselves, called *granularity*, the subjective appearance of which is called *graininess*, and consists of fine-grain noise; (b) random quantum absorption of X-ray energy in the intensifying screens (coarse-grain noise); (c) screen structure fluctuations; and (d) noise due to random neural processes in the eye and brain while viewing.

The various sources of radiographic noise are often called *mottle*; their powers and their *coarseness* are usually described in the spatial-frequency domain in the form of the power or Wiener spectrum.[36, 44] Figure 1.24 shows typical noise spectra for a selection of screen-film combinations (Cowen, unpublished). Noise tends to obscure desired signals and is thus a very important feature. In clinical radiography the various noise sources make very roughly equal contributions to the total.

The transduction of information from X-ray quantum interactions to light flashes is described on page 18. Each quantum interaction is described as a 'unit of information', and their random fluctuations are described as 'noise'. Noise in a visual image is a random phenomenon that tends to obscure the 'signal', i.e. the structure that is desired to be seen. The two words originated in the earlier part of this century in the world of communication engineering; the signal was obviously the message that it was desired to transmit and the noise described the random fluctuations that tended to obscure the signal. If an electric current, consisting of a random flow of electrons, is passed through earphones or a loud speaker, it results in a characteristic hissing sound that is commonly called noise. If the same current is passed into a television receiver, it results in a characteristic speckled

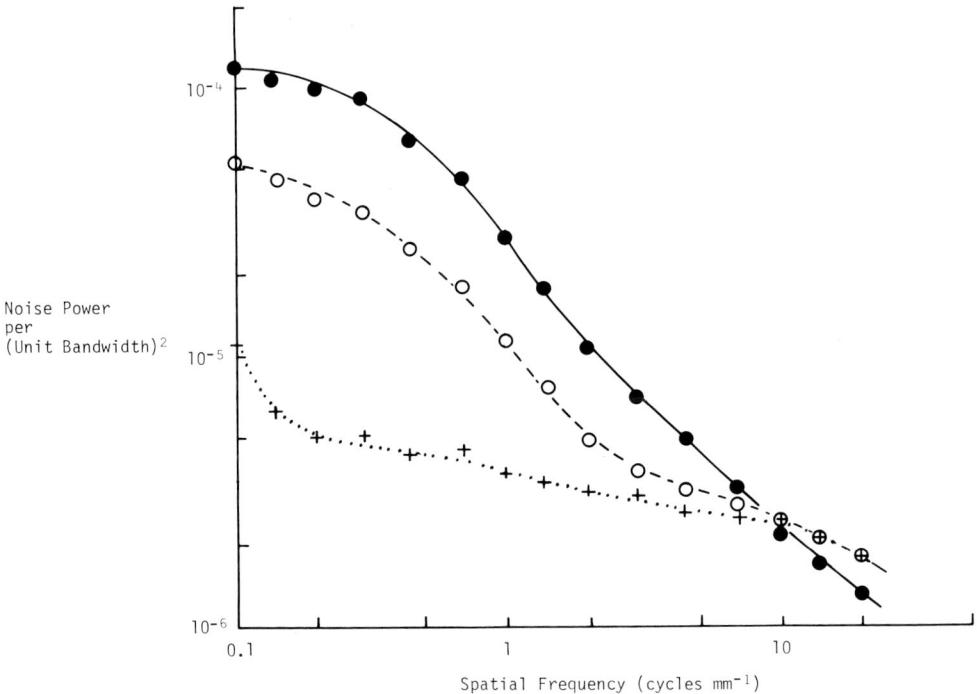

Fig. 1.24 Showing the power spectra of the noise (mottle) of different screen-film combinations. ●—●—●— a high-speed rare-earth screen-film system; --○--○-- a high-speed calcium tungstate screen-film system, and ··+··+·· the film alone exposed to light. The preponderance of low-frequency energy in the screen-film combinations is due to the unsharp X-ray quantum noise. The sudden rise at very low frequencies in the film alone is due to processing irregularities.

two-dimensional pattern that, by analogy, is also called 'noise'.

It may not be immediately clear how, in the case of the image, the same phenomenon, i.e. the X-ray quantum interactions, can at the same time both convey information and destroy it. However, it is the mean number of the quantum interactions that constitute the signal and the fluctuation about that mean that constitutes the noise. Figure 1.25 demonstrates this principle in the case of a diametrical cross-section through two disc-shaped objects of high and low contrast respectively.

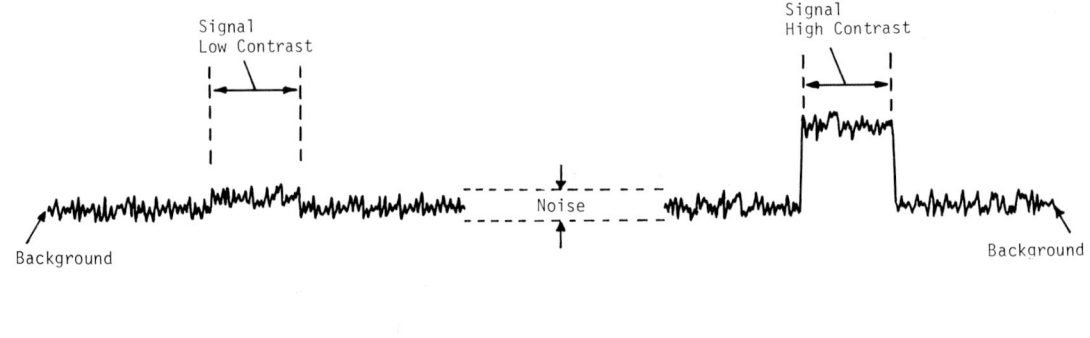

Fig. 1.25 A diagrammatic representation of the relation between high- and low-contrast signals on the one hand and noise on the other. The signal is the difference between the averages of numbers of quanta per given area per unit time, and the noise is the root-mean-square fluctuation about those averages. It is evident how a low-contrast signal might be 'lost in the noise'.

It is usually the relative standard deviation (the coefficient of variation) of the number of events in any given area that is significant. For example, if in a given area, say 1 mm², the mean number of X-ray quantum interactions is N, then the absolute standard deviation of root-mean-square fluctuation of events is $N^{1/2}$ (assuming a Poisson distribution of numbers of events), and the relative standard deviation is $N^{1/2}/N = N^{-1/2}$. Hence the larger the number of events, the smaller is the effective noise and the better is the image quality. This is in accordance with the idea that one event represents a unit of information, for then the larger the number of events the larger is the amount of information and the better is the image quality.

Rare-earth screens

Conventional screen radiography today for the most part makes use of intensifying screens of calcium tungstate (Table 1.2), a material that has been in use for many years. Since the early 1970s, however, there have been moves to substitute other materials which are usually classed together as *rare-earth* screens. Table 1.2 shows one example of this type of screen, gadolinium oxysulphide. Controversy rages as to the desirability or otherwise of these screens for clinical work; their physical properties, however, are in the main well understood, and an attempt is made here to show how these properties might affect their clinical use.

The advantages of the rare-earth screens over calcium tungstate are: (1) moderately improved fractional X-ray absorption (without increased unsharpness); and (2) greatly improved conversion efficiency of absorbed X-rays to light (Table 1.2). The former naturally increases the amount of information extracted from the X-ray beam, which can only be beneficial; the latter, for a given film speed, enables the X-ray exposure to the cassette, and hence the patient dose, to be reduced by a factor of as much as five times. This may seem at first sight to be a wholly desirable end, until it is realised that the very reduction in X-ray exposure is accompanied by a reduction of information, in this case by a factor of $\sqrt{5}$ (see p. 25). Because this is accompanied by an increase in the relative standard deviation ($N^{-1/2}$), the perceptible noise would appear to be increased by the same factor. The quality of the radiograph is thus inferior to that made with the slower screens. It is evident that a compromise has become possible in radiography between patient dose and image quality. A way in which this compromise can be implemented is to use a slower film, thus necessitating a larger X-ray exposure for the same density. Thus a moderate reduction in patient dose may be made for a small loss in image quality. Indeed, the colour of the light emitted from some of these new screens is green, thus necessitating a special green-sensitive film anyway; others, however, (not shown in Table 1.2), for example lanthanum oxybromide, emit blue light and can be used with conventional film.

It is not clear at the present time how this conflict may be resolved. Some departments, especially the dose-conscious, have changed over completely to rare-earth screens. Others, concerned at the increased noise (mottle), have rejected them after short clinical trials. It seems likely that the best compromise is achieved by using the rare-earth screens for techniques, such as obstetric studies, in which dose reduction is of paramount importance, while conventional calcium tungstate screens are retained for techniques where the ultimate in image quality is desired, and dose-reduction is of secondary importance. To this end it seems logical to choose rare-earth screens that are blue-emitting so that the same film stock can be used for both types of screen.

Measurement of transducer characteristics

The physical characteristics such as noise, unsharpness etc of transducers, in particular of radiographic screen-film systems, are not difficult to measure; an indication is given in this section how this is achieved in the laboratory. Despite much experimentation, however, it is not at present clear how to interpret the objective physical properties of systems in terms of their subjective clinical performance. Certain broad principles can be laid down (pp. 36–42) but we are very far indeed from the stage at which clinical performance can be predicted from physical properties.

The unsharpness of screen-film systems is usually measured in terms of the line spread-function, which Fourier-transforms into the modulation transfer function (see p. 15). The cassette is exposed to X-rays through a narrow slit in lead or platinum sheet; a width of 10 μm is typical. The resultant blackening on the film is a measure principally of the LSF of the screen-pair, because the sharpness of the film itself (and hence its MTF; see Fig. 1.19) is very good. This blackening is scanned by an optical slit about 5 μm wide in a scanning microdensitometer (see p. 21); the resultant LSF cannot be directly Fourier-transformed because it is the result of the nonlinear characteristic of the film. Therefore it is first corrected for the latter, and expressed in terms of equivalent X-ray exposure. This yields the same function as the light distribution from the screens, because the screens are truly linear. The corrected distribution is then Fourier-transformed to give the MTF of the screen-film system. It is noteworthy that this MTF is a notional function only, and cannot be used to predict density distributions in the film as a result of other patterns of exposure, because of the film non-linearity. This reveals one grave disadvantage of the concept of MTF, as already mentioned on page 15.

The noise is usually measured in the form of the Wiener or power spectrum.[36, 44] A narrow collimating slit is imaged on a rotating disc of the film concerned. The light transmitted by the film is collected by a compound microscope and collimated by a second measuring slit; a photomultiplier then collects this light and converts it into an electrical signal. The electrical signal is analysed by a temporal-frequency analyser into a spectrum that relates amplitude to temporal frequency. The temporal frequency is then converted into the corresponding spatial frequency via the effective relative linear speeds of the film and the slit. An alternative method of noise measurement[45] makes use of a conventional microdensitometer that makes many evaluations of density in a constant but moveable area of the film; the output of the microdensitometer is on line to a computer that assesses the autocorrelation function of the noise. From this the power spectrum can be obtained by Fourier transformation. A typical set of power spectra is shown in Figure 1.24.

Within the limits of exposure used in radiography, intensifying screens are linear. It is always necessary to determine the characteristic curve of the film, however, and this necessitates producing a range of exposures, which can be done in several ways. The two most important ways are by intensity variation and time variation. Time variation is not a suitable method in this context, because in conditions of visible light exposure, such as obtained in a cassette, the blackening of a film, for a given exposure, depends on the exposure rate and hence on the exposure time (failure of reciprocity law).[18] For this reason, intensity variation is chosen. For routine monitoring purposes, a step wedge consisting of graded thicknesses of X-ray attenuator such as aluminium can be used, but this has the disadvantage that the X-ray spectrum changes with the absorber thickness. Therefore, for sensitometric purposes it is usual to vary intensity by varying the distance between the X-ray focus and the cassette, the inverse-square law holding sufficiently accurately for most applications. The mA.s product for the X-ray tube is held constant; for the most accurate work it is not sufficient to rely on generator stability but to monitor each exposure with an ionisation chamber type of exposure meter.

Radiography is a relatively sensitive process; a typical screen-film combination requires an exposure of only about 1 mR (2.58×10^{-7} C kg^{-1}) to the cassette to produce a density of one. It yields only a static image; when it is necessary to observe dynamic processes one must have recourse to fluoroscopy.

X-RAY IMAGE TRANSDUCERS; FLUOROSCOPY AND IMAGE INTENSIFIERS

Traditional fluoroscopy

Traditional fluoroscopy, or *screening*, made use of a simple fluorescent screen. This was viewed by the radiologist through a thick layer of lead glass to give him protection against the X-ray energy transmitted through the screen. Fluoroscopy has the outstanding advantage that movement of organs is in principle perceptible; in its traditional form, however, it has several disadvantages. In the first place, for a reasonable exposure rate to the patient the screen luminance is extremely low, so low in fact that the radiologist found it necessary to dark-adapt his vision for at least 15 min prior to fluoroscopy. Even when so dark-adapted, however, the information perceptible on the screen is far less than that available from a radiograph of the same patient. For many years this deficiency was attributed to screen unsharpness, until it was shown,[6] by photographing the fluoroscopic screen, that there is much more information inherent in the screen image than is perceptible to the unaided eye, even when dark-adapted. The inference is that the known deficiencies of fluoroscopy are entirely a result of the poor performance of the eye at such low light levels. This conclusion has now been given theoretical support,[41] the essence of the argument being given later.

In the meantime, however, means were sought to improve the quality of the image in fluoroscopy. The dose to the patient was already at what was considered then as a tolerable maximum (and now thought to be excessive), so the X-ray exposure rate could not be increased. A device was required that would increase the luminance of the fluoroscopic screen without increasing the X-ray exposure rate, and the answer was found in the X-ray image intensifier.[8, 42]

X-ray image intensifiers

Figure 1.26 shows a cross-section of a modern X-ray image intensifier. The X-ray image falls on a fluorescent screen that is in intimate contact with a photocathode. The X-rays produce visible light, which in turn produces photoelectrons from the photocathode. These photoelectrons are accelerated and focused through an electron lens system on an output fluorescent screen. The latter is backed by a thin layer of aluminium, which serves to transmit the electrons yet prevents feedback of light from output to input; it also acts as an electrode. The electrons are accelerated by a constant potential difference of about 25 kV between the photocathode and the aluminium layer; focusing is achieved by intermediate potentials being applied to intermediate electrodes. The input fluorescent screen is typically 225 mm in diameter, and the output screen is about 20–25 mm in diameter, hence a gain in luminance of about 100 is obtained by the consequent reduction in area (the so-called *minification*). A further factor of about 50 is attained by the acceleration of the electrons. The result is a total luminance gain of the order of 5000. The gain of a modern intensifier, however, is not normally expressed as a dimensionless factor,

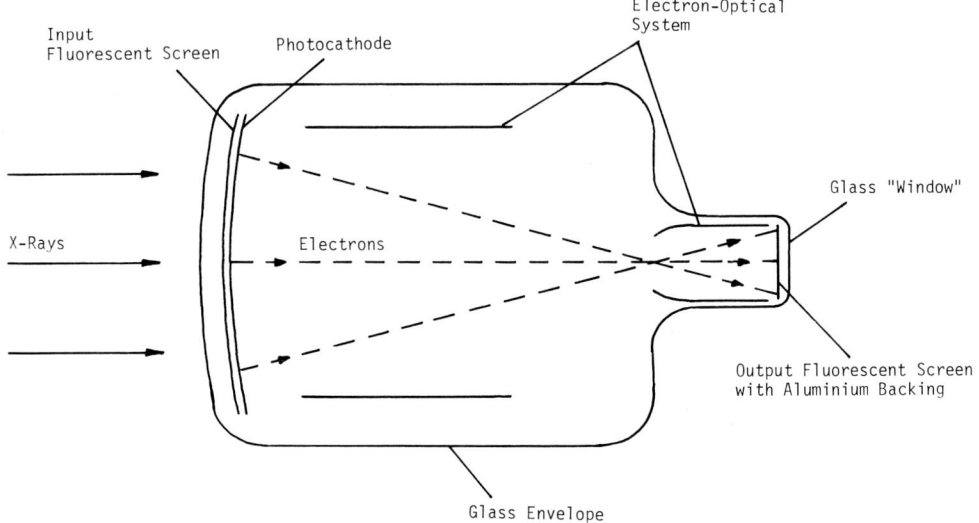

Figure 1.26 A simplified cross-section of a typical X-ray image-intensifier tube. The aluminium backing of the output fluorescent screen is held at a potential of 25–35 kV relative to the photocathode, and the intermediate electrodes in the electron-optical system are held at intermediate potentials to satisfy focusing and minification requirements. A considerable fraction of X-rays is absorbed in the input glass window.

but in terms of the output luminance of the screen in cd m^{-2} mR^{-1}s. A typical value is 100 cd m^{-2} mR^{-1}s.

The output of an image intensifier, an image of about 25 mm in diameter, was originally viewed through a simple magnifier. Though such a viewing device is in practice highly inconvenient, it serves for the purpose of demonstrating the fundamental properties of the image intensifier. Although the image is only 25 mm in diameter, it can be made to appear to be 250 mm in diameter by reducing the viewing distance to a value of about 25 mm. At this distance, however, the eye is out of focus; this must be corrected by the interposition of a magnifying glass, which, because it forms a virtual image, does not result in any decrease in brightness. Thus the use of the image intensifier results in an increase in brightness of the fluoroscopic image by a factor of about 5000 times; we now explore the significance of this gain for clinical fluoroscopy.

When the X-ray image intensifier was first devised, it was thought by many that the increased brightness would result in a transmission of information far beyond that experienced in radiography. That this would not be so was soon pointed out,[41] and at the same time the reason for the inferiority of the eye's performance in traditional fluoroscopy was correctly deduced.

Figure 1.27 shows a conventional fluoroscopic screen, viewed by the radiologist's eye and brain at a distance of about 300 mm. For a typical zinc-cadmium sulphide fluorescent screen, one absorbed X-ray quantum produces an average of about 2000 visible light quanta usefully emitted forwards into a solid angle of 2π (see p. 18). Only a very small fraction, however, (viz about 10^{-4} of these) are collected by the pupil of the eye at its viewing distance of 300 mm. Of these, only about one-tenth produce a visual sensation, due to the inefficiency of the retina. As all these processes are stochastic in nature, it can be calculated that an average of 50 absorbed X-ray quanta are required to produce one visual sensation. This represents a serious loss of information; clearly it is the geometrical inefficiency of the eye combined with its retinal inefficiency that results in its poor performance at low light levels.

The image intensifier is a fundamental advance over traditional fluoroscopy because it substitutes the vastly superior light-gathering property of the photocathode in contact with the fluorescent screen for the extremely poor geometrical efficiency of the human eye at its normal viewing distance.

From this type of calculation it was originally estimated that brightness gains of about 100 would enable the whole of the information inherent in the input fluorescent screen to be perceived, but later estimates set this value at about 500. This indeed was the brightness gain of the first image intensifiers, the increase to the present-day value of 5000 being solely in terms of convenience. The above type of calculation also shows clearly why the early hopes that high factors of intensification would result in

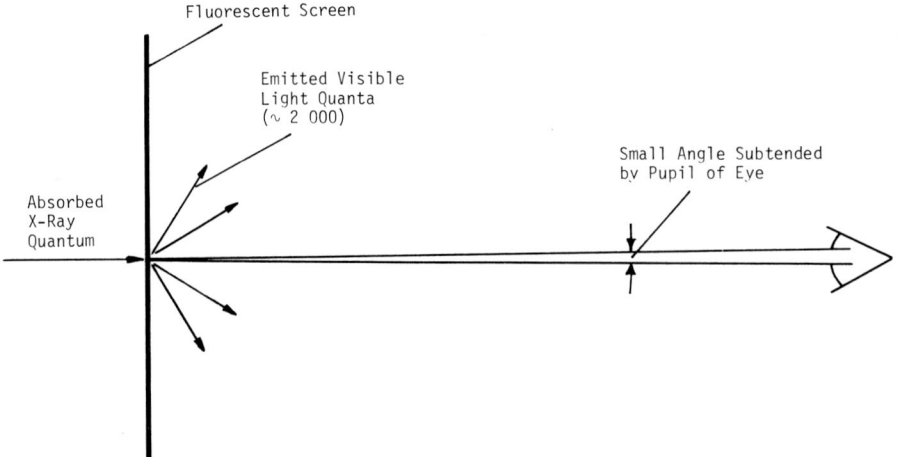

Fig. 1.27 Showing how the eye at a normal viewing distance accepts only a very small fraction ($\sim 10^{-4}$) of the visible light quanta emitted into 2π by a fluoroscopic screen.

almost indefinite gains of information were doomed to disappointment; as soon as the gain of the image intensifier is sufficient for each absorbed X-ray quantum to be perceptible, no further gain of information is to be expected (because of the X-ray quantum limit, discussed on p. 18). The situation is analogous to the viewing of the newspaper photograph that is built up of discrete dots. As soon as the dots themselves are perceptible, no further gain of information can be expected from increased illumination, magnification or from any other means.

In the years between 1949 and about 1970, other configurations of image intensifier were developed and manufactured,[12] but these are now obsolescent, and have given way to the original type of X-ray image intensifier tube described previously.

Methods of viewing and recording the image intensifier output

A magnifying glass is an extremely inconvenient means of viewing the output of an image-intensifier tube for clinical purposes. For a short time, binocular microscopes and similar optical systems with large exit-pupil mirror viewing were in use, but in the early 1950s the small industrial type of closed-circuit television camera system had been developed, and this was soon adapted to the output of the image intensifier. It was claimed for the television system that not only would viewing be possible on the television monitor in full room lighting, but also that many other television techniques such as image enhancement, video-tape recording, etc., would be applicable to the X-ray image. Moreover, by imaging the output of the intensifier on a small-format still or cine film, a permanent record of the X-ray image, either static or dynamic, could be made. The static record, the so-called *spot film*, would have the advantage that a much smaller dose to the patient would be required than in the case of full size radiography, though of course the image quality would be inferior.

Figure 1.28 shows a functional diagram of a typical clinical X-ray image intensifier television system with small-format film and/or cine recording facilities. It might be argued that only a single lens is necessary for the optical coupling between the intensifier and, say, the television camera. However, this would necessitate a lens designed for a 1:1 object-to-image size ratio, with aberrations corrected for the appropriate distances. Such lenses are not common and are not easy to design, most lenses being corrected to work with object or image at infinity. Hence, the coupling between the intensifier on the one hand and the television, spot-film or cine camera on the other is always made via a 'tandem pair' of lenses. Each lens is focused at infinity, and its focal length is designed to be appropriate for the size of the object or image it is designed to work with. This arrangement is important, for to achieve maximum light transfer the lenses have very larger apertures of f 1·0 or greater; thus any feature that reduces their aberrations is much to be desired.

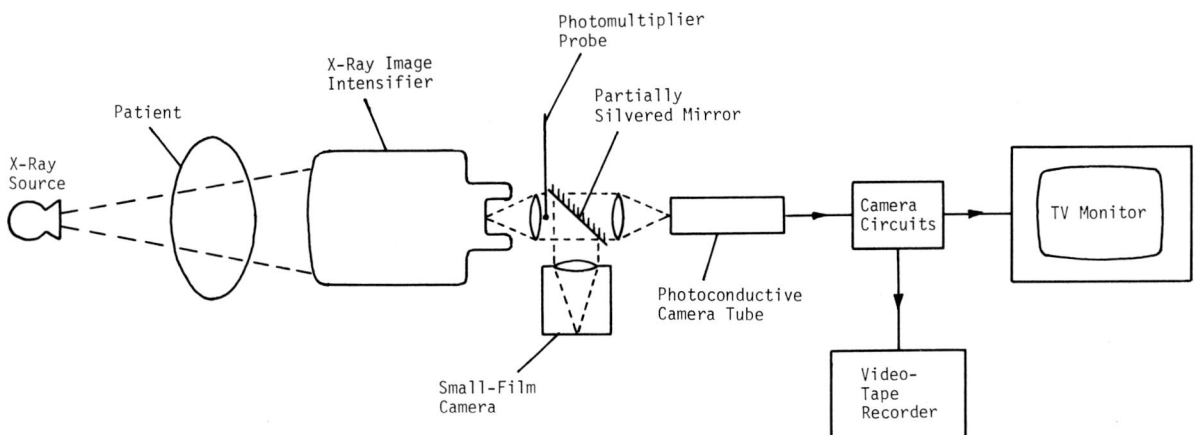

Fig. 1.28 A typical modern X-ray image-intensifier-television system with provision for video-tape recording and for small-film- or cine-fluorography. For further explanation see text.

The photomultiplier probe shown in Figure 1.28 is for the purpose of sampling the light output of the image intensifier. The resulting electrical signal can be fed back to the X-ray generator to control the mA and/or the kV, thus compensating to a certain extent for different patient thicknesses and ensuring a constant television output brightness or a constant spot-film density. This servo system is generally known as an *automatic brightness control* (ABC) or *automatic density control*.

X-ray television systems

Figure 1.29 shows a cross-section of the commonly-used photoconductive television camera pick-up tube. The light image is focused, through a transparent metallic signal plate, on the photoconductive layer which is situated at the front of the tube, and which becomes conducting roughly in proportion to the light falling on it. An electron gun at the back of the tube projects a low-velocity beam of electrons on the back of the photoconductive layer. The electron beam is magnetically focused and also magnetically deflected in the manner of the familiar television raster, and falls on the back surface of the photoconductive layer. In the absence of light, the electron beam charges this surface to the potential of the cathode of the electron gun (regarded as zero). The signal plate has a positive potential of between 10 and 50 V applied to it; when light falls on an area of the photoconductive layer it is rendered conducting and electrons flow through it to the signal plate, leaving the back surface positively charged. When the electron beam scans this area, electrons are deposited almost instantaneously on the surface, giving rise to a positive induced signal on the signal plate and hence a flow of electrons from the signal plate. The latter is connected via a blocking capacitor to an amplifier that amplifies the signal corresponding to the illuminated area. If this amplified signal is fed to a television monitor whose scanned raster is in synchronism with that of the camera pick-up tube, a light area is displayed on the monitor corresponding to that originally falling on the camera tube. The voltage fed to the monitor is called the *video signal*; the two rasters are kept in synchronism by synchronising pulses that are transmitted along with the video signal, the whole being termed the composite television waveform.

The functioning of the camera pick-up tube may be considered in two parts. First, positive signals are continuously and relatively slowly accumulated or stored on the back of the photoconductive layer. Second, this positive image is relatively rapidly scanned or evaluated by the scanning electron

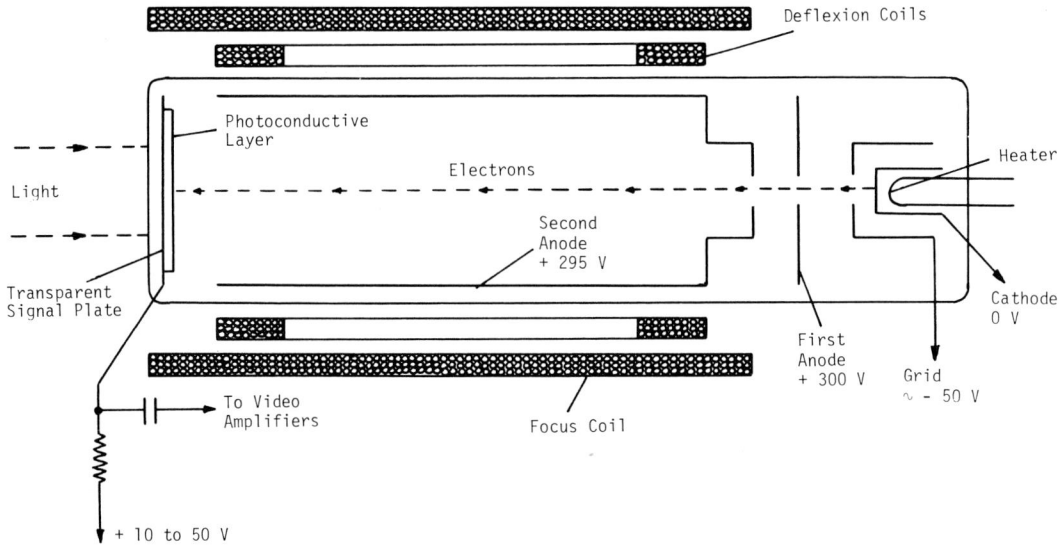

Fig. 1.29 Cross-section of a typical photoconductive television camera tube. The electron gun comprises the heater, the cathode, the grid and the first and second anodes. For a description of its operation see text.

beam. This scanning takes place at the rate of 25 pictures (or *frames*) per second (each frame being divided into two interlaced *fields* in the customary manner). In each frame there are 625 lines (in the European standard). The process of scanning or evaluating the positive charge image also discharges it, resulting in a relatively high frequency signal (the video signal) appearing at the signal plate. The tube is thus said to operate in a storage mode, an important fact that ensures its relatively high sensitivity, for the electron beam does not evaluate only the light that exists in the brief fraction of a second during which it passes over a picture element, but collects all the charge that has been stored in that element during the whole frame time (40 ms, again in the European system).

Until quite recently, two types of photoconductive tube were available. The first, historically, called the *vidicon*, has a photoconductive layer of amorphous antimony trisulphide (Sb_2S_3). This material has three characteristics that are important in radiology. First, it has a tendency to conduct when no light is present (the so-called *dark current*); this dark current is apt to be non-uniform thus producing irregular shading in the dark parts of the image. (Modern vidicons are much superior in this respect.) Second, the stored image is not proportional to the incident light, but the current is approximately proportional to $(light)^{0.7}$. Thus the gamma of the vidicon (compare with a film emulsion, discussed on p. 19) is about 0.7, and the X-ray contrast is reduced by that factor. Third, the conduction of the antimony trisulphide layer is not instantaneous, but suffers from lag, due to solid-state processes within the layer. Hence movement unsharpness is apparent in moving objects. X-ray quantum noise is moving, however, and hence a vidicon with appreciable lag tends to reduce the quantum noise level, with a consequent advantage for stationary objects. A slow vidicon is unsuitable for cardiac studies, but may well be a better choice for abdominal work where organ movement is usually slow. Vidicons today tend to be much faster than formerly.

The second type of photoconductive tube, called the plumbicon, has a photoconductive layer of lead oxide (PbO). The layer is not amorphous, however, but is in the form of a semiconductor P–N junction; it is this fact that confers on the plumbicon its unique properties. It has three advantages over the vidicon. First, its dark current is practically zero, hence it can be used with relatively large signal-plate voltages with a resultant large increase in sensitivity. Second, it is linear; i.e. its gamma is 1.0. Third, its lag is almost negligible. Thus the plumbicon is the tube of choice for fast-moving objects such as the heart; it does not degrade the X-ray contrast though it tends to give a somewhat noisy picture compared with that of a slow vidicon.

Very recently, many new types of photoconductive tube have appeared, all with claims of improved performance. As these are only just at the time of writing beginning to appear in clinical equipment, it is perhaps too early to evaluate their advantages.

Television monitors, video-tape recorders and storage devices

The television camera pick-up tube is a very important component in the radiological system; an almost equally important component, together with its operating conditions (though it is not often sufficiently recognised), is the television monitor. This contains a picture-type of cathode-ray tube having at the back an electron gun that projects a high-velocity beam of electrons on a fluorescent screen at the front of the tube, where it produces a light image. Controls in the monitor enable the brightness (dark parts of the image) and contrast (light parts of the image) to be adjusted at will. The gamma of the television monitor is about 2.5, due to the characteristics of the electron gun. When television systems were first introduced into radiology, it was claimed that images could be satisfactorily produced in full room lighting, resulting in large gains of convenience in techniques such as cardiac catheterisation where much ancillary apparatus and staff were needed in the fluoroscopy room.

It was soon discovered, however, that high ambient lighting conditions result in large losses in displayed contrast (compare the effect of room lighting on the screen image produced by a slide projector). Fluoroscopy room lighting was then soon fitted with dimmers so that a suitable compromise could be achieved between image contrast and operating convenience. Some manufacturers fitted light shields and tinted glass to the fronts of their monitors to reduce the deleterious effect of room lighting. Moreover, the higher the room light level the higher must be the luminance (brightness and contrast settings) of the monitor. This results in an electron beam of higher density that causes defocusing of the scanning beam and consequent loss of sharpness. It has been recently revealed[17] that monitors vary widely in their susceptibility to this effect. It is thus necessary first, to choose a good monitor and second, to use it at the lowest value of screen luminance consistent with operational convenience.

Another component that has not altogether fulfilled its early promise in clinical use is the videotape recorder. This functions very much in the same manner as the domestic tape recorder, except that the relative speed between recording or reproducing head and tape is much higher. Video-tape recorders are of course in universal use in professional television studios, but there they have skilled personnel to operate them. It is our belief that such should also be the case in the radiological context, except perhaps for the latest models; a video-tape recorder does not give of its best unless there is someone whose duty it is to operate it. This may be an engineer or a dedicated radiographer; undoubtedly useful recordings for teaching and reference purposes, etc, are being produced by such means. It seems that the recorder that is just 'pushed into a corner' and expected to function with little careful attention, however, does not produce results worthy of the technique.

The exposure to the patient in traditional fluoroscopy is about 100 mR s^{-1} maximum. In image-intensifier-television fluoroscopy the exposure rate varies from 300 μR s^{-1} for thin body sections to 10 mR s^{-1} and upwards for thick body sections. This represents a worthwhile saving in patient dose; nevertheless, attempts are currently being made to reduce patient dose by pulsing the X-ray beam (thus decreasing the exposure time to the patient) and storing the transient image so produced. Some storage devices operate with a digital store and record only one television frame, while others use analogue storage tubes and can store a number of frames from 1–25. If only one frame is stored, there is an increase in apparent X-ray quantum noise because the human eye and brain in continuous viewing stores for 100 ms or more. On the other hand, the displayed quantum noise can be materially reduced by storing a number of frames; then there may be a limitation to perceptibility caused by movement unsharpness and by background variations in the storage tube. Storage devices are not yet in widespread clinical use and it is too early to attempt to evaluate their efficacy, though they can undoubtedly be of value in techniques such as hip-pinning where high image quality is not essential.

The X-ray television system as an imaging device

The conventional X-ray image-intensifier television system exhibits in some degree most of the possible defects of an imaging system: (1) unsharpness (PSF); (2) noise, arising from random X-ray quantum absorptions, also occurring in television camera amplifiers; (3) variable backgrounds due to various causes; (4) contrast loss, arising mainly in the intensifier tube and the television monitor; it can be regarded as resulting from the skirts of the PSF, as shown in Figure 1.17; (5) lag, a term used to describe the inability of the system to follow rapid changes of X-ray input; it arises mainly in the vidicon television camera tube (p. 32); (6) non-linearity; the monitor has a gamma of about 2·5 (p. 33) the vidicon 0·7 and the plumbicon 1·0 (p. 32); (7) distortion, arising mainly in the intensifier and the lens system; (8) vignetting, a reduction in energy transfer in the periphery of the field of view; and (9) anisoplanasy: the properties, e.g. the PSF of the system, vary over the field of view.

Added to such a formidable list of defects is the complication that most of these properties interact with each other. Two examples suffice: (1) X-ray quantum interactions, being almost infinitesimal, should appear as points of light in the output image. The PSF of the system spreads their energy, however, so that the X-ray quantum noise appears coarse in structure; its power spectrum has lost its high spatial-frequency components. (2) Lag in a vidicon would appear to be wholly deleterious as it causes movement unsharpness in the images of non-stationary objects. X-ray quantum noise also is moving; hence the lag of the vidicon helps to reduce the effective noise power and to increase the signal-to-noise ratio.

Fluorography and cine-fluorography

The output of the image intensifier is often recorded on film in a still or cine camera (p. 31). These techniques are known as fluorography and cine-fluorography respectively. An optical beam-splitter (Fig. 1.28) directs the output of the intensifier to a still or cine camera.

In the case of the still camera, typical film sizes are 70 mm square, 100 mm square or 105 mm square, the latest preference being for the last size. Such *fluorograms*, whose quality can be predominantly quantum limited, can be produced at a patient exposure of the order of one-tenth or less of that of a full-size radiograph.[10] Many radiologists believe that the quality of such films is not adequate for clinical use (but see [39]); this belief may be linked with the optical difficulty of viewing smaller films, particularly by the elderly! The quality of fluorograms is much superior to that of the television image; for example, in a typical 230 mm image intensifier the limiting resolution (see p. 36) of the whole system including the fluorographic camera might be 2·5 cycles mm^{-1}, whereas that including television might be only 1·0 cycles mm^{-1}. Fluorograms are best viewed via some sort of projector; an aspect of this that is not generally mentioned is the possibility of the improvement in contrast caused by the different mode of illumination of the film compared with the standard viewing box (see p. 21).

Cine-fluorography can make use of either 35 mm or 16 mm film. In both cases the image quality is much inferior to still fluorography because of the increased effect of film granularity; it is assisted by the extended storage time of the eye which in the projected image of the film integrates both film noise and quantum noise over several frames. Cine-fluorography is of great value in studying rapidly-moving organs such as the heart; in the case of a child's heart very high frame rates may be contemplated, but it seems fruitless to attempt rates above about 200 s^{-1} because the response time of the image intensifier (about 10 ms) is then the limiting factor.

Improvements in X-ray image intensifiers

The traditional X-ray image intensifier made use of a curved input screen of zinc-cadmium sulphide in contact with a caesium-antimony photocathode; the electron optical system was of relatively rudimentary design and the electrons were focused on a flat output fluorescent screen laid on a thick, flat glass window. Its performance was mediocre in terms of unsharpness, contrast loss, distortion and overall gain. Since these early beginnings, the performance has been improved out of all recognition, in the following respects:

1. The electron optics has been subjected to computer design, assisted by certain configuration changes, described later.

2. The zinc-cadmium sulphide input screen has been replaced by one of evaporated caesium iodide (Table 1.2).[23,1] This material forms into long, thin crystals, each of which has a long absorption path for X-rays yet acts in the manner of a thin light guide that is optically separated from its neighbours, thus ensuring a small PSF. The PSF of the caesium iodide screen is at least twice as good as that of the zinc-cadmium sulphide screen, yet its X-ray absorption is markedly superior (Table 1.2).

3. The photocathode has been changed to one of tri-alkali type, thus ensuring enhanced efficiency.

4. In the earliest image intensifiers, the PSF exhibits relatively large skirts, giving rise to a large-area contrast loss, described in the frequency domain as a *low-frequency drop* (Fig. 1.19). This is predominantly caused by internal light reflection in the output window of the tube. It has been reduced in later tubes by making the output window of tinted glass, but a more radical solution has been to use an output window consisting of a fibre-optic light guide, in which lateral spread of light is significantly curtailed. Moreover, if desired, the fibre-optic output window could be incoherently coupled to the fibre-optic input window of a special camera tube, thus eliminating the aberrations and the vignetting of the optical system.

A recent and, from the point of view of fluorography, a most desirable development has been the design[24] of a 350 mm diameter input image intensifier, with optional 250 mm and 150 mm modes. This tube has many radically new features; it is made of stainless steel, and has a concave titanium input window with exceedingly low X-ray absorption. The output window is a fibre-optic bundle with a plane outer surface and a concave inner surface, the latter facilitating the computer design of the electron optics. It is believed that this tube, with its large input diameter and small low-frequency drop should for the first time enable fluorography to rival large-film radiography, but at a much lower patient dose.

IMAGE DETECTION AND PERCEPTION

Visual detection, perception and pattern recognition

Compared with the major technological advances that have produced modern X-ray equipment, the study of the visual detection and perception of the resulting visible light images is at a rudimentary stage.

The task of the radiologist is broadly twofold: the detection of details that are very small or very faint (threshold detection), and the recognition of patterns in images, the details of which are already above threshold. A little work has been done on the former; the latter has been scarcely explored. The reason for this situation is clearly that both tasks involve the physiology and the psychology of the eye and the brain, subjects whose difficulties are formidable.

Threshold detection: limiting resolution

In threshold detection, it is generally accepted that the detectability of an image detail depends on a comparison of the desired signal with the interfering noise. In an image composed of random X-ray quantum events, the signal is the mean spatial distribution of events and the noise is the fluctuation about that mean. Further noise may be added by physical systems or in the visual system itself. The difficulty is to specify what aspects of the signal and the noise are to be compared.

Before discussing possible visual mechanisms, the widely-used concept of *limiting resolution* must be referred to. It is explained on page 15 how spatial functions may be resolved by Fourier analysis into spatial frequency functions; such functions are ideally infinitely long sinusoidal distributions of intensity, etc., with varying spatial frequency and peak intensity. This concept gives rise to the idea of using such functions as test objects. Test objects for X-rays with sinusoidal distributions are difficult to make, but an adequate substitute consists of a thin lead plate having repetitive patterns of rectangular transmission instead of sinusoidal transmission cut in it. The spatial frequency may vary from group to group or it may be continuously variable. An example of each type of pattern is shown in Figure 1.30.

In use, the test object is placed as near to the image transducer as possible, usually in the centre of the field, and low kV and high mA conditions chosen so as to produce as high a contrast as possible with as little quantum noise as can be achieved. The predominant noise should then be that of the visual system itself. The highest spatial frequency at which the repetitive pattern can be resolved is then called the limiting resolution. Any convenient viewing distance may be chosen; in radiography and fluorography a magnifying lens may even be used, as the object is to test the properties of the physical system rather than those of the visual system.

The limiting resolution is widely quoted as a measure of image quality, yet it is not always a very important property. Figure 1.31 shows its relation to a typical modulation transfer function of an image-intensifier-television system, from which it can be seen that it specifies only approximately the upper limit of the function and reveals nothing of the important aspects of the remainder of the curve such as the low-frequency drop and the course of the function at medium frequencies. Nor can it be a measure of the noise properties of the system; it is true that if X-ray quantum noise is allowed to increase, the limiting resolution decreases, but this gives no information as to how the system responds to clinically realistic images.

Test objects for X-ray image transducers

In studying threshold detection, it is difficult to use patients, because their structures are irregular and therefore difficult to quantify. Instead, some kind of test object or *phantom* is interposed in the X-ray beam. The test object is usually designed to yield details having a wide range of contrasts; for simplicity, circular details are often chosen. The earliest type of phantom of this nature was made of

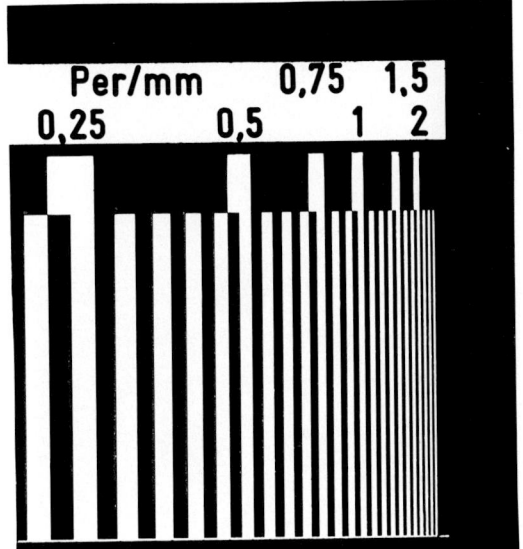 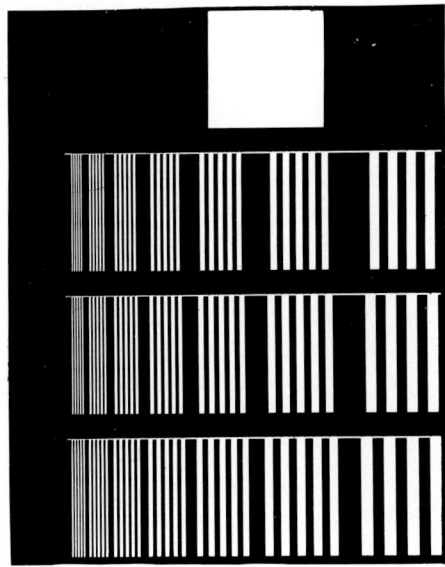

Fig. 1.30 Two common limiting-resolution test objects for X-ray use, made from lead foil 50 μm thick. The right-hand type is preferable because it includes groups of constant spatial frequency, whereas the other presents a continuously variable spatial frequency and moreover is less easy to 'read'.

a block of thick Perspex having holes of various diameters and depths drilled in it.[5] To avoid the complications of scattered radiation and geometrical unsharpness, the Burger phantom was developed into a planar test-object.[14] Figure 1.32 shows a positive print of a non-screen radiograph of the so-called 'Leeds' test object (type TO6) i.e. as it would appear on a perfect fluorescent screen. The test object consists of a plate of Perspex on which are mounted a number of discs of aluminium, lead

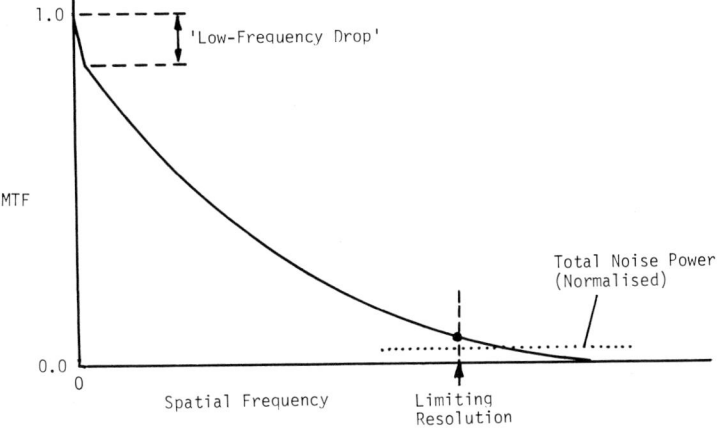

Fig. 1.31 The modulation transfer function of a typical X-ray transducer system, illustrating the concept of 'limiting resolution'. The contrast of the resolution test object is approximately unity; the limiting resolution of the system is found at that spatial frequency at which this contrast is reduced to about twice the total noise level. Also shown is the 'low-frequency drop' that results from Fourier transformation of the long low-amplitude 'skirts' of the line spread-function. (Note that the signal level corresponding to the limiting resolution is ($k \times$ noise), where $k \sim 2$.)

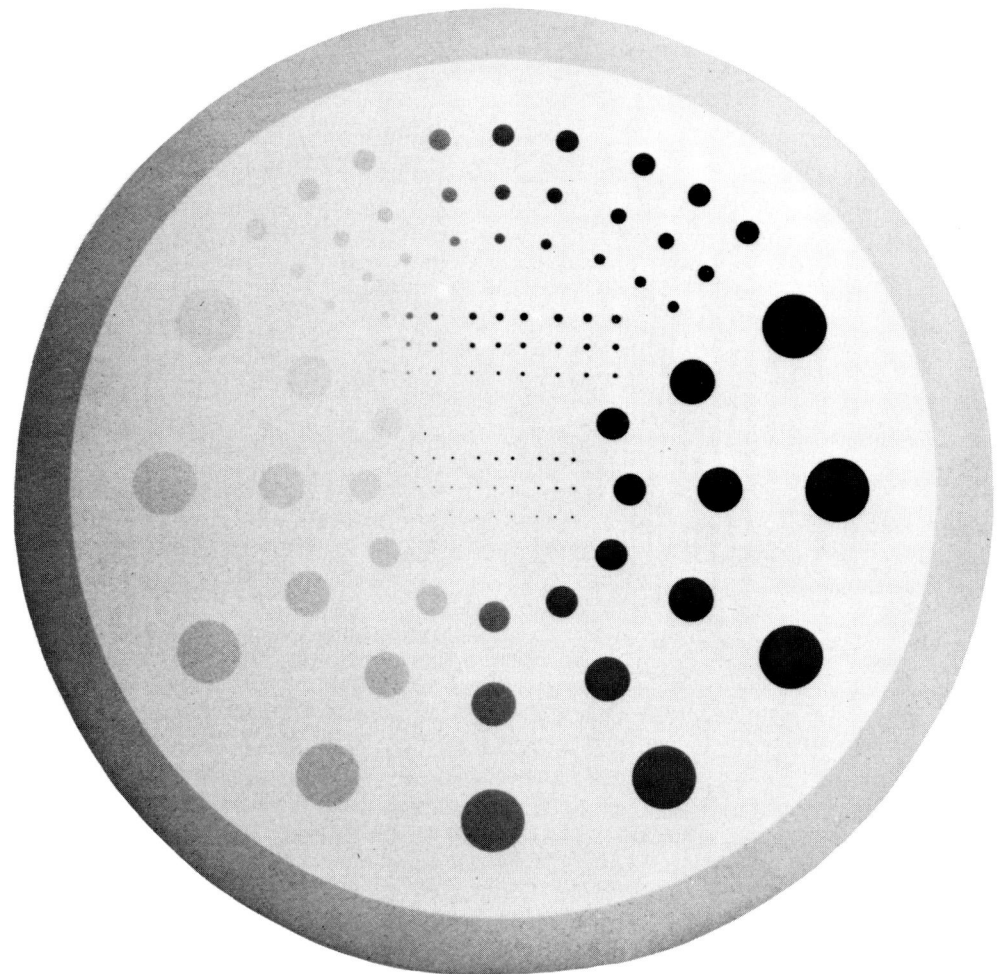

Fig. 1.32 An X-ray test object (Leeds type TO–6) designed to yield (with radiation of the appropriate quality) a wide range of detail sizes and contrasts. By its use the familiar contrast-detail diagram can be readily derived (see Fig. 1.33).

and copper which, in conjunction with an X-ray beam of known kVp and filtration, yields a large number of circular signals with a wide range of accurately known sizes and contrasts. In use, the test object is placed in the appropriate X-ray beam, and the threshold contrast for each size of disc is determined. If $-\log C_T$ (threshold contrast), is plotted against $-\log d$ (diameter), the result is the well known contrast-detail (C–d) diagram. Figure 1.33 shows typical C–d diagrams for two image-intensifier-television systems, one with a ZnCdS tube, the other a CsI tube. It is clear that the image quality of the latter is superior to that of the former; this illustrates one important application of such a test object, viz the testing of systems in the field, as well as in the laboratory. Such tests can reveal the gross deficiencies in the setting-up of these complex systems that are frequently encountered.

The $C - d$ diagram reveals other facts, however, for example that large objects are more readily detectable than are small objects. This, of course, is a matter of common experience, but it is relevant to enquire why this is so. Moreover, it would be of interest and value to know how small or how faint a signal could be detected in any given conditions of unsharpness, noise etc. An appropriate theoretical model and analysis might reveal the possible manner in which the eye and brain function at threshold.

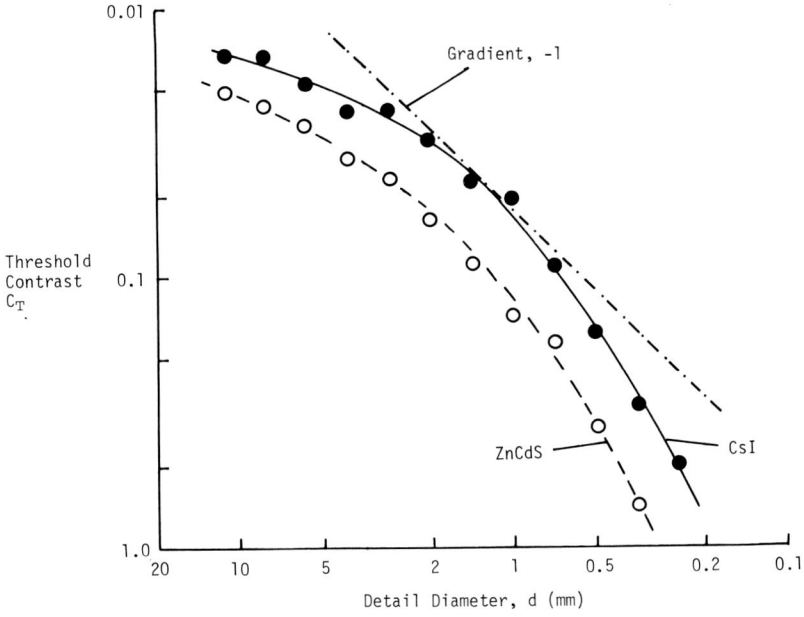

Fig. 1.33 Typical 'contrast-detail' (C–d) diagrams for two image-intensifier-television systems: one having a zinc cadmium sulphide intensifier of inferior performance, the other having a modern caesium iodide intensifier. The straight line shows the shape to be expected from the model of visual detection described by Equation 1.12.

A model of visual threshold detection

Figure 1.34a shows an image field with a background of n quanta mm^{-2} s^{-1} in which is a detail having $(n + \Delta n)$ quanta mm^{-2} s^{-1}. The contrast between the two for the present purpose may be defined as $C = \Delta n/n$. (It is noteworthy that contrast defined in this way, for the small contrasts common in radiology, is approximately equal to the definition $C_r = \ln((\Delta n + n)/n)$ (p. 7). This would not be so if logs to the base 10 were used to define X-ray contrast.)

To calculate signal and noise from the quantum flux density, it is necessary to define an area and a time over which the absorbed quanta are integrated. For conventional images,[34, 35, 43] and further for X-ray images,[41] it has been proposed that both signal and noise should be integrated over the area of the signal. The integrating time is assumed to be identical with the storage time of the brain (see p. 6). No probable anatomical location for the hypothetical integrating area has been suggested, although it has been proposed that there could exist, in the visual cortex of the brain, neural receptive fields that would fulfil this function.[15] There is considerable physiological evidence for the existence of such receptive fields in the visual cortex, at least for edges and bars. These assumptions lead to the following model.

Let d mm be the diameter of the signal, and τ s be the storage time of the system. Then the signal is given by

$$S = \Delta n d^2 \tau \pi / 4$$

In order to calculate the noise, it is now necessary to assume that the quanta are integrated over the same area as the signal (scaled, of course, to the visual cortical area). Then the noise N is given by

$$N = (nd^2\tau\pi/4)^{1/2},$$

because the noise is associated with the total background n, and the fluctuation is the square root of the average number of events, assuming a Poisson distribution.

Now let us assume that, for threshold detection,

$$S = kN,$$

where k is a constant (usually approximately equal to 2, but dependent on the degree of certainty with which the detail is detected).
Then

$$\frac{\Delta n d^2 \tau \pi/4}{n} = \frac{k(nd^2\tau\pi/4)^{1/2}}{n}$$

hence

$$C_T d = k\,(\tau n)^{-1/2}\,(\pi/4)^{-1/2}, \qquad (1.12)$$

where C_T is the threshold contrast.

This equation leads to three important conclusions: (1) for constant τ and n, $C_T \propto d^{-1}$; (2) for constant τ and d, $C_T \propto n^{-1/2}$; and (3) for constant n and d, $C_T \propto \tau^{-1/2}$.

Conclusions (1) and (2) are shown graphically in Figures 1.34b and 1.34c. Figure 1.34b correctly

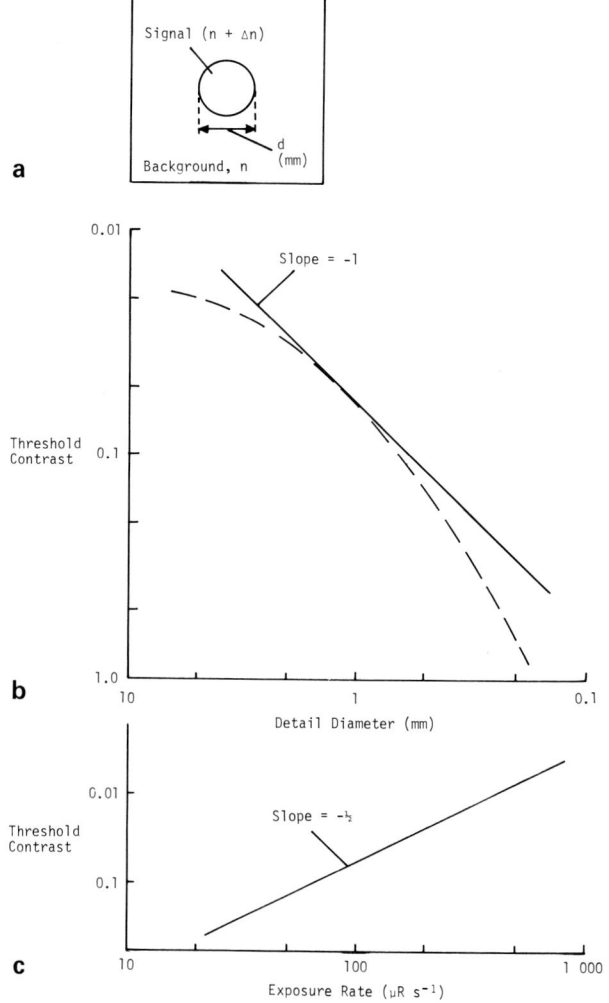

Fig. 1.34 (a) Showing a wanted signal of $(n + \Delta n)$ quanta mm^{-2} s^{-1} and diameter d mm against a background of n quanta mm^{-2} s^{-1} (compare Fig. 1.25). (b) —, the theoretically predicted function $C_T.d$ = constant from Equation 1.12; – – – –, a typical experimentally determined contrast-detail curve (compare Fig. 1.33). (c) the theoretically predicted function $C_T \propto n^{-1/2}$, showing how image quality improves slowly with increase of exposure rate (compare Fig. 1.35).

predicts the general trend of experimentally determined $C - d$ diagrams, though the practical results, as shown, deviate from the theoretical for both large and small detail, requiring modifications to the theoretical analysis. Figure 1.35 shows $-\log C_T$ plotted against exposure rate (which is proportional to n) for a panel-type image intensifier (Hay and Cowen, in preparation); the gradient of ½ denoting the square root law is evident. Clearly image quality improves with exposure rate, though the change is somewhat slow, and the law is often complicated by factors such as changing storage time (of television camera tubes) and the presence of neural noise in the visual system. In a similar fashion, image quality improves with storage time, which is the reason for the superiority of the images of stationary objects produced by a vidicon.

Visual effects important in radiology

Apart from the effects described on page 39, the visual system has properties that profoundly influence the viewing of radiological images.

The eye and brain have great difficulty in judging the small differences in luminance between areas that are separated by a considerable distance. If these areas are brought together so that they have a common boundary, however, quite small differences, of the order of 2 per cent, can be detected. This is of great advantage in radiology in detecting the boundary between areas of differing radiopacity. It is assisted by two properties of vision.

First, the eye appears to have the ability to integrate along a long boundary. Thus if a just-de-

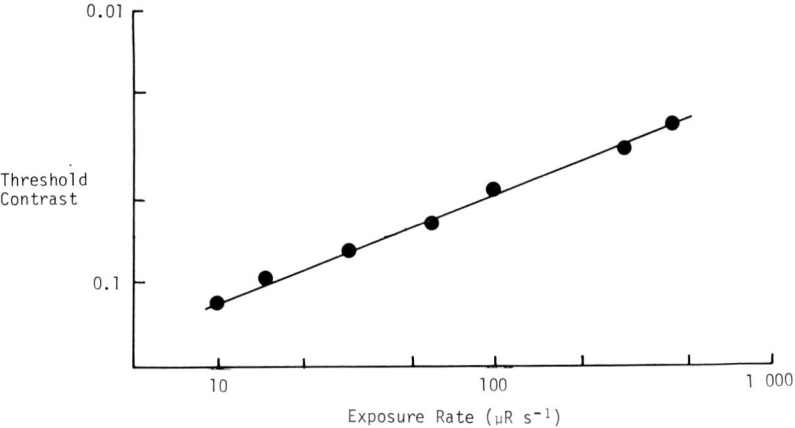

Fig. 1.35 Showing the decrease in threshold contrast for large disc-shaped signals (improvement in performance), resulting from increased exposure rate, for a panel-type proximity image intensifier. The curve approximates a half power law, which is predicted by Equation 1.12.

The deviations of practical $C - d$ curves from the theoretical ideal can be explained in a variety of ways. For small detail, it is almost certain that unsharpness is implicated. By varying the unsharpness[7] of an optical projection system or of an X-ray television system, the expected change in the lower end of the $C - d$ curve results. This has been confirmed by Cowen (unpublished), and an explanatory mechanism has been suggested.[15] The large area departure is not so easy to explain, and at the time of writing no valid mechanism for this region has been proposed. Much further work is desirable in this field.

tectable long boundary is presented, then if the length of the boundary is curtailed, the difference in brightness between the two areas disappears. The reason for this ability is not known.

Second, the eye performs a spatial differentiation that assists in the detection of boundaries. Figure 1.36a shows a radiograph of a step wedge (see p. 27) in which the luminance of the image has a rectangular form as in Figure 1.36b. Because of the presence of inhibitory neural connections in the retina, the step wedge is perceived with a characteristic 'fluted' appearance. This is known as the *Mach effect*. It has the effect of accentuating

42 SCIENTIFIC BASIS OF MEDICAL IMAGING

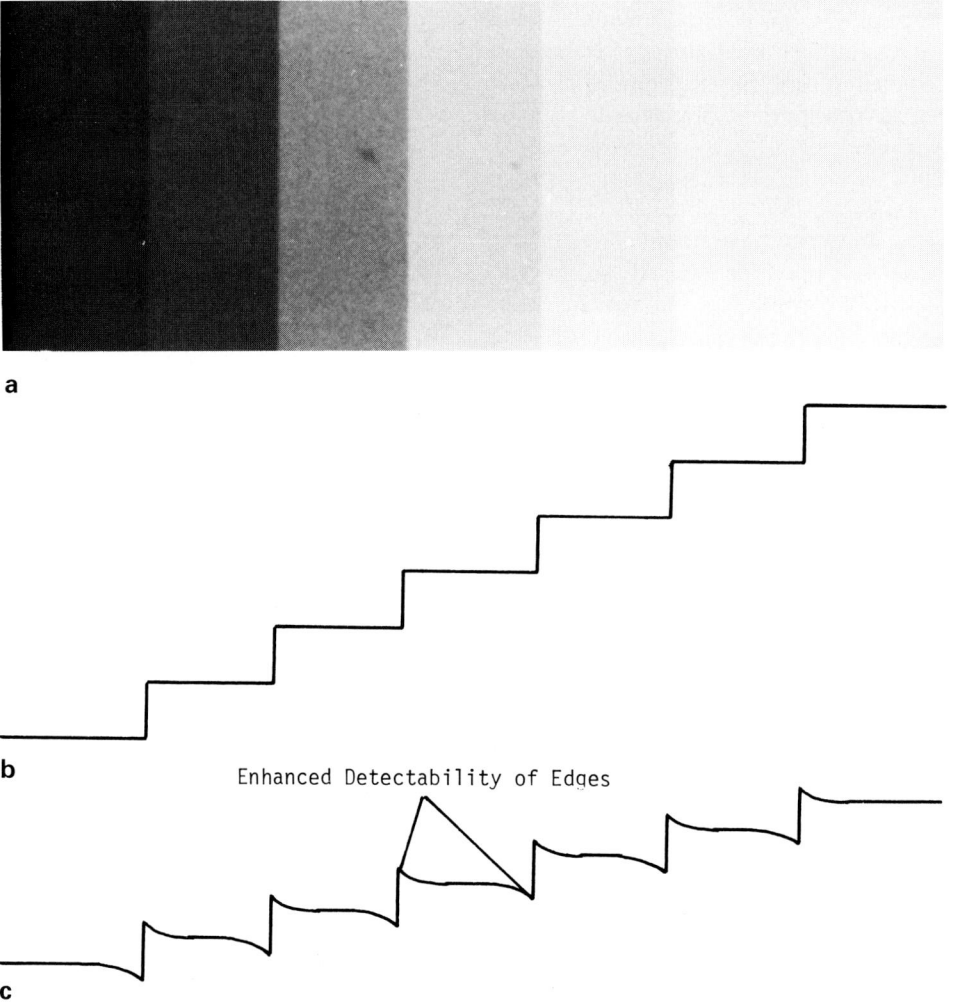

Fig. 1.36 (a) A radiograph of an aluminium step-wedge. (b) The luminance (= light emitted) distribution of (a). (c) The brightness (= subjective appearance) of (a), in which inhibitory neural connections in the retina perform a spatial differentiation process, thus enhancing the detectability of the edges.

boundaries and of compressing the gray scale of the image. A similar effect, though much more pronounced, is obtained from xeroradiography (see p. 44). This effect naturally depends on the viewing distance, and the wise radiologist views his films from various distances in an attempt to detect the feature of interest.

Pattern recognition

A considerable part of the radiologist's task is occupied with pattern recognition. As previously pointed out, the X-ray image is a two-dimensional representation of a three-dimensional object; a large part of the radiologist's training consists of learning how to interpret this representation in terms of patient structures. In this he is assisted overwhelmingly by his memory, which, in some way yet unknown, stores a wide variety of images and enables him subsequently to recognise patterns that the untrained observer cannot see at all. Because of the complexity of this subject, analytical treatments of pattern recognition in radiology are almost completely lacking.

IMAGE ENHANCEMENT

The processing of images so that threshold detection or pattern recognition might be enhanced has always seemed an attractive possibility. Many attempts have been made, but only one, viz image subtraction, is used routinely, and that only at relatively few centres. This statement, of course, excludes the extremely powerful technique of CT scanning (Ch. 2), which may be regarded as a form of image enhancement.

Threshold detection

If threshold detection is regarded basically as a signal-to-noise ratio determination, it might be argued crudely that whatever process enhances the signal also enhances the noise, resulting in zero gain. No doubt the processes involved are more subtle than would be indicated by such a simple analysis. The fact remains, however, that all attempts to enhance threshold detection where the noise and the signal arise at the same point (as in X-ray quantum limited images) have been broadly unsuccessful. They have resulted only in gains of convenience and in aesthetic improvement.[11] When the noise arises at a point after the signal, however, for example in conventional vision, significant gains are possible. This accounts for the well known efficacy of spectacles! It may be, however, that this somewhat pessimistic view is a result of attempts to perform the enhancement by analogue methods; the greater flexibility of digital methods (p. 45) may yet lead to significant gains in threshold detection. It is probable that such gains could accrue only as a result of a much fuller understanding of human visual processes than we have at the present time.

One example of image enhancement that purports to improve the detectability of isolated structures partly obscured by noise is called image *smoothing*. Essentially this consists of a controlled increase in unsharpness of the system. The power spectrum of the noise is assumed to extend to higher spatial frequencies than does the spectrum of the signal. Hence an increase of unsharpness tends to remove the excess noise frequencies without affecting the signal. This, it is argued by its protagonists, must necessarily improve the detectability of the signal, but it is known[15] that noise frequencies in general tend to obscure only similar component frequencies of the signal. Hence it might be argued that the removal of these noise frequencies has little or no effect on the lower frequencies that constitute the signal. Again, the visual mechanisms are not fully understood, and there is considerable controversy as to whether this technique affords real gains of detectability or simply gains of convenience and aesthetics.[11] A recent description of image smoothing in CT scanning,[20] in which the processing is performed digitally by a computer, makes claims of real gains in detectability. In this case, however, because of the filtered back-projection type of computer reconstruction employed, the noise is non-white, being deficient in low spatial frequencies. This fact may profoundly influence the visual mechanisms involved. (Note that this paper also includes a useful bibliography of image smoothing in general.)

Another example of image enhancement that is intended to assist in the threshold detection of edges and which results also in a compression of the gray scale and hence in a wider latitude is the technique known as *harmonisation*. This is essentially a spatial differentiation process similar to that which occurs in the eye and in xeroradiography; it may be performed in an analogue mode by special radiographic techniques or by television methods. In radiography, a blurred negative copy is made of the radiograph and the copy and the original are then viewed simultaneously in spatial registration. The effect is to enhance edges and to compress the gray scale. A similar result is attained by viewing the same radiograph through two television cameras, one being deliberately and grossly set out of focus. The two electrical outputs are then subtracted and the result viewed on a television monitor. An instrument performing the latter function has been available commercially for many years, yet little clinical use has been made of it. It may again be that the greater controllability of digital methods of processing would lead to worthwhile gains.

Pattern recognition

Where pattern recognition is concerned, image enhancement can result in very large gains of perceptibility. Consider two X-ray exposures, between which a small change has taken place that is normally difficult to distinguish against the background of all the extraneous detail. For example, the first exposure could be one of an arterial system without contrast medium; the smaller arteries are below threshold contrast. The second could be the same exposure after the injection of contrast medium. If the image of the first phase is subtracted from the image of the second, the element of change will become clearly visible in the difference. Procedures of this sort are known as *subtraction* techniques. The mode of operation of this type of technique depends on removing the vast amount of redundant information from the original image. The technique has been described for radiography[47] and for image intensifier television.[28] It is also referred to on page 45.

NEW TYPES OF TRANSDUCER

New types of transducer fall into two categories: those that function with the conventional two-dimensional X-ray image, and those that function with completely different geometry. The former category includes xeroradiography, ionography, multi-wire proportional chambers and digital radiography; these are described later. The latter category is represented by an extremely powerful new technique called computed tomography which is dealt with in Chapter 2.

Xeroradiography

In this technique, a thin layer of amorphous selenium laid on a metal backing plate is given a uniform surface charge by a corona-charging device. The initial potential difference is several hundred volts. The layer is then exposed to the X-ray image, and, since it is a photoconductor, charge is dissipated in exposed regions thus leaving a charge image on the selenium surface. This charge image is then developed by exposure to a cloud of fine powder particles from an aerosol.

The sensitivity of the xeroradiograph depends on the layer thickness and on the development process, but successful clinical images can be made at X-ray exposures of the order of 10 times that of the average radiograph. The limiting resolution of the layer is extremely high, of the order of at least 10 times that of a screen radiograph. The display of fine detail is also enhanced by the behaviour of the developing powder in seeking out regions of high field strength which occur at boundaries. This phenomenon also results in great sensitivity to small contrasts by virtue of the edge enhancement so produced. Additionally, because of the spatial differentiation effect of the same phenomenon, the xeroradiograph exhibits a marked compression of the gray scale and therefore an extremely wide exposure latitude. The general behaviour is analogous to that of the eye (the Mach effect p. 41) but is much more marked.

The peculiar advantages of xeroradiography make it of special value in mammography, in arteriography and venography and in radiography of bones and joints.[2] Of these, only the first has so far found considerable clinical application.

Ionography

This technique is similar to xeroradiography but makes use of ionisation in a gas to produce the charge image on an insulating foil. The X-ray energy is absorbed either in the ion chamber walls[31] or in the gas itself.[3] Sensitivities and limiting resolutions approaching those of screen radiography are possible but depend critically on the difficult engineering design features. Ionography is not expected to rival radiography in the foreseeable future.

Multi-wire proportional chambers

The chamber is bounded by two planar cathodes, each consisting of a grid of conductors. The two grids are at right angles to each other. Midway between the cathodes is an anode composed of thin conductors held at a few kilovolts with respect to the cathodes. The chamber is filled with a high-atomic-number gas such as xenon. Absorption of an X-ray quantum produces a photoelectron in the gas which results in an electron avalanche and a signal at both cathodes. The wires of each cathode are connected to a delay line; thus by electronic timing the position of the avalanche in the chamber can be signalled as a function of two orthogonal coordinates.[29] From this information a computer can construct a two-dimensional image on a television monitor.

For X-ray imaging the chamber has an absorption efficiency of about 0·15 but its limiting resolution cannot compare with that of radiography. Its advantage lies in its quantitative digital output. No routine clinical applications can at present be foreseen.

Digital radiography

Conventional radiography suffers from a number of limitations. First, a single radiograph should be so exposed that it results in the structure of interest falling in the region of maximum gamma. If attention is directed to another structure of differing radiopacity it may well be found in a region of unfavourable gamma, thus necessitating a further exposure using different mA and perhaps kV, with the undesirable result of additional patient doses. Second, the photographic emulsion itself, despite its great advantages, has limitations, principally of contrast sensitivity and limited latitude. Third, despite the relatively sophisticated performance of the human eye, it is deficient in respect of contrast sensitivity, gray-scale differentiation etc.

In principle, a system can be envisaged in which an X-ray exposure could be made, with appropriate measures for the maximum reduction of scattered radiation, at a value of kV that would yield optimum X-ray contrast. The resulting X-ray image could be received by a two-dimensional transducer that converted each elementary area (*pixel*) of the image into an electrical signal that represented the original X-ray exposure in digital form. The ensemble of digital signals could then be stored in a computer and then subjected to any desired form of image manipulation, in a manner similar to that employed in the existing CT scanner (Ch. 2). Image enhancement techniques could be employed in a much more flexible form than is possible by the analogue methods which are discussed on page 43. The resulting digital image could then be displayed on a printer or converted back to analogue form on an electronic X-Y display unit. It is possible to envisage that the various forms of image manipulation or enhancement could be under the direct control of the radiologist, who, after a degree of familiarisation with the system's potentialities, could then display to greatest advantage the desired structures.

Such a device is not available at the present time, but a few pilot studies have been made of the possibilities of this technique, making use of readily available components. Two examples of such studies, using widely differing components, are now briefly described.

The first example[21] makes use of the X-ray source and the detector system of a CT body scanner (Ch. 2). A highly collimated fan beam of pulsed X-rays, only 1·5 mm wide, is used in conjunction with a linear array of highly collimated high-pressure xenon ion-chamber transducers. The patient is moved the requisite distance through this arrangement at a constant linear speed of 6 cm s^{-1}. The use of such apparatus, in conjunction with the resulting patient-transducer air gap, results in a very high degree of reduction of the scattered radiation that normally results in serious loss of contrast as explained on page 8. The use of xenon transducers results in a very high dynamic range, of the order of 10^4, giving full scope for subsequent computer manipulation. The general performance of the system is intermediate between CT scanning and conventional radiography. It is at its best for thick sections and objects >3mm; conventional radiography is superior for thin sections and small objects. For thick sections a considerable saving in dose amounting to a factor of about 20 in incident exposure to the patient is achieved. The disadvantages are long exposure time (7 s for a 42 cm field), which seriously limits its use for moving structures, and poor limiting resolution (high unsharpness) because of the size of the X-ray scanning beam.

The second example[22] avoids these disadvantages to a certain degree, but introduces others. In this system, a conventional X-ray tube operating at 100 kVp, 8–50 mA, or 60 kVp, 150–300 mA is used in conjunction with a conventional caesium iodide 230/150 mm image intensifier followed by a plumbicon television camera tube. The video information from the latter is collected at standard television rates, amplified logarithmically (to accommodate the desired gray scale), and digitised to 8 bits every 100 to 200 ns. After digitisation, data can be stored in one of three memories in which temporal integration of up to 32 video fields can take place. After computer processing of these images, the data are reconverted to analogue form and displayed on a video monitor. It is clear that this system avoids some of the disadvantages of the first example, viz slow response and poor limiting resolution, but substitutes other disadvantages, such as inferior rejection of scattered radiation and reduced dynamic range. It may be questioned why it is not possible to subtract the effects of scattered radiation in the computer. It *is* possible to subtract the mean value, but, as pointed out on page 8 scattered radiation carries with it the inevitable fluctuation or noise associated with the random absorption of X-ray quanta, and this, being random, cannot be subtracted. The system described has been used principally for time-dependent studies. In one mode, the so-called *mask* mode, the image of the heart of a dog is integrated over 32 television fields; this provides the time- and space-integrated mask from which subsequent fields, either single or integrated up to three or four fields, may be subtracted. The resulting image reveals the change that is produced by the injection of contrast medium into the heart; it is an example of a subtraction process (p. 43). The mask mode technique is sensitive to respiratory motion. An alternative mode that avoids this disadvantage is *time interval difference* imaging, which differs from the mask mode in that the two images that are subtracted are both formed in relatively short periods, which results in a higher noise level. Studies have been made in dogs also without contrast medium and the results are promising but the authors conclude that the technique is ready for trial using human volunteers only with contrast medium.

The above two examples show the kind of advantage that is to be gained by the use of digital radiographic techniques. It seems likely that an apparatus especially designed for such an application, using for example a conventional X-ray beam with an array of collimated solid-state transducers might combine the advantages of both examples. Conventional radiographic techniques are so firmly entrenched in the routine clinical department, however, that in the author's opinion* it will be a long time before digital techniques become routinely accepted. There is a long time interval between the laboratory experiment and the final engineered clinical equipment, especially when the fundamental gains to be achieved are not outstandingly obvious, as they were in the case of CT scanning.

CLINICAL APPLICATIONS

There is hardly any region of the human anatomy in which traditional X-ray imaging techniques have not been applied to advantage. In many regions, the new technique of CT scanning (Ch. 2) has enormously extended the contrast sensitivity of the X-ray imaging process, but at the time of writing, by far the greater part of routine radiology makes use of traditional techniques. Because of their relative simplicity and low cost, this situation is likely to persist for many years to come.

Fluoroscopy, radiography and fluorography

Fluoroscopy has the outstanding advantage that it enables movement to be observed, and, using video-tape or cine techniques, to be recorded. Especially since the development of high-performance image-intensifier-television systems, many diagnoses of pathological conditions, for example in the digestive system and in gross skeletal changes, can be made from the television image itself, without the need for any subsequent radiograph. It is usually felt necessary to make a permanent record of the image for future reference, however, and this is traditionally carried out by full-size radiography. The advent of fluorographic recording of the image-intensifier output has made it possible to make record films ('spot films') which are of adequate image quality at a small fraction of the cost and silver requirement of full-size radiography.

In applications where the image quality of the television system is inadequate for final diagnosis, for example in arteriography and in studies of cardiac function, the television system can be used to great advantage in suitably positioning the patient

---

*The author has kindly agreed that the editor may express a contrary view. It is the editor's opinion that digital radiographic techniques will rapidly gain acceptance. He thinks that many conventional machines will be replaced by digital systems as they wear out, particularly because of high cost of silver used in conventional radiography, and because of the enormous advantage of intravenous angiography.

ready for the subsequent radiograph or radiographs. In such cases, it may be that the very recent advances in image intensifier design (p. 35) will result in adequate image quality for diagnosis from 105 mm fluorography, thus rendering the high cost and large silver requirement of the full-size radiograph unnecessary. This, of course, will also be accompanied by a welcome reduction in dose to the patient (p. 35). In the further future, perhaps one may look forward to the potentialities of digital radiography (p. 45) to rival both fluorography and full-size radiography.

Because of the breadth of application of traditional X-ray imaging techniques, a detailed list of their applications would be both voluminous and tedious. Many such applications have been used above to illustrate specific physical techniques, but there are several broad applications of these techniques that can be singled out for specific mention, as follows.

Techniques using unusual values of kV

The great majority of radiological techniques use values of kV between 60 and 100, at which optimum contrast is obtained. There are situations, however, where markedly increased or decreased kV may be used to advantage.

High-kV radiography has been mentioned as a means of increasing the effective latitude of a radiograph, for example in displaying both bone and soft-tissue detail on the same film. It has other secondary advantages: (1) because of the rapid variation of exposure with kV ($E \propto kV^4$), the mA.s product is greatly reduced resulting in a decrease of exposure time and of movement unsharpness; (2) because of the greater efficiency of X-ray production, X-ray tube heating is reduced; (3) because of the lower mA.s possible, a fine-focus tube may be used; and (4) the radiation dose to the patient (i.e., total absorbed energy) is reduced.

To set against these advantages is the over-riding consideration that contrasts as a whole are reduced (see p. 7), and may not be sufficient for adequate diagnosis.

For radiography of soft tissues, particularly in relatively thin sections, for example in radiography of the breast (mammography), it is essential to increase the contrast by operating over a kV region where the photoelectric type of interaction predominates (p. 4). This necessitates operation in the region of 25–35 kVp. The small contrasts so produced may be rendered even more perceptible by increasing the edge sharpness of boundaries, either by using non-screen radiography or by xeroradiography. In the interests of patient dose reduction, however, it is customary today to use screen-film techniques, with films and screens especially designed for mammography.

Serial radiography

This technique makes use of a rapid succession of exposures to study time-dependent phenomenena such as events in the circulatory system as revealed by the rapid injection of iodine-carrying contrast medium into an artery or into the heart chambers. This procedure is known as *angiography*.

Serial radiography in general can make use of several types of apparatus. For slow changes, hand operation of cassettes may be adequate. Otherwise, machines known as *serial changers* are used, producing 8 or 10 exposures consecutively at short intervals. These may operate in two dimensions (*bi-plane* serial changers). Alternatively, small-film fluorography or even cine-fluorography may be used, the X-ray exposures being synchronised with the film movement. In all cases it is essential to ensure that the X-ray generator is capable of delivering the necessary energy within a short space of time, and also that the X-ray tube is capable of dissipating the large amount of heat so produced without excessive damage to its target.

Stereoscopic radiography

It is well known that binocular vision produces a three-dimensional impression of a scene. A similar result may be attained in radiography by taking two exposures between which the X-ray tube has been moved through the interpupillary distance, usually about 6 cm. The radiographs are then viewed via a mirror system on a double viewing box. Stereoscopic radiography is not widely used, but is most frequently employed for the sacro-iliac joints and for certain views of the skull.

Macroradiography

The technique of macroradiography is used on page 14) to illustrate the complex interplay of factors in X-ray image formation. The usual method of implementing this technique is to maintain the source-to-patient distance constant and to increase the source-to-transducer distance. Indeed, it is often said that reduction of source-to-patient distance must not be used, as it would result in an increase of patient dose. This view is fallacious, however, as in that case the source-to-transducer distance would be unchanged and the X-ray tube output would not have to be increased.

Macroradiography is used mainly for skeletal structures, for chest radiography (lung pathology), for eye studies and for radiography of various glands.

Tomography

Tomography is described on page 11 as a form of selective unsharpness. For the purpose of demonstration, linear tube-film movement is often assumed, but many different forms of movement are advocated as being superior. The principal disadvantages of the technique are the need for precision engineering in the equipment and complete lack of movement in the patient, for the tube-film movement may occupy several seconds. Moreover, the blurred images of the overlying structures cause loss of contrast in the wanted plane; therefore, it is necessary to maintain as low a kV as possible consistent with adequate penetration of the patient. Multisection tomography makes use of a multilayer cassette which usually contains five pairs of screens, thus enabling five planes to be selected simultaneously. This results in a reduction of patient dose (compared with that for five separate exposures), also the advantage that all planes are imaged at the same phase of respiration. The applications of tomography are numerous.

Foreign body localisation

Radiography can be used to locate foreign bodies by reference to well-established anatomical landmarks. Often only a single film is sufficient, but a bi-plane exposure might be helpful. It is important that final radiography should immediately precede surgery for removal, as foreign bodies can move considerable distances in some circumstances. Foreign bodies in the eye are more difficult to locate and special geometrical techniques are necessary.

Contrast media

Contrast media can have either high atomic number, for example barium and iodine, or low atomic number, such as air. Many body structures, for example the intestine, the lungs and the paranasal sinuses already contain air. In other cases the contrast medium must be either ingested or injected. Contrast media must be non-toxic, must produce adequate contrast, must have a suitable viscosity, must have a suitable persistence, and must be either miscible or immiscible with body fluids, as appropriate. The administration, particularly the injection, of contrast media is always accompanied by clinical risk and inconvenience and steps must always be taken to minimise these disadvantages. For example, in the case of a barium enema it is no longer thought necessary completely to fill the intestine with a suspension of barium sulphate but merely to inject sufficient of a compound that will outline the walls of the intestine. Similarly, it was originally hoped that the high contrast sensitivity of the CT scanner would render contrast media, particularly in the head, unnecessary, but such appears not to have been the case, though concentrations may be considerably reduced.

Figures 1.37 and 1.38 show a typical clinical use of contrast medium in which an iodine compound is used to render more perceptible the bronchial tree. The use of postero–anterior (PA) and lateral views enables the anatomy to be recognised and analysed more easily.

Further clinical examples

Figures 1.39 and 1.40 show respectively a normal (lumbar) spine and an arthritic (cervical) spine. The fusing together of the vertebrae in the case of arthritis is clear. Figures 1.41 and 1.42 show respectively fractures of the tibia and fibula and of the pubis. These four examples of full-size radiography of the skeleton are of applications in which 105 mm fluorography might be adequate for diag-

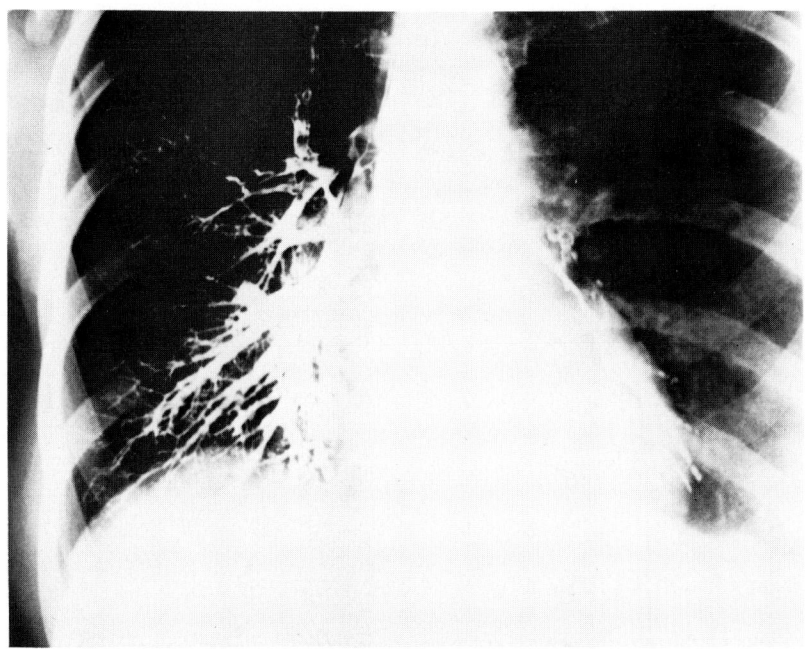

Fig. 1.37 Postero-anterior bronchogram showing the use of contrast medium for rendering more perceptible the bronchial tree.

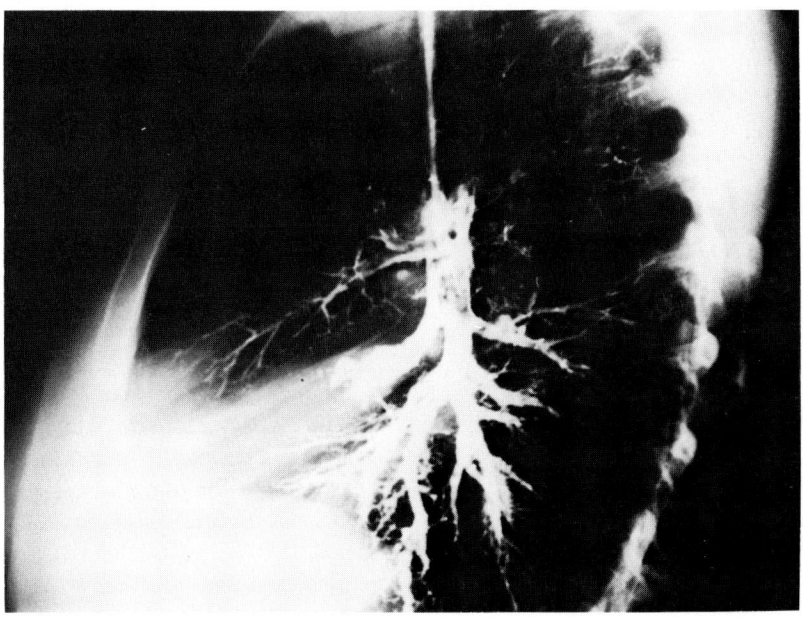

Fig. 1.38 As Fig. 1.37, but lateral view.

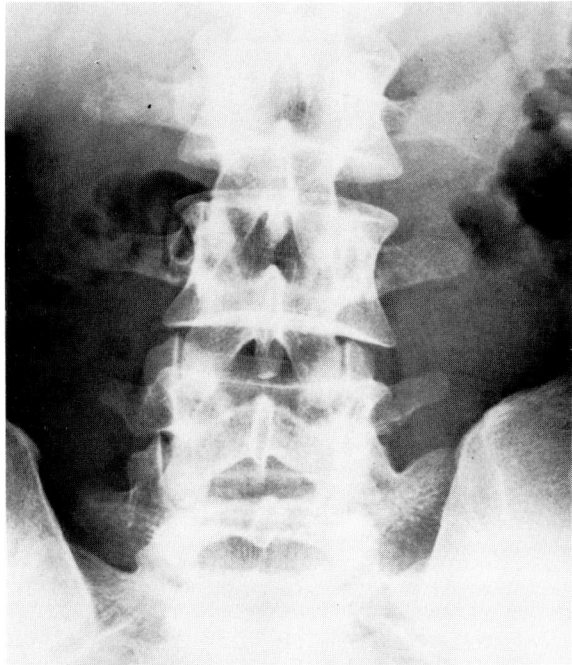

Fig. 1.39 Normal lumbar spine showing normally articulated vertebrae.

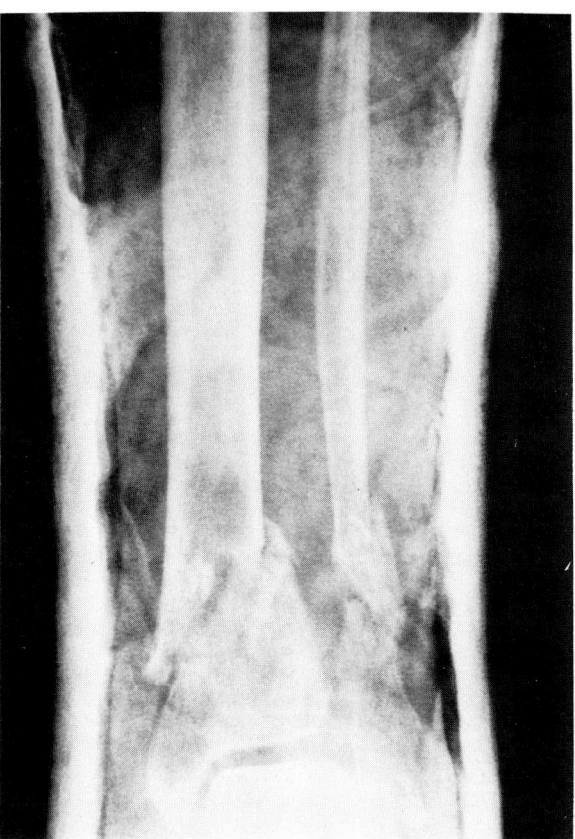

Fig. 1.41 Fractures of the tibia and fibula.

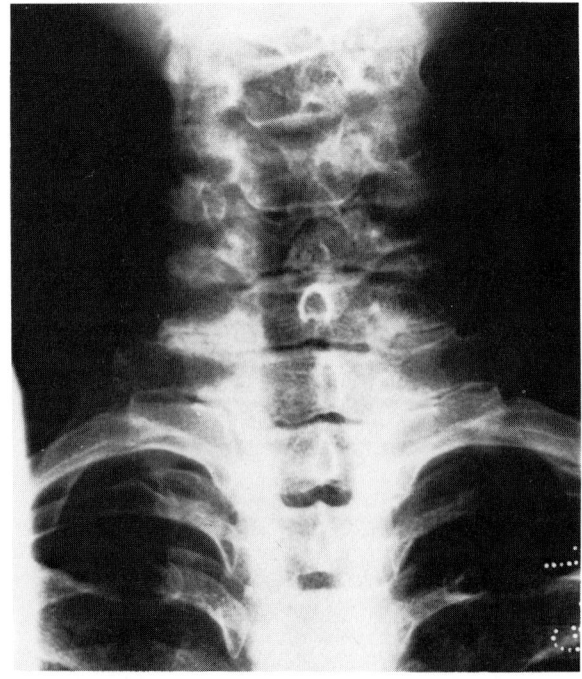

Fig. 1.40 Cervical spine showing the fused vertebrae of arthritis.

nosis. Figure 1.43 shows a Charnley prosthesis for replacement of a hip joint — clearly a case in which 105 mm fluorography would present entirely adequate image quality for diagnosis. Indeed, orthopaedic surgeons are now beginning to use electronic image stores for such examinations, with a saving in patient dose and an even greater saving of expense in terms of money and of silver.

The remaining three clinical examples show full-size radiographs in which perhaps the inferior image quality of the 105 mm fluorogram may not be adequate for diagnosis. Figure 1.44 is a lateral chest radiograph showing a heart valve replacement; this is clearly visible on the original radiograph but may not be so clear in the half-tone reproduction. It is a matter of speculation whether or not the fluorogram would yield adequate image quality for this application; it probably would not

TRADITIONAL X-RAY IMAGING 51

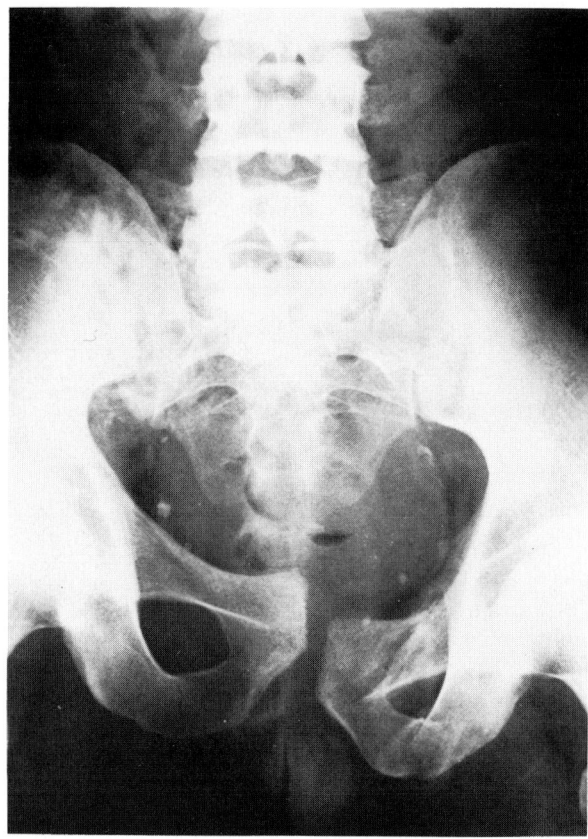

Fig. 1.42 A dislocated pubis.

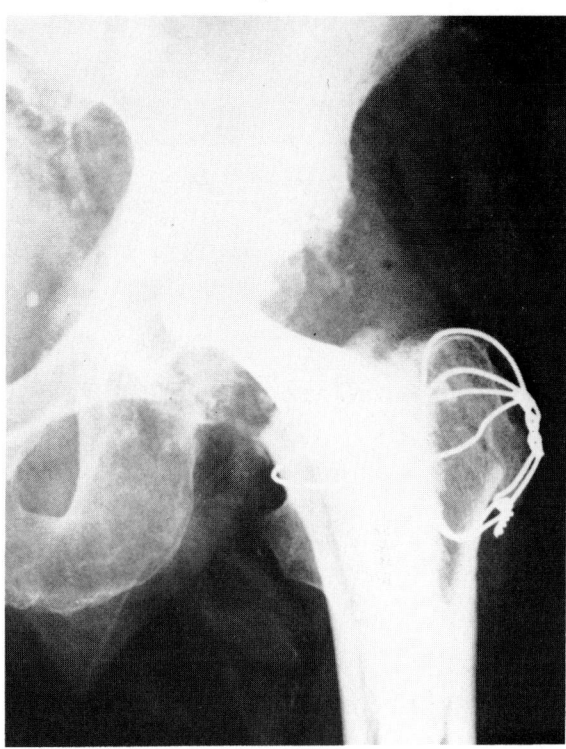

Fig. 1.43 A prosthesis (metal) for the replacement of a hip joint.

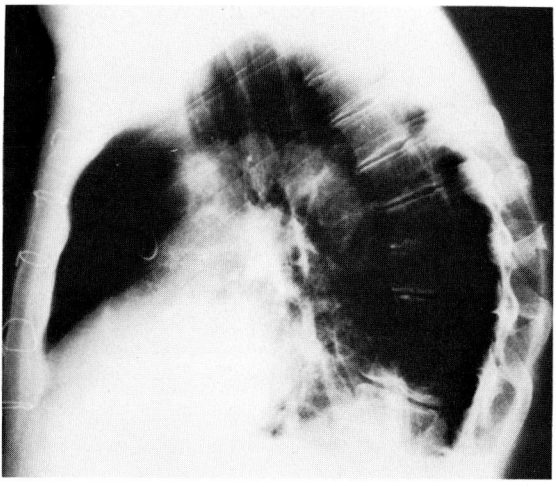

Fig. 1.44 Lateral chest showing a heart valve replacement.

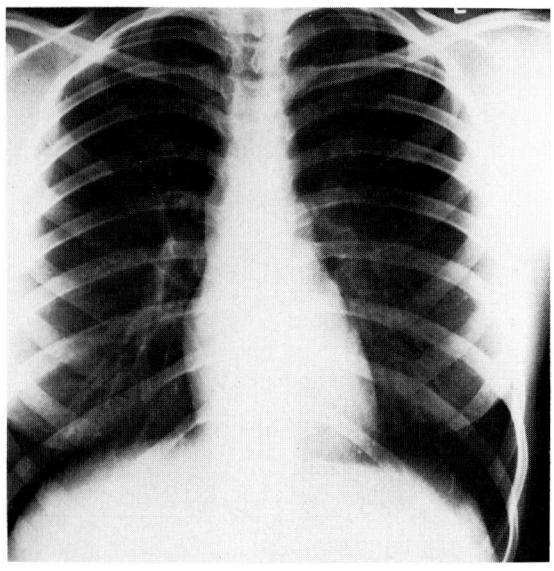

Fig. 1.45 PA view of a chest showing normal lung structure.

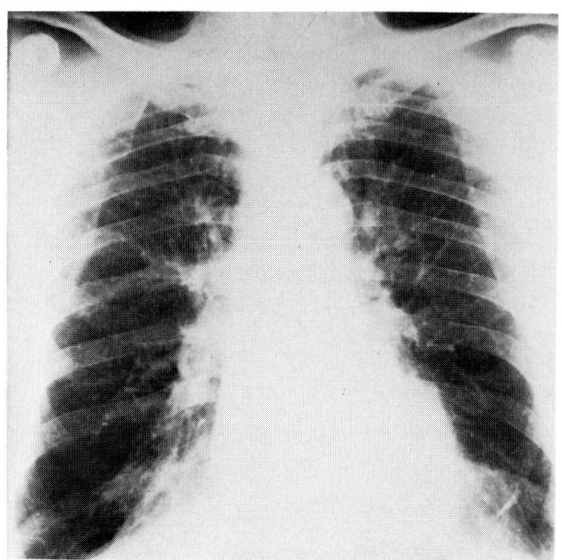

Fig. 1.46 PA view of a chest showing bronchitic lungs: a case where pattern recognition is all-important to the radiologist.

for the detection of, for example, some calcifications in heart valves.

Figures 1.45 and 1.46 show respectively a normal chest (with normal lung structure) and a bronchitic chest. This is a good example of a situation in which the radiologist must distinguish between two different patterns. Again, the patterns are clearly differentiated in the original films; they may not be so clear in the half-tone reproduction, but it is entirely a matter of opinion whether or not they would be distinguishable in a 105 mm fluorogram, even with the most recent design of image intensifier. The radiologist's visual system and brain are conditioned predominantly to function with full-size radiographs; any departure from this technique, whether it be in the direction of image-intensifier fluorography or of digital radiography, will demand a new set of learned skills.

Acknowledgement

It is my pleasure to acknowledge the assistance of the Staff of the Department of Diagnostic Radiology in the General Infirmary at Leeds in obtaining the clinical radiographs which illustrate this chapter.

REFERENCES

1. Birken, H. & Bejczy, C. I. (1973) A new generation of image intensifiers. *Medicamundi*, **18**, 120–7
2. Boag, J. W. (1973) Xeroradiography. *Phys. Med. Biol.*, **18**, 3–37.
3. Boag, J. W., Barish, R. J. & Seelentag, W. W. (1976) Ionography. In *Medical Images*, ed. Hay, G. A., pp. 3–19. London: Wiley.
4. Bracewell, R. (1965) *The Fourier Transform and its Applications*. New York: McGraw-Hill.
5. Burger, G. E. C. (1950) Phantom tests with X rays. *Philips techn. Rev*. **11**, 291–8.
6. Chamberlain, W. E. (1942) Fluoroscopes and fluoroscopy. *Radiology*, **38**, 383–413.
7. Chesters, M. S. (1973) The influence of visual noise on visual detection thresholds. *PhD. Thesis*. University of Leeds, England.
8. Coltman, J. W. (1948) Fluoroscopic image brightening by electronic means. *Radiology*, **51**, 359–67.
9. Evans, R. D. (1968) In *Radiation Dosimetry*, ed. Attix, F. H. & Roesch, W. C. vol I, 2nd edn, p. 138. New York: Academic Press.
10. Feddema, J., Vijverberg, G. P. M., Monté, G. L. A. & Proper, J. (1974) X-ray exposures in intensifier fluorography. *Medicamundi*, **15**, 55–7.
11. Fuchs, W. A., Messerschmid, U., Herren, U, & Steck, W. (1972) Electronic detail enhancement in roentgen television. *Invest. Radiol.*, **7**, 140–6.
12. Gebauer, A., Lissner, J. & Schott, O. (1967) *Röntgen Television*. New York: Grune and Stratton.
13. Hårdstedt, Ch., Rundelius, B. & Welander, U. (1976) Photographic subtraction. *Acta radiol. (diagn.)*, **17**, 101–6.

14. Hay, G. A. (1964) A physical assessment of the Cinelix electro-optical image intensifier in television fluoroscopy. *Radiology*, **83**, 86–91.
15. Hay, G. A. & Chesters, M. S. (1976) Threshold mechanisms in the presence of visible noise. In *Medical Images*, ed. Hay, G. A., pp. 208–19. London: Wiley.
16. Hay, G. A. & Hughes, D. (1978) *First-Year Physics for Radiographers*, 2nd edn. London: Baillière-Tindall.
17. Hay, G. A., Cowen, R. A. & Coleman, N. J. (1980) The importance of some characteristics of television monitors to the overall performance of image-intensifier systems. *DHSS Report STB/2/80*.
18. Herz, R. H. (1969) *The Photographic Action of Ionizing Radiations*. New York: Wiley-Interscience.
19. Jaffé, C. & Webster, E. W. (1975) Radiographic contrast improvement by means of slit radiography. *Radiology*, **116**, 631–5.
20. Joseph, P. M., Hilal, S. K., Schulz, R. A. & Kelcz, F. (1980) Clinical and experimental investigation of a smoothed CT reconstruction algorithm. *Radiology*, **134**, 507–516.
21. Katragadda, C. S., Fogel, S. R., Cohen, G., Wagner, L. K., Morgan III, C. Handel, S. F., Amtey, S. R. & Lester, R. G. (1979) Digital radiography using a computed tomographic instrument. *Radiology*, **133**, 83–7.
22. Kruger, R. A., Mistretta, C. A., Houk, T. L., Riederer, S. J., Shaw, C. G., Goodsit, M. M., Crummy, A. B., Zwiebel, W., Lancaster, J. C., Rowe, G. G. & Flemming, D. (1979) Computerized fluoroscopy in real time for non-invasive visualization of the cardiovascular system. *Radiology*, **130**, 49–57.
23. Kühl, W. (1969) X-ray image intensifiers today and tomorrow. *Medicamundi*, **14**, 132–7.
24. Kühl, W. & Schrijvers, J. E. (1977) A new 14″ image intensifier tube. *Medicamundi*, **22**, 9–10.
25. Meredith, W. J. & Massey, J. B. (1972) *Fundamental Physics of Radiology*, 2nd edn. Bristol: Wright.
26. Metz, C. E. & Doi, K. (1979) Transfer function analysis. *Phys. Med. Biol.*, **24**, 1079–106.
27. Mika, N. & Reiss, K. H. (1973) *Tabellen zur Röntgendiagnostik*, vol. II. Erlangen: Siemens.
28. Oosterkamp, W. J. & van't Hof, A. P. M. (1974) Colour radiography and subtraction. *Medicamundi*, **19**, 116–8.
29. Reading, D. H. (1976) Multiwire proportional chambers. In *Medical Images*, ed. Hay, G. A., pp. 39–50. London: Wiley.
30. Reichmann, S. & Helander, G. G. (1974) High-voltage radiography. *Acta radiol. (diagn.)*, **15**, 561–9.
31. Reiss, K. H. (1965) Die bildmäßige Darstellung ionisierender Strahlen durch elektrostatische Speicherung von Elektronenlawinen. *Z. Angew. Phys.*, **19**, 1–4.
32. Röntgen, W. K. (1898) Über eine neue Art von Strahlen. *Ann. der Phys.*, **64**, 1–37.
33. Roesch, W. C. & Attix, F. H. (1968) *Radiation Dosimetry*, vol I, 2nd edn., ed. Attix, F. H., & Roesch, W. C., pp. 7–10. New York: Academic Press.
34. Rose, A. (1942) The relative sensitivities of television pick-up tubes, photographic film and the human eye. *Proc. Inst. Radio Engrs*, **30**, 295–300.
35. Rose, A. (1948) Sensitivity performance of the human eye on an absolute scale. *J. opt. Soc. Am.*, **38**, 196–208.
36. Rossmann, K. (1963) Spatial fluctuations of X-ray quanta and the recording of radiographic mottle. *Am. J. Roent.*, **90**, 863–9.
37. Rossmann, K. (1969) Point spread-function, line spread-function and modulation transfer function. *Radiology*, **93**, 257–72.
38. Schnitger, H., Dietz, H. & Geldner, E. (1975) Focal-spot intensity distribution and its influence on loadability and geometrical image blurring. *Proc. S. P. I. E.: Medical X-ray Photo-optical Systems Evaluation*, vol 56, pp. 181–3. SPIE, Palos Verdes.
39. Skucas, J. & Gorski, J. W. (1976) Comparison of the image quality of 105 mm film with conventional film. *Radiology*, **118**, 433–7.
40. Stevels, A. L. N. (1975) New phosphors for X-ray screens. *Medicamundi*, **20**, 12–22.
41. Sturm, R. E. & Morgan, R. H. (1949) Screen intensification systems and their limitations. *Am. J. Roent.*, **62**, 617–34.
42. Teves, M. C., & Tol, T. (1952) Electronic intensification of fluoroscopic images. *Philips tech. Rev.*, **14**, 33–43.
43. de Vries, H. L. (1943) The quantum character of light and its bearing upon threshold of vision, the differential sensitivity and visual acuity of the eye. *Physica*, **10**, 553–64.
44. Wagner, R. F. & Weaver, K. E. (1973) Assortment of image-quality indices for radiographic film-screen combinations. *SPIE*, **35**, 83–94.
45. Wagner, R. F. & Weaver, K. E. (1975) Noise measurements on rare-earth intensifying screen systems. *SPIE*, **56**, 198–207.
46. Wagner, R. F. & Weaver, K. E. (1976) Prospects for X-ray exposure reduction using rare-earth intensifying screens. *Radiology*, **118, 183**–8.
47. Ziedses des Plantes, B. G. (1961) *Subtraktion*. Stuttgart: Thieme Verlag.

2

X-ray computed tomography

Malcolm Davison

INTRODUCTION

Normal tomographic procedures (see p. 11) attempt to isolate a layer from a three-dimensional object by a synchronised movement of the X-ray tube and film, but the structures of overlying and underlying strata remain as blurred shadows on the film reducing the overall contrast. In the special technique of *transverse axial tomography* developed in the 1950s a plane perpendicular to the axis of an erect patient is recorded by using an X-ray beam inclined at an angle of 20° to the horizontal and a horizontally placed film, with both the patient and the film rotating synchronously about vertical axes during the exposure, as illustrated in Figure 2.1. Making the angle of inclination smaller and smaller limits the volume irradiated and increases the radius of blur for points out of the plane of interest. In the limit the superimposition of the blurred shadows from unwanted planes could be completely avoided by irradiating only the plane to be imaged. The X-ray tube, the plane of interest and the film would all be in the one plane. Rotating the patient may not always be convenient and the same effect could be achieved by rotating the X-ray tube and the film together around a stationary patient, provided the film was held with its right hand edge always pointing to the right, as shown in Figure 2.2. This simple technique was in fact suggested by Watson in 1940 but not pursued at the time. It is a difficult practical arrangement with the X-ray beam parallel to the film surface, and it is not

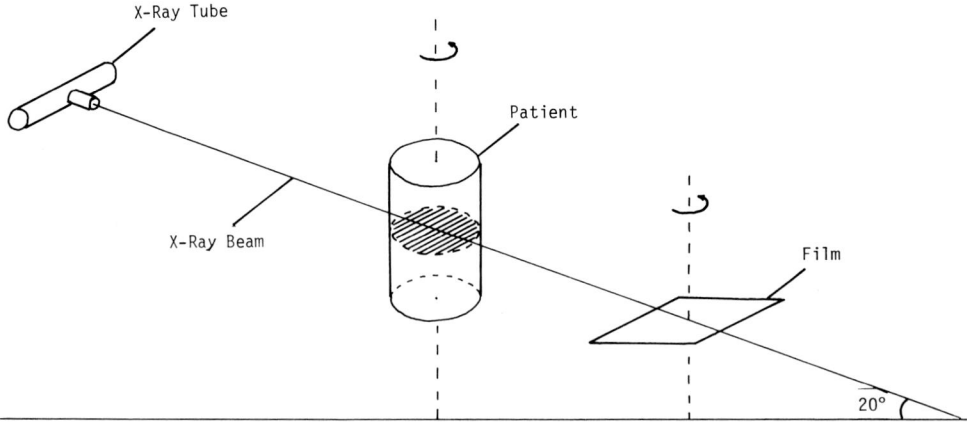

Fig. 2.1 The technique of transverse axial tomography using a synchronised rotation of the patient and film with a 20° inclination between the X-ray beam and the film plane.

obvious what happens to the image in this extreme case.

Look at the geometry of image formation with the small angle transverse axial tomograph, as illustrated in Figure 2.3. The shadow of a sphere in the focal plane is a circle at the correct location in

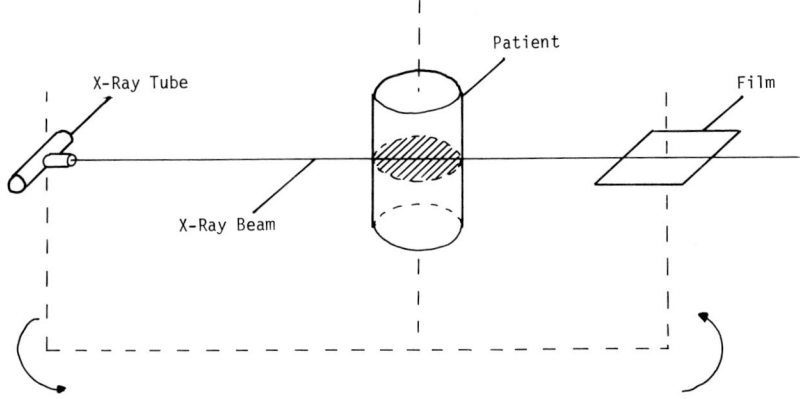

Fig. 2.2 Zero angle transverse axial tomography with a stationary patient and synchronised rotation of the X-ray tube and the film.

the field. As the angle is decreased the image of the object in the focal plane should remain of the same appearance. But in the limit, when the angle is zero, the object casts a shadow completely across the film in all orientations throughout the exposure. Surprisingly this still produces an image, although one of low contrast. How it does this involves the theory of *back projection* and is the basis for the production of images by *reconstruction* or *computed tomography*. Since the information to produce a sharp cross-sectional image of the thin plane is in the beam leaving the patient, it is only necessary to solve the problem of recording, rearranging and displaying it.

Reconstruction by a film analogue method is possible but not exact, as explained later. If, however, data from a number of orientations or views are collected and analysed mathematically then in theory it is possible to calculate precisely the way in which the X-rays were attenuated as they passed through the plane under investigation. The complexity of the calculations requires the use of a computer and hence the more common terminology of computed tomography (CT) has been adopted. Although in theory the image reconstruction can be precise, in practice compromises and simplifications have to be adopted, and a number of different mathematical approaches can be used.

An average film radiograph is capable of displaying objects of dimensions as small as 0·25 mm with a contrast of 10 per cent, allowing for film resolution, geometric blur, movement blur and scattered

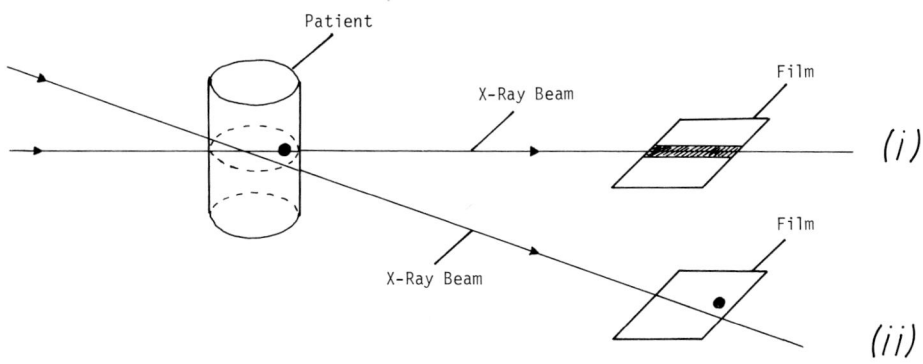

Fig. 2.3 Shadow of a small spherical object. (i) Zero angle protection. (ii) Small angle projection.

radiation. If the picture were to be divided into a matrix of picture elements in the way that a newspaper picture is broken up by the printing screen then a mesh size of four elements per millimetre would be required to display the radiographic picture without further blurring. For a picture of dimensions 30 × 30 cm this implies a total of 1200 × 1200 picture elements, or *pixels* as they are usually called. Therefore, to reconstruct a plane giving an image with the same spatial resolution as a radiograph would mean the solving of 1·44 million independent simultaneous equations derived from the data collected in 1200 independent views for a complete solution. Without a computer this would be virtually impossible and even with currently available computers it would take too long to be of any practical value. A working system has to compromise by reducing the number of pixels in the reconstructed picture (reducing the resolution), and by using approximations to the reconstruction theory to reduce the calculation time (with the introduction of artifacts). The contrast limit in radiography is very much dependent on the characteristics of the recording medium, that is the film, and is dependent on the emulsion graininess and other non-uniformities. These fluctuations can be considered as a form of detector noise. The CT process, however, is capable of much finer contrast discrimination as a result of using detectors with very high signal-to-noise ratio, the limit being related to the detected X-ray intensity. In addition, restricting the irradiation to the plane of interest reduces the detection of scattered radiation thus giving further increased contrast.

The appearance of a conventional radiograph is judged on the basis of pattern recognition where changes in opacity in the film are related to changes in density or thickness of tissue. No attempt is made to relate the film blackening to the physical properties of the tissue in a quantitative way. In order to reconstruct or compute a tomograph, however, consideration has to be given to numerical data even though the final image is likely to be viewed again purely as a pattern recognition problem. The available information is the intensity of the transmitted X-ray beam and the parameter that forms the basis of the calculations is the linear attenuation coefficient of a small volume element in the patient.

RECONSTRUCTION PRINCIPLES

The initial discussions presented here are all in terms of a plane of reconstruction and area elements (pixels), but it must be remembered that the plane has a small but finite depth and the pixel really represents a volume element (a *voxel*), which is small enough for the assumption of uniform density and atomic number to be valid. That is uniform attenuation coefficient through the pixel. Now considering a narrow beam of monochromatic or single energy X-rays passing through the patient, scattered radiation is minimised because of minimum volume, and the intensity transmitted I is related to the incident intensity I_0 by the normal exponential attenuation formula:

$$I = I_0 \exp(-[\mu_1 + \mu_2 + \mu_3 + \ldots]w) \quad (2.1)$$

where μ is the linear attenuation coefficient at the particular energy and the subscripts refer to the tissues in the different pixels of length w traversed by the beam (Fig. 2.4). This can be rewritten as:

$$\log(I/I_0) \propto \mu_1 + \mu_2 + \mu_3 + \ldots \mu_i + \ldots \mu_n$$
$$= \sum_{i=1}^{i=n} \mu_i \quad (2.2)$$

Hence a measure of the transmitted intensity is related to the sum of the attenuation coefficients of the pixels traversed in that particular ray. This is called the ray sum (p) and it is the basic information from which the image can be reconstructed.

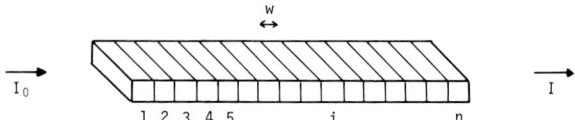

Fig. 2.4 Attenuation of ray passing through n pixel elements, each of width w.

It is obviously not possible, however, to distinguish the attenuation coefficients of the individual pixels from the one ray sum measurement when these are all different. For an object of four pixels the ray sum $p = 20$ could be a result of summing 5+5+5+5, or 2+7+9+2, or some other combination. Further information in the form of ray sums is required before a complete solution can be found. If the plane to be reconstructed is split into a matrix array of n by n pixels a total of n independent measurements of the transmitted intensity have to be recorded from different directions traversing the matrix. This can be done simply by moving the X-ray source and detector in a linear traverse across the matrix to record n successive intensity values I_1 to I_n, as shown in Figure 2.5.

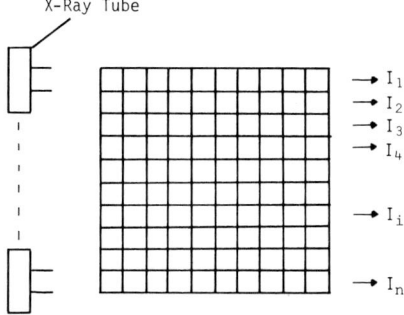

Fig. 2.5 Profile of intensity measurements I_1 to I_n following a linear traverse across the scan plane matrix.

The sequence of intensities or the corresponding ray sums p_1 to p_n is known as the intensity or ray sum *profile* for that particular view. If then the X-ray source and detector are rotated together through a small angle, a second linear traverse can be carried out generating a second profile of intensity values which can also be recorded.

The X-ray beam, although narrow, has to have a finite width and this can be taken to be the same as the width of the pixel w. In the first traverse there is no doubt as to which pixels contribute to the attenuation of the individual readings, but in the oblique cases it can be seen from Figure 2.6

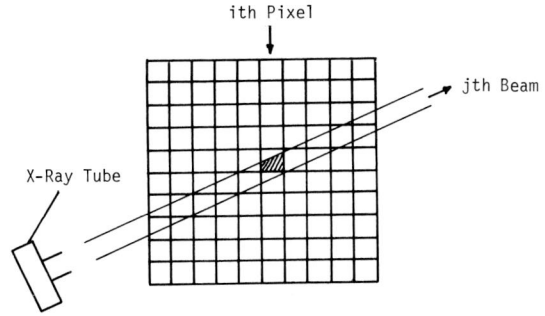

Fig. 2.6 Contribution of the i_{th} pixel to the j_{th} ray in an oblique view. The ray is in fact a beam of width w, the same as the pixel width.

that various fractions of pixels are traversed by the beam at any one time. The contribution of any one pixel i is a function of the area w_{ij} of the pixel actually intersected by the beam j. Therefore the ray sum p_j is given by:

$$p_j = \sum_{i=1}^{i=n} w_{ij} \mu_i \qquad (2.3)$$

Further rotations and traverses are carried out until sufficient data in the form of ray sum profiles have been recorded to permit an analysis and reconstruction of the attenuation coefficients of the individual pixels.

In more general terms if we take a co-ordinate system (x,y) for points in the image and a co-ordinate system (r,s) for the ray paths rotated through angle ϕ from the y axis, then the ray profile described by $p(r,\phi)$ represents ray sums p_1 to p_n in a particular view at angle ϕ, and is given by the line integral of the attenuation coefficient distribution $f(x,y)$.

$$p(r,\phi) = \int_{r,\phi} f(x,y)\, ds \qquad (2.4)$$

Not all ray sums are in fact independent. For example, take the simple case of a 2×2 matrix where the attenuation coefficients of the pixels are 3,4,1 and 8, as illustrated in Figure 2.7. The first

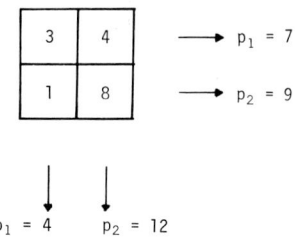

Fig. 2.7 Ray sums for horizontal and vertical views through a four element matrix.

horizontal view gives $p_1 = 7$ and $p_2 = 9$, and the vertical view gives $p_1 = 12$ and $p_2 = 4$. Although we have four unknowns and four equations, only three of these equations are independent and no singular solution can be found without extra information. The matrices 1,6,3,6, 2,5,2,7, 3,4,1,8, and 4,3,0,9 all satisfy the four ray sums. Therefore, in order to obtain sufficient independent data points

58 SCIENTIFIC BASIS OF MEDICAL IMAGING

it is normally necessary to scan more than n views. The complete data set then consists of m views spaced at equal angles, each consisting of n ray sums at intervals w.

Theories of reconstruction go back to 1917 when Radon first solved the problem of determining functions in a plane from their integrals,[22] and the first practical techniques were developed by Bracewell in 1956 for an application in radio astronomy mapping solar microwave activity from a series of strip detector signals. The first clinical use of reconstruction techniques, however, was an application for radionuclide imaging using the most basic scheme known as *back projection*.[14] Although this technique has not been used in any practical transmission CT units it is useful to consider the theory and its limitations as a first step to understanding the more complex reconstruction principles.

Back projection

The profile data is simply projected back into the matrix plane by taking the value in each ray sum and applying it to the pixels traversed by that ray. Then for each pixel the contributions from the different projections are added together. That is

$$\hat{f}(x,y) = \sum_{j=1}^{j=m} p_j \, \Delta\phi \qquad (2.5)$$

where $\hat{f}(x,y)$ is the distribution of attenuation coefficients obtained by back projection and summation of m projections spaced at angles $\Delta\phi$ apart. This summation technique can be implemented either by computer or by non-computer methods, and it can be illustrated both ways. Suppose we start with the simple unknown matrix 3,4,1,8 as illustrated in Figure 2.8. With the first projection the ray sums for the horizontal view are measured as $p_1 = 7$, $p_2 = 9$. Back projection puts these numbers into the pixels traversed by the two rays. Suppose now the second projection is at an angle of 45° to the first. The ray sums are $p_1 = 4$, $p_2 = 11$ and $p_3 = 1$, and these values are added into the relevant pixels. The third projection vertically gives $p_1 = 12$, $p_2 = 4$ and these are projected back and added giving a new total. Fourthly a second oblique projection with ray sums $p_1 = 8$, $p_2 = 5$ and $p_3 = 3$ are added back to the pixels giving a final total of 25,28,19,40. If now as a last step a background of 16 is subtracted from all values and

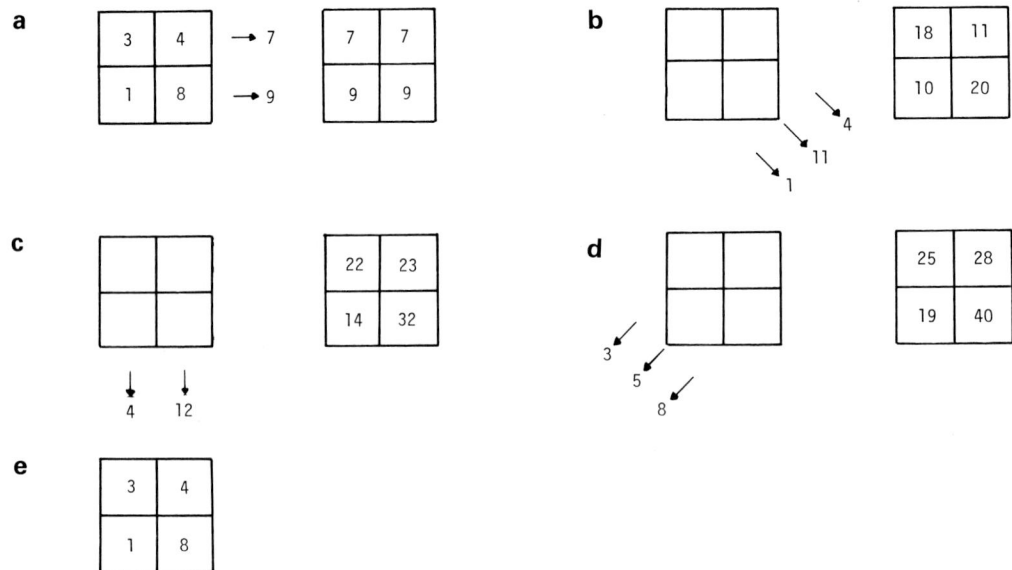

Fig. 2.8 Back projection applied to a four element matrix. (a) Ray sums from the horizontal view placed in the corresponding pixels. (b) to (d) Ray sums from the following views added in. (e) Subtraction of a uniform background and rationalisation of pixel values.

the resultant sums divided by 3 the answer is seen to be 3,4,1,8. Thus we have the required values. This oversimplification is too good to be true in practice. The limitations become apparent if we consider the back projection in an analogue way for a single small dense object in the plane to be reconstructed. Each profile used projects back a stripe of high optical density across the matrix (as can be seen in Fig. 2.9), resulting in a star artifact measured ray sums. As a starting point a uniform value is assumed for each pixel in the image and the ray sums are calculated for a given view. These sums are then compared with the measured values and the differences are used as corrections to the pixels contributing to the particular ray sums. The simplest correction is to divide the difference equally among the pixels in a ray and to add this to the assumed values. The process is repeated for

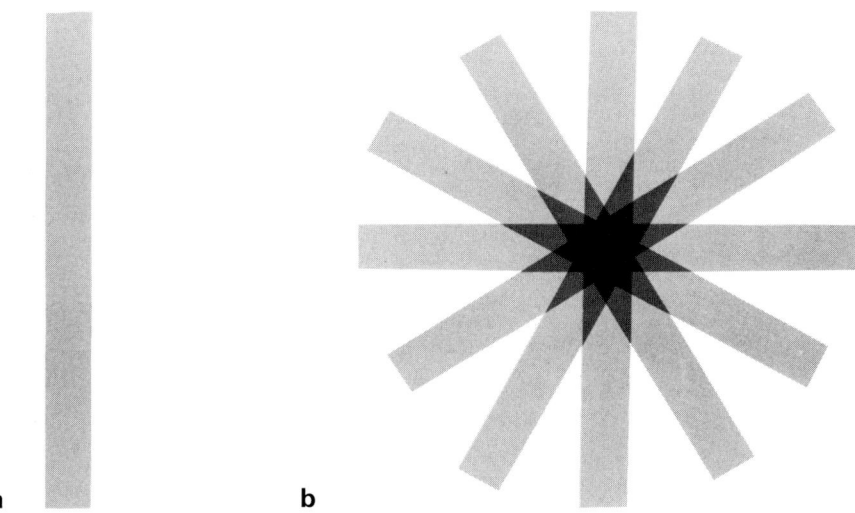

Fig. 2.9 Analogue back projection. (a) Single view profile of a small object back projected into the image matrix. (b) Summation of six equally spaced profiles showing a star artifact with 12 spokes.

with 2 m spokes for m projections. As the number of projections is increased the separate spokes become indistinguishable and the appearance is that of a central spot of high density corresponding to the original object with a surrounding background blur with density falling off with distance from the centre of the object. For most practical purposes this would give unacceptable picture quality (but see p. 73). Since the image matrix can be considered to be made up of a number of high density pixels each with its own blur pattern the problem of reconstruction is to derive appropriate correction factors to be applied during the back projection process.

Iterative reconstruction techniques

The next simplest technique uses a ray-by-ray process to correct the calculated attenuation coefficients and provide a better match with the each view to complete one iteration. The whole procedure is then repeated comparing the new calculated values with the measured values of the ray sums. For example, taking the four pixel matrix 3,4,1,8 as illustrated in Figure 2.10, if the initial assumption is a uniform 4,4,4,4 then the first horizontal projection gives calculated ray sums $p_1^c = 8$, $p_2^c = 8$ and measured ray sums $p_1^m = 7$, $p_2^m = 9$. Therefore, the correction to the elements of p_1 is $\frac{1}{2}(p_1^m - p_1^c) = -\frac{1}{2}$, and to the elements of p_2 it is $\frac{1}{2}(p_2^m - p_2^c) = +\frac{1}{2}$. This gives a new assumed matrix. For the first oblique projection $p_1^c = 3\frac{1}{2}$, $p_2^c = 8$, $p_3^c = 4\frac{1}{2}$, and $p_1^m = 4$, $p_2^m = 11$, $p_3^m = 1$, leading to a second corrected matrix. Further corrections are made following the vertical projection and the second oblique projection to complete the first iteration. The result looks something like the original. It might be hoped that repeating this procedure would give an answer approaching closer and closer to the true values. The values could tend to

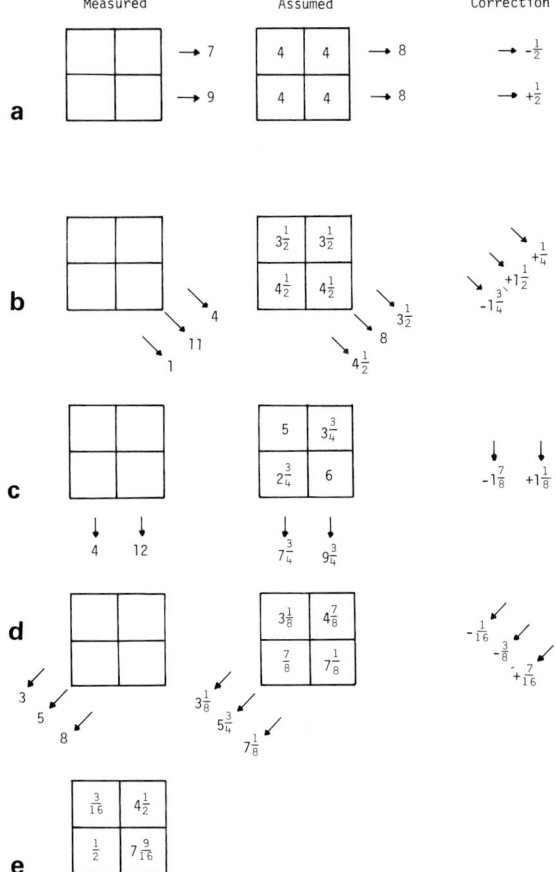

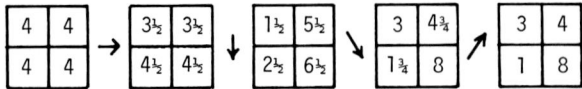

Fig. 2.10 Algebraic reconstruction technique (ART) applied to a four element matrix. (a) Correction factors derived from the horizontal view. These are then added into the assumed matrix. (b) to (d) Corrections from the following views applied to the assumed values. (e) The final reconstructed values.

however, does tend to converge rapidly to start with but can be confused in the final stages by the presence of noisy or faulty data.

It is difficult to illustrate this technique in an analogue way as was done for back projection of a single dense object. But since each projection adds in a correction term, which may be positive or negative, rather than the ray sum itself, the effect is to reduce the intensity of the star artifacts, but it can not avoid them entirely. This technique is known as an *algebraic reconstruction technique* (ART).[10]

Other iterative sequences are also possible with different convergence characteristics. A point-by-point correction technique takes all the rays passing through an individual pixel and applies a correction factor to the measured value, and then proceeds to do the same for each pixel in the picture in turn to complete the first iteration. This is known as *simultaneous iterative reconstruction technique* (SIRT). And in another method, differences between the assumed ray sums and the measured ray sums of all the views can be calculated at the same time and the corrections applied simultaneously to all the pixels for the first iteration; the same procedure is then repeated, comparing these calculated values with the measured values. Using our example again, it is seen that over-correction each time does not allow convergence.

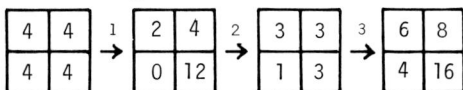

After three iterations we are no nearer to the correct values. But a damping factor can be applied to the corrections, and in this simple example if the corrections to each pixel are halved the correct answer is in fact obtained in only one iteration. Goitein[12] chose a damping factor which gave a least squares best fit to the data after each iteration so the method became known as *iterative least square technique* (ILST). This allows convergence of noisy data, although in practice not converging as fast as the algebraic reconstruction technique. Obviously a combination of the two techniques would be preferable with ART used first, quickly to give values close to the true ones, followed by ILST to optimise the result.

Calculations may be speeded up by the use of constraints since the attenuation values can never

wander, however, particularly when large numbers of projections are taken in sequence and over-corrections may be repeated. In practice convergence takes place more rapidly when large angles are used between successive correcting projections. If in the above sequence the horizontal projection is followed by the vertical then the first oblique and finally the second oblique projection the results will be

It is a bit fortuitous that the correct answer is achieved after only one iteration. Normally five or more iterations would be required. The sequence, go negative, and can never rise above the known values for bone. With iterative techniques all the data has to be collected before processing can begin. Therefore, there is a time delay before a picture can be displayed. It was, however, the method used in the original EMI Head Scanner.

Simple back projection is imprecise and iterative reconstruction is slow. Neither has the elegance of an exact mathematical solution to the basic equation.[4] All practical scanners now use some form of analytical solution, and the only approximation that is required to avoid excessive computational time is a limit to the spatial frequencies involved. This allows reconstruction on an array of points using discrete Fourier series rather than the integrations of Fourier transforms.

Convolution techniques

The simple back projection technique fails because each point in the object plane gives rise to a blurred image. This blurred pattern can be described as the *point spread function* $h(x,y)$. Back projection and summation by integration over a semicircle for a unit point impulse $\delta(x,y)$ gives

$$h(x,y) = \int_0^\pi \delta(x) d\theta = \int_0^\pi \delta[r \cos(\phi - \theta)] d\theta = r^{-1}$$

(2.6)

The system is behaving as any other imaging system whether it be a simple lens, image intensifier or a gamma camera, since all of them produce blurring of point objects in the image to a greater or lesser extent. This blurred image can be considered as the correct image convolved with the point spread function. This is a mathematical way of saying that each point in the image has been blurred according to the point spread function. If $f(x,y)$ is the set of attenuation coefficients for the pixels in the x,y plane, $F(u,v)$ is the Fourier transform of $f(x,y)$ with spatial frequency components u and v, and $H(u,v)$ is the Fourier transform of the blurring function $h(x,y)$ with the symbol ˆ added to denote representations of the blurred image. Then

$$\hat{f}(x,y) = f(x,y) \star h(x,y)$$

Since convolutions in real space are equivalent to multiplications in Fourier space then

$$\hat{F}(u,v) = F(u,v) H(u,v)$$

and by rearranging

$$F(u,v) = \frac{\hat{F}(u,v)}{H(u,v)}$$

and since the Fourier transform of the blurring function r^{-1} is the inverse of the spatial frequency, that is $|R|^{-1}$, then

$$F(u,v) = |R| \hat{F}(u,v) \qquad (2.7)$$

All that is necessary to deconvolve the blurred image is to take its Fourier transform, multiply each value by its distance from the origin in frequency space, then take the inverse Fourier transform and obtain the true image.

Alternatively the blurred image can be thought of as being produced as a result of the poor transmission of high spatial frequencies and the enhancement of low frequencies. Any procedure that reverses this emphasis helps to deblur the image. This approach is useful in analogue reconstruction methods and can be carried out optically. It is related to the radiographic subtraction technique which enhances fine detail by a copying process in which an unsharp reversal copy of the original is used as a mask. It is also related to the television enhancement technique (proposed by Siemens) called *harmonisation*.

The data consisting of profiles taken at a finite number of views is not adequate for Fourier transform application. Starting from the Fourier transform of each profile, it is possible to derive the complete two dimensional transform of the image by interpolation, and this can then be retransformed into the required image. The method of interpolation is based on the central section theorem. This states that if the Fourier transform of a profile at angle ϕ is calculated, then the values obtained are the same as those obtained from the two dimensional Fourier transform of the distribution by looking along a line at angle ϕ to the u axis. If $p(r,\phi)$ is the profile at angle ϕ and $P(R,\phi)$ is its Fourier transform, with $|R|$ the magnitude of the spatial frequency given by $R^2 = (u^2 + v^2)$, then

$$F(u,v) = P(R,\phi) \qquad (2.8)$$

As illustrated in Figure 2.11, the image is reconstructed on an array of points spaced $1/2R_{max}$ apart, where R_{max} is the maximum spatial frequency that is allowed.

gative components cancel out the star artifacts for points outside the true image. The filtered profile which back projects to give the true image is derived from the measured profile multiplied by the

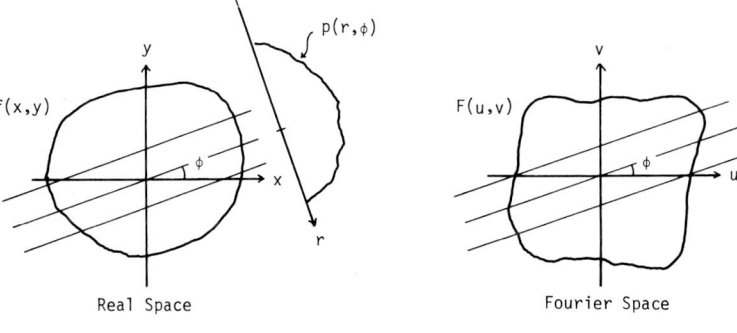

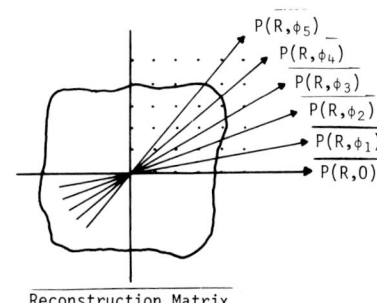

Fig. 2.11 Derivation of the two dimensional transform from discrete profiles. According to the central section theorem the values of the Fourier transform of a profile $p(r,\phi)$ at angle ϕ are the same as those obtained from the two dimensional Fourier transform of the distribution viewed at the same angle ϕ. $F\{p(r,\phi)\} = P(R,\phi)$. Values on a rectangular array are then obtained by interpolation, with points spaced $1/2R_{max}$ apart.

The technique for removing the r^{-1} blurring function can be achieved in both one and two dimensions. In practice the filtering can be applied to individual profiles before using the back projection, or it may be applied to the complete image array following back projection. As applied to individual profiles, it is known as *filtered back projection*, and this is the technique used in most if not all '20-second' scanners. In order to obtain the true $f(x,y)$ distribution instead of the blurred $\hat{f}(x,y)$, it is necessary to replace the profiles $p(r,\phi)$ in Equation 2.5 by the filtered profiles $p^\star(r,\phi)$. Then $f(x,y) = \Sigma\, p^\star(r,\phi)\Delta\phi$. If a circular object gives an unfiltered profile as shown in Figure 2.12, the filtered profiles take a form with negative components as well as the central positive components. These ne-

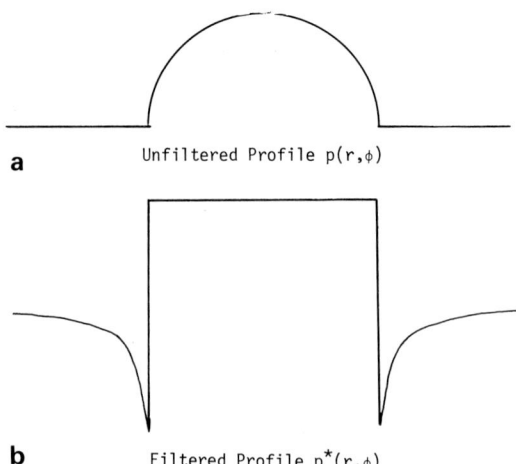

Fig. 2.12 Filtered back projection. (a) Unfiltered profile $p(r,\phi)$ from a circular object. (b) Filtered profile $p^\star(r,\phi)$.

magnitude of the spatial frequency. This can be done in various ways. In Fourier space

$$P^\star(R,\phi) = |R| \, P(R,\phi)$$

and

$$p^\star(r,\phi) = \int_{-\infty}^{+\infty} |R| \, P(R,\phi) \exp(2\pi i R r) dR$$

$$= \frac{1}{2\pi^2} \int_{-\infty}^{+\infty} \frac{p(r',\phi) \, dr'}{(r-r')^2} \quad (2.9)$$

This integral contains a singularity $r = r'$ and has to be integrated by parts. Solutions to this type of equation were first found by Radon[22] to solve gravitational equations. In the more common solution of convolution filtering the singularity is overcome by using a frequency cut-off making $|R|$ zero for $R > R_{max}$, which leads to

$$p^\star(r,\phi) = R_{max} \, p(r,\phi) - \int_{-\infty}^{+\infty} p(r',\phi) \frac{\sin^2[\pi R_{max}(r-r')]}{\pi^2 (r-r')^2} dr' \quad (2.10)$$

And this can be solved as a summation with points spaced $w = 1/2 \, R_{max}$ apart.[23] With this technique the computation is carried out on each projection as the data are being accumulated. This saves on computer core space, and also means that the resulting picture is available immediately scanning stops.

Two dimensional Fourier reconstruction is faster overall if the computer capacity is available; it may be the method of choice for the fastest scanning times. In this case Equation 2.7 is solved directly. The true image is obtained from the back projected image by taking its Fourier amplitudes, multiplying by the magnitude of the spatial frequency and then taking the inverse transform. In other words, the high spatial frequencies are enhanced to make up for the deficiencies of the blurred image. A more detailed discussion of the various reconstruction techniques is given elsewhere.[4]

SCANNING INSTRUMENTS

The principles of reconstruction tomography from transmitted rays were demonstrated by Oldendorf in 1961 and Cormack in 1963 without generating much interest, and it was not until 1971 that Hounsfield of EMI produced a clinically useful machine applied to head scanning. The technique was then immediately seen to be useful and the demand created an explosive development, with the scan field size increasing to cover the whole body cross section, and scan times dropping from minutes down to only a few seconds. Specialised units were also developed for breast, bone and cardiac applications.

The first machines employed what is known as a *translate rotate* system of scanning, in which a single collimated X-ray source and detector mounted in a gantry are moved together in a linear traverse across the scan field taking a series of intensity measurements. The whole gantry is then rotated through a small angle (usually 1°) and the traverse is repeated in the opposite direction. This procedure is continued to cover 180° of rotation about the patient. With 160 readings per traverse a total of 28 000 values can be accumulated in about 4 min. Some of the time is required for the reversal and rotation movements, but about 5 ms is required to accumulate the data for each measurement of a ray sum.

To speed up the actual scanning time the first development was the use of a *fan beam* of X-rays falling on an array of detectors. The EMI 5005, for example, uses 30 detectors with a 10° fan. With this arrangement the data can be collected much faster and the rotation angle can be increased to 10° between traverses so that the overall scan time can be reduced to about 20 s for a whole body machine scanning over 180°. Since slower scans are feasible for head scanning because of the lack of patient movement, a smaller number of detectors in the fan can be used resulting in a lower cost unit. In these cases it is usual to collect data for two scan slices simultaneously to reduce the overall investigation time.

The next logical step in reducing the scan time is to employ a fan with many more detectors, so that the beam more than covers the scan field at any one time. It is then only necessary to use rotational movement and scan times down to 2 s are possible. Most machines of this type use a bank of detectors rotating with the X-ray tube, but a complete ring of stationary detectors is also utilised. Rotation of these machines is normally through 360° (Fig. 2.13).

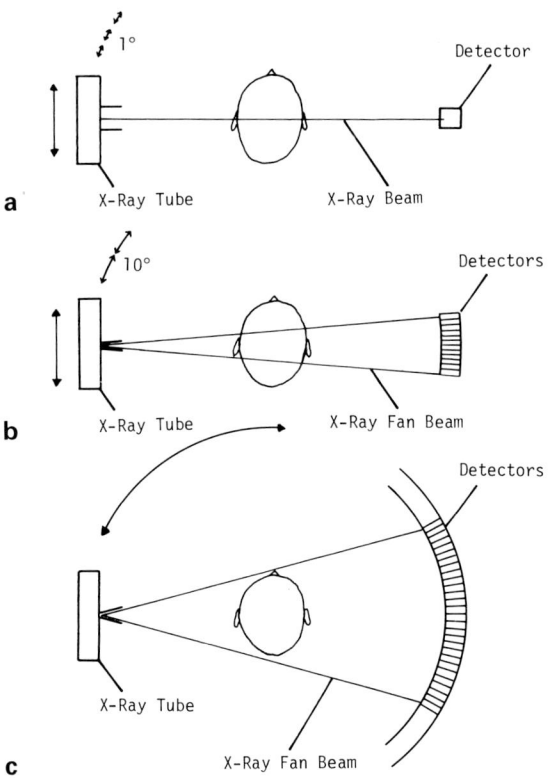

Fig. 2.13 Scanning principles. (a) First-generation translate-rotate machine with a single detector. (b) Second-generation rotate-translate machine with fan beam. (c) Third-generation rotate-only machine with wide angle fan beam.

Fan beam reconstruction

The convolution procedures described for the parallel beams of a simple translate-rotate system can be adapted to fan beam geometries, but require much more computing effort because the rays back-projected into an image matrix are all in different directions. In fact, the convolution is calculated for a number of points along the rays of the fan in one view, and this is then converted to data on a rectangular array of points by extrapolating from the surrounding four points (Fig. 2.14). The attenuation coefficient for a particular pixel is then found in the normal way by summation of the contributions from all the views.

Analogue methods

A number of instruments have been constructed using film or image intensifier detectors and relying on optical methods of image processing and reconstruction. While not strictly computed tomography, they are based on the same principles and are discussed on page 73.

X-ray sources

All clinical transmission scanners use X-ray tubes as the radiation source, although these give polychromatic beams with a spectrum of energies, which complicates the reconstruction since the theory is based on the attenuation of an X-ray beam of a single energy. There is no suitable radioactive source in terms of γ-ray energy, activity and long half-life, although a simple low cost machine using a Caesium 137 source has been described by Monahan.[20]

Translate-rotate machines operate with an industrial-type fixed anode X-ray tube with a line focus typically of 2 × 16mm. Oil cooling is necessary to permit continuous exposures with factors of 100–160 kVp and about 30 mA for the duration of the scan time; the power is typically 4 kW. The X-ray intensity is low and the signal has to be integrated for a period of about 5 ms for each reading. Since the X-ray tube and detector assembly is continuously moving there is a displacement of the order 1·6mm during each reading. The beam is filtered by 3·5–4·5mm aluminium.

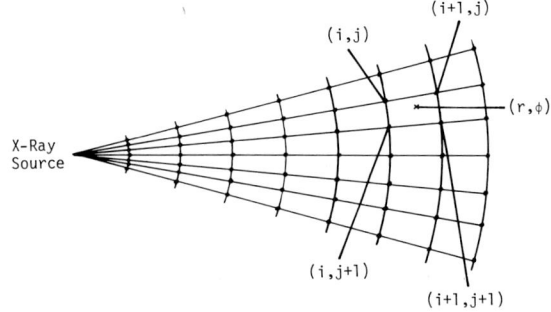

Fig. 2.14 Fan beam reconstruction. Convolutions are calculated for a limited number of points on each ray. The convolution at any other point (r,ϕ) is then determined by extrapolation from the four surrounding points.

As scan time is reduced and scan field diameter and resolution are increased, higher X-ray intensities are required. All fast third-generation scanners use special small focal spot rotating anode tubes of high power-handling capability. Most of these employ pulsed operation to make efficient use of the X-rays with exposures of 2–3 ms. The latest developments use graphite anodes run at high speed with monitoring of anode and housing temperatures, some with metal centre sections to the tube envelopes to give longer stable tube life. Seventy-five kW is a typical power rating. The beam is filtered by a minimum of 3·5–4·5mm aluminium, together with specially shaped filters to improve the dynamic range, and in many cases an additional 0·5mm copper to give a harder, more nearly monochromatic, beam. With a rotation of 360° in 3 s and a new view every 1°, a measurement has to be taken every 8 ms.

The X-ray beam is collimated at the X-ray tube to reduce the irradiated volume and to minimise the overlap of successive scans. Originally set with a slice thickness of 13mm only, the later machines give an option of thicknesses between 2–15mm. The thinner slices are used to help to resolve small objects, such as the optic nerve, where they might be lost when the data are averaged over the volume of a pixel. The smaller slice thicknesses make it easier to pick out an object of density different to the background, but since the number of photons detected from the pixel elements is reduced the noise in the picture increases. Measurements of patient dose with the early machines revealed an unnecessary dose due to overlap of the edges of the beam from adjacent scans. A simple collimator allows a significant amount of penumbra to form from the finite length of the focus, giving a beam profile much wider than the scan slice thickness. One way of improving the situation (adopted by EMI) is to add a beam splitting plate between the X-ray tube focal spot and the collimator aperture, giving a much sharper cut-off outside the main beam.

Constant potential generators are used to minimise fluctuations in the output. The X-ray intensity varies approximately as $(kV)^3$, and a ripple of 0·1 per cent in the voltage gives a 0·3 per cent change in the output. This is not good enough for the highest precision, and special generators have been built with the ripple as low as 0·01 per cent. Reference detectors are also used to monitor the direct output of the X-ray tube so that measurements can be converted to the ratio of the transmitted to incident intensity. This is a separate detector close to the X-ray tube in a first- or second-generation machine, but is one of the detectors at the edge of the fan beam in a third-generation machine. This means that changes in intensity across the fan can not be compensated for if they occur during a scan and are likely to lead to artifacts in the picture. Such changes have to be minimised by careful design and choice of components.

Detectors

It is essential to avoid the detection of scattered radiation. This is better done by good collimation at the detector than by the use of pulse height analysis to discriminate in terms of energy. It has been estimated that for the EMI head scanner the detector collimation accepts less than 0·2 per cent of the non-primary radiation. There are additional advantages of doing it this way because the electronic circuitry is simplified and the cost reduced, and the actual signal detected can be increased if interactions other than the photo-peak can be used. This reduces the problem of small detector dimensions with the inherent difficulty of a large fraction of escaping secondary photons. Since pulse counting is difficult at the high count rates encountered, it is normal to use a current mode with the analogue signal being related to the energy deposited in the detector.

For accuracy of measurement it is desirable that the detector itself should not add any noise to the signal. The requirements are a high detection efficiency, good stability and fast response, with a small cross-section to provide the required spatial resolution. The traditional X-ray detector is a sodium iodide thallium-activated crystal optically coupled to a photomultiplier tube, and if it is thick enough it can have a detection efficiency approaching 100 per cent. This is used in all the early scanners. But it has limitations as a result of after-glow following high radiation intensities, and also a limited dynamic range. It also is a deliquescent crystal and has to be very carefully encapsulated. The dark currents from the photomultipliers are zeroed out in the translate-rotate scanners by measuring the signal behind a lead plate at the end of each traverse as part of the calibration procedure.

Calcium fluoride doped with europium is a scintillation crystal with only 60 per cent of the efficiency of sodium iodide, but it does not suffer from after-glow effects, and is used in some of the early scanners. Bismuth germanate combines high efficiency with low after-glow, a very good dynamic range, and long term stability. It is used in the current Technicare Deltascan machines. A more recent development is the use of caesium iodide thallium-doped scintillation crystals coupled with silicon semiconductor photodiodes. This is the approach favoured by EMI and Siemens for their fast scanners to get wide dynamic range and close detector spacing with high efficiency, avoiding the need for high voltage power supplies.

A different principle of detection has been employed by CGR, GE, Philips and Varian in their scanners. This is based on the use of very high pressure xenon or xenon-krypton ionisation chambers. By using one continuous gas chamber with separating plates of tungsten it is possible to combine the features of close detector spacing with built-in scatter rejection as in a Bucky grid. The tungsten plates, pointing towards the focal spot of the X-ray tube, absorb the oblique rays without producing significant ionisation (Fig. 2.15). The depth of pressurised gas absorbs the primary rays

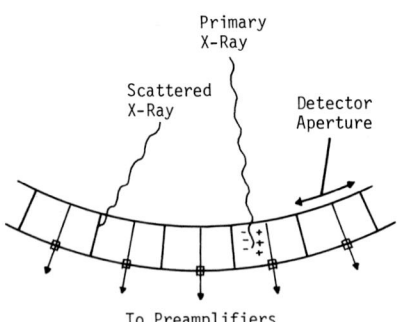

Fig. 2.15 Xenon ionisation chamber detectors. Tungsten plates act as collimators and detector separators. Central collecting electrodes are taken to individual preamplifiers.

producing ions that are collected on intermediate plates connected to individual amplifiers. A polarising potential of about 500 volts is used. The gas, being common to all detectors, gives good reproducibility of response between detector cells. Individual calibrations can be used, but by careful manufacture the differences in sensitivity are kept small. Working in an ionisation mode, the current is independent of the polarising voltage and hence stability is superior to scintillator photomultiplier tube detectors. Detector efficiency is only about 50 per cent, but in practice the apertures in front of scintillation detectors are reduced to improve spatial resolution, and the corresponding efficiency is also of the order of 50 per cent. The energy responses of all the different types of detector used are similar. With third-generation machines using a fixed fan, stability is most important because it is not possible to calibrate the individual detectors during a scan. This can be done with the fixed ring of detectors, each of which is used for only part of the scan while for the rest of the time it is available for calibration checks.

Dynamic range

To measure attenuation values to 0·5 per cent requires the detection of more than 4×10^4 photons in each ray sum. With an attenuation of about 6000 in the thicker parts of the abdomen, this means handling signals of 24×10^7 photons in the primary beam around the edge of the patient. This wide dynamic range would impose problems with the computer. The first scanners used a water bag technique to ensure that all the rays traversed the same path length in tissue and water. This technique was inconvenient, and scanners now incorporate shaped wedge filters designed to compensate as nearly as possible for the curvature of the body. Different wedges are used for head and body sections.

Gantry and couch

The X-ray tube and detector assembly are mounted within a scanning gantry. This is a frame provided with an aperture within which the body plane to be scanned can be positioned. It contains the mechanisms for driving the source and detector precisely through the scanning movements and is provided with the sensors to pick off the position coordinates to be fed to the computer. One of two or more scan times can normally be chosen depending on the requirement of short exposure time or high resolution. In many types of machines, the complete gantry frame can be angulated 15–20° either side of the vertical to allow the reconstruction of planes other than that perpendicular to the long axis of the patient. Scan fields of 40–50cm are now available for whole body units to cover the largest expected patient diameter, but more limited apertures are used in head-only machines.

The couch is a table with motorised movements and a radiolucent top allowing the required body plane to be positioned accurately in the scan plane. Manual positioning can be by means of light beam markers, and the longitudinal movement can normally be set remotely for carrying out a series of scans at known intervals. With the latest machines it is possible to take the equivalent of a normal radiographic film, a *scanogram*, by using the X-ray tube in a fixed position and moving the patient through the fan beam. The detector signals are then used to modulate the display directly producing a truly orthogonal image showing anatomical detail with all the positional co-ordinates stored in the computer. In order to produce a reconstructed plane or planes the operator has only to mark the required positions by means of a moveable cursor superimposed on the image and the computer then automatically controls the scanning procedure, including the necessary couch movements. In this way the scans are produced exactly at the planes set from the anatomical markers, and there is no need to estimate the positions of the planes from external features.

Computer arrangements

All clinical scanners follow the same general principles, although the faster scanners require much more sophisticated systems to handle the large amount of data collected in the shortest possible time. Data processing is carried out in three phases: (1) collection; (2) reconstruction; and (3) display. In the collection phase, the detector signal current is integrated or summed over a finite measuring time. It is then converted with high precision (14 bit or more) into a digital form appropriate for computer processing. The first processing step is to take the ratio of each signal to the reference signal, and then to calculate the logarithm of the ratio and normalise it to some appropriate scale. In practice absolute values of linear attenuation coefficient are not used, but a scale of CT numbers expressed as integer values is derived with water set at zero, air at -1000 and bone varying from $+100$ to more than $+1000$. The CT number is in fact related to the attenuation coefficient by the equation

$$\text{CT} = K \left(\frac{\mu_{\text{tissue}}}{\mu_{\text{water}}} - 1 \right) \qquad (2.11)$$

with K normally equal to 1000 (but with a value of 500 for those machines using the EMI scale).

The data from individual profiles have then to be stored. The second phase is reconstruction by one of the filtered convolution techniques followed by back projection and then image arrangement to give the corrected image data. Again these data are put into store. Finally the picture can be displayed in a number of different ways and various methods of picture processing can be applied. Speed is achieved by carrying out several tasks simultaneously using a multi-computer system (Fig. 2.16). A *pipeline computer principle* is the name given to a system taking the data through a series of processing steps in stages. With a second-generation type of machine, where linear traverses are followed by rotation, the data from one traverse are preprocessed and passed to the first storage file in the time interval at the end of the traverse. With a third-generation machine, rotation is continuous and measurements are taken from a number of detectors simultaneously every few milliseconds. To cope with this, it is normally necessary to process the information from each projection in the time between successive exposures. Following an exposure, the data from the several detectors are multiplexed and fed sequentially through the preprocessing stage and into the first store file. With both types of machine the data are then handled in a similar way although following different time scales. As data for the second view are taken through the preprocessor the first set of data is passed through the convolution processor. Then with the following views the first data set is back projected and finally passed into the image store where successive projections are added until the final picture is built up and becomes available for display as a gray-tone picture. The various processing steps are controlled and monitored by a standard mini-computer, which additionally is used to control all the aspects of scanning and display in response to commands given by the operator. An essential feature of the operator's control unit is a *video display unit* which can not only display the picture but can also be used in conversational mode to provide the operator with prompts regarding the current status of the machine with requests where further information is required. An example is given in Figure 2.17. The video display is also used by the maintenance engineer for running diagnostic tests to check machine performance and to locate faults. Both operating programmes and image data ready for viewing are stored on magnetic disc. In some of the more elaborate systems the main computer may be used to monitor the heat input to the X-ray tube, and hence it can calculate the shortest possible cooling time between scans. It may also be used automatically to set the X-ray factors, the scan and the patient position to a predetermined programme selected by a single command instruction, or to carry out performance checks and correction routines where this would be impracticable by manual methods on a large number of detectors.

Images are normally reconstructed once only. Several types of machines, however, give the option of a number of reconstruction algorithms for different parts of the body depending upon the amount of included bone, and for enhancing the different features being studied. When the raw data are not stored the choice of algorithm must be made before scanning is initiated. In machines with very short scan times, however, where mass memory facilities of megabytes of storage are provided, a number of reconstructions may be tried after scanning is completed without the need for collecting further data. Developments of the computer to cope with decreasing total scan-plus-processing time make use of specially developed array processors and hard wired fast Fourier transforms (where speed is achieved by parallel pipelined operation). These allow calculations to be carried out on a complete array of data at one time rather than point-by-point. Consequently the mapping of array data from one coordinate system to another, and Fourier transforms or convolutions, can be carried out with a single computer instruction.

Display and recording facilities

The various options open for storing and viewing the images are standard for all computer imaging

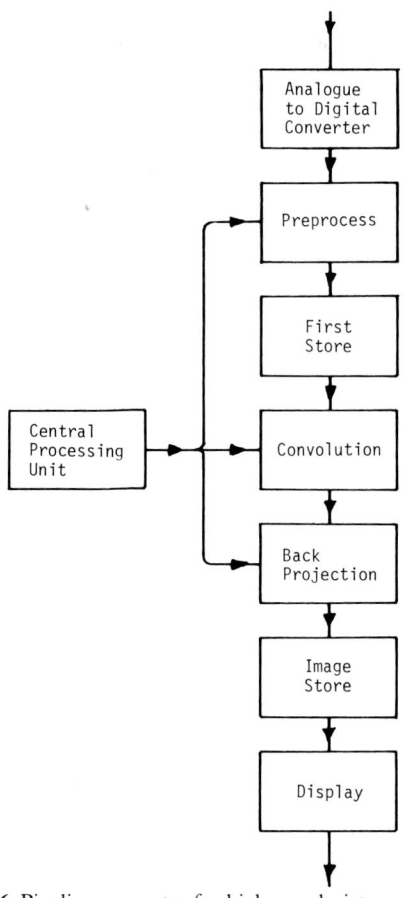

Fig. 2.16 Pipeline computer for high speed picture processing.

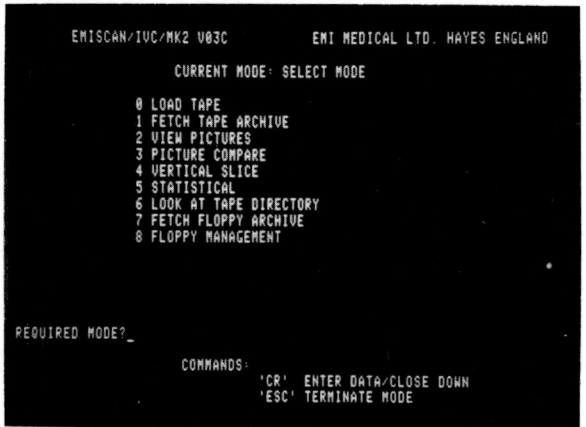

Fig. 2.17 Video display unit showing instructions to the operator.

systems. Long term storage is provided either by magnetic tape or floppy discs. Hard copy records are provided by Polaroid pictures from the display monitor, by bromide paper prints, or by using a multi-format camera with several images on one X-ray film. The actual numerical values of the individual attenuation coefficients can also be printed out on a line printer, but this is not found to be diagnostically helpful, although it is of some value for test purposes.

The computer calculates CT numbers for each pixel of the image matrix in a scale normally of 2000 values. It is not possible for any display system to present this enormous range as discrete gray-tones without exhibiting some saturation effects or requiring picture processing. Even if the display could cope, the person viewing the image could not distinguish more than about 20 values at any one time. Because the computer stores all the picture data it is possible to recall it in different ways without requiring further X-ray exposures, and effectively to alter the contrast of the displayed picture. A band of CT numbers can be selected by choosing a particular window width and the CT numbers within the band can be displayed as a full range of gray-tones. The position of the displayed band of numbers within the full scale can be set by adjusting a window level control. Figure 2.18

level control and noting its value when that part of the picture changes from black to white. This can be of help in identifying the nature of unknown lesions by a comparison with known tissues. Information such as the value of window width and level is normally automatically displayed superimposed on the edge of the picture display together with patient identification data keyed in by the operator.

It is also standard practice for the operator to be able to select a small region of interest from the picture by means of a joystick or tracker-ball control, and then to obtain the average CT number and standard deviation for the pixels within that region. This again is of help in trying to determine the exact nature of particular tissues. The area of the selected region can also be displayed so that measurements of organ size may be obtained.

The picture information stored on magnetic tape or floppy disc can be replayed remotely from the scanner, but requires the use of another computer and disc store to allow picture processing. Independent display consoles allow a full range of image processing and recording capabilities but cannot change the initial reconstruction algorithm unless the facility for transferring raw data on disc is provided. This would only be possible with the very fast sophisticated systems.

The value of picture smoothing or edge enhance-

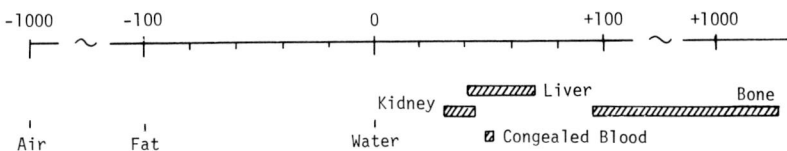

Fig. 2.18 Scale of CT values for a range of tissues.

illustrates CT numbers for some typical tissues. Thus, with a window width of 200, a level of $+10$ would be used for viewing liver tissues, a level of -400 for lung tissues and a level of $+100$ for studying bone. The effect is demonstrated in Figure 2.19. A wide window decreases contrast and allows differences in bone and soft tissue to be seen simultaneously.

In the extreme, when the window width is reduced to one CT unit, all gray-tones are eliminated and the picture is bistable or black and white only. It is then possible to determine the precise CT number at any part of the picture by adjusting the

ment is uncertain. Filtering or smoothing can be used to reduce the effective noise level since picture noise is associated with high spatial frequencies. This increases the detection of low contrast differences at the expense of resolution, and may be useful, for example, in picking out brain tumours (Fig. 2.20) or large liver mesastases that can be difficult to visualise. Nine point smoothing in which the data from nine adjacent points are averaged, or Wiener filtering, may be appropriate as in nuclear medicine imaging. Noise and resolution are related by the expression $\sigma^2_\mu \propto w^3$ (see Equation 2.18), where σ_μ is the standard deviation in the

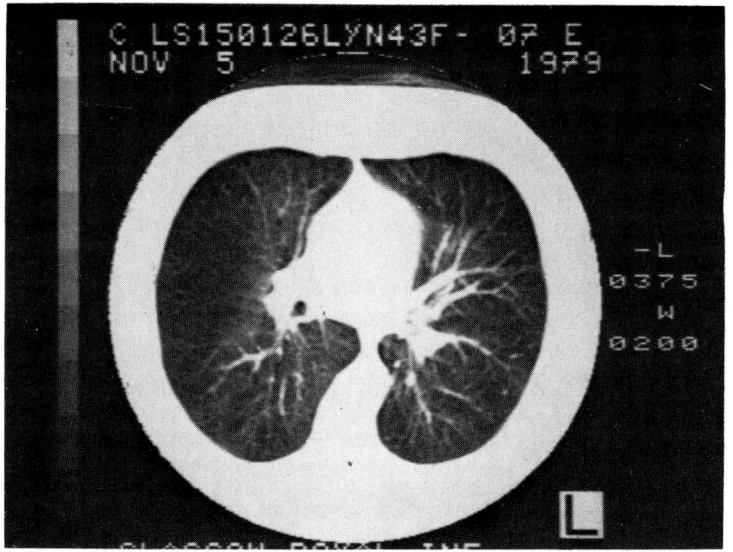

a

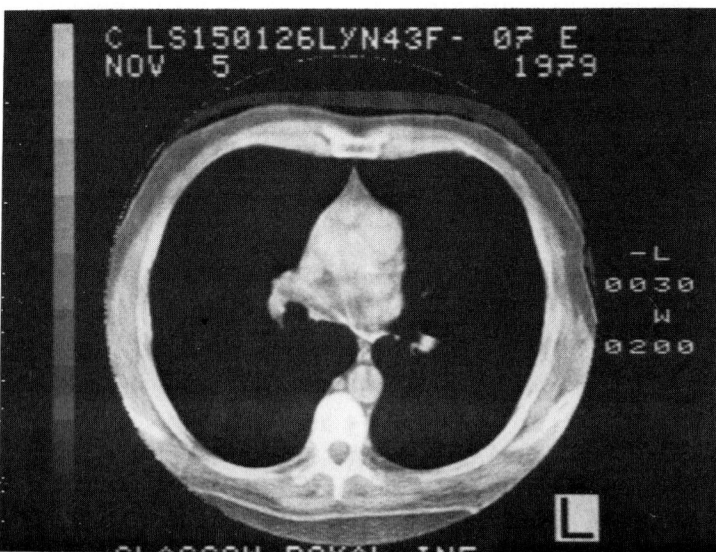

b

Fig. 2.19 Pictures illustrating the effect of changing display window level with a fixed width of 200. (a) Level at − 375. (b) Level at − 30.

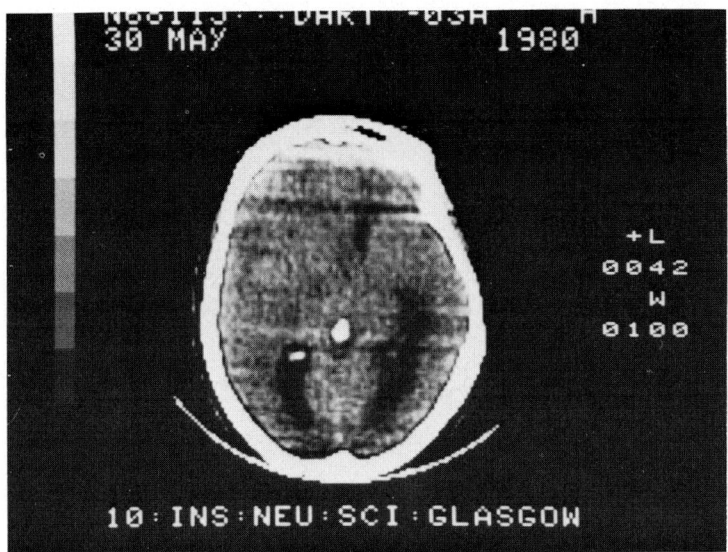

a

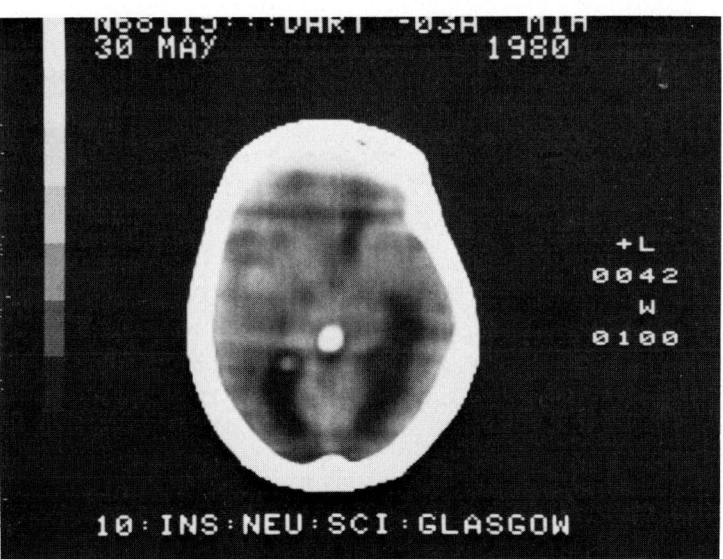

b

Fig. 2.20 Pictures illustrating the effect of different display filtering. (a) High resolution. (b) Low noise, with averaging over a 5 × 5 matrix.

72 SCIENTIFIC BASIS OF MEDICAL IMAGING

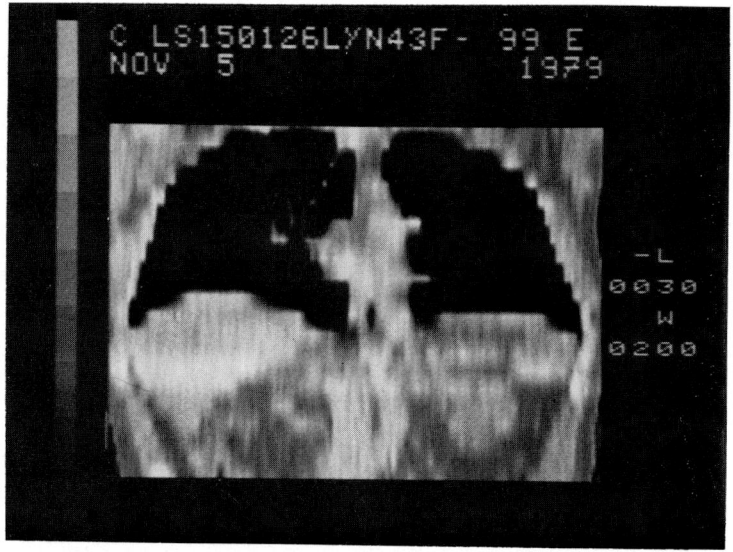

a

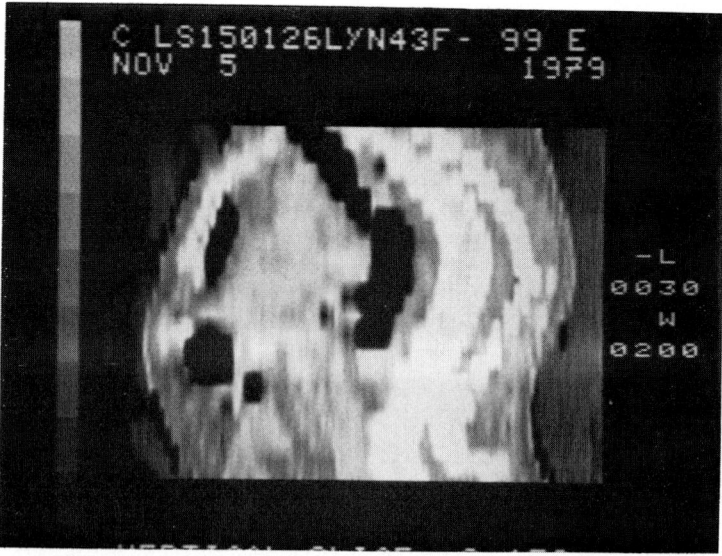

b

Fig. 2.21 Reconstructed chest section from a number of adjacent axial planes. (a) Coronal plane. (b) Sagittal plane.

attenuation coefficient and w is the pixel width of the display matrix. Thus, an image might give σ_μ = 0.5 per cent with a 160 × 160 matrix or σ_μ = 1.4 per cent with a 320 × 320 matrix. It is also possible to carry out image subtraction following the injection of contrast medium. A more useful processing procedure seems to be the reconstruction of saggital, coronal and even oblique planes from a series of axial planes (Fig. 2.21). The required plane is selected by positioning a cursor onto a view in the axial plane. The computer then extracts the relevant picture information from each of the axial planes available, records it and displays rather time consuming processes. Using films or image intensifiers as detectors leads to high resolution capabilities at the expense of contrast, the limits being set by the properties of the film emulsion or the intensifier screen used for detecting the transmission profiles.

The simple one-step process of unfiltered back projection on to film suggested by Watson, originally considered to be impracticable, has been shown[16] to give good images of moderate to high contrast objects after careful geometrical adjustment of the apparatus. If the X-ray tube, the object plane to be reconstructed and the film are all placed

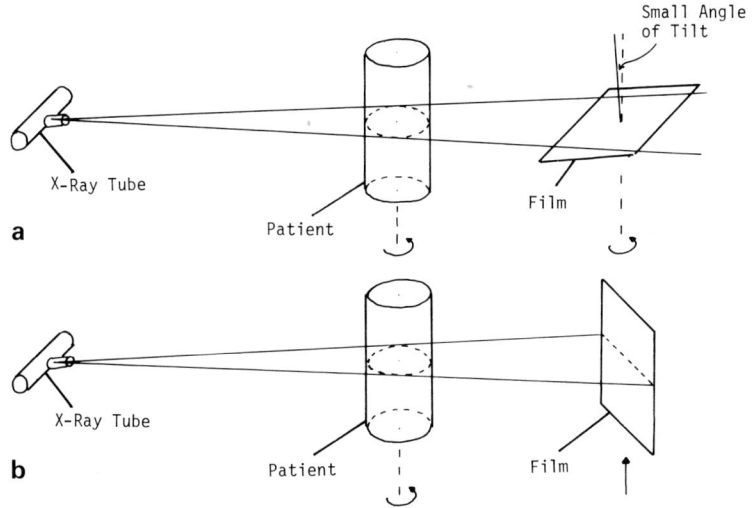

Fig. 2.22 Analogue reconstruction techniques. (a) A simple one step process giving an unfiltered back projection. (b) The recording of a sinogram as the first step towards a filtered back projection.

it in the correct geometrical position. The axial planes may be overlapping or non-overlapping, in which case the computer can generate linear interpolations for the missing data. Longitudinal section resolution depends upon the thickness of the scan slices (8–13mm normally), and upon the distance between individual slices. Interpolation of widely separated slices gives rise to a streaky appearance.

Analogue reconstruction methods

The techniques of back projection and spatial filtering are not restricted to computers but can be carried out in analogue form although they are in one plane, then the X-ray projection is effectively back projected across the complete width of the film. When the object and the film are synchronously rotated the different back projections are correctly summed on the film. In the ideal case for a thin section the radiation is parallel to the film emulsion and is very strongly absorbed. But a small tilt of the film results in a uniform exposure across its surface. At 100 keV the half value thickness for absorption in the emulsion is 7 mm and a tilt of 10^{-3} radians is sufficient to image an object of 100 mm radius with a slice thickness of 0.2 mm, as shown in Figure 2.22. With the narrow effective collimation of the small viewing angle the effect of

Compton scatter is negligible. The r^{-1} blurring factor, however, cannot be avoided and results in an overall fogging reducing the contrast in the image.

A more sophisticated version of this technique records the profiles on a film placed perpendicular to the irradiated slice, the film being moved in a direction parallel to the axis of rotation as the object is rotated. Under these conditions each point in the object records a sinusoidal trace on the film. For this reason this type of image is sometimes called a *sinogram*. Spatial filtering of the image can now be carried out by means of a superimposed compensation mask[8] and back projection is achieved in a third stage, moving the convoluted sinogram in front of a slit light source which projects through a cylindrical lens onto a final film rotated in the same way as the object during the initial recording of the profiles.

A commercial version using this principle with an image intensifier television system replacing films has been developed by Oldelft as an addition to their radiotherapy planning simulator (Simtomix). In this case the patient is fixed and the X-ray tube and image intensifier rotate through 360°.

SYSTEM PERFORMANCE

In order to evaluate or compare the diagnostic effectiveness of different CT scanners it is necessary to select certain parameters that can be measured under test conditions. The final assessment is made on the basis of clinical diagnosis, but it is not appropriate to use patients for comparative tests in view of the radiation hazard associated with X-rays and the need to keep exposures to the minimum consistent with obtaining a diagnosis.

Image quality

The images produced by CT scanners can be considered in terms of the normal parameters used for image assessment, noise, contrast scale and spatial resolution. In addition it is important that the presence of artifacts should be recognised and their cause identified.

Precision

When scanning a water bath the picture should appear as a uniform shade of gray, but generally it shows a speckled appearance which can be called *picture noise* (Fig. 2.23). This noise can be quantified if the values of CT numbers are printed out in the form of a histogram, when a distribution will be found (Fig. 2.24). The distribution can be described in terms of its mean value, which should be zero for the water bath, and a standard deviation. Such a distribution is of the type known as a Gaussian distribution, and it arises from the random process associated with the finite number of X-ray photons detected in each measurement. For n detected photons, Poisson statistics indicate a standard deviation of $(100/\sqrt{n})$ per cent. This corresponds to 3 per cent for 10^3 photons and 1 per cent for 10^4 photons. An ideal scanner introducing no other noise would produce a distribution with a standard deviation dependent only on the number of detected photons. The greater the value of the standard deviation, the more noise is apparent in the picture, and the more difficult it is to distinguish tissues with small differences in attenuation coefficient. Additional noise is added to this intrinsic photon noise as a result of fluctuations in the output of the X-ray tube caused by instabilities in the filament, and as a result of noise added in the detector electronics.

The precision of measurement is thus related to the statistical noise in the number of detected photons in each pixel. Although the physical parameter imaged by the CT scanner is the attenuation coefficient, for convenience the display is scaled in CT values. For comparing on an absolute scale, the CT values should be converted to attenuation coefficients. Then the standard deviation of the distribution of attenuation coefficients for a water bath phantom is a measure of the precision of that particular machine, which can be compared with subsequent measurements or with values for other machines. To change the CT values to the coefficients it has been found convenient to use the fact that the average linear attenuation difference between perspex (plexiglass) and water is a constant 0·024 cm^{-1} for 100–150 kVp and moderate filtration. Consequently, a measure of CT numbers for water and perspex averaged over a small area of

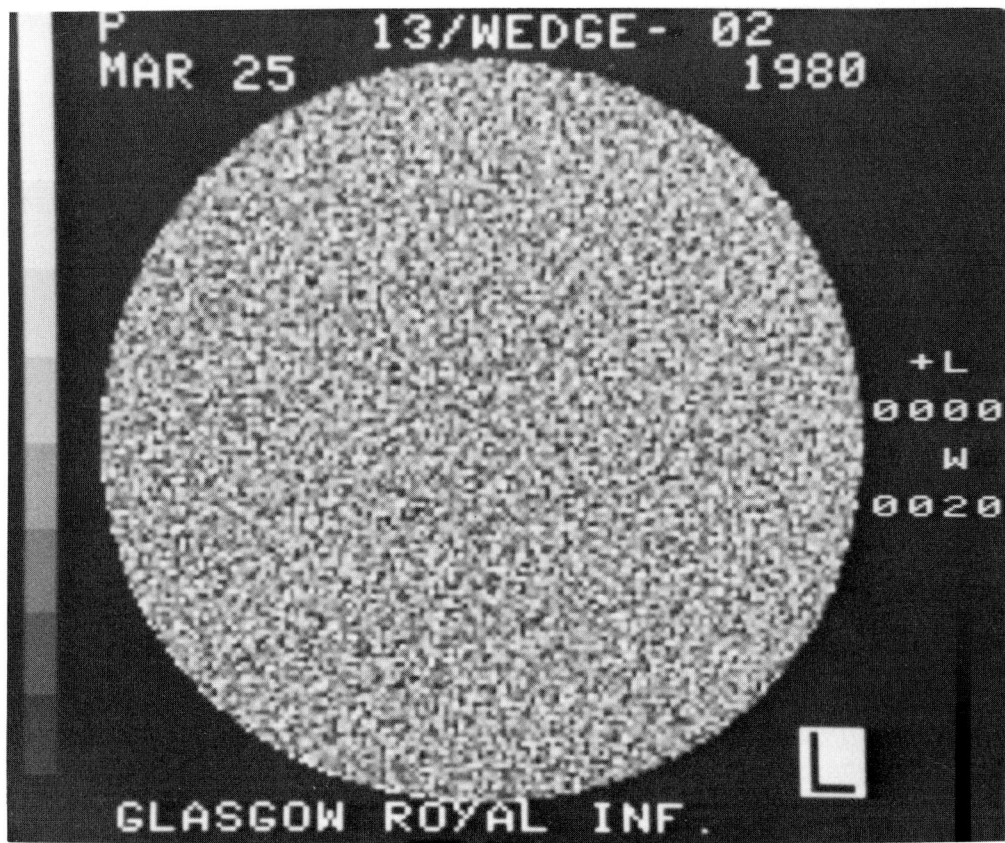

Fig. 2.23 Scan of water bath phantom displayed with narrow window width to show picture noise.

about 25 pixels at the centre of a water bath can be used to set the *contrast scale* (CS) relating CT numbers to attenuation coefficients:

$$\text{CS} = 0.024/(\text{CT}_{\text{perspex}} - \text{CT}_{\text{water}}) \quad (2.12)$$

per cm per CT number; and precision, expressed as a percentage of the attenuation coefficient of water, is given by:

$$\%\sigma_\mu = \sigma \, \text{CS} \, 100/\mu \quad (2.13)$$

Precision refers to the spread in values which are all expected to be the same. Accuracy on the other hand is an indication of the difference between the mean value of a set of readings and the theoretical value under the conditions of the measurement (effective energy and scanned object size). The diagnosis or detection of small contrast differences depends upon the precision but not upon the accuracy. This is because diagnosis is normally carried out on the basis of relative differences, and there does appear to be a considerable range in attenuation coefficients for the same pathological and normal tissues both between patients and within the same patient. Nevertheless it is most desirable that the expected CT values should not vary by more than one or two standard deviations with changes in operating conditions of kVp and scan size, and change of position within the scan field.

Resolution

The size of the smallest high contrast object that can be seen on a reconstructed picture depends on three factors: (1) the combination of the width of the detector aperture and the focal spot size; (2)

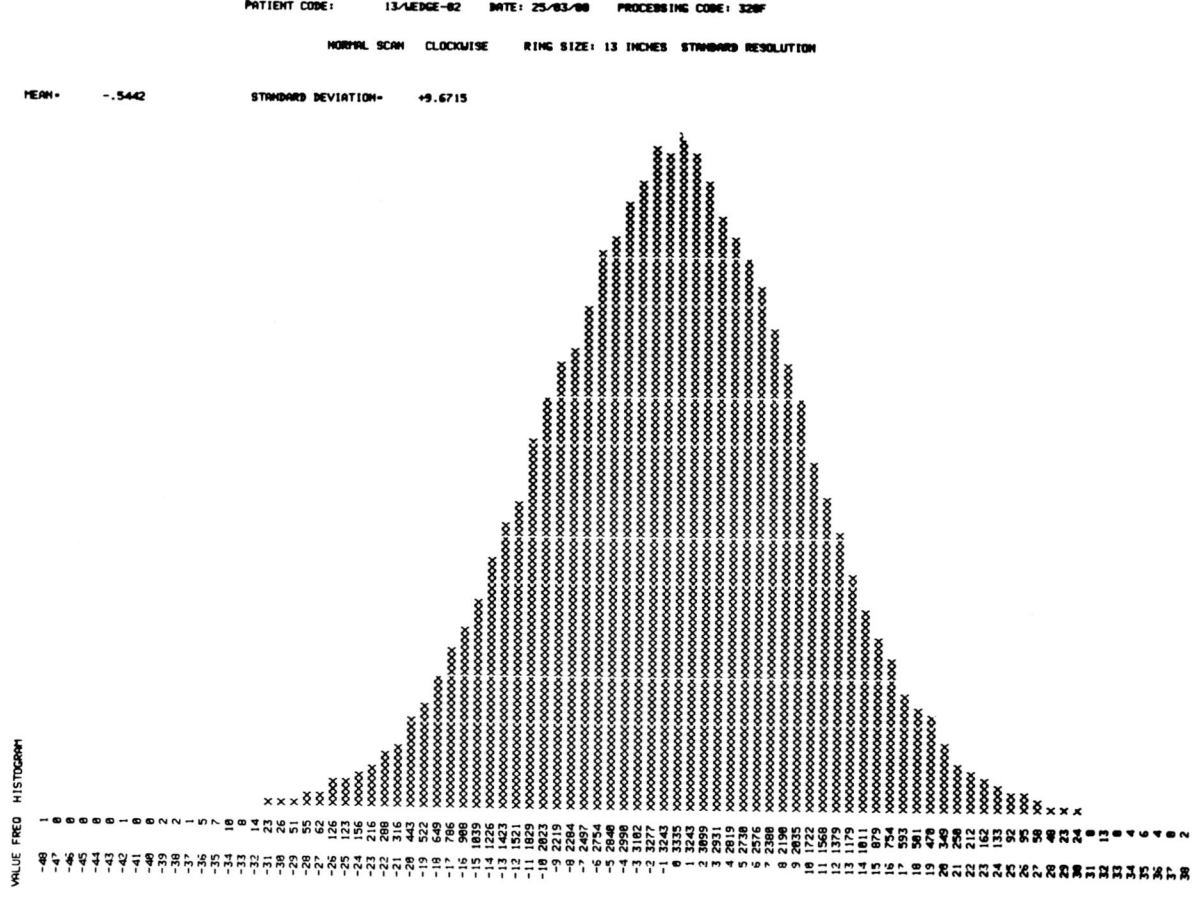

Fig. 2.24 Histogram of CT numbers corresponding to the water bath scan illustrated in Figure 2.23.

the separation of the measurement points; and (3) the display pixel size. One standard way of describing the ability of an optical system to resolve image detail is in terms of a *modulation transfer function*. This can be measured by observing the response of a small detector as it is moved across a periodic line object containing different spatial frequencies. An *aperture transfer function* can be determined in a similar way by observing the response of a finite sized detector moved across line objects of different spatial frequencies. The response depends upon the detector aperture a, the magnification factor M and the focal spot size A with a relationship in the form:

Aperture transfer function
$$= \frac{\sin \pi f a/M}{\pi f a/M} \cdot \frac{\sin \pi f A(M-1)/M}{\pi f A(M-1)/M}$$

The limit of this is given when the function first falls to zero, and this happens with either $\pi f a/M = 1$ or $\pi f A(M-1)/M = 1$. For most machines the effect of the focal spot is not as important as the effect of the detector aperture itself. Obviously when the object dimensions are greater than the detector aperture the response or modulation is a maximum, but as the object size is decreased the response falls until it reaches zero when the width of one line pair of the object equals the width of the detector.

Not only is the size of the detector aperture relevant to the smallest detectable detail, but so also is the separation between measurement points. With the rotating detector design of scanner, the separation depends upon the physical separation between adjacent detectors. For periodic objects that are large compared with this distance a fully modulated signal is obtained. But the detectors must sample at least twice for each periodic object to get a true representation. So the maximum frequency that can be reproduced (known as the *Nyquist* frequency) is half the sampling frequency, and the limiting frequency in line pairs per cm is given by $f_n = 1/2d$, where d is the sample separation distance in cm. Figure 2.25a shows that, for the GE machine with 511 detectors in a fixed 30 fan beam necessary for a whole body scan, the ray spacing at the centre of rotation is 0·8mm, and this is unaltered for smaller scan field diameters, so that $f_n = 6·2$ line pairs cm^{-1}. Philips in their Tomoscan machine move the centre of rotation towards the X-ray source for the smaller scan diameters so that the ray spacing is reduced and the value of f_n is increased. With the stationary type of detector the separation between detectors is not the important factor. Each detector sees the X-ray source and gathers data as the source passes round the patient, so that each view is a collection of rays whose numbers and spacing are determined by the rotation rate and the time between measurements. This detector sampling frequency can be varied to suit the size of object being scanned. With the Technicare Δ2020 (Fig. 2.25b) a scan can be made with 512 rays and 0·5 mm spacing at the centre of rotation for a head scan of 25 cm diameter, or with the same number of rays and 1 mm spacing for a 50 cm body scan.

Displayed resolution also depends on the number of pixels in a given scan field (Fig. 2.26). The maximum displayed frequency is $1/2w$, where w is the pixel width at the centre of rotation. For a 25 cm head field a 320 pixel matrix has a pixel size of 0·8 mm, whilst a 160 pixel matrix has a pixel size of 1·6 mm and a 512 pixel matrix has a pixel size of 0·5 mm.

The various limits are summarised in Table 2.1.

Table 2.1 Resolution limits for 25 cm scan field with typical CT scanners

	Technicare Δ2020	GE CT/T 8800
Limits in line pairs per cm:		
Aperture transfer function limit	6·2	13
Data sampling frequency limit	10	6·2
Display resolution limit	10	6·2
Magnification M	2·5	1·4
Aperture size a, mm	4·0	1·05
Focal spot size A, mm	0·6	1·2

Since all these limits apply, the displayed resolution is set by the lowest limit in each case. It can be seen that the overall resolution for the 25 cm scan field is similar for the different scan principles

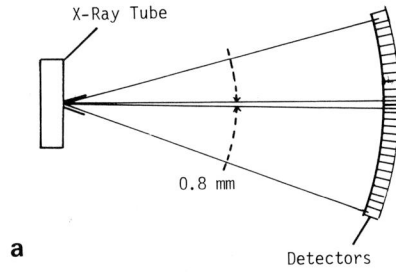

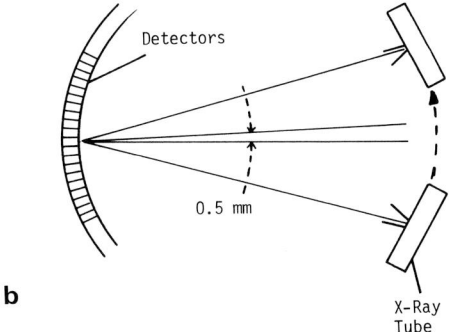

Fig. 2.25 Ray spacings for third generation machines. (a) GE rotating detector system with 30° fan. Ray spacing 0·8 mm at the centre of rotation. (b) Technicare Δ2020 fixed detector system. Ray spacing 0·5 mm at the centre of rotation.

used in the third-generation machines.

In common with other medical imaging techniques there is no universally accepted way of measuring spatial resolution. It is fashionable to

78 SCIENTIFIC BASIS OF MEDICAL IMAGING

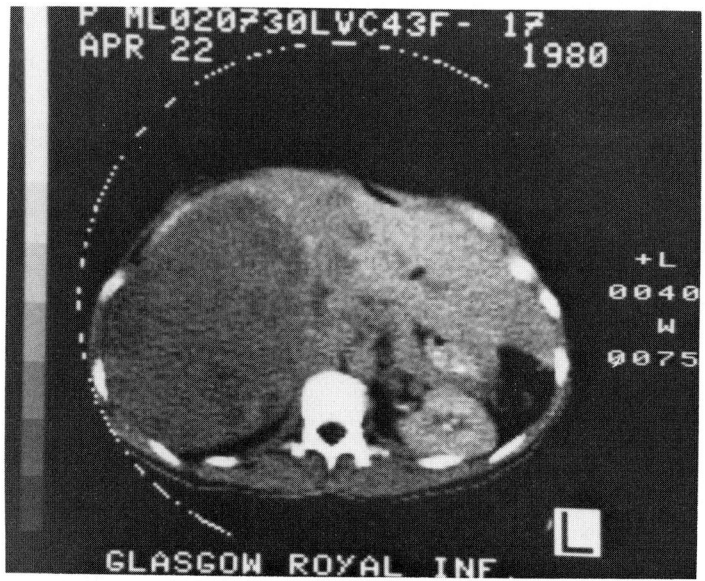

a

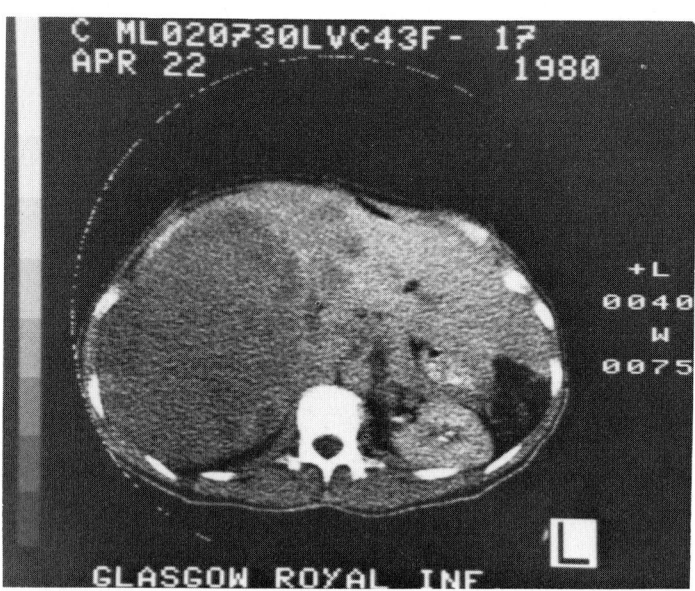

b

Fig. 2.26 Images showing the effect of changing the number of matrix elements in the display. (a) 160 × 160. (b) 320 × 320.

quote the modulation transfer function measured from star or bar patterns, but noise and picture processing confuse the interpretation of spatial resolution patterns except when measured at high contrast. An acceptable way of checking the resolution limit is to find the smallest group of holes and spaces in a perspex and water phantom. A group of 5 or more holes of diameter and spacing ranging from 0·75–2·5mm is appropriate to cover the currently available systems.

Artifacts

The precision and resolution of an image are set by fundamental design features and represent the optimum conditions. The picture quality may be further degraded, however, by the introduction of a number of artifacts arising from machine faults or limitations in the reconstruction algorithms. It is important that the source of these artifacts should be recognised and that either due allowance should be made in the picture interpretation or the most appropriate algorithm chosen where this is possible.

Aliasing

Where spatial frequencies higher than the Nyquist sampling frequency occur in any object then these frequencies can be subject to spurious detection and appear as lower frequencies. The effect is normally unnoticeable except at boundaries of high contrast, such as the edges of bone, which being sharp have intense high spatial frequency components. The effect shows up as streaks from the bone edges (Fig. 2.27). Aliasing is reduced in the GE system by the technique of scanning for the second half of the 360° with the detectors offset by half the scanning aperture to cancel out the artifacts produced in the first 180°. It can also be reduced by the form of filtering used in the convolution reconstruction. As explained on page 63, a high frequency cut-off at R_{max} is introduced to overcome the singularity in the integration (see Equation 2.10). However, a straight cut-off can be too crude and can introduce other artifacts such as overshoot or ringing at sharp boundaries. This is known as the *Gibbs phenomenon* and may be seen as a low density ring inside a high density skull image. If the high frequencies are cut-off gradually rather than abruptly above R_{max} in the filtering process, the ringing can be avoided and the aliasing reduced. Different filter windows can be used depending on the object to be studied. The *Hanning window*,[7] for example, replaces the simple value of $|R|$ used to filter in Fourier space (Equation 2.9) by the more complex $|R| [1 + \cos(\pi R/R_{max})]$ for $|R| < R_{max}$ with $|R| = 0$ for $|R| > R_{max}$. A certain amount of overshoot may, however, be beneficial in giving edge enhancement. Alternatively it may be desirable to give smoothing with a reduction in

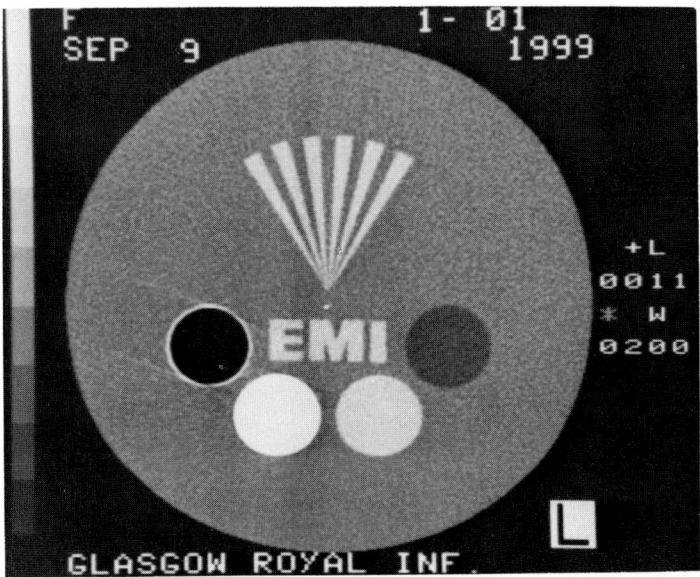

Fig. 2.27 Image showing streaking from simulated bone-air interface.

Beam hardening

The reconstruction process assumes initially that monoenergetic photons are used so that Equation 2.2 is valid. X-ray tubes produce polychromatic beams, however, with a range of energies from a lower limit set by the tube filtration up to the maximum set by the applied kilovoltage. The spectrum from an X-ray tube operating at 120 kilovolts peak and filtered by 4 mm aluminium is equivalent to a monoenergetic source of 56·5 keV when measured in terms of its half value thickness of aluminium. As the X-rays pass through the patient being scanned the lower energy photons are preferentially absorbed and the beam becomes harder, the absorption being a result of the energy dependent photoelectric effect and Compton scattering. In this case the measured log I/I_0 is not a linear function of absorber thickness. In the early water-bag scanners the path length in tissue and water is the same for all rays so that the effect of the beam hardening is not noticeable in the different rays unless the amount of bone present varies appreciably. Where no water bag is used the different tissue path lengths through the edges and centre of the body are sufficient to give disturbing beam hardening effects even without the presence of bone, with the result that CT numbers in the centre of the picture are lower than they should be. This is the so-called *cupping* effect. To some extent this is reduced by the use of shaped filters over the X-ray tube, designed also to reduce the dynamic range of the signals passing through the centre and edges of the body (see p. 66).

Further reduction in the beam hardening effect is achieved if the beam is initially hardened by increasing the filtration at the X-ray tube. The radiation output of the stationary anode tubes is limited, but the rotating anode tubes used in the fast scanners give sufficiently high outputs to permit the addition of 0·5 mm copper in the beam increasing the effective energy from 56·5–71 keV for 120 kVp applied. The radiation output is not high enough to permit the use of selective K edge filtering with thulium filters to enhance the tungsten characteristic radiation at 59 keV.

In practice, a combination of hardware and software solutions is used, and a convenient method is to assume that the patient is water equivalent, ignoring the bone for a first approximation. If a water phantom of approximately the same shape and size as a patient is initially scanned and the transmissions determined for the different rays, then non-linear corrections can be applied to the patient data before carrying out the reconstruction. This is called *linearising* the data. This is sufficient where very little bone is present, but a further refinement can then be made by identifying the bony parts of the reconstructed picture with pixels above some threshold CT value. The attenuation coefficients for bone vary with energy in a different way to those for tissue and knowing the ratio between μ_{bone} and μ_{water} averaged over the energy spectrum of the transmitted beam it is possible to calculate exactly the influence the detected bone would have on the measured signals, and to correct for the effect with a second reconstruction.

Complete correction would be possible during the processing stage if two separate scans were carried out with different applied kilovoltages on the X-ray tube giving two different energy distributions. Then the Compton scatter and the photo-electric absorption contributions could be separately determined. This is inconvenient, however, and may not be generally necessary since in practice the photoelectric absorption is less important than the Compton scatter.

Streak artifacts

Registration artifacts can be caused either by mechanical misalignments or by patient movements. Both show up as streaks from high contrast details. The machine-induced artifacts can be readily recognised when scanning a small aluminium pin in a water bath. The appearance of a streak in the form of a tuning fork pattern is associated with a misalignment of the optical graticule used to measure the translational movement in a first- or second-generation scanner. Since the collection of data from the various rays has to be accurately related to positional co-ordinates r,ϕ and matrix co-ordinates x,y, very careful adjustment of the graticule is necessary and precision in the manufacture of the rotational movements is of great importance.

Movements during scanning of the patient, either as a whole or of individual organs, can lead to severe streaking or star pattern artifacts from high contrast objects such as air and bone and to detail blurring of lower contrast objects. This is illustrated in Figure 2.28. Because of the complex way in which the measured data values lead to the picture, the artifact can effect image quality over parts of the picture distant from the moving object.

ation movement artifacts, a scan time of two seconds appears to be desirable, and to stop cardiovascular motion requires scan times very much less than this. For known movements or misalignments it would not be impossible to make corrections during the reconstruction process.[15]

Ring artifacts

Ring patterns may occur with any scanner. In translate-rotate machines they can be caused by

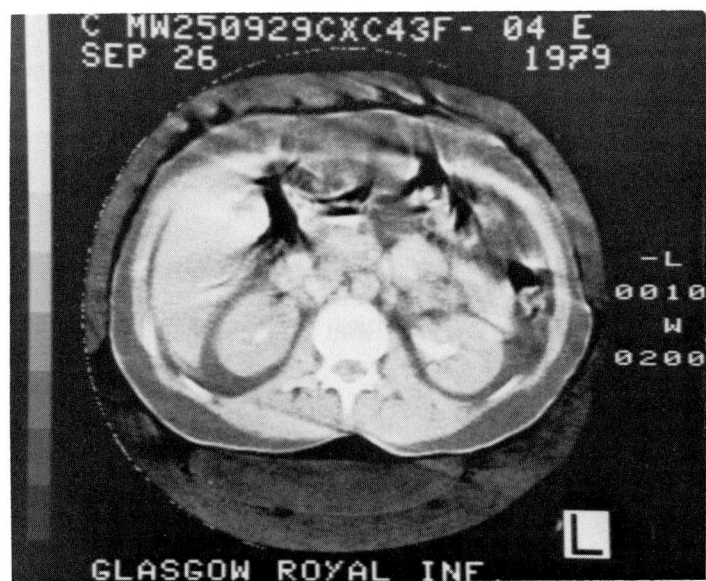

Fig. 2.28 Image showing effect of patient movement.

For sudden movements the streaks appear in a direction perpendicular to the rays being measured at the instant the movement occurred, but for slow movements the difference is detected only on completion of the scan cycle and normally causes streaking in the direction of the starting beam.

Movement artifacts are obviously minimised with shorter scan times, but also by scanning more projections than are necessary and averaging out the redundant information. The frequencies of muscular motion may be up to 10 cycles per minute, peristaltic motion up to 20, respiration up to 30 and cardiovascular motion up to 150 cycles per minute.[2] To avoid muscular, peristaltic and respir-

mechanical imperfections, vibrations or detector lag. In fan beam rotating-detector systems such artifacts are caused when certain detectors of the array differ slightly in sensitivity or energy response. A drift of 1 part in 5000 can cause problems since it is not possible to carry out calibrations during a scan, and in fixed-detector systems time-varying X-ray beam intensities can cause similar problems. The solution to all these problems is precision construction and frequent calibration.

Partial detection

In third-generation machines using a small focal

spot rotating anode tube the beam is divergent and it is possible that an object may not be seen when it is near the X-ray tube, but yet can be seen clearly when it is near the detector. In the case of a high contrast object the inconsistency instead of being averaged out can lead to a streaking artifact.

Similar artifacts are not normally found in the second generation machines where the broader focal spot with suitable source and detector collimation leads to more uniform beam geometry. But in those machines that give two scan slices simultaneously, the two beams are inclined and the artifact may then occur.

The effect of non-uniform beams is not only to introduce artifacts but also to lead to uncertainties in the detection of small objects when making consecutive scans displaced by the nominal beam width. Information regarding the slice geometry can be obtained with a simple phantom incorporating a 0·88 mm thick strip of Teflon 25 mm wide mounted at an angle of 45° inside a perspex phantom block 20 or 30 cm in diameter.[5] The contribution of the strip towards the attenuation coefficient of a particular pixel depends on the partial detection at that point. The effective thickness of the strip perpendicular to the slice is constant so that the resulting attenuation coefficients reflect the beam sensitivity at each point. Quantitative displays can then be obtained from numerical print-outs giving a graph of slice profiles at selected points. The beam width (FWHM) can be measured from the profiles both in the centre and at the edges of the scanned field.

Partial detection of low density objects may also produce an artifact not readily visible but possibly leading to a misinterpretation. The CT values of a small cyst lying within liver tissue, for example, may be as high as +10 whereas the same cyst situated on the liver surface and imaged in the same plane as lung tissue could show a value as low as −10. Such an effect is less likely to occur with thinner scan slice thickness and small pixel size.

Extracted data

The derived CT numbers expressed on the scale ±1000 (or any other arbitrary scale) are not absolute values of linear attenuation coefficient, but are calculated with respect to reference materials air and water. The true CT number (the *Hounsfield number*) for a particular tissue is derived by normalising the attenuation coefficient for the tissue to water, subtracting 1 and multiplying by 1000. This gives a scale with the CT value for water equal to zero and with each unit representing 0·1 per cent of the attenuation of water. Thus:

$$H = 1000\ (\mu_{tissue}/\mu_{water} - 1) \quad (2.14)$$

In practice the measured values for a given scanner may not exactly match the true scale, and they are to some extent dependent on the tissues in the beam due to beam hardening effects. In this case calibration with water and air is carried out using a realistic phantom to give comparable effects. Then:

$$H = 1000\ (CT_{tissue} - CT_{water})/(CT_{water} - CT_{air}) \quad (2.15)$$

The actual attenuation coefficient cannot be uniquely obtained from the CT or Hounsfield numbers because these are relative scales and the value of the coefficient depends on the effective energy of the X-ray beam. CT values for a blood sample fall with increasing kV from a value of 83 at 100 kVp to 79 at 120 kVp and 75 at 140 kVp, whilst a sample of subcutaneous fat gives values rising from −114 at 100 kVp to −103 at 120 kVp and −95 at 140 kVp. The different behaviour is explained by the effect of the photoelectric component of the attenuation coefficient. Fat has a lower effective atomic number than water, and blood has a higher effective atomic number. This differing response with kV provides a method of estimating the atomic number of a tissue. It is, however, important to verify that the CT number is linearly proportional to the attenuation coefficient for a given kVp and this has been shown to be valid by a number of different workers over the range of clinical interest.[29]

If test samples of materials of known composition are scanned it is possible to calculate the attenuation coefficients and hence the CT numbers for particular photon energies. A comparison of the measured CT numbers, usually averaged over a number of pixels, with the calculated values indicates the effective photon energy of the beam under the conditions of the test. Variations are to be expected with phantom diameter and the presence or absence of simulated bone. Suitable test materials developed by White are mixtures of ethanol and carbon tetrachloride in various proportions, immersed in a water tank. The effective energy of the EMI 5005 scanner operated at 120 kVp using a 20 cm phantom has been shown to be 70 keV when bone is present and 67 keV without bone. Using a different phantom with polystyrene, nylon, lexan and perspex inserts in water, a value of 77 keV has been obtained.[19]

The linear attenuation coefficient has two components when photon energies in the diagnostic range are used. The photoelectric component μ_{pe} predominates at low keV, and the Compton component μ_c predominates above 60 keV.

$$\mu_{pe} \propto \rho\, n_o\, \tilde{Z}^{3.4}\, E^{-3.1} = a_1 E^{-3.1} \quad (2.16)$$

$$\mu_c \propto \rho\, n_o f(E) = a_2 f(E) \quad (2.17)$$

where ρ is the density, n_o is the electron density, $\tilde{Z}$ is the effective atomic number and E is the incident photon energy. $f(E)$ is a decreasing function of energy.

The photoelectric effect is dependent on atomic number, whereas the Compton effect depends on the electron density, or, for most materials, the mass density. To separate these effects could possibly lead to additional information because a tissue of increased attenuation coefficient may be of increased density or of increased atomic number due, for example, to the incorporation of calcification. By scanning twice and obtaining measurements of attenuation coefficients at two energies, 100 kVp and 140 kVp, it has been shown to be possible[26] to determine electron density to 0.5 per cent and effective atomic number to 3 per cent when averaging over an area of 25 pixels. The sensitivity can be increased either by averaging over a larger number of pixels or by using energies further apart, but the technique has yet to find a clinical application.

Dose

The precision of measuring the attenuation coefficient, the resolution in the image and the X-ray exposure or patient dose are all interrelated. The precision can only be increased by recording an increased number of photons in each ray sum, and this can be done either by increasing the X-ray tube output, increasing the scan time or by increasing the detector aperture. This effect is illustrated in Figure 2.29. The standard deviation in the attenuation coefficient due to statistical noise in the detected photons is given by

$$\sigma_\mu \propto B^{1/2}\, w^{-3/2}\, h^{1/2}\, D^{1/2} \quad (2.18)$$

where B is the attenuation through the patient, w the pixel width, h the slice thickness and D the patient skin dose. For fixed resolution the dose must be quadrupled to improve the precision by a factor of two, and to reduce the pixel width by two requires eight times the dose for a given level of precision.

The skin dose that is received by the patient during a CT study, and the dose distribution within the patient, depend upon the radiographic factors chosen (as in conventional radiography), and also depend on the scanning motion, the beam profile, the number of scans in the study and on the required picture quality. The dose distribution can be described in terms of a maximum skin dose, a set of isodose curves in the scan plane and a set of beam profiles perpendicular to the scan plane.

For a scanner that rotates through exactly 360° with a constant X-ray output, the patient's skin dose within the slice is approximately the same at all points, and the dose contours follow the body contours. But for the rotate-translate scanners covering only 180°, the dose contours are appreciably 'U' shaped with the minimum skin dose 20–25 per cent of the maximum value. For the same image quality it would be expected that the maximum skin dose for a 180° scanner would be twice that for a 360° scanner, giving the same total number of transmitted photons. In either case the attenuation across the body is very much less than in conventional radiography using a fixed beam direction, so that only a limited amount of dose sparing of superficial organs (eyes, thyroid, breast) is possible by choice of scan start position. The beam profile, ideally sharp-edged, is in practice rounded by effects of penumbra and scattering so that beam overlap in a multiple scan study increases the doses above the single scan values. An increase of 1.6 times is typical for scan spacings equal to the full width at half maximum of the single scan profile. Beam profiles can be demonstrated using a photographic film wrapped around the surface of a patient phantom (Kodak X-Omat R therapy verification film is suitable). Relative dose values

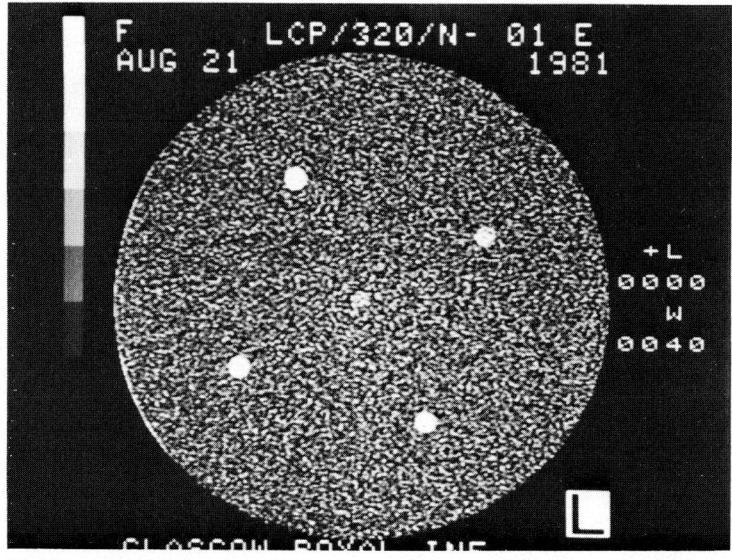

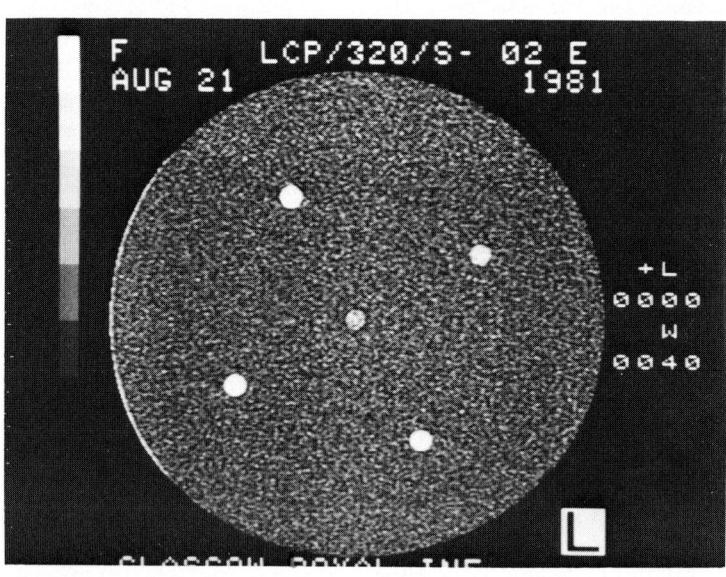

Fig. 2.29 Images showing effect of scan speed on precision. (a) Normal fast scan. (b) Slow scan, showing improved quality.

are easily obtained but absolute values require a calibration of the response at the appropriate energy. Because of the small beam cross-section accurate measurements with standard ionisation chambers are not possible, and the use of small thermoluminescent dosimeters is appropriate. Lithium fluoride (TLD – 700) has an energy dependence that varies only a few per cent over the expected range of beam effective energies 40–80 keV. Chips of dimensions $3 \times 3 \times 1$ mm can be positioned side-by-side in a strip across the wider beams, or face-to-face across the narrow beams. Calibrations of response can be carried out either at the same effective energies, or at high energies applying a correction factor of 1·3.

Since most scanners can be operated in a number of different modes with various scan times and noise levels, any comparison of machines must be carried out under similar conditions. Using a 22 cm diameter perspex cylinder for head scanners and a 20 × 33 cm elliptical phantom for body scanners, single scan maximum dose values between 14 mGy (1·4 rad) and 65 mGy (6·5 rad) for rotate-translate machines in the normal mode and up to 350 mGy (35 rad) for a low noise multiple scan mode have been measured.[18] Rotate-only machines can be operated at such a wide range of kV, mA and time values that comparison is not easy. For similar image quality an important parameter is the overall detection efficiency. Both rotating xenon detectors and fixed scintillation detectors using aperture restriction to improve spatial resolution have an efficiency of about 50 per cent compared with the 85–90 per cent efficiency achieved in the rotate-translate machines. This compensates for the factor two in maximum doses expected between 180° and 360° scanners so that in practice there appears to be no dose advantage with either scan principle.

Although the patient dose follows the expected relationship to kV and mA, it does not necessarily do so with scan time. For example, increasing the scan time by a factor 3·5 increases the dose by a factor 5 in a typical rotate-translate machine,[28] since a significant period of time is occupied with gantry rotation and this remains the same for the slower scan.

It is difficult to compare doses received in particular examinations between CT and conventional radiography because of the differences in dose distribution within the patient. Energy imparted may be a more useful concept and it has been calculated[28] that the energy deposited from a brain study with eight scans in the normal mode (50–70 mJ) is equivalent to two conventional skull radiographs, and the energy imparted with eight scans to the torso in the normal mode is roughly double this but less than the energy associated with a barium meal. The somatic risks of CT studies in the normal fast-scan mode are comparable with those accepted in conventional diagnostic radiology, whereas the selection of a higher accuracy mode increases the dose and hence the risk towards the top end of the conventional range.

Doses to surrounding areas arise from leakage and scattered radiation. The leakage levels are similar to those from diagnostic X-ray tube housings, but the scattered radiation levels are quite small because only a small area of skin is irradiated in each slice. Since the normal patient investigation includes a number of scans, however, the levels expected are of the order a few tens of μGy at 1 m from the scan circle. The workload and the position of the control area determine the necessary protection for the operating staff.

Quality control

It is important to keep a check on the performance of any imaging system. In normal radiography this may simply be a matter of assessing the diagnostic value of the films as they are reported. With a system as complex and expensive as a CT scanner, however, where frequent calibrations and adjustments are necessary, a regular programme of quality control should be followed. A number of phantoms are available either supplied by the manufacturers of the scanner machines or designed by groups interested in comparative tests (AAPM Task Force, DHSS CT Users' Group).

A basic protocol should measure precision and accuracy daily, and this can be done using a simple water bath scanned with rotations in both directions, where this is done in clinical practice. A print-out of the mean values and standard deviations indicates if further action is necessary. A non-zero mean value could require a repeat wedge correction procedure, and an increase in the standard deviation could indicate a failing X-ray tube or a noisy detector. A more detailed look at the unprocessed data can be carried out weekly, to look for detector and integrator uniformity, noise and speed corrections, and spatial uniformity. Monthly checks of contrast scale and alignment can be carried out with the use of a composite phantom that includes blocks of various plastic materials and an aluminium pin in a water bath. Perspex and water are used to determine the contrast scale, but the addition of polyethylene, polystyrene, nylon and lexan make it possible to carry out a check of linearity and to estimate the effective energy of the beam. More detailed checks such as beam profile and dose measurements can be carried out at 3-monthly intervals following the more extensive preventive maintenance schedule.

CLINICAL USES

CT is a relatively new technique that has still to find its place as a diagnostic tool in relation to the other more established techniques of radiography, tomography and ultrasound. Radionuclide imaging is rather different in that it produces images related to function within an organ rather than to structural anatomy.

Conventional X-radiographs are shadows with images of various structures overlapping, and, in the case of bone, masking overlying details. This is particularly a problem in the brain where all the structures are covered by the skull. But conventional X-radiography is relatively cheap and can be extensively used. This means a service coping with a large throughput of patients can be run by a reasonably small number of radiographers and radiologists.

Tomography, computed tomography and ultrasound are more directly comparable in that they all image thin sections, so that a complete picture of the organ has to be built up from a number of adjacent slices. This inevitably means that such procedures are time-consuming, and, therefore, can only be applied to selected groups of patients. They also demand much more of the radiologist's time in interpreting the results. Conventional tomography is never used before conventional radiography, and although it is useful for bony structures and solid lesions, it fails to distinguish healthy and diseased tissues. Ultrasound can be used on its own, and being less hazardous and cheaper to run than CT should be used where possible as the method of first choice. But ultrasound does require skill and perhaps some artistry to produce diagnostically useful images, and since ultrasound radiation is almost totally reflected by bone or air interfaces it is of little value in scanning the head and lungs, and can be limited in the abdomen by the presence of bowel gas.

Computed tomography, however, produces clear anatomical sections virtually automatically but does require an experienced radiologist to interpret the results. Although capable of high precision in directly distinguishing tissues with small density differences, the use of dilute contrast agents of high atomic number can in many cases help with the identification of organs and vascular pathology. Since a normal examination may consist of eight or more scan slices with or without contrast medium each examination can be a time-consuming process.

Patients for CT scanning must be carefully selected and prepared because of the limited throughput in a day and because patient movement may lead to pictures of no diagnostic value. It is essential carefully to explain the procedure to the patient beforehand and to sedate those who are restless or apprehensive. For abdominal scans suitable low residue diets must be prescribed for the previous 24 hours to reduce the formation of bowel gas, and relaxants must be given where peristalsis is likely to be a problem. Ideally a slit beam radiograph or scanogram should be taken to help locate the scan planes in relation to anatomical or external markers. With some machines it is necessary to use bolus bags around the patient to simulate a more circular cross section and so reduce the dynamic range to be handled by the computer.

CT images are displayed by convention as if the scan planes were viewed from below the patient.

Head

CT scanning was first applied to the brain partly because the early machines required the use of a compensating water bath, which cannot be conveniently applied to body scans, but mainly because there was a great need for improving the diagnostic techniques available to the neuroradiologist. CT was immediately seen to be an accurate and reliable non-invasive procedure. Very quickly it proved to be of value in demonstrating cerebral abnormalities such as abscesses, angiomas, contusions, haematomas, hydrocephalus and tumours, almost entirely replacing the invasive techniques of cerebral angiography, air encephalography and ventriculography. As time went on it was found that the accuracy of delineating small lesions or detecting small tissue density differences could be improved by the use of contrast agents such as intravenous injections of water-soluble iodine compounds to enhance the vascular system or inhaled xenon, which crosses the blood-brain barrier, to diffuse into brain tissue. Diagnosis is normally on the basis of recognition of a space occupying lesion, although an analysis of CT numbers can be useful in assessing regional cerebral blood volume[13] provided allowance is made for partial volume detection effects.

Ultrasound is of limited application to the adult brain although it could be more widely used with neonates. It is, however, useful as a preliminary method in ophthalmic diagnosis to be followed by CT particularly where there might be bone involvement or a deep lying lesion.

Body

The extension of machines to cover whole body scan fields was a logical step by the equipment manufacturers. Experience has now shown that CT can image transverse axial planes, and a limited range of oblique planes, of virtually every part of the body. Its superiority over conventional radiography in picking out small contrast differences makes it an appropriate diagnostic tool for investigating soft tissues, while its inferior resolution capability limits its use for studies of fine detail. Patient movement is a problem and ill patients cannot easily hold their breath for the 20 s scanning periods of the second-generation machines especially if repeated, as they usually are, for a number of scan planes. Even the fast 2 s scanners cannot stop cardiac movements.

CT has been found to be particularly useful for the thorax and pleura where it can demonstrate smaller lesions than is possible with conventional tomography, and for the diagnosis of mediastinal masses. Ultrasound is of limited value in the thorax because of the air boundaries, and radionuclide scanning is a complementary technique in that it displays function and not anatomy.

It is in the abdomen that a body scanner may be of first choice. Although ultrasound can be very good for outlining solid lesions there are times where the technique proves impossible. Ultrasonic penetration through obese patients is difficult, and yet these provide the best CT pictures with the abdominal organs outlined by adipose tissue. The extent of disease involving the pancreas, retroperitoneal space and lymph nodes can be shown and widespread abdominal masses are also clearly seen.

As scanners of improved resolution are introduced, studies of the spinal cord will prove useful. It is also possible to use the scanner both to help in the localisation of biopsy sampling, and even for in vivo tissue analysis from the CT numbers. Microcalcifications can be inferred from the average CT number even though their detail can not be resolved, and the dual energy method has been used to estimate the iron content in the liver.[6]

Radiotherapy treatment planning

The ability of CT to demonstrate all structures from air to bone within a patient's cross section precisely both in terms of tissue density and position makes the technique of great significance for the staging and monitoring of malignant disease. It permits the determination of the size and shape of a lesion and shows any dissemination or invasion of neighbouring organs. Although only one cross section can be displayed at a time, a series of adjacent scans obviously contains the three dimensional information necessary for accurate planning of radiotherapy treatment even of deep seated tumours. CT planning takes place in stages using an interactive facility: (1) is the display of anatomical topography; (2) is the delineation of the tumour and of surrounding critical organs; (3) is the calculation of the dose distributions for the selected treatment modality; and (4) is the specification of the treatment machine parameters. These stages are discussed in more detail in the following paragraphs:

Stage 1

The only requirement during scanning is to reproduce the conditions imposed on the patient's position during the treatment. The couch top has to be the same shape as that of the treatment couch, and external pressures from such as bolus bags, which might distort the skin contours, have to be avoided. Exact localisation of internal structures with regard to surface markers is helped by the use of the scanogram film and by the use of laser marker beams and polypropylene rods taped to the skin.

Stage 2

An interactive display using a light pen or trackerball allows the radiotherapist to outline the patient's skin, skin markers, the tumour and any critical organs to be spared and to feed this information to the planning computer.

Stage 3

Internal calculations are complicated by tissue inhomogeneities such as lung tissue, bone and air gaps. A simple approach gives an average attenuation coefficient to perturbing features, which have been outlined, but this does not make use of the detailed information available in the individual CT numbers. A pixel-by-pixel method can be used to calculate the effect of varying tissue absorption.[21] But first consideration must be given to the possible presence of movement and partial volume artifacts. If the data are satisfactory, then the next problem encountered is due to the fact that the CT numbers are derived using diagnostic X-ray energies and the properties at therapy beam energies are required. The attenuation coefficient of a particular tissue derived from the scanner X-ray spectrum is not related in a simple way to that in the megavoltage energy range, because of the influence of photoelectric effect, as explained on p. 82. For most tissues the Compton effect predominates and this is dependent on the electron density of the tissue. Where this is not the case, a relative electron density may be determined and used to give an effective path length. Figure 2.30 shows the results of an experimental determination of the relationship between CT numbers and electron density. For a particular operating kilovoltage a linear relation covers lung and soft tissues up to a CT number of 130. A different relation is found for bone and bone-related structures.

Inhomogeneity corrections are based on effective path lengths, CT numbers are converted by means of the experimentally determined relation to relative electron density values and the equivalent distance at any point of a treatment beam is obtained from a sum of effective path lengths of pixel elements. Further complications might be considered in which improved algorithms could correct for electron non-equilibrium at tissue boundaries, and eventually could give planning in three rather than two dimensions.

Stage 4

The optimised dose distributions and the treatment machine parameters required to give these distributions are normally displayed superimposed on the relevant scan. It would not be impossible to carry the interactive process a stage further with the computer either controlling or simply verifying the treatment as it is carried out. As yet this has not been done in a routine procedure.

Bone studies

CT may not be the method of choice for studying skeletal disorders, but it is capable of displaying complex fractures in cases where conventional radiography proves difficult, such as at the base of the skull, and it is probably the most sensitive method available for demonstrating small sclerotic deposits in bone. But CT can go beyond the simple imaging of bone structures and can provide quantitative information with regard to the mineral distribution within any bone. Osteoporosis is a disease of the bone resulting in demineralisation and a drop in bone density. Conventionally this change has been investigated by radiographic film densitometry or by gamma densitometry, but Pullan has shown that the CT numbers produced by an EMI head scanner from an area of bone are a much more sensitive index for detecting changes in mineral content.

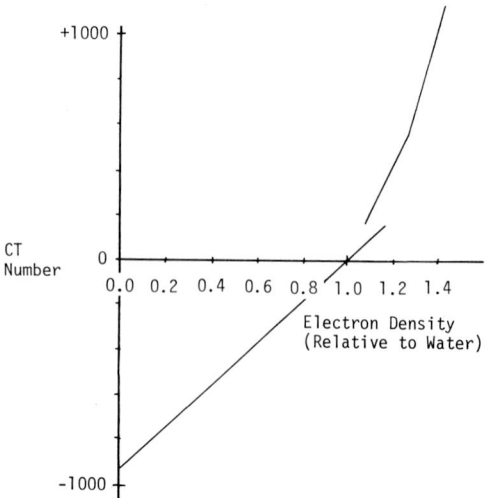

Fig. 2.30 Relationship between CT numbers and electron density (relative to water).[21]

A special purpose scanner using an iodine-125 γ-ray source has been built[25] to produce a high resolution scan of the forearm with a possibility of separately quantifying the mineral content of the compact and trabecular bone. Some of the whole body scanners now can give high resolution images over a limited scan area and so make it possible to investigate the mineral content not only in the bones of the forearm and femur but also in the spine.

FUTURE TRENDS

There are pressures to push the development of CT scanners in two directions. On the one hand there is a requirement for an improvement in resolution and a reduction in scan time, and on the other hand there is a desire for a reduction in the capital and running costs of the system. Of course these two objectives are not compatible, since an improvement in resolution implies more detectors and a reduction in scan time implies faster processing, both involving greater expense. The only ways in which the costs might be reduced are by accepting a more limited specification in terms of resolution and scan time or by selling in much larger quantities. The specification of a unit for a radiotherapy department might, for example, be acceptable with a resolution of only 5 mm, a precision no greater than 1 per cent, a scan time of 20 s and utilising the same computer for both image reconstruction and treatment planning purposes. Or the demand might increase for a unit giving a high throughput of patients if it were able to replace conventional radiographic and tomographic units in a moderate sized X-ray department.

All these trends are apparent, but to try accurately to predict the final place of CT scanners in the diagnostic armamentarium is not possible. Developments are of course taking place simultaneously with the automation of ultrasonic machines and the cost difference between an ultrasonic unit incorporating a dedicated computer and a basic whole body scanner is now quite small.

A greater range of both hybrid and special purpose scanners is likely in the future. Dedicated bone scanners and breast scanners have already been designed. Work is also in progress using image intensifiers as input devices to a computer system where each video line scan is in effect a profile of high spatial resolution. In theory it would be possible to use a conventional screening unit coupled to a computer. Rotation of the patient in a period of 5–10 s in front of the image intensifier would then give enough data to permit the reconstruction of a number of adjacent scan planes, of good spatial resolution but of limited precision for detecting low contrast differences. It is obviously possible to produce pictures equivalent to conventional radiographs, as is done with the scanogram in setting up the scan planes, so that in the future a multipurpose unit could be used for both plain radiography and computed tomography, thus increasing the flexibility of the system.

There is still scope also for improvements through software developments, and new reconstruction algorithms could give much greater flexibility in diagnostic capability. If for example only a part of the normal scan field is reconstructed then for the same resolution a picture of half the diameter would permit the dose, the scan time and the reconstruction time all to be reduced by a factor two. Whereas a reconstruction to improve the resolution is also possible, it would inevitably lead to some increase in the dose, scan time and processing time. There can be no compromise in the relation between precision, dose and resolution (see Equation 2.18). It is interesting to note that for the same dose, in theory at least, a picture may be reconstructed to give a precision of 0·5 per cent on a 160 × 160 pixel matrix, or a precision of 11 per cent on a 1200 × 1200 pixel matrix, and this latter image would be very comparable with the quality of a conventional film radiograph.

New techniques in data reduction could be developed, to permit higher processing speeds. Various methods of bandwidth compression have been suggested[11] that would be able to cope with increased rates of data collection. Ultimately a full three dimensional display can be envisaged with the ability to focus immediately on any desired plane as required.

As the CT techniques develop so also will those of ultrasound and radionuclide emission tomography. It will be necessary continually to review the relative merits of the different approaches.

Cardiac applications

Ultrasound is the method of choice for studying the movement of the heart walls and valves. CT might have a part to play in the measurement of the chamber sizes and investigations of the myocardium if it were possible to overcome the limitations of the current range of scanners, which with a single X-ray source are unable to freeze heart movements. Some attempts have been made to gate the recording system from ECG and respiratory transducers. Static pictures could be built up corresponding to one phase of the cardiac cycle, but would require a period of several minutes with a second generation scanner. Any arrhythmic cycles would have to be rejected. An alternative method available with rotate-only scanners would be to record the ECG signal correlated with the angular position of the scanner so that subsequently projections recorded at a particular delay following the R-wave could be reconstructed. In this way several images through a heart cycle could be obtained from a scan of less than a minute. This is not the optimum way of dealing with the problem. Further attempts aimed at dynamic reconstruction propose to produce up to 60 images per second by using multiple X-ray sources. Thus, a *Dynamic Spatial Reconstructor* (DSR)[24] which uses 28 pulsed X-ray sources and imaging systems has been constructed. The X-ray sources are rotating anode tubes arranged around a semi-circle below the patient, and the imaging systems are fluorescent screens and associated image intensified television cameras arranged in an opposing semi-circle above the patient. The system can record on video disc 28 television pictures each of 240 video lines within a period of 10 ms, repeated either 60 times per second (mains frequency) for one or two heart cycles, or at a rate of 4 per second over one or two respiratory cycles. Subsequently the data are processed by computer to give up to 60 adjacent cross sections reconstructed for each 10 ms period of operation. The display can be set to show a selected cross section in real-time so as to produce images of a beating cross section of the heart.

One problem associated with these attempts at dynamic reconstruction is the production of artifacts as a result of the limited number of projections used for each image. This problem is avoided in normal scanning by taking 300 or more views. If the angular intervals are too small compared with the desired spatial resolving power, a star pattern of artifacts appears from high contrast edges. Typically the number of angular intervals should exceed the number of pixels in the width of the display, although a suitable choice of reconstruction algorithm can minimise the effect of an under-determined image.

Cost effectiveness

CT scanners are expensive both to buy and to run, and cannot cope with high patient throughputs. Therefore, it is relevant to look at the ways in which they can be used in a health care service, and to consider the implications for resource allocation.

Data on the costs, locations and uses of scanners are readily obtained, whereas data on the clinical efficacy are not. A review of published papers shows that most studies are reported in terms of diagnostic accuracy. The necessary implications of efficacy have been considered by the Institute of Medicine, Washington, who derive a hierarchy of five levels.[9] These are: (1) technical capability: an accurate representation of the area scanned; (2) diagnostic accuracy: provision of information that contributes to the formulation of correct diagnoses; (3) diagnostic impact: the extent to which CT scan information replaces other diagnostic procedures, including diagnostic imaging, surgical exploration and biopsy; (4) therapeutic impact: change in disease management that would not have taken place without the information from the scan; and (5) patient outcome: the effect of CT scan information on patient morbidity and mortality.

The hierarchy might well be taken a stage further to consider the impact of CT scanning on the overall health of the population served by the scanner.[27] The levels (1) to (3) have now been well evaluated. It is fairly clear that CT gives a primary imaging approach to intracranial disease and here it may represent the definitive diagnostic method.[1] The major application of CT to the body appears to be in the localisation and therapeutic management of mass lesions in the abdomen. It appears never to be a primary imaging approach other than to the brain, and must be used in conjunction with complex X-ray techniques, radionuclide imaging and ultrasound. It does not seem possible that the use of CT could reduce the number of these other examinations to a level where such units would not be needed. The way in which CT can affect the therapeutic impact and the patient outcome is not known. Neither, it should be said, is it known for any other diagnostic technique. The earlier detection of disease may have little effect on the treatment, it might increase the length of treatment, or it might shift the emphasis from surgery to drugs. It has been suggested that the majority of CT body scans have no effect on patient management. It is clear that further clinical trials need to be carried out in a rigorous and controlled way to provide the information to place CT in its true perspective.

Acknowledgements

The author gratefully acknowledges the help given to him in the preparation of this manuscript by the Department of Radiology, Glasgow Royal Infirmary and by the Division of Neuroradiology, Glasgow Institute of Neurological Sciences.

REFERENCES

1. Abrams, H. L. & McNeil, B. J. (1978) Medical implications of computed tomography (CAT scanning). *New Eng.J.Med.*, **298**, 255–61 and 310–8.
2. Alfidi, R. J., MacIntyre, W. J. & Haaga, J. R. (1976) The effects of biological motion on CT resolution. *Am.J.Radiol.*, **127**, 11–5.
3. Baker, C. & Way, L. W. (1978) Clinical utility of CAT body scans. *Am. J. Surg.*, **136**, 37–44.
4. Brooks, R. A. & Di Chiro, G. (1976) Principles of computer assisted tomography (CAT) in radiographic and radioisotope imaging. *Phys. Med. Biol.*, **21**, 689–732.
5. Brooks, R. A. & Di Chiro, G. (1977) Slice geometry in computer assisted tomography. *J. Comput. Asst. Tomog.*, **1**, 191–9.
6. Chapman, R. W. G., Williams, G., Bydder, G., Dick, R., Sherlock, S. & Kreel, L. (1980) Computed tomography for determining liver iron content in primary haemochromatosis. *Br. Med. J.*, **280**, 440–2.
7. Chesler, D. A., Riederer, S. J. (1975) Ripple suppression during reconstruction in transverse tomography. *Phys. Med. Biol.*, **20**, 632–6.
8. Edholm, P., Hellstrom, L. G. & Jacobson, B. (1978) Transverse tomography with incoherent optical reconstruction. *Phys. Med. Biol.*, **23**, 90–9.
9. Fineberg, H. V., Bauman, R. & Sosman, S. (1977) Computerised cranial tomography: effects on diagnosis and therapeutic plans. *J. Am. med. Ass.*, **238**, 224–7.
10. Gordon, R., Hermann, G. T. & Johnson, S. A. (1975) Image reconstruction from projections. *Sci. Am.*, **233**, no. 4, 56–68.
11. Gordon, R. (1977) High speed reconstruction of the finest details available in X-Ray projections. In *Reconstruction Tomography in Diagnostic Radiology and Nuclear Medicine*, ed. Ter-Pogossian, M. M., Phelps, M. E., Brownell, G. L., Cox Jr, J. R., David, D. O. & Evans, R. G., pp. 77–83. Baltimore: University Park Press.
12. Goitein, M. (1972) Three dimensional density reconstruction from a series of two dimensional projections. *Nucl. Instr. Meth.*, **101**, 509–18.
13. Kendall, B. E., Radue, E. W. & Zilka, E. (1978) Xenon enhancement in computed tomography. *Xtract*, **4**, 7–12.
14. Kuhl, D. E. & Edwards, R. Q. (1963) Image separation in radioisotope scanning. *Radiology*, **80**, 653–61.
15. Kowalski, G. & Wagner, W. (1977) Artefacts in CT pictures. *Medica Mundi*, **22/3**, 13–7.
16. Lindegaard-Anderson, A. & Thueson, G. (1979) Simplified highly efficient apparatus for photographic transaxial X-Ray tomography. *J. sci. Instr.*, **12**, 924–6.
17. McCullough, E. C., Payne, J. T., Baker, H. L., Hattery, R. R., Sheedy, P. F., Stephens, D. H. & Gedgaudus, E. (1976) Performance evaluation and quality assurance of computed tomography scanners, with illustrations from EMI, ACTA and Delta scanners. *Radiology*, **120**, 173–88.
18. McCullough, E. C. & Payne, J. T. (1978) Patient dosage in computed tomography. *Radiology*, **129**, 457–63.
19. Millner, M. R., Payne, W. H., Waggener, R. G, McDavid, W. D., Dennis, M. J. & Sank, V. J. (1978) Determination of effective energies in CT calibration. *Med. Phys.*, **5**, 543–5.
20. Monahan, W. G. (1977) Computer tomography using a Cs 137 source. *IEEE Trans. nucl. Sci.*, **NS-24**, 567–9.
21. Parker, R. P., Hobday, P. A. & Cassell, K. J. (1979) The direct use of CT numbers in radiotherapy dosage calculations for inhomogeneous media. *Phys. Med. Biol.*, **24**, 802–9.
22. Radon, J. (1917) On the determination of functions from their integrals along certain manifolds. *Ber. Sachs. Akad. Wiss.*, **69**, 262–77.
23. Ramachandran, G. N. & Lakshminarayanan, A. V. (1971) Three dimensional reconstruction from radiographs and electron micrographs. application of convolutions instead of Fourier Transforms. *Proc. Nat. Acad. Sci. U.S.A.*, **68**, 2236–40.
24. Ritman, E. L., Sturm, R. E. & Wood, E. H. (1977) Needs, performance requirements and proposed design of spatial reconstruction system for diagnostic and investigative studies of cardiopulmonary and circulatory dynamics. In *Reconstruction Tomography in Diagnostic*

Radiology and Nuclear Medicine, ed. Ter-Pogossian, M. M., Phelps, M. E., Brownell, G. L., Cox Jr, J. R., David, D. O., & Evans, R. G., pp. 431–5. Baltimore: University Park Press.
25. Rüegsegger, P., Elsasser, U., Anliker, M., Gnehm, H., Kind, H. & Prader, A. (1976) Quantification of bone mineralisation using computed tomography. *Radiology*, **121**, 93–7.
26. Rutherford, R. A., Pullan, B. R., & Isherwood, I. (1976) Measurement of effective atomic number and electron density using an EMI scanner. *Neuroradiology*, **11**, 15–21.
27. Stocking, B. & Morrison, S. L. (1978) *The Image and the Reality*. Oxford: Oxford University Press.
28. Wall, B. F., Green, D. A. C. & Veerappan, R. (1978) The radiation dose to patients from EMI brain and body scanners. *Br. J. Rad.*, **52**, 189–96.
29. White, D. R. & Speller, R. D. (1980) The measurement of effective photon energy and 'linearity' in computerised tomography. *Br. J. Rad.*, **53**, 5–11.

3

Radionuclide imaging

D. A. Weber and R. E. O'Mara

INTRODUCTION

Radionuclide imaging is the general term used to describe those external counting procedures in nuclear medicine which detect and display the distribution of administered radioactive materials in the human body. The procedures are conducted in patients to obtain diagnostic information on the presence or absence of a disease process, the extent of disease and changes in tissue or organ function and metabolism. Depending on the medical problem presented, a particular radioactive tracer, termed a *radiopharmaceutical*, is selected for administration to the patient and an imaging procedure is subsequently performed.

Radionuclide imaging (also referred to as *radioisotope scanning*), includes many procedures useful in the study of both localised and systemic disease processes. Its use in assessing function and metabolism, in addition to morphological changes, makes it an important procedure in monitoring treatment. Acute changes in structure and function can be repeatedly assessed and different therapy modalities tested, using radiopharmaceuticals containing short-lived radionuclides. Depending upon the specific radiopharmaceutical administered and the imaging procedure performed, problems involving changes in metabolism, physiology or function can be investigated and regional pathology such as metastatic or primary bone tumour, pulmonary emboli, liver metastasis, renal function, brain tumour or thyroid pathology can be studied. The radionuclide imaging procedure is especially useful in determining the presence and extent of occult disease.

Procedures are available for the study of the skeleton, thyroid, lungs, heart, kidney and several other organs and tissues. The imaging procedure may require only the assay of the static distribution of a radiopharmaceutical that has been deposited or which is slowly passing through a tissue compartment or organ, or it may require special physiological gating or an imaging device to assess the uptake and clearance of a radiopharmaceutical through an organ or tissue. In the latter case, combined morphological and physiological or functional changes may be evaluated using physiological signals from the patient to control the acquisition time of the imaging equipment. An example of this is the use of the electrocardiogram to limit image acquisition time of myocardial images to selected portions of the cardiac cycle.

These imaging procedures are performed with a variety of different instruments, ranging from a basic detector system that employs one or two collimated NaI(Tl)* scintillation detectors, motor driven in a raster pattern over the patient to detect and provide two-dimensional images of the distribution of radioactivity within the body, to more advanced systems. The latter include, for example, systems which employ banks of collinearly opposed NaI(Tl) detectors, or opposed single crystal scintillation detectors that rotate about the patient, obtaining the necessary counting data to produce three-dimensional images of the distribution of radioactivity. Although each instrument is designed to detect individual decay events and to record the distribution of radioactivity, variations in system design and in performance capabilities are sufficient to restrict the performance of some procedures to certain specified instruments. The

*Thallium – activated sodium iodide crystal.

basic imaging system which is driven in a raster pattern over the patient, for example, cannot be used for dynamic imaging studies. The system is designed to assay the static distribution of radioactivity in the whole body or some part of the body by moving the detector over the patient. Distribution data can only be recorded when the detector moves and thus cannot allow the measurement of regional clearance of radioactivity where an entire organ or region of the body must be viewed continuously. Similarly, variations in the performance characteristics of these systems can preclude their use in certain other procedures. For example, variations in sensitivity, which is the number of events detected per unit of radioactivity present, or in spatial resolution, which is a measure of an instrument's ability to record accurately and to display the positions of detected X or gamma ray events from a source distribution of radioactivity, can dramatically change the image quality and influence the type of information which can be gained from the procedure.

The radionuclide imaging procedure is a powerful tool in capable hands. Optimum use of the procedure by itself, or in conjunction with other diagnostic imaging procedures, first requires that a careful assessment of the clinical problem should be made. This information, along with a comprehensive understanding of the available radiopharmaceuticals and instrumentation, provides the basic tools for the nuclear medicine specialist. A similar approach is used when planning a new laboratory or expanding an existing one; the anticipated procedure load and imaging requirements are first established and then instrumentation specifications are defined. In the material which follows, several different areas are presented which are important to the understanding of the basic principles and the use of radionuclide imaging.

RADIOPHARMACEUTICALS

Radionuclide imaging procedures depend upon localisation and clearance properties of administered radiopharmaceuticals to obtain diagnostic information. Administered to patients primarily by the intravenous route, and less frequently by the oral, intrathecal, intramuscular and other routes of entry, radiopharmaceuticals are characterised by several important qualities. Historically, major emphasis was placed on the decay scheme and the physical characteristics of a radionuclide proposed for use in imaging. Unlike those radioactive materials used for in vitro assay procedures, however, the biochemical, physiological and pharmacological properties of these agents must be considered as equally important to the chemical and physical characteristics of specific radionuclides and associated chemical compounds. These materials include only those radioactive tracers which use sufficiently low levels of radionuclide and associated carrier molecules to make them safe and acceptable for human use. The various properties now recognised as important in the development, design and selection of radiopharmaceuticals are listed in Table 3.1.

Table 3.1 Important radiopharmaceutical properties

Radionuclide	**Biological behaviour**
Decay scheme	Localisation
Photon and particle emissions	Kinetics
Energy	
Abundance	**Pharmacology**
Half-life	Sterility
Production methods	Pyrogenicity
Specific activity	pH
Radionuclidic purity	Chemical toxicity
Cost and availability	Pharmacologic response
	Isotonicity
Chemistry	
Formulation and labelling methods	**Radiation dose**
Radiochemical purity	
Chemical stability	

The important properties of radiopharmaceuticals can be described in five major subject areas. These include characterisation of the radionuclide, chemistry of the carrier molecules and the radiopharmaceutical, biological localisation and kinetics, pharmacological properties, and absorbed radiation dose. Each of these different factors must be considered when new radionuclides or carrier molecules are investigated.

A good understanding of radionuclide decay schemes frequently prevents wasted time and effort when selecting new radioactive materials for developing a radiopharmaceutical. As a rule of thumb, a radionuclide emitting X or gamma rays within the energy range of 25–511 keV is considered useful for imaging purposes. Within this range, further constraints may be placed as a result of the type of instrumentation available for imaging. The design and operating characteristics of the single crystal scintillation camera result in the camera being most effective for imaging photons having energy of 75–300 keV, whereas the rectilinear scanner can be most effectively used for imaging photons above and below this energy range. By definition, positron emission tomography instrumentation must be able to detect the 511 keV photons released during positron annihilation.[18]

The different types of radioactive decay processes which may yield X or gamma ray photons within this energy range are listed in Table 3.2.

Table 3.2 Radioactive decay processes

Primary decay process	Symbol	Secondary emissions
Alpha emission	α	γ, IC e$^-$, X-ray, Auger e$^-$
Beta emission	β$^-$	γ, antineutrino, IC e$^-$, X-ray, Auger e$^-$
Positron emission	β$^+$	γ, neutrino, IC e$^-$, X-ray, Auger e$^-$
Electron capture	EC	γ, neutrino, internal bremsstrahlung, IC e$^-$, X-ray, Auger e$^-$
Isomeric transition	IT	γ, IC e$^-$,
Internal conversion	IC	X-ray, Auger e$^-$

Although suitable energy gamma photons can accompany alpha particle decay, the radiation dose resulting from the total absorption of the high linear energy transfer (LET) particles by the body makes their use unsuitable for diagnostic studies.[51] Despite almost total absorption of beta emissions by the body, the lower LET beta particles present less hazard to the patient. As a result, selected radionuclides which decay by beta emission can be used for radiopharmaceutical preparations when a high gamma ray yield accompanies the beta decay and the radionuclide has useful biological clearance properties. Two examples of radionuclides demonstrating these characteristics are iodine-131 (^{131}I) and xenon-133 (^{133}Xe). ^{131}I decays by beta-minus decay with a 8·06 day half-life and a 364 keV gamma photon that is released in 82 per cent of the disintegrations.[27] ^{133}Xe decays by beta-minus decay with a 5·31 day half-life and an 81 keV gamma photon that is released in 36 per cent of the disintegrations.[27] ^{131}I as sodium iodide has been an important radionuclide used in the study of thyroid disease and ^{133}Xe as a gas or in saline is frequently used to study blood flow and regional pulmonary function. Several radionuclides which decay by the release of positively charged electrons, termed positrons, are used for tomographic imaging studies. Examples of these include the 20·3, 10·0 and 2·1 min half-life carbon-11 (^{11}C), nitrogen-13 (^{13}N), and oxygen-15 (^{15}O) radionuclides used for pulmonary imaging studies, and the 109 min half-life radionuclide of fluorine-18 (^{18}F) used for bone and brain imaging.[27]

As a general rule, it is preferable to use radionuclides which deposit only small amounts of energy in the patient, while providing high photon yields within the energy range suitable for imaging, i.e. radionuclides with a high photon yield to radiation dose ratio. Radionuclides which can best approach these requirements are those which decay by isomeric transition or electron capture; an example of each of these radionuclides follow. The radionuclide most frequently used for diagnostic imaging studies, technetium-99m (^{99m}Tc), decays by isomeric transition. Administered for imaging purposes in several different chemical forms, ^{99m}Tc serves as the radioactive component in the majority of radiopharmaceuticals administered for diagnostic imaging procedures. Technetium-99m has a 6·03 h half-life and emits a 140·5 keV gamma photon in 88 per cent of its disintegrations.[27] Gallium-67 (^{67}Ga) citrate is used for the localisation of inflammatory processes and tumours.[45] Gallium-67 decays by electron capture and releases three different gamma photons: 93 keV in 38 per cent of its disintegrations, 185 keV in 24 per cent and 300 keV in 16 per cent.[27]

In addition to having an efficient supply of photons of acceptable energy, the half-life of the radionuclide must be sufficient to allow localisation and imaging of the radiopharmaceutical in the tissues of interest, without contributing unnecessary radiation dose to the patient.[48, 110] Radionuclide purity must be sufficiently high to maintain radiation dose to the patient at an acceptable level and to prevent degradation of image quality. Specific activity, the ratio of the amount of activity per unit mass of radioactive and nonradioactive atoms of the same element in the preparation, must be known in order to evaluate possible chemical effects on the radiopharmaceutical or its biological uptake and clearance. The remaining radionuclide properties which require examination include problems of general availability, ease of production and cost.

The chemistry involved in the formulation and labelling of suitable chemical carriers is a second major category of radiopharmaceutical properties. Even if it has a useful decay scheme, a radionuclide has little value if it cannot be placed in the appropriate chemical form to achieve tissue or organ specificity. Similarly, the chemical methods must be both time- and cost-efficient. The final radiopharmaceutical must demonstrate an acceptably high chemical purity and shelf life stability.

The pharmacological properties of radiopharmaceuticals must fulfill many of the requirements placed on unlabelled pharmaceuticals used in the diagnosis or treatment.[58] Administered intravenously and by other routes of entry, these materials must be sterile, pyrogen-free and at suitable pH. Only small amounts of chemical carrier and radionuclide can be present, and the radiopharmaceutical should not present any problems in chemical toxicity or pharmacological reaction or response.

The assay of biological behaviour in terms of target to nontarget localisation and the rates of deposition and clearance from target and nontarget tissues indicates how effective a radiopharmaceutical is for the evaluation of various medical problems. A variety of biological and biochemical mechanisms affect the localisation and clearance characteristics of the different radiopharmaceuticals. Variations in distribution and clearance occur according to particle size, biological compartment size, rates of excretion and detoxification, abnormal permeabilities, sulhydryl binding and metabolic involvement of small ions and molecules. Mechanisms of localisation include active cellular transport, phagocytosis, cellular sequestration, capillary blockade, simple diffusion, physicochemical adsorption and compartmental localisation.[67] A thorough understanding of the different properties of radiopharmaceuticals and the mechanisms of localisation and clearance must be possessed by the nuclear medicine specialist to make optimum use of these different materials.

If a radiopharmaceutical appears adequate in terms of all these properties, the major consideration remaining is the radiation dose to the patient resulting from the use of the preparation. Radiation dose estimated from the localisation and clearance characteristics of a radiopharmaceutical must be as low as possible, using only that amount of radioactivity necessary to obtain adequate information for diagnosis. Table 3.3 shows examples of the radiation dose received from a few radiopharmaceuticals used in conventional imaging studies. The radiopharmaceuticals included in this Table are only a small percentage of the total number of those currently available for use in radionuclide imaging. In recent years, there has been a trend towards the greater use of short-lived radionuclides for imaging procedures. These materials allow more frequent repetitive trials to evaluate short-term function or disease processes and allow for greater administered activity doses, frequently yielding improved image quality at a lower or the same radiation dose as that received from a longer lived material. As more attention is given to these materials, it is expected that gradually more shorter-lived radionuclides will be introduced and used for diagnostic imaging purposes. Consistent with the continuing advances in cyclotron and radionuclide generator technology, very short-life radionuclides such as ^{11}C ($t\frac{1}{2}=20\cdot3$ min), ^{13}N ($t\frac{1}{2}=10\cdot0$ min), ^{15}O ($t\frac{1}{2}=124$ s), ^{81m}Kr ($t\frac{1}{2}=13\cdot0$ s) and others are expected to play a much larger role in nuclear medicine imaging in the future.[38, 61, 99]

INSTRUMENTATION

Two basic types of imaging systems account for the majority of external counting procedures in nuclear medicine. These two systems are the rectilinear scanner and the single or multiple crystal scintillation camera. Historically, the prototype of the current day rectilinear scanner was introduced in the literature in 1951 by Cassen;[22] the first single crystal scintillation camera was described by Anger in 1958;[4] and the first multicrystal scintillation camera was described in 1960 by Bender and Blau.[11] Since their introduction, each of these

Table 3.3 Radiopharmaceuticals used for selected imaging procedures

Procedure (Activity dose)	Radiopharmaceutical	Dose ($\times 10^{-2}$ Gy)	Target organ	Reference
Liver/Spleen (185 MBq)	^{99m}Tc sulphur colloid	0.8–1.7 1.1–2.1 0.1–0.4	Liver Spleen Red marrow	72
Thyroid (3.7 MBq)	^{123}I sodium iodide	1.3 (25% uptake)	Thyroid	73
Tumour/Inflammation localisation (111 MBq)	^{67}Ga citrate	1.7 1.4 1.2 2.7	Marrow Liver Kidneys Lower large intestine	71
Brain (555 MBq)	^{99m}Tc sodium pertechnetate	0.8–3.8 2.0	Stomach wall Thyroid	74
Lung Ventilation (370 MBq)	^{133}Xe gas	0.065–0.11 0.009–0.014	Lung Total body	7
Perfusion or Perfusion-Ventilation (370 MBq)	^{133}Xe in saline	0.07–0.16 0.009–0.021	Lung Total body	7
Bone (555 MBq)	^{99m}Tc pyrophosphate ^{99m}Tc methylenediphosphonate ^{99m}Tc (1-hydroxyethylidene) diphosphonate	0.48–1.02 0.12–0.24	Skeleton Total body	111 112

instruments has undergone a series of dramatic changes in design and performance. Initially, those imaging systems which required movement of the detector in order to obtain an image (also termed a scan), were referred to as *scanners*, while those systems which acquired images with position information provided electronically without detector motion were referred to as *scintillation cameras*. The introduction of camera or imaging platform motion to achieve larger field of view images, better resolution, or changes in other performance characteristics, eliminated this distinction. In the sections which follow, the general performance characteristics of these and other types of radionuclide imaging systems and the basic mode of operation of representative instruments are presented.

General performance characteristics

The different instruments used for radionuclide imaging show a wide range of performance and operating characteristics. These performance characteristics depend on the type and dimensions of the detector, the associated signal processing and electronics, collimation, shielding, and the type of image display system. Major design and operational differences separate and distinguish the different systems. Since these differences can affect the type of procedure which can be conducted with an instrument, careful attention must be given to the performance and operational characteristics of a system.

The performance specification most frequently cited is *spatial resolution*. Spatial resolution is a term used to describe the instrument's ability accurately to reproduce an observed activity distribution in its output display.[94] Spatial resolution is affected by the type of collimator and the amount of scattered radiation in the activity distribution observed by the detector. In the single crystal gamma camera, it is further affected by the electronic positioning circuitry which is used to reproduce the relative position of detected events in the image. The specification for spatial resolution is generally expressed as the full-width-at-half-maximum count rate (FWHM) of the counting profile obtained for a small diameter line source or a point source of radioactivity placed beneath the detector. The spatial resolution of focused collimators used in rectilinear scanners is usually specified for the focal plane of the collimator. Since scintillation camera systems provide positional information in a different manner, two different types of spatial resolution are specified; these are *intrinsic* and *system* spatial resolution. Intrinsic spatial resolution is the resolution measured without a detector collimator, whereas system resolution refers to measurements made with a particular collimator. All values are normally expressed for the line or point source placed directly beneath the detector, or at a specified distance from it. Spatial resolution may be expressed as the *modulation transfer function* (MTF); however, this term has been used less frequently to describe these systems in recent years. The MTF measures the ability of the imaging system to transfer the source activity modulation to an image modulation.[94]

Depending on the type of instrument, other important factors which relate directly or indirectly to system performance include: (1) sensitivity; (2) deadtime; (3) field uniformity and size; (4) detector energy resolution; (5) spatial distortion and linearity; (6) detector shielding; and (7) design engineering. A few brief comments about these factors and how each relates to the different systems are given next.

Sensitivity is a measure of the counting efficiency of an instrument. It is normally expressed in counts per second per unit of activity for a known volume of radioactivity at a specified position in the detector field. The size and type of detector, the type of collimator and the width of the pulse height energy window are major factors which affect sensitivity. It is difficult directly to compare efficiencies of all systems; it can be stated as a rule of thumb, however, that single crystal scintillation camera systems are more efficient than rectilinear scanner systems over the energy range of approximately 75–300 keV. The rectilinear scanner generally shows increased sensitivity and other advantages outside this energy range due to the scintillation crystal thickness and the method for obtaining position information of detected events.

Different systems exhibit variations in the processing and display or recording time of detected events. These variations can translate into significant count rate losses in procedures where high counting levels are observed. The amount of time between events during which a new event cannot be registered is termed *deadtime*. The count rate dependence of different systems may be paralysable, nonparalysable or a combination of both. With a paralysable system, a fixed amount of time between successive photopeak events is required before a new event can be counted; the recovery time of an instrument is reset to the deadtime increment if an event occurs during the recovery stage. These systems paralyse or the count rate decreases with increasing radioactivity, approaching a zero count rate response to count rates above the resolution capacity of the system. With a nonparalysable system, events occurring during the processing time of an event do not effect deadtime. As activity continues to increase above the resolution of a nonparalysable system, the count rate levels off, but the system does not exhibit paralysis. Typical deadtimes observed for current generation scintillation cameras range from 1·5–8 µs.

Field uniformity is a term which applies principally to scintillation camera systems. It refers to the variations in count rate response across the field of view of the detector to a uniform field irradiation. System uniformity refers to the response with a collimator in position, whereas intrinsic uniformity refers to the response without a collimator. Field uniformity is typically expressed as a percent deviation from the mean count rate seen by the crystal. Typical camera uniformity specifications on the current systems are $\leq \pm 5$ per cent.

Field size, another specification pertinent only to camera systems, refers to the maximum dimensions which can be imaged without moving the camera or the imaging platform. Field sizes on single crystal scintillation cameras, for example, vary from 24–53 cm.

The *energy resolution* of the NaI(Tl) scintillation detectors used in the different imaging systems provides an assay of the statistical fluctuations introduced in the various stages of the X or gamma ray detection process that contribute to a characteristic broadening of the photopeak portion of the energy spectrum. The breadth of characteristic photopeaks of selected radionuclides, for example, ^{99m}Tc and ^{57}Co with scintillation cameras, and ^{137}Cs with a rectilinear scanner, are used to assay energy resolution. The width of the characteristic photopeak measured in energy units (keV) at one half maximum count rate observed in the peak, or the full width at half maximum is normally expressed as a percentage of the characteristic X or gamma ray energy. Expressed in such a manner, the larger the FWHM, the poorer the energy resolution.

Typical resolution characteristics of rectilinear scanners for ^{137}Cs range from 7–9·5 per cent; on camera systems, the energy resolution for ^{99m}Tc is typically of the order of 12–16 per cent. An important part of the detection process, the energy resolution of a system can affect spatial resolution, sensitivity and field uniformity.

Spatial distortion and linearity are also important system performance factors. They refer to the accuracy of the instrument's electronics to translate and correctly to position events from a radioactivity distribution beneath the camera to a final image. Various types of phantoms including both radioactive emission and lead bar-type transmission sources are used to test this specification.[94]

Two remaining factors are *detector shielding* and *design engineering*. The adequacy of detector shielding or the thickness of the shell surrounding the detector in each imaging system, determines the energy range of X and gamma ray photons which can be imaged with the instrument. An undershielded detector allows X and gamma photons from outside the field of interest to contribute to the background noise in an image. This results in deterioration of spatial resolution and uniformity, degrading overall image quality. Similarly, design engineering can affect the manoeuvrability and ease of operation, directly influencing the type, number and quality of images which can be obtained with a specific instrument.

The consideration of each of these factors is necessary when selecting or evaluating radionuclide imaging systems. The optimum use of the different instruments depends on a thorough understanding of these different properties.

Radionuclide imaging systems

Rectilinear scanner

The first rectilinear scanner used a small collimated calcium inorganic tungstate crystal to detect X and gamma photons.[22] The crystal was moved in a raster pattern over the patient by means of a motorised drive and an image was recorded by activating a pen which in turn made marks on a sheet of paper. Reported in the literature in 1951, this represented a major advance. Contemporary work primarily depended upon manually placing a Geiger-Müller detector at selected positions over a patient for counting and recording count levels by hand. This initial instrument was quite different from the modern rectilinear scanner. Innovative work in the field of NaI(Tl) scintillation crystal detectors,[79] focused collimators,[33] pulse height analysers,[2,33] photoscan image displays,[59] and computer assisted data acquisition, processing and display[113,115] has greatly influenced and changed the design of this instrument.

Present rectilinear scanners use one or two collimated NaI(Tl) scintillation detectors which are moved over and/or under the patient to obtain images of the distribution of administered radiopharmaceutical. The block diagram in Figure 3.1 shows the layout for a single probe scanner and Figure 3.2 shows a photograph of a dual probe scanner.

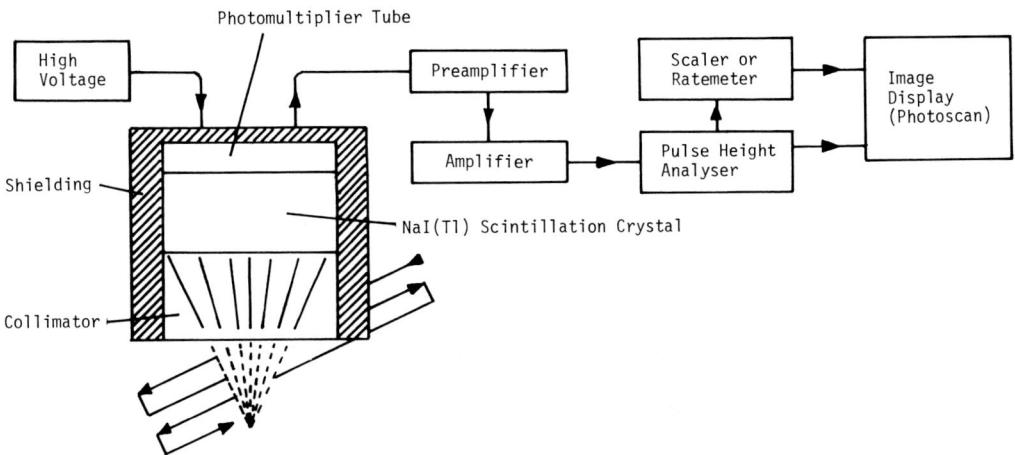

Fig. 3.1 Block diagram of a single probe rectilinear scanner.

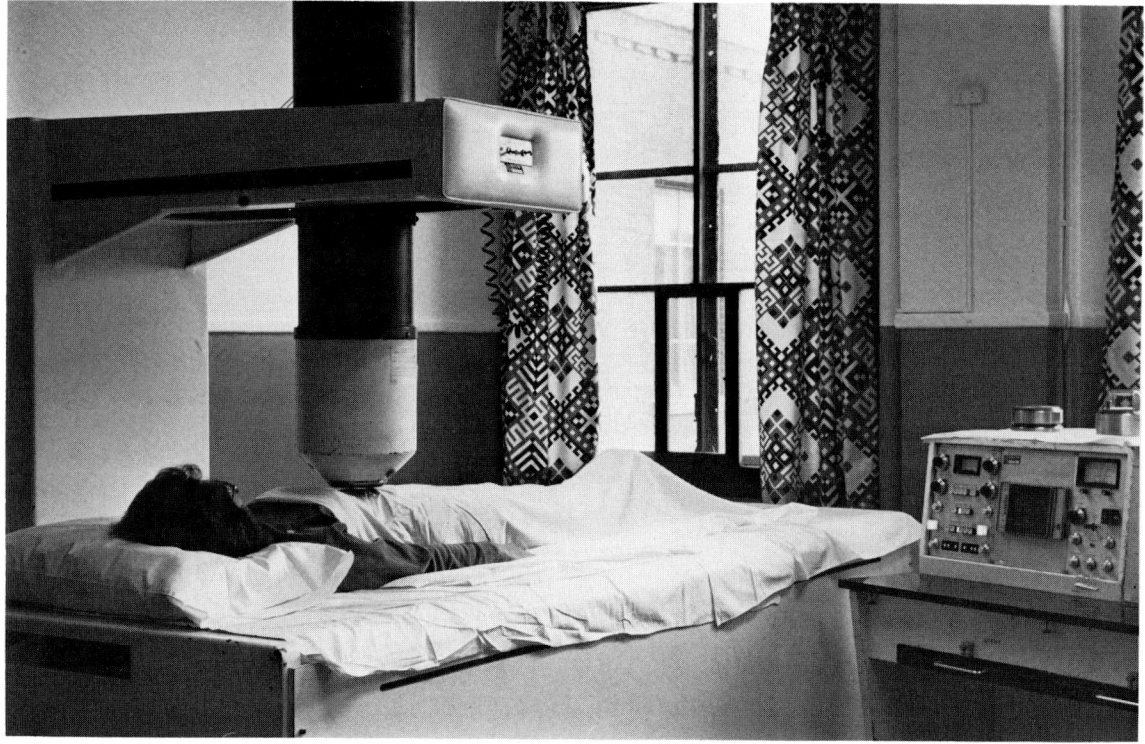

Fig. 3.2 A dual probe rectilinear scanner and associated electronics and display console. Two shielded scintillation detectors, 127 mm in diameter by 64 mm thick are collinearly opposed, one above and one below the imaging platform. A focused collimator defines the field of each detector.

The major difference between the two types of systems is that the dual probe scanner can supply two simultaneous views, e.g. anterior and posterior, whereas the single probe unit can provide only one view at a time. With the dual probe system, there are two detectors, one above and one below the patient imaging platform; imaging or scan times for many conventional procedures are reduced to one-half.

The NaI(Tl) scintillation detectors conventionally used in scanners are 127 mm in diameter by 51–76 mm thick. The sides and back of the detector are shielded with lead and a multihole focused collimator is placed immediately adjacent to the face of the scintillation crystal. The collimator defines the field of view, a small resolution element beneath the detector, and the detector is moved in a raster pattern in order to scan or image a radioactivity distribution. The collimator typically is a lead cylinder with concentric rings of tapered holes that converge at a distance of 4–15 cm beyond the collimator. The number of holes in a collimator and their length and diameter are chosen to obtain necessary spatial resolution and sensitivity characteristics for different energy gamma photons over the range of 25–510 keV and more. As a result of the variations in radionuclide distribution with depth in the body, collimators with different focal lengths are used for different procedures. The spatial resolutions of these detector systems typically show a FWHM of 5–15 mm; improved spatial resolution can be gained at the expense of decreased sensitivity or a decrease in the depth of field over which resolution remains relatively constant. The variations in spatial resolution, sensitivity, focal length and depth of field for focused collimators used with different instruments can be found in the literature.[28, 44] The light released from a X or gamma photon absorption in the scintillation crystal (detected events) is converted to an electronic signal by the photomultiplier tube (PMT). The electronic processing of these signals by the preamplifier, amplifier and pulse height analyser provides the means by which unscattered photons absorbed by the detector are counted and contribute to the final image of the radioactivity distribution. Scanner images are produced by exposing radiographic film to a collimated light source which is flashed at a frequency proportional to the count rate observed by the detector. A two-dimensional image of the activity distribution is produced by moving the photoscan light source in synchrony with the scanner detectors, i.e. moving continuously in one axis, and step wise in the perpendicular direction over the structure to be visualised.

The rectilinear scanner served as the major instrument for radionuclide imaging until approximately 1970; since then, it has been gradually replaced in most centres by the scintillation camera. In comparison with the camera, the rectilinear scanner is: (1) unable to provide dynamic images; (2) less efficient for imaging X and γ photons in the energy range of 75–300 keV, frequently having a less desirable collimator response which shows deterioration in spatial resolution both above and below the focal plane; and (3) less manoeuvrable for special views, generally requiring a more time-consuming set-up. As a result, the rectilinear scanner has generally assumed a backup role in many laboratories, or it is used primarily for imaging radiopharmaceuticals whose high energy or very low energy gamma photons are not measured efficiently by camera systems.

Single crystal gamma camera

The single crystal gamma camera was first described in the literature by Anger in 1958.[4] Designed as a stationary imaging device which could be used to image large areas in the body or whole organs without requiring detector motion, the introduction of this method was a major milestone in the field of nuclear medicine. Providing the means by which dynamic images of radiopharmaceutical deposition and clearance can be investigated and, also, a more efficient instrument than the rectilinear scanner for imaging gamma photons in the energy range of 75–300 keV, this device now plays a dominant role in radionuclide imaging.

The initial camera designed by Anger could image only small regions of the body. The sensitive detector was a 102 mm diameter by 6·4 mm thick NaI(Tl) crystal; seven 38 mm photomultiplier tubes (PMTs) in a hexagonal array were used to detect the position of light emitted from X and gamma absorption events. By the time the first commercial version of the single crystal Anger camera became available, the design had been revised to use a 279 mm diameter by 13 mm thick scintillation crystal backed with a hexagonal array of nineteen 76 mm PMTs.

The basic operation of the Anger camera shows many similarities to the rectilinear scanner, despite a totally different approach to obtaining position information. Like the rectilinear scanner, a scintillation crystal is used to detect X and gamma photons. The energies of the different photons absorbed by the camera are sorted using a pulse height analyser and only those pulses within an acceptable energy range contribute count and position information to an image. The major difference between gamma cameras and rectilinear scanners is the approach used to obtain positional information. Whereas the rectilinear scanner looks at a single small volume element beneath a collimated detector, requiring detector motion to see different regions, the gamma camera looks at a relatively large region continuously and provides two-dimensional distribution information without requiring any detector movement.

With the aid of the block diagram in Figure 3.3, the operation of this system is explained. Gamma photons pass through holes in the collimator and are absorbed by the scintillation crystal, resulting in the release of light. The detection of the amount of light released and the position of this light is the initial stage of the electronic processing procedure which identifies the energy and position of absorbed photons in the crystal. Some cameras use an optically coupled light pipe between the crystal and the PMTs to improve the efficiency of light collection and the distribution of light to individual PMTs; this has not been found necessary, however, in all systems. The photocathode of the PMT directly above the position where the gamma photon was absorbed in the crystal receives the largest amount of light and lesser amounts of light reach the surrounding PMTs. The electronic processing of the signals from the PMT array provides both the energy and position information needed to form an image of a radioactivity distribution.[90]

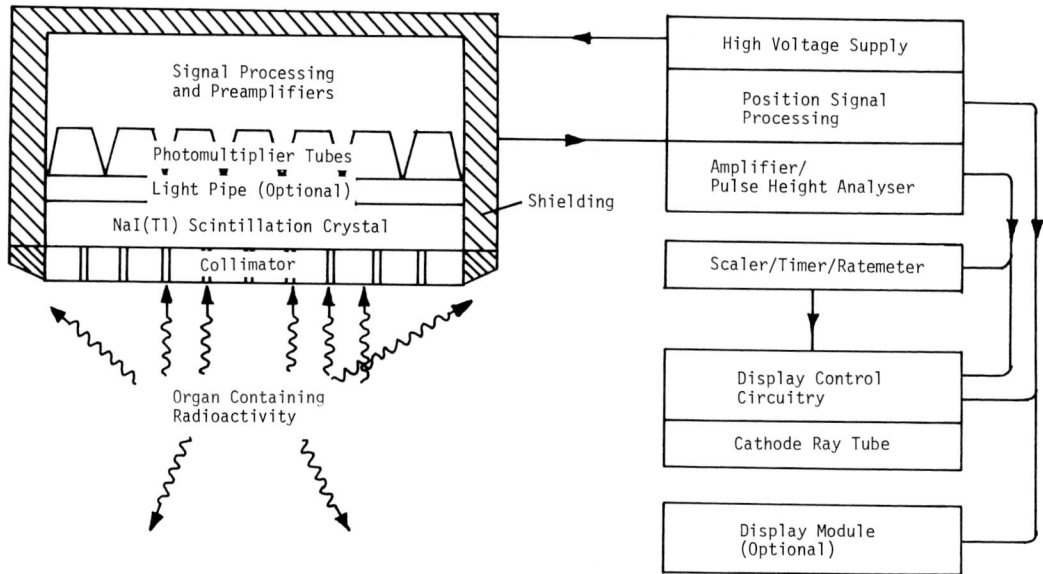

Fig. 3.3 Block diagram of a single crystal scintillation camera (Anger camera).

Typically, the processed signals control the position and on-time of a cathode ray tube (CRT) electron beam. A photographic exposure of the CRT display screen with positive or negative film provides the image of the radioactivity distribution. Alternatively, the electronic signals from the camera can be processed using a computer to provide quantitative image acquisition processing and display.[113, 115]

Several advances in gamma camera technology have been made since 1960.[44, 90] As a result of these developments, current systems offer larger image fields, shorter deadtimes, improved spatial resolution, whole body imaging capabilities, portability, improved collimators, multiple photopeak counting options and improvements in display module technology. Initially, commercially available gamma cameras used NaI(Tl) crystals, 25–30 cm diameter, providing useful crystal diameter or field of view of approximately 23–27 cm in diameter. Large field of view (LFOV) gamma cameras became available in the mid-1970s. These systems provided useful fields of view ranging from 37–42 cm. More recently, even larger systems have entered the market; one manufacturer now distributes a camera with a 53 cm diameter useful field of view. Changes in photocathode materials used in the photomultiplier tubes, thinner scintillation crystals in portable cameras, improvements in signal processing, circuitry and light optics have improved the intrinsic spatial resolution and deadtime of these systems. Current standard field of view (SFOV) cameras provide intrinsic resolutions of the order of 3–6 mm for ^{99m}Tc at the face of the scintillation crystal. Whereas the initial stationary single crystal cameras could only image limited regions in the body, innovations in design have extended the use of cameras to whole body imaging. Another development has been the introduction of the portable or mobile gamma camera, used for providing emergency imaging services to patients unable to come to the nuclear medicine laboratory. SFOV and LFOV gamma cameras have been assembled in several different mobile configurations. The systems are driven or pushed from the nuclear medicine laboratory to the patient's room.

Figures 3.4 through 3.6 show the basic types of single crystal gamma camera systems currently in use. Figure 3.4 shows a mobile gamma camera system. In this system, a SFOV gamma camera, a multiformatter image display module and a computer are all contained in a compact, DC motor driven unit. Figure 3.5 shows a photograph of a LFOV gamma camera. The multiformatter shown is used to record images on X-ray film. The motor driven platform or table positioned beneath the detector is an accessory which can be used to obtain total body images. In this particular model, the gamma camera is stationary and the imaging platform moves to obtain a total body scan. Other commercially available units use stationary platforms and move the camera; these instruments require less floor space.

SFOV camera, account for the majority of radionuclide imaging procedures now conducted in the field of nuclear medicine.

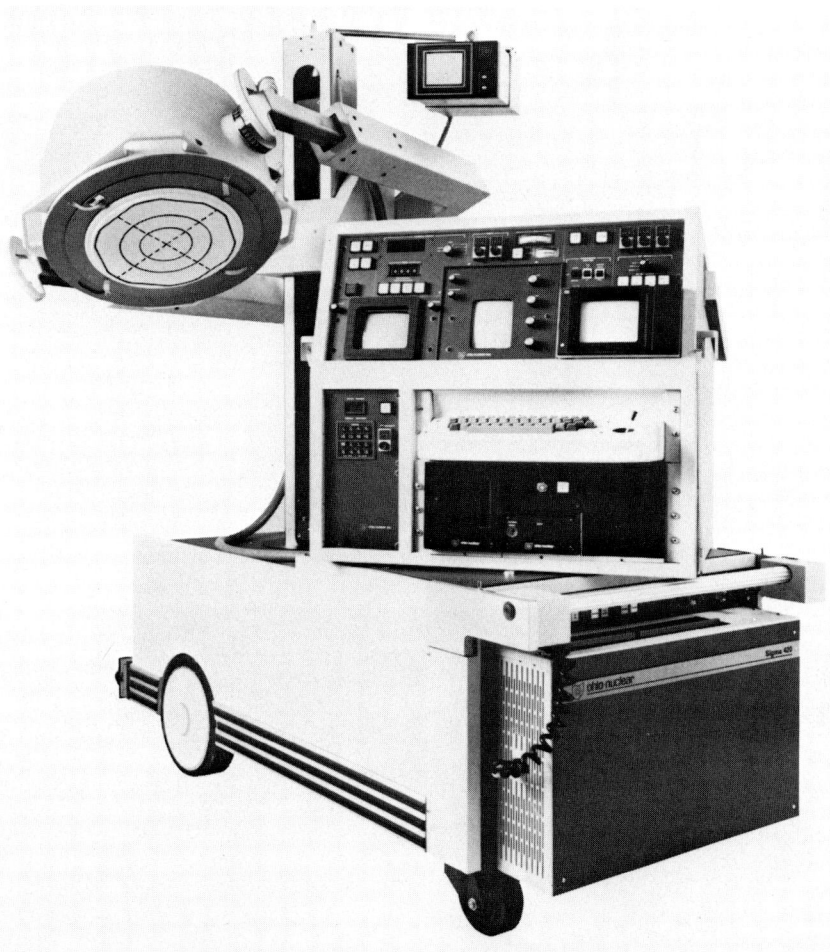

Fig. 3.4 Portable standard field of view (SFOV) scintillation camera and associated processing and display modules. (Spectrum One, Technicare Corporation.)

One of the major advantages of the larger useable image fields is to reduce both the number of images and the time required to conduct most procedures. The camera which currently provides the largest field of view is shown in Figure 3.6. This unit uses 60 cm diameter by 12·7 mm thick NaI(Tl) crystal, providing a 53 cm diameter useful field of view. The different types of camera systems shown in Figures 3.4–3.6, in addition to the conventional

Multicrystal scintillation camera

The multicrystal scintillation camera introduced by Bender and Blau was initially called an *autoflouroscope*.[11] Unlike the Anger camera in detector design, the prototype system consisted of a rectangular array of 20 small collimated NaI(Tl) scintillation crystals coupled to photomultiplier tubes. Like the gamma camera, this instrument

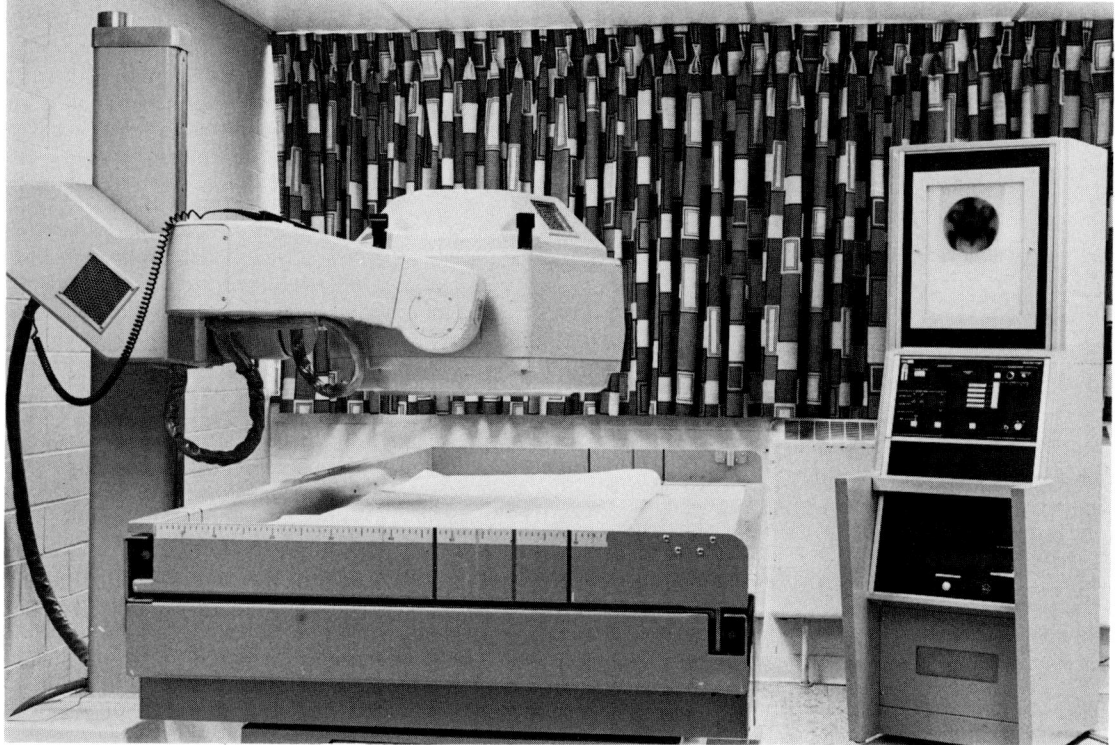

Fig. 3.5 Photograph of a large field of view (LFOV) scintillation camera and total body imaging platform. A multiformatter image display module is seen to the right of the imaging platform.

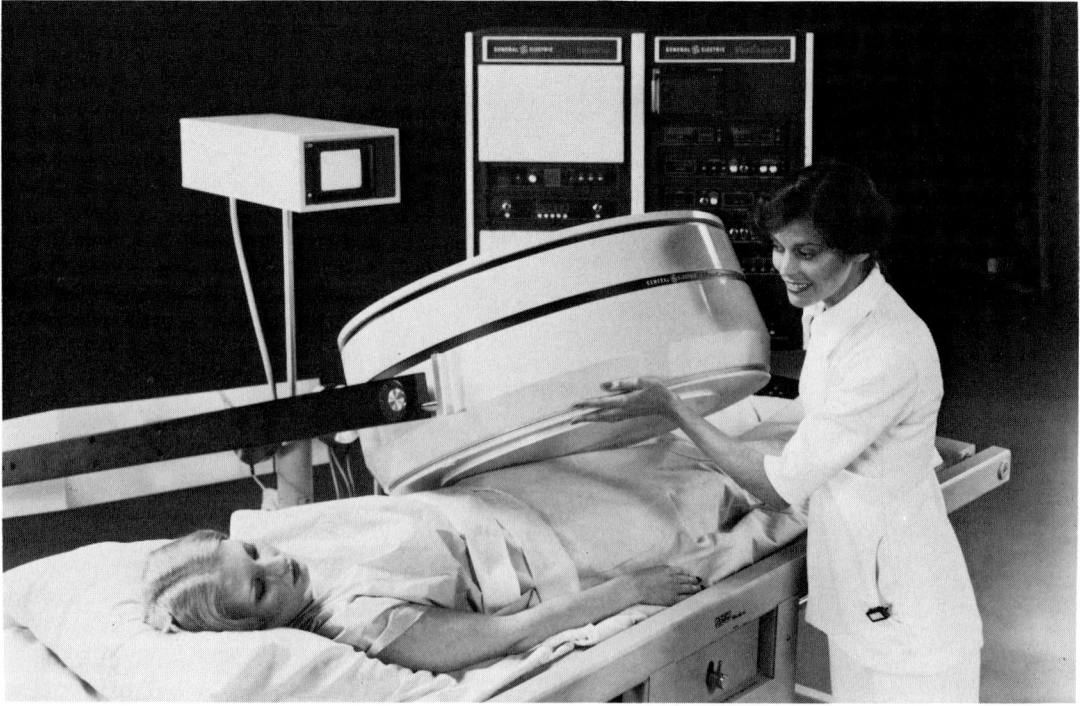

Fig. 3.6 Large field of view camera which provides a 53 cm field of view. (Maxi-Camera 535, General Electric Company.)

was designed to assay the regional distribution of administered radiopharmaceuticals without requiring movement of the detector.

The basic operation of the multicrystal scintillation camera is described using the block diagram shown in Figure 3.7. The present system uses 294 NaI(Tl) crystals assembled in 14 by 21 array, each crystal being 8 mm square by 3·8 cm long. With a 11 mm centre-to-centre spacing, the crystal array provides a useful field of view of approximately 15 by 23 cm. Using somewhat unconventional light optics compared to the camera systems previously described, each crystal employs a split light guide or light pipe which is connected to one row (row 1, 2 . . . 14) and one column PMT (column 1, 2, 3 . . . 21). The PMT signals are processed by 35 linear amplifiers. The output signals from each of these amplifiers passes through a lower level discriminator (LLD); following appropriate signal processing and pulse height analysis, photon absorption events within a preselected energy range are stored in a quantitative format in a memory location corresponding to the crystal in which the absorption event took place. The position of a gamma photon absorption event in a specific crystal is defined uniquely by its detection by one row and one column PMT. Each event stored in memory satisfies three conditions. These conditions include: (1) simultaneous detection on an event by a row and column PMT; (2) the energy dissipated in a single scintillation crystal must fall within the energy range selected on a single channel analyser; and (3) only a single pair of row and column detectors can simultaneously detect a valid absorption

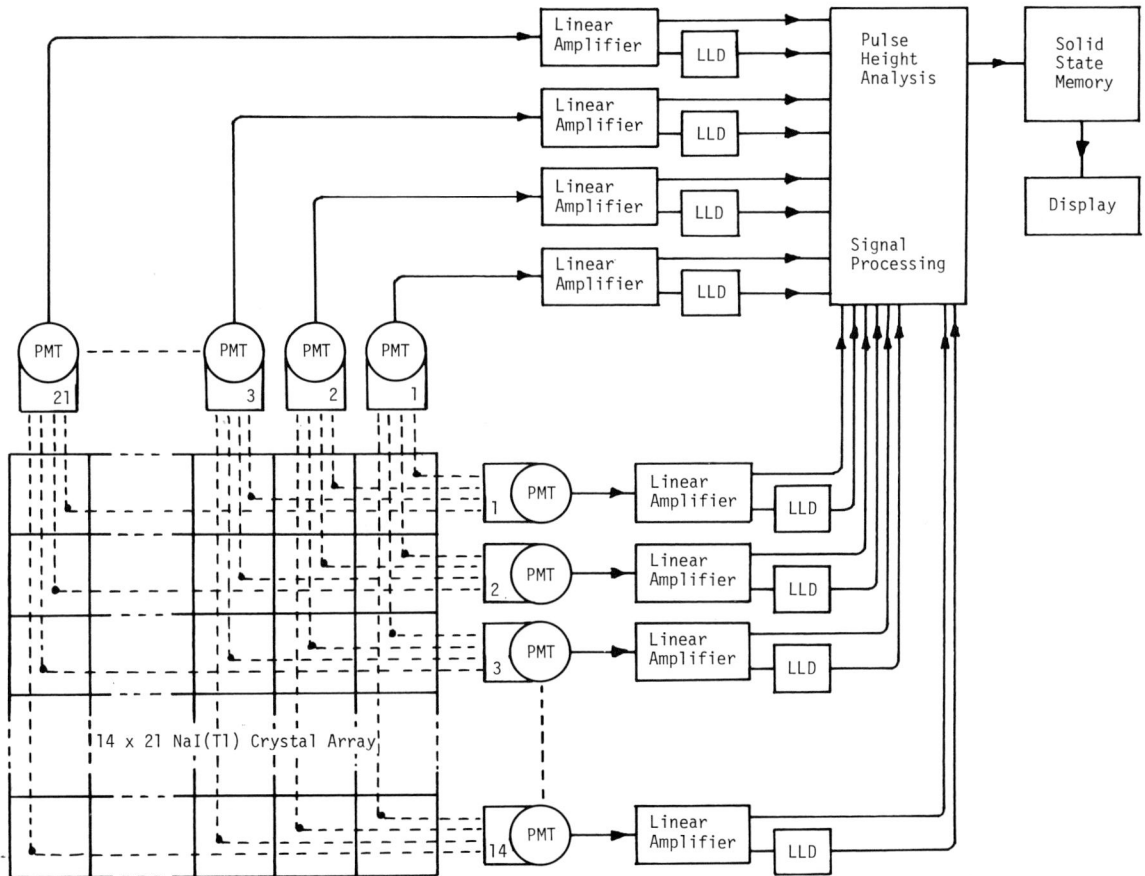

Fig. 3.7 Block diagram of the multicrystal scintillation camera. (PMT: photomultiplier tube; LLD: lower level discriminator.)

event, i.e. anticoincidence logic inhibits the recording of events which occur simultaneously in more than one crystal.

The multicrystal camera can operate at higher count rate levels than single crystal camera systems as a result of the independent determinations of the position and energy of detected events. Spatial resolution depends primarily upon the collimator and detector configuration. In comparison with the single crystal camera systems, the thicker crystals used in this system provide increased sensitivity at higher gamma ray energies. Disadvantages of the system include: (1) intrinsic resolution is limited by the cross sectional size of the crystals and image field size is small unless the camera head or the patient is moved; (2) energy resolution of the detector assembly is poor as a result of light loss in the light pipes between the crystals and the PMTs; and (3) sensitivity at high gamma ray energies is less than might be expected, as a result of a decreasing fraction of photoelectric absorption events at higher photon energies. Although the use of these systems for general imaging has been limited as compared to Anger cameras, interest in the system continues as a result of its high count rate capabilities. Here the short deadtime characteristics have made the instrument particularly useful in high counting rate dynamic procedures. Most recent interest has centred around its use for the first pass determination of cardiac ejection fractions.[12]

Other imaging systems

Although the majority of nuclear medicine procedures are conducted using the different imaging systems already presented, several other instruments and approaches to imaging the distribution of radioactivity from administered radiopharmaceuticals have received increasing attention in the last few years. These are expected to play a larger role in nuclear medicine in the future. They include: (1) single photon and annihilation photon computed tomographic imaging systems; (2) a seven-pinhole, a rotatable parallel slant-hole, and other collimators designed to be used with conventional SFOV or LFOV cameras for tomographic imaging of selected regions in the body; (3) a scanner which employs two gamma camera type detectors which can be used for tomographic imaging of individual organs or the entire body; (4) a high spatial resolution germanium detector gamma camera; (5) a cadmium telluride matrix gamma camera; and (6) a high efficiency multicrystal scanner. Although space does not allow a broad discussion of these systems here, a few remarks about the basic operation of each and references to pertinent literature are given. Each of these systems was designed and developed from interests in improving certain aspects of acquiring, processing and display of radionuclide images. These systems are particularly important since trends in imaging instrumentation design will be strongly affected by the successes and failures observed with them.

The first three types of instrumentation just mentioned refer to tomographic imaging systems. These systems are designed to image and display the distribution of radionuclides at various depths within a subject. This type of imaging is termed *emission computed tomography* (ECT). Displaying several similarities to X-ray transmission computed tomography (see Ch. 2), ECT provides a qualitative or quantitative mapping of the distribution of radioactivity at a specified depth within a particular region of the body, analogous to the mapping of attenuation coefficients using transmission CT. As such, these instruments provide information in three-dimensions as opposed to the two-dimensional information gained from conventional cameras and scanners.

Two major types of ECT systems have dominated development in this area thus far. These are *single photon tomography* (SPT) and *annihilation photon tomography* (APT, also called *positron tomography*).[18, 20, 87] SPT involves the imaging of conventional radiopharmaceuticals where a single photon is released in a single disintegration, whereas APT involves the detection of coincident annihilation photons emitted in positron annihilation following radioactive decay by positron emission. Cameras with specially designed collimators, scanners with camera type detectors, rotating single or dual opposed gamma cameras, multicrystal detector arrays and opposed proportional chambers have been used for ECT. Regardless of the type of detector, the subject is viewed from several different angles in SPT to obtain projections or count rate profiles of the radioactivity distribution. The image data from the multiple views are processed with a computer to produce final tomographic images (tomograms) by a method called tomographic reconstruction. Collinearily opposed detectors are used to detect the 511 keV photons released from positron annihilation events in APT; image data collected in this manner are processed by a computer to reconstruct tomograms.

It is anticipated that the additional information obtained with these systems will greatly increase and improve the diagnostic utility of certain imaging procedures. These instruments are further expected to play a more significant role in nuclear medicine as experience is gained with them and as design parameters and image reconstruction procedures are improved. It is not possible at this time accurately to predict whether SPT or APT will dominate the field of ECT. The advantages and disadvantages of each have been presented and investigation in each area continues.[19, 40, 82, 87, 105]

Numerous complete imaging systems have been designed for SPT or APT over the last several years. Examples of representative systems are listed in Table 3.4. The listing describes the detector configurations used on the different systems and

Table 3.4 Emission computed tomography systems

Single photon tomography	Detector type	Detector dimensions	References
1 Mark IV Scanner	Four detectors in a square array, each a NaI(Tl) matrix	Eight crystals/detector each 76 mm high × 25 mm wide × 25 mm deep	(1976)[60]
2 (a) Univ of Michigan Humongotron	Rotating γ-camera, NaI(Tl)	SFOV	(1977)[54]
(b) Searle Radiographics-Baylor Univ	Rotating γ-camera, NaI(Tl)	SFOV	(1977)[50]
(c) General Electric, Model 400T	Rotating γ-camera, NaI(Tl)	LFOV	(1977)
(d) Univ of California, Berkeley	Rotating γ-camera, NaI(Tl)	SFOV	(1977)[20]
3 Aberdeen Scanner – J & P Engineering	Four detectors in a square array, each a NaI(Tl) matrix	—	(1973)[14] (1977)[87]
4 Univ of California, San Francisco	Germanium gamma camera	HP Ge detector, 64 mm × 32 mm × 10 mm	(1980)[83] (1977)[30]
5 Dynamic Computer Assisted Tomograph (DCAT)	Four detectors in a square array, each a NaI(Tl) matrix	16 crystals/detector, 14 cm × 2 cm × 13 mm NaI(Tl)	(1980)[100]
6 Searle Whole-Body Single-Photon Emission Computed Tomography System (SPECT)	Dual opposed rotating γ-cameras, NaI(Tl)	LFOV	(1979)[49]

Annihilation photon tomography			
1 MGH Transverse Section Positron Camera Cyclotron Corporation Model 4200	Dual opposed multiple NaI(Tl) crystal arrays	12 × 12 crystals/array, each 2 cm diameter × 4 cm long	(1977)[17] (1978)[18]
2 Washington University PETT III, Ortec ECAT	Hexagonal opposed multiple NaI(Tl) crystal arrays	11 crystals/array each 38 mm diameter × 76 mm long	(1975)[105]
3 Searle Positron Camera	Dual opposed gamma cameras, NaI(Tl) crystals	Each 42 cm diameter × 25·4 mm thick	(1977)[76]
4 Washington University PETT IV	Hexagonal opposed multiple NaI(Tl) crystal arrays	8 crystals/array, each 5 cm thick × 17 cm long	(1977)[87] (1977)[106]
5 Brookhaven-Montreal Circular Tomograph	Circular array of NaI(Tl) crystals	32 crystals, each 32 mm diameter × 25 mm thick	(1973)[91]
6 UCLA Circular Ring Traverse Axial Positron Camera	Circular array of NaI(Tl) crystals	64 crystals, each 2 cm diameter × 38 mm long	(1977)[24]
7 Univ of California, Berkeley, Ring Array	Circular array of NaI(Tl) crystals	280 crystals, each 8 mm × 3 cm × 5 cm deep	(1977)[20]
8 Univ of California, San Francisco	Dual opposed proportional chambers	48 × 48 cm chamber, filled with 70% argon and 30% methane gas mixture	(1975)[63]
9 UCLA Bismuth Germanate Positron Camera (Proposed System)	Circular array of $Bi_4Ge_3O_{12}$ crystals	<2 cm diameter × 38 mm long	(1977)[25]
10 Time of Flight Positron Camera (Proposed System)	Two opposed and orthogonally skewed cylindrical plastic scintillators	—	(1978)[80]

indicates the somewhat diverse approaches which have been used to obtain emission tomograms. No one system as yet has been demonstrated to be clearly superior to the others. As a result, research in instrument design and clinical trials continues on a wide scale. Unlike the tomographic scanner and the specially designed collimators described later, the majority of the SPT systems are designed to provide transverse tomographic images (image plane or section perpendicular to the face of the detector). The APT systems usually provide longitudinal and transverse tomographic sectioning capability as well as conventional two-dimensional images. Some of the systems listed in Table 3.4 are one of a kind; others are or will be available commercially. Figure 3.8 illustrates an example of a SPT system which can be obtained commercially.

systems have been a major asset in the development of ECT, supplying the image storage, processing and display capability needed in each of the SPT and APT systems. Of interest to many laboratories, these systems provide the storage and computational capabilities needed with the collimators designed for tomographic imaging with conventional gamma cameras. This development has given nuclear medicine laboratories the opportunity to conduct regional tomographic imaging without purchasing new imaging systems. Requiring either a SFOV or LFOV scintillation camera as the detector and a computer for data acquisition and image processing, a laboratory can add tomographic imaging capability by acquiring one of these collimators and the corresponding computer software needed for image reconstruction. Tomographic im-

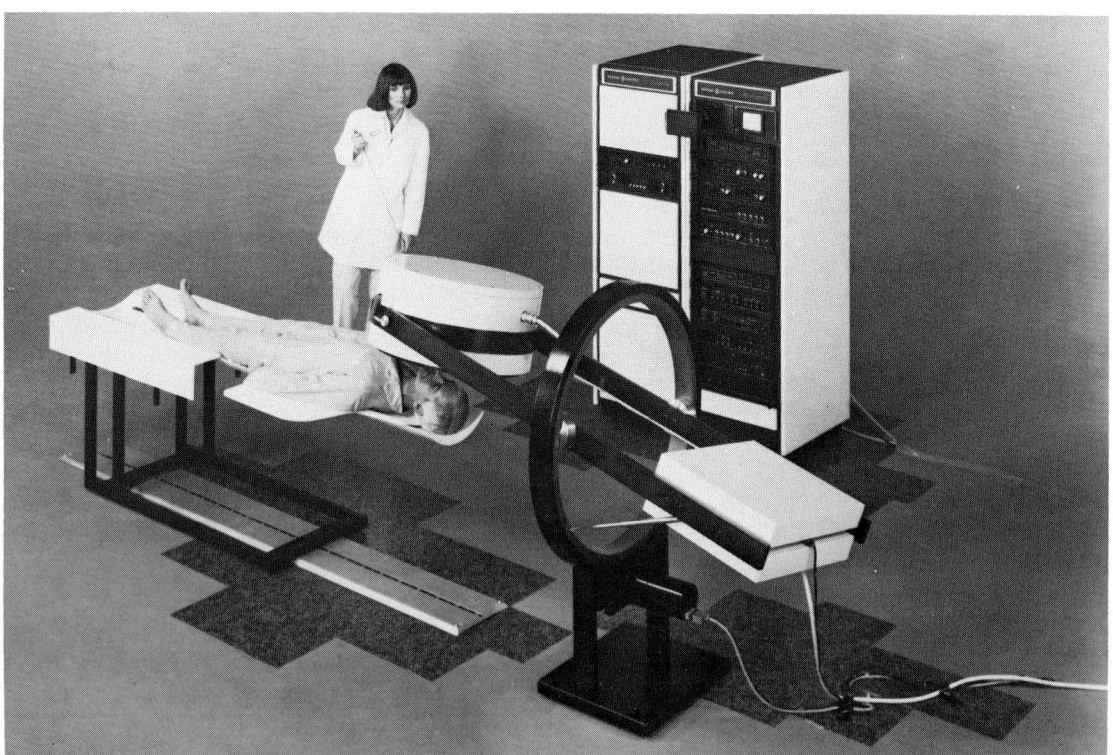

Fig. 3.8 Single photon tomography system which employs a large field of view (LFOV) scintillation camera mounted on a rotatable gantry. (Maxi-Camera 400T, General Electric Company.)

A growing number of nuclear medicine facilities maintain a dedicated computer system in the laboratory, of the type shown in Figures 3.9 and 3.10.[113, 115] Used for imaging and nonimaging applications in the nuclear medicine laboratory, these

ages can thus be obtained from existing camera systems for relatively low cost as compared to the systems outlined in Table 3.4. Collimators investigated for this purpose have included a seven pinhole collimator,[15, 39, 108] a rotating slant hole

RADIONUCLIDE IMAGING

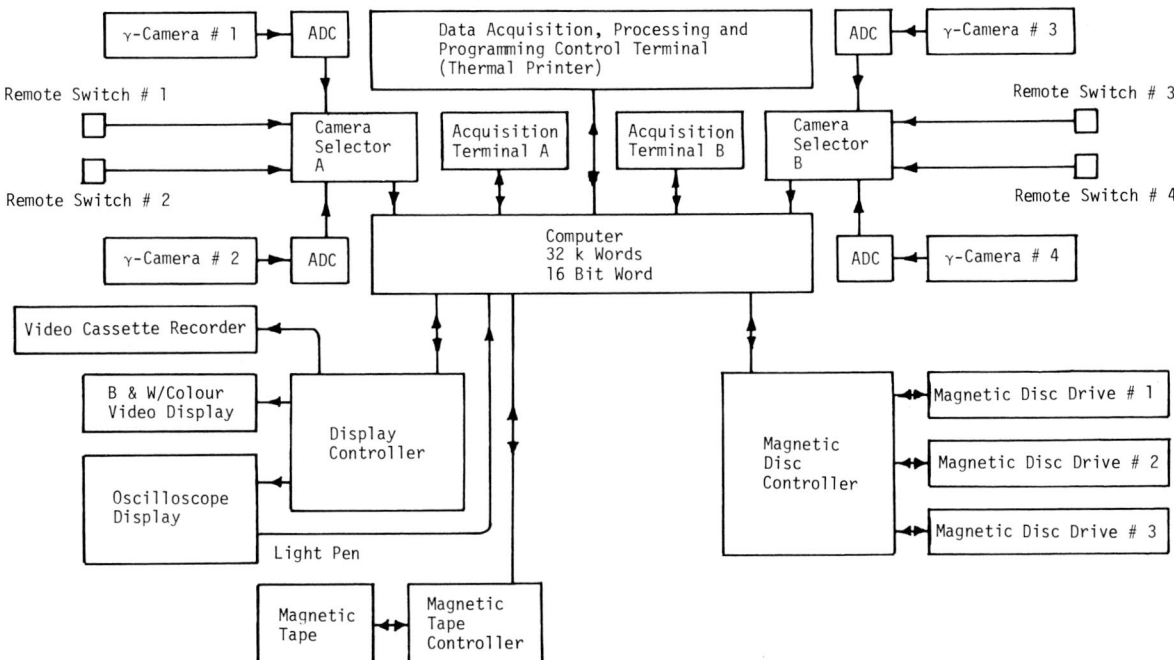

Fig. 3.9 Block diagram of a minicomputer system dedicated to nuclear medicine imaging, associated data processing, record keeping, teaching, quality assurance and display used in the Division of Nuclear Medicine at the University of Rochester Medical Center. Systems of this type are used for conventional two-dimensional image acquisition and processing and for tomographic image acquisition and reconstruction.

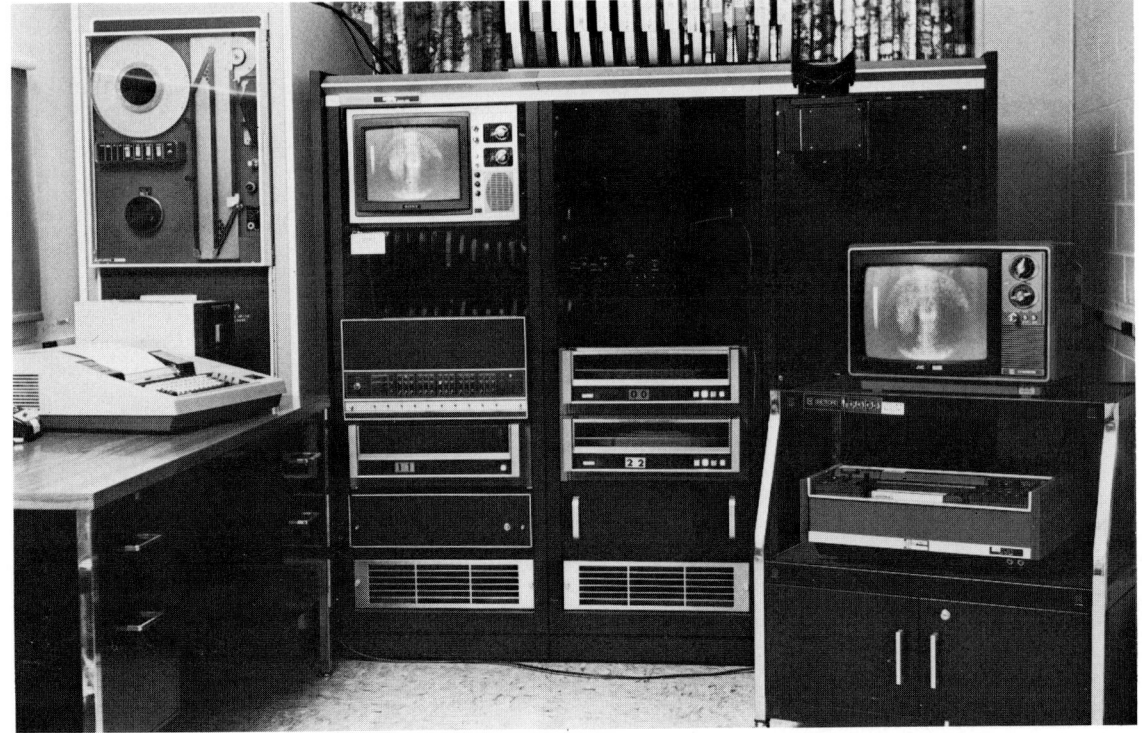

Fig. 3.10 Photograph of computer system shown in the block diagram in Fig. 3.9

collimator,[39, 75, 97] and various other coded aperture collimators.[8, 23, 57, 89, 93] Currently, two of these collimators, the seven pinhole and the rotating slant hole collimator, are available commercially for tomographic imaging. The seven pinhole collimator displays horizontal spatial resolution of ≤ 1 cm and a vertical spatial resolution of ≤ 15 mm for distances up to 127 mm from the collimator face over a 12 cm diameter field when used with a LFOV camera. Similar specifications have been reported for the rotating slant hole collimator. There is debate over the optimum design and the trade-offs between spatial resolution and such quantities as sensitivity, distortion, field size and acceptance angle.[39, 97] As these problems are resolved, a clearer definition of the utility of this approach to tomographic imaging should emerge. Initial clinical trials with these collimators have been encouraging.[16, 26, 109] Tomographic images of myocardial thallium-201 perfusion with the seven pinhole collimator, for example, were reported to show improved detection sensitivity as compared to those obtained with a conventional parallel hole collimator.[109]

Thus far the longitudinal plane tomographic scanner has been the principal imaging system dedicated to tomography that has been commercially available on a broad scale. Two detectors, each consisting of a single NaI(Tl) crystal viewed by an array of PMTs mounted on a scanner platform provide the means by which whole body and regional tomograms can be obtained. Each detector resembles a single crystal scintillation camera in its physical and electronic design. Fitted with focused collimators and moved in a raster pattern over the patient, these detectors provide the information used to obtain longitudinal tomographic images (images with focal planes parallel to the long axis of the body). The design for this instrument was introduced by Anger in 1966.[5, 6, 40] Originally designed to employ two NaI(Tl) detectors, each 216 mm in diameter by 25 mm thick coupled to seven PMTs, and more recently redesigned to use two 236 mm by 13 mm NaI(Tl) detectors coupled to nineteen 51 mm PMTs, this instrument combines advantages of the rectilinear scanner and the gamma camera to provide tomographic displays of radionuclide localisation. Figure 3.11 shows the commercially available system. Several reports suggest that the multiplane tomographic scanner is particularly useful for imaging radiopharmaceutical localisation in deep-seated structures and in thick organs.[41, 118] The findings from continuing clinical trials with the redesigned detector configuration, and improvements in the methods for reducing unwanted activity from adjacent regions lying above and below the focal plane, are expected strongly to influence the future role of this instrument.

The use of high energy resolution semiconductor materials as the detectors for gamma imaging systems is expected significantly to improve spatial resolution and image quality available for two-dimensional and tomographic imaging procedures. Although the documentation and the experience with these systems are limited as compared with other systems described in this Section, some reports on a germanium detector configuration,[30, 53, 83] and more recent studies on a cadmium telluride (CdTe) detector[3, 66] suggest that high energy resolution semiconductor material may be used effectively in small field of view gamma cameras, offering greatly improved spatial resolution and a promise of true portability. Improvements in detector technology, newer methods of assembling detector arrays, and reduced costs in fabrication could make their use an attractive alternative to NaI(Tl) detectors.

The last instrument noted at the beginning of this Section is the multicrystal scanning system. Unlike the other instruments in this Section, this unit was designed primarily to offer conventional two-dimensional imaging capabilities while maintaining levels of spatial resolution equal to or better than that obtained with a rectilinear scanner. The Cleon Whole Body Imager* is an example of this type of system. Using two collinearly opposed detectors, each consisting of 10 collimated rectangular NaI(Tl) crystals, 61 mm wide by 114 mm long by 25 mm thick, image acquisiton time is reduced while spatial resolution is maintained as compared with conventional dual probe rectilinear scanners. One detector is mounted above the platform and a second detector is mounted below. The central axes of each of 10 focused collimators on each detector are separated by a distance of approximately 61 mm.[117] A 61 cm wide scan can be made

*Raytheon Medical Systems, Stamford, Connecticut, USA.

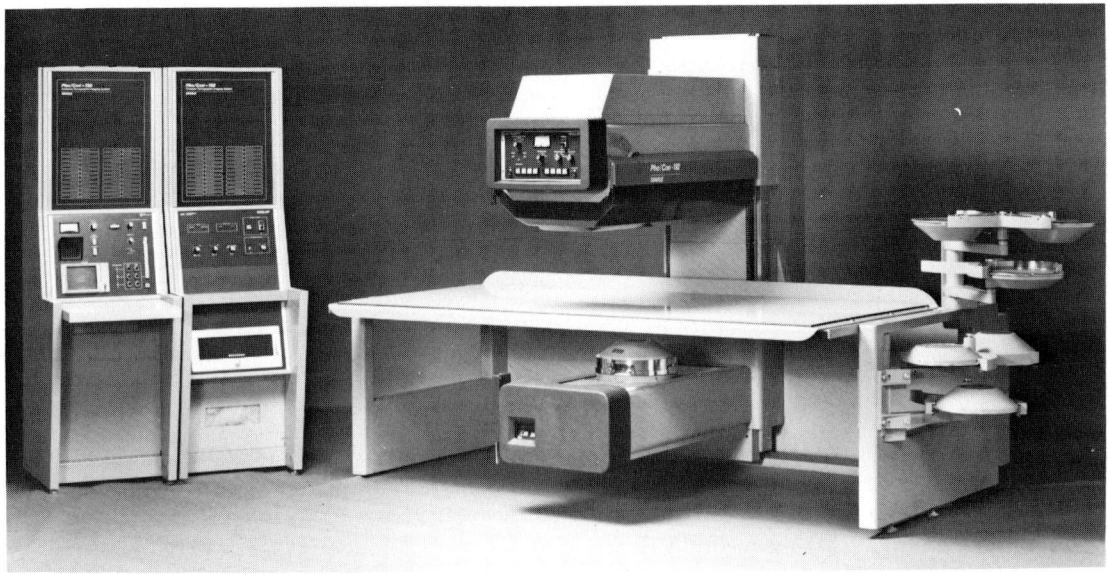

Fig. 3.11 Longitudinal plane tomographic scanner. (Pho/Con 192, Siemens Gammasonics.)

by moving the detector 61 mm in the transverse direction as the detectors move in a longitudinal motion over the patient. Similar in its basic design to the rectilinear scanner, the instrument cannot be used for dynamic studies and the parabolically focused collimators show variations in spatial resolution with depth characteristic of this type of collimation.

CLINICAL APPLICATIONS

As evolution has occurred in the areas of basic instrumentation and radiopharmaceutical development, changes in clinical application of radionuclide imaging techniques have also occurred. The main thrust of this change has been to move away from static organ imaging to determine anatomical pathology, to a more functional approach in organ system pathology. This change in clinical application has responded to the need for answers to specific questions about medical problems involving the biochemical or physiological properties in specific pathological processes. This Section briefly presents the current major clinical applications of radionuclide imaging based on an organ system scheme.

Central nervous system

Brain imaging and perfusion

Studies of the brain have undergone major changes in approach and application due to the development of X-ray transmission computed tomography, as discussed in Chapter 2. The CT imaging process has replaced, for the most part, the use of radionuclide brain imaging for evaluation of space occupying pathology such as tumour, abscess, trauma and cystic disease. This is a result of better anatomic delineation of lesions such as primary or secondary brain tumours and the improved anatomical information that may be gained about the relationship of a lesion to the normal anatomy in the CT procedure.[1] Nonetheless, the radionuclide brain scan still plays an important role in a variety of clinical applications.[21, 32]

The brain imaging procedure involves a bolus injection of radiopharmaceutical and the recording of serial dynamic images to evaluate cerebral perfusion in the early arterial and the mixed capillary-venous phases; immediate and delayed static images of multiple projections of the head are obtained subsequently.[34]

The clinical indications for brain imaging include: (1) the evaluation of neoplasms, especially in those cases where CT imaging may be equivocal or normal in the face of clinical symptomatology, or in institutions where CT imaging is not available; (2) the evaluation of vascular diseases of the central nervous system, including cerebral vascular accident (both haemorrhage and infarction); (3) infectious diseases, including brain abscess, encephalitis and meningitis; and (4) trauma, including subdural haematoma and cerebral contusion or haemorrhage.

Currently, three radiopharmaceuticals are widely used for evaluation of the brain. These are: ^{99m}Tc pertechnetate and ^{99m}Tc labelled diethylenetriaminepentaacetic acid (DTPA) and glucoheptonate. The latter two offer several advantages over pertechnetate. Predosing patients with perchlorate or potassium iodide is not necessary to block uptake in the choroid plexus; higher lesion-to-brain ratios are obtained at earlier times following tracer administration; and neither tracer localises in the parotid and submandibular glands. Each of the radiopharmaceuticals is administered intravenously; typical activity doses range from 370–740 MBq and most studies of the brain are conducted using a SFOV gamma camera. A normal study shows a uniform distribution of radiopharmaceutical within the vascular spaces in the brain in the arterial, capillary and venous phases of blood flow. In the later static images of the brain, only minimal activity is seen in normal brain tissue while lesions, when present, show accumulation of administered radiopharmaceutical in the lesion as a result of disruption of the blood-brain barrier. Various disease entities present several combinations of findings which can be useful in differentiating disease processes.[81] These include: (1) the majority of primary neoplasms: these frequently cause increased arterial flow extending through the venous phase in the area of neoplastic involvement (Fig. 3.12); (2) cerebral vascular accidents: these are generally characterised by a zone of decreased perfusion in the arterial phase; increased activity is seen in the late venous phase as a result of collateral circulation present in the area of abnormal radio-

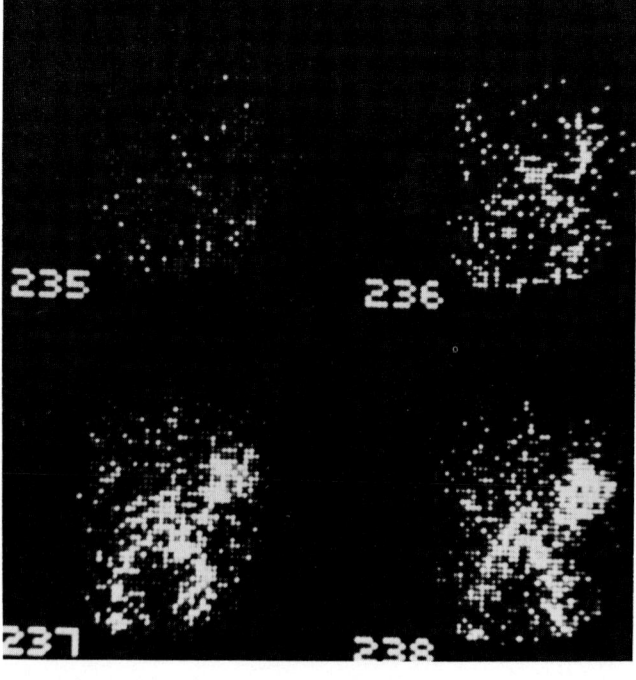

a

Fig. 3.12 Anterior cerebral perfusion study performed after intravenous administration of 555 MBq of ^{99m}TC DTPA. Gamma camera images demonstrate increased perfusion in the distribution of the left middle cerebral artery seen in the (a) early arterial and (b) mixed and late venous phases. Posterior static view (c) shows increased activity in a lesion located in the posterior parietal lobe. At operation, a grade IV astrocytoma was found.

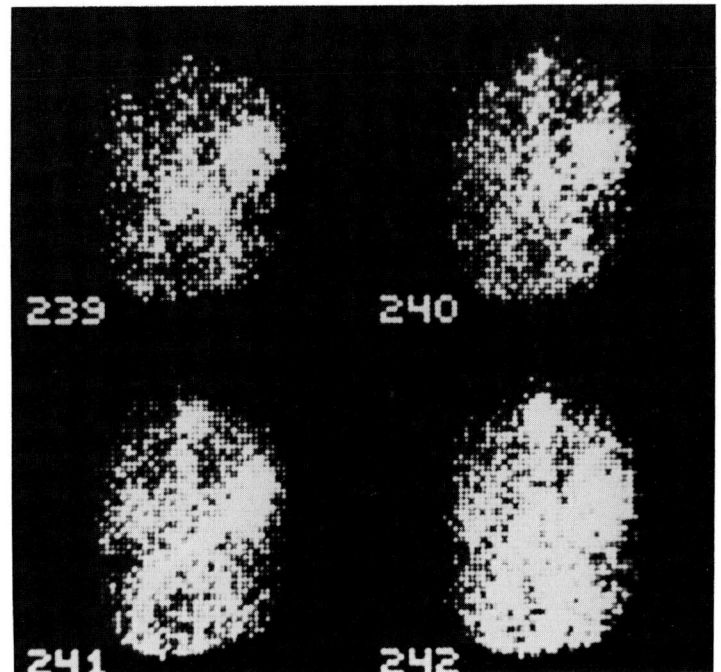

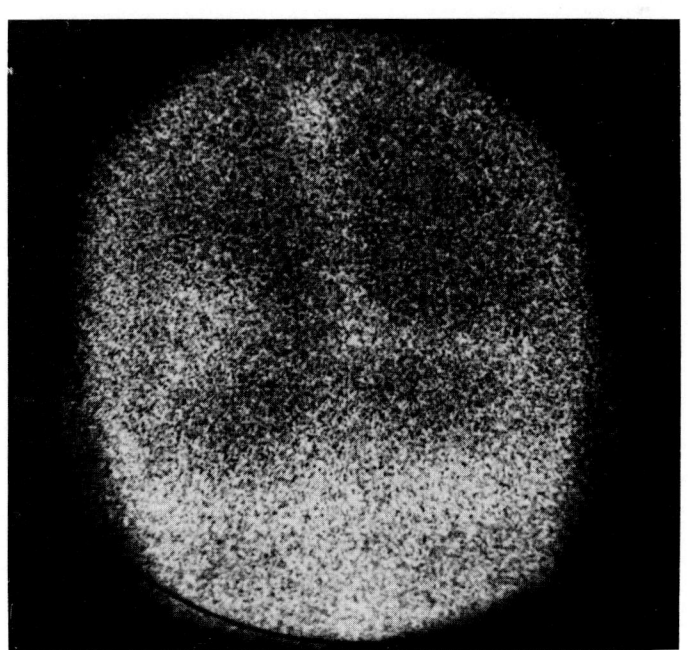

114   SCIENTIFIC BASIS OF MEDICAL IMAGING

nuclide accumulation (Fig. 3.13); (3) subdural haematomas: these present a peripheral convex zone of decreased perfusion which persists during the perfusion phase and are associated later with increased peripheral activity seen on the static images; and (4) infectious diseases: these offer a

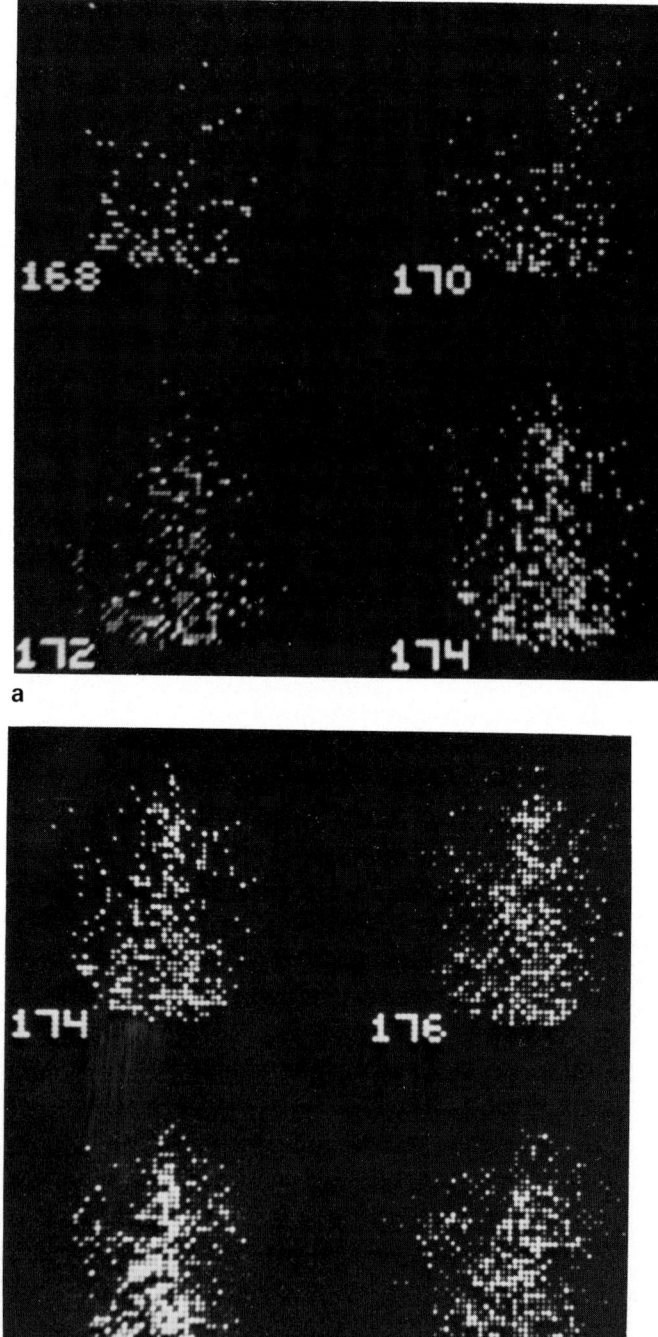

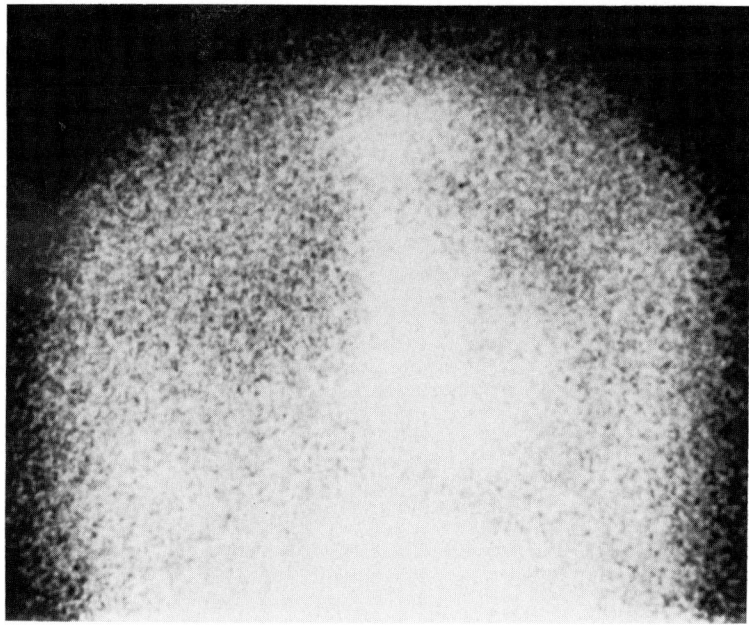

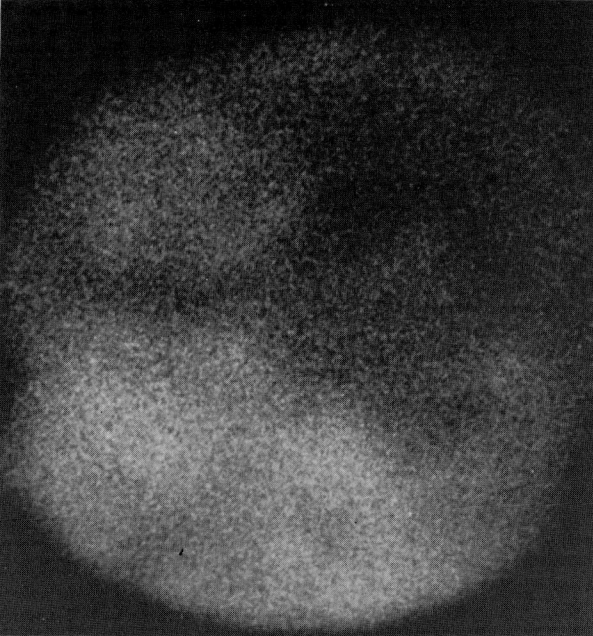

Fig. 3.13 Cerebral perfusion study (a and b) demonstrates decreased flow in the neck vessels (frames 170–174) associated with decreased perfusion through the distribution of the left anterior and middle cerebral arteries, followed by later increased activity as a result of collateral circulation (frame 180). Static images in the (c) anterior and (d) left lateral views obtained 2 h after the bolus administration of 555 BMq of ^{99m}Tc pertechnetate demonstrate a large area of increased activity. A large area of cerebral infarction was observed in the frontal and parietal lobes at autopsy.

variety of changes depending upon the state of development of the infectious process; once the primary condition has been established in all of the disease entities, the radioisotopic technique may be used to assess the adequacy of a therapeutic regimen.

Cerebral spinal fluid dynamics

In the evaluation of cerebral spinal fluid dynamics, a radiopharmaceutical is administered intrathecally via puncture directly into the ventricles or into the subarachnoid space, usually in the lumbar region. Serial images are performed over several days utilising a SFOV or LFOV gamma camera. Radiopharmaceuticals currently used are ytterbium-169 (^{169}Yb) DTPA or indium-111 (^{111}In) DTPA.[29, 92] (The latter has the advantage that it allows a reduced radiation dose if there is significant cerebral spinal fluid trapping in either the spinal canal or brain without affecting image quality.) The major clinical applications of this type of study are: (1) to test for the presence of normal or low pressure hydrocephalus; here the entry of an intrathecally placed radiopharmaceutical into the ventricular system is seen, marked by slow clearance from the ventricular system and slow clearance from the normal pathway above the surface of the cerebral convexities; (2) detection of communicating hydrocephalus; (3) detection of cerebral spinal fluid leaks through the ear or nasal cavities; most commonly this is a result of trauma; here the accumulation of the radiopharmaceutical in nasal or auditory canals on the images is seen or its presence is demonstrated by evaluating the amount of absorption of radiopharmaceutical in pledgets placed in these anatomical regions; and (4) the evaluation of the patency of cerebral spinal fluid shunts postoperatively; here the radiopharmaceutical is placed into the shunting reservoir and the patency and effectiveness of the afferent and efferent loops of the shunt are determined.

Pulmonary imaging

Pulmonary imaging usually evaluates two components of pulmonary physiology. These are regional perfusion and regional ventilation. Regional perfusion is best studied using the intravenous administration of radioactive particles, 10–15 μm in size. These are injected into a peripheral vein where they mix uniformly with the blood, pass through the right heart, and then are trapped in the pulmonary arteriolar or capillary bed. The most commonly used radiopharmaceuticals are ^{99m}Tc labelled serum albumin macroaggregates or microspheres.

Regional ventilation is most commonly assessed by having the patient inhale a relatively insoluable radioactive gas. Xenon-133 (^{133}Xe) is the most frequently used radioactive gas due to its physical and biological properties, and its ready availability. A typical procedure includes the recording of static images for the initial breath ^{133}Xe distribution and of the equilibrium distribution after ^{133}Xe rebreathing, followed by serial images of the ^{133}Xe washout. Shorter lived radionuclides such as krypton-81m (^{81m}Kr) are sometimes used for ventilation imaging.[62] Another group of agents used to evaluate inhalation is the radiolabelled aerosols. The distribution and clearance of such aerosols may be used to study lung ventilation and permeability.[42] The most widely used aerosols are prepared from ^{99m}Tc DTPA, ^{111}In DTPA and ^{99m}Tc sulphur colloid.[64, 88] These studies are usually carried out with either SFOV or LFOV gamma camera systems, although multicrystal imaging devices may also be used to evaluate lung perfusion and ventilation.

The more common clinical applications include: (1) the evaluation of pulmonary embolic phenomenon: here the ventilatory capacity is normal when embolisation occurs without infarction (Fig. 3.14) while the perfusion pattern demonstrates defects caused by the presence of blood clots;[69] (2) the evaluation of chronic obstructive lung disease or acute obstructive lung disease such as may be seen with emphysema or asthma; (3) the diagnosis of an aspirated foreign body, especially in the paediatric age population; (4) the evaluation of lung function in order to predict pulmonary capability before pneumectomy or lobectomy is planned; (5) the evaluation of chronic lung diseases such as bronchiectasis and cystic fibrosis; (6) the assessment of congenital pulmonary abnormalities and cardiac abnormalities such as shunts and the effect of corrective surgical procedures; and (7) the early evaluation of respiratory burns.

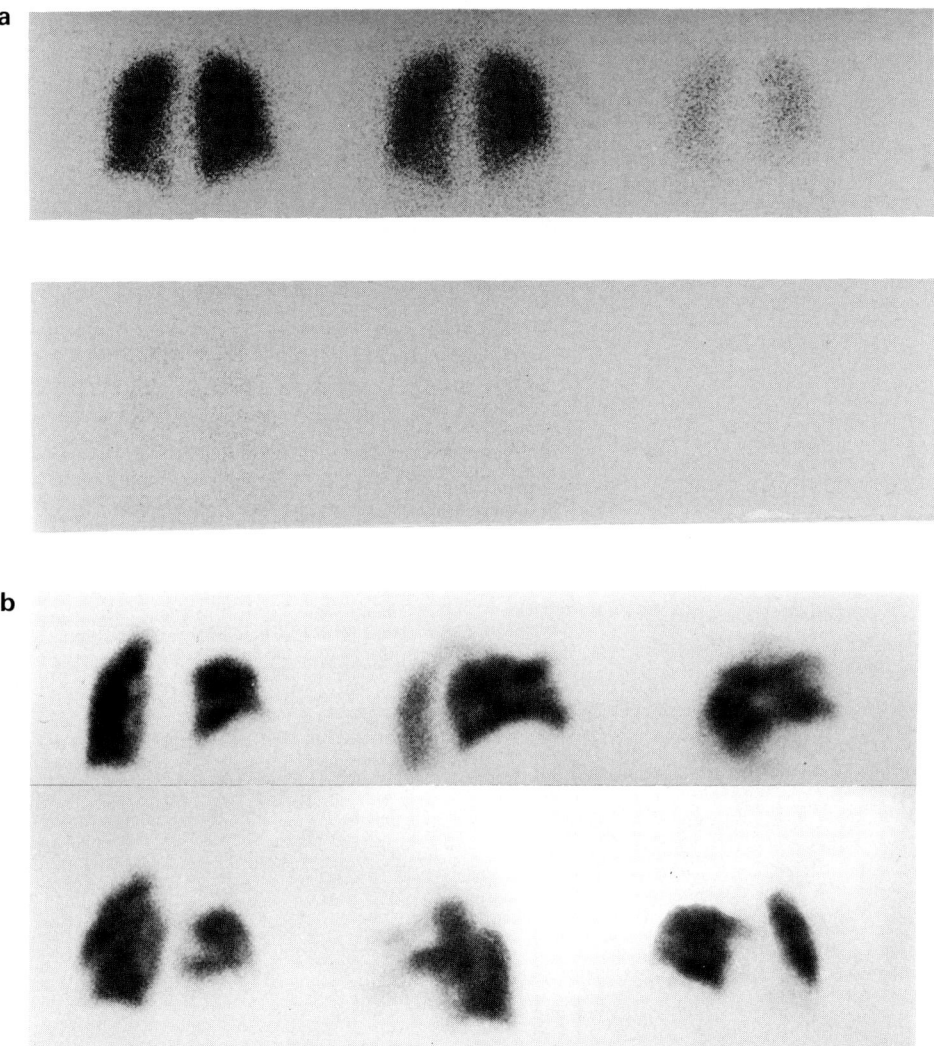

Fig. 3.14 (a) Xenon-133 ventilation study shows normal single breath inhalation, equilibration and early washout (top row) with complete washout by 60 s after equilibration (bottom row). (b) Pulmonary perfusion images performed following adminstration of 111 MBq of ^{99m}Tc MAA. Posterior, right posterior oblique, right lateral (top row), left posterior oblique, left lateral and anterior projections (bottom row) views demonstrate multiple perfusion defects in the lungs of this 57 y old female with proven pulmonary embolism.

Cardiovascular studies

A wide variety of clinical applications are conducted in this area,[84] and a discussion of these follows.

Avid imaging ('hotspot')

The radiopharmaceutical used for this type of study is ^{99m}Tc pyrophosphate (^{99m}Tc PPi). ^{99m}Tc PPi localises in damaged myocardial cells around recent infarction as well as in other areas of infarction including the brain, peripheral muscles and the bowel.[85] The study is usually carried out with either a SFOV or LFOV gamma camera and is most commonly performed in the evaluation of questionable recent myocardial infarction (Fig. 3.15). The vast majority of these cases are diagnosed using ECG and serum enzyme level changes. The procedure is particularly useful in patients whose clinical setting and laboratory findings are equivocal, and in those with postmyocardial infarction who have chest pain reccurrence. The procedure is helpful in evaluation of cardiomyopathies, coronary artery disease, drug toxicity, and rhabdomyolysis.

Radiopharmaceutical deficient lesion imaging ('coldspot')

The current radiopharmaceutical of choice for performance of this imaging procedure is thallium-201 (^{201}Tl) chloride. Demonstrating biological clearance characteristics similar to that of potassium and providing a decay scheme more suitable for imaging than that available from radioactive isotopes of

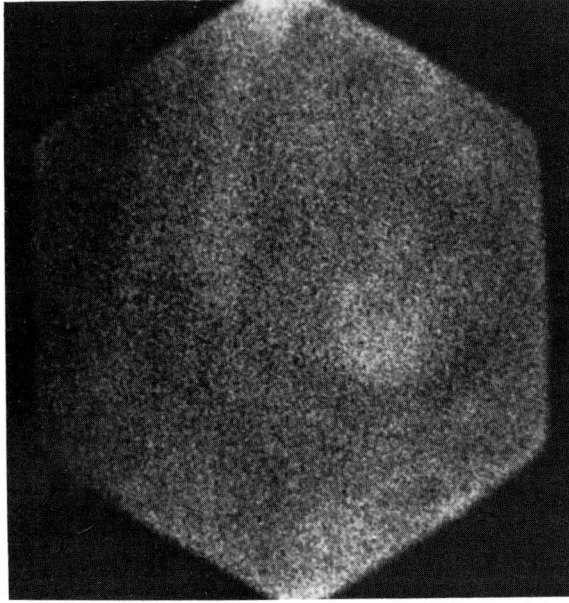

Fig. 3.15 Left anterior oblique view of a myocardial imaging study performed after the intravenous administration of 444 MBq of ^{99m}Tc pyrophosphate. The abnormal, large accumulation in the left ventricle is diagnostic of a myocardial infarction present in this 61 y old male. This was later confirmed by ECG and enzyme changes.

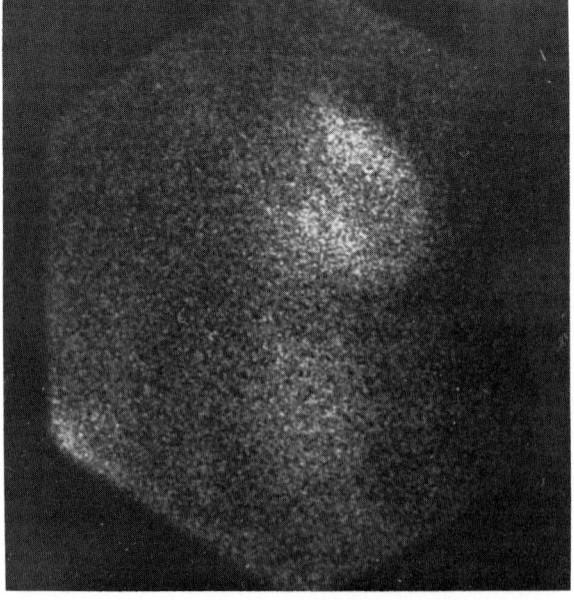

a

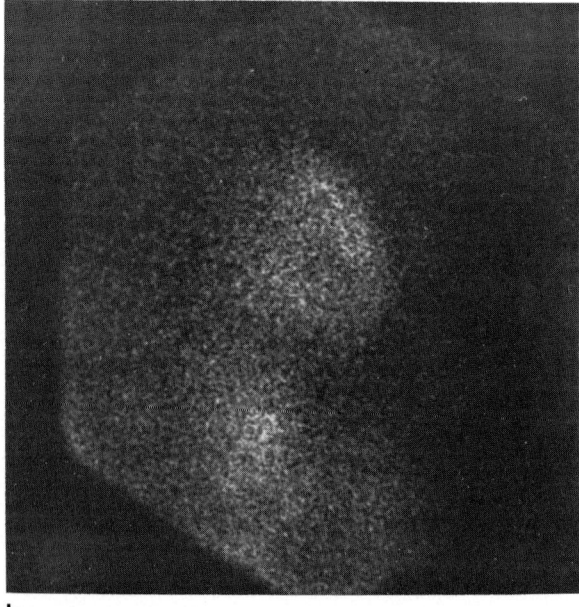

b

Fig. 3.16 Right anterior oblique cardiac images performed after the intravenous administration of 56 MBq of ^{201}Tl chloride. Images were obtained at (a) maximum stress and (b) after 2 h of rest in a 51 y old male with severe angina. The large defect seen at stress and persisting into the resting, recirculation phase is indicative of marked myocardial damage, as a result of severe coronary artery disease which was confirmed at coronary angiography.

potassium, ^{201}Tl is currently the radionuclide of choice for myocardial perfusion studies. Thallium is extracted from the blood and is transported by the sodium-potassium pump intracellularly. It is distributed evenly throughout the myocardium; usually only the left ventricle of the heart is visualised, however, due to its large muscle mass.[101] The clinical indications for these studies include: (1) evaluation of patients with suspect damaged myocardium resulting in angina: this is usually accomplished as a two-part study with injection of the radiopharmaceutical performed while the myocardium is stressed by exercise, or cold pressor techniques, and then a later evaluation observing redistribution (Fig. 3.16); the distribution pattern evolved is then used in the workup of the patient for possible coronary vessel bypass surgery; (2) evaluation of the postoperative status of the myocardium following bypass surgery; and (3) evaluation, extent and sizing of myocardial infarction and ischaemia.

These studies are usually performed on a stationary or portable SFOV or LFOV gamma camera. The portable cameras are especially useful for these cardiac studies since they allow the procedure to be carried out in the cardiac intensive care unit or in conjunction with other exercise studies performed in cardiac evaluation centres.

Ventricular dynamic measurements

These studies are generally conducted using one of two imaging procedures.[31] These are the *multiple gated acquisition* (MUGA) and *first pass* procedures. The MUGA procedure involves the measurement of ventricular function following equilibration of

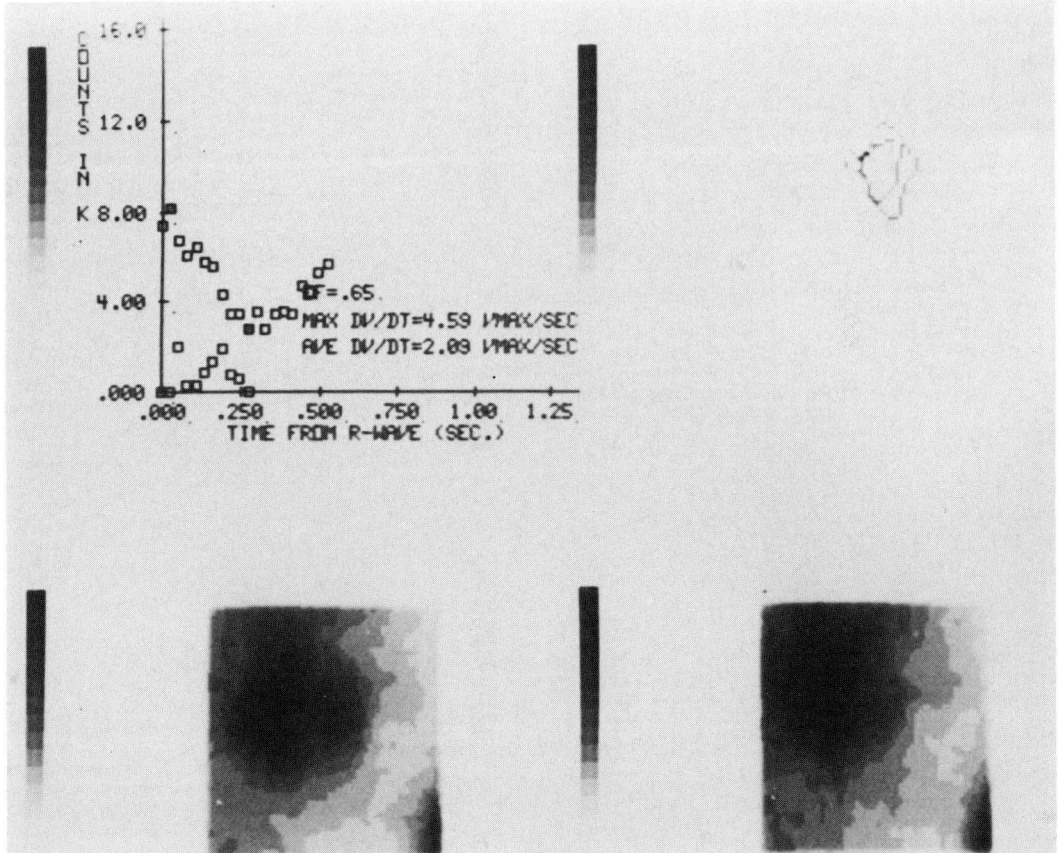

Fig. 3.17 Results from a cardiac blood pool study in a 54 y old male with a recent myocardial infarction involving the inferior and apical walls of the heart. The ejection fraction (top left) is normal at 0·65. The left anterior oblique projections of the summed end diastolic (bottom left) and end systolic (bottom right) images are normal as is the computer-generated image of the ventricular motion edges (top right).

blood pool tracers (e.g. ^{99m}Tc labelled red blood cells or human serum albumin) in the vasculature.[102] A series of images is recorded during the patient's cardiac cycle by using the patient's ECG to gate or control image acquisition. High spatial resolution images of the heart for different segments of the cardiac cycle are obtained by summing images of identical time segments from consecutive cardiac cycles. The images, which are usually stored in computer memory during acquisition, can be processed to assess regional wall motion, ventricular ejection fraction, ejection rate, ventricular volume, and other related parameters. This type of study is usually carried out using a SFOV or LFOV camera system. The second procedure is the first pass assay of cardiac dynamics. In this procedure, the ventricular system is evaluated during the initial passage of the radiopharmaceutical (e.g. ^{99m}Tc pertechnetate or ^{99m}Tc sulphur colloid) through the heart. Again, this study is conducted in conjunction with the patient's ECG in order that appropriate segments of the cardiac cycle can be evaluated. Although this technique may be accomplished with the standard camera system, the use of a multiple crystal imaging device offers an advantage because of the higher counting rates this instrument can handle.[13] The multiple gated techniques offer advantages when repetitive studies are desired since they can be carried out using only a single dose of radioactivity. This is particularly helpful when it is desired to evaluate ventricular function following medicinal or interventional therapeutic regimens. The first pass technique has been found to be particularly useful in the study

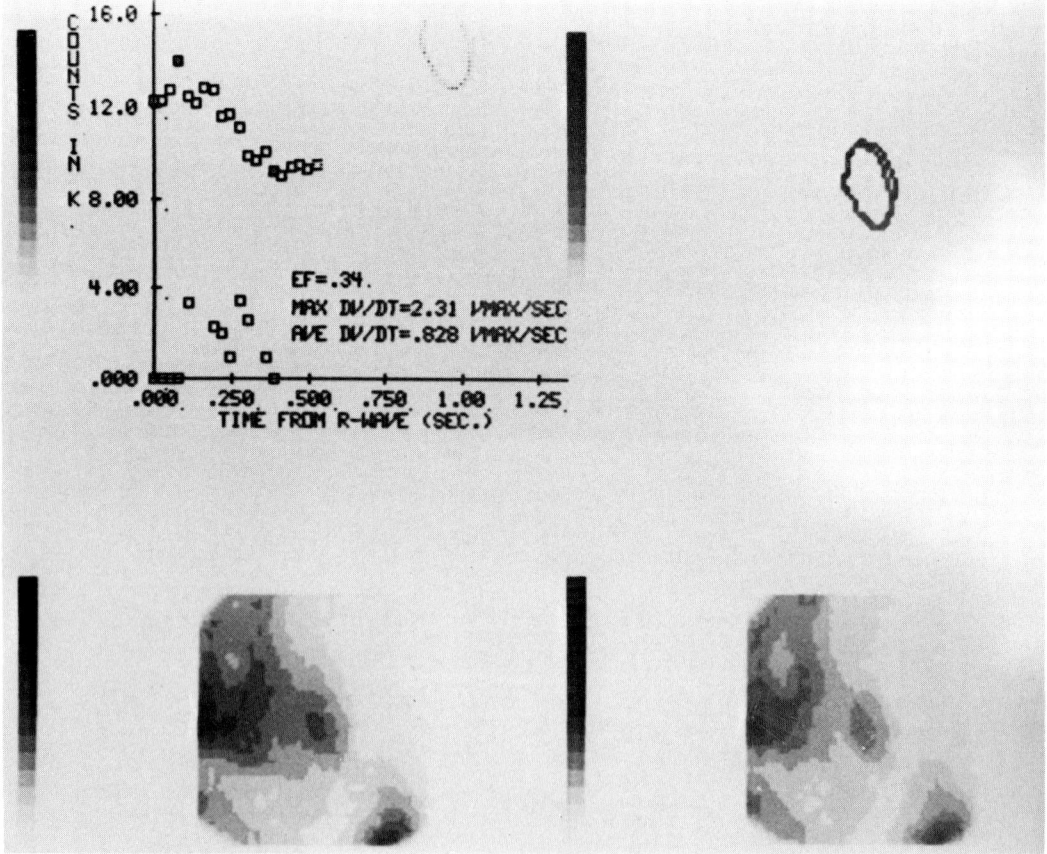

Fig. 3.18 Gated cardiac blood pool study in a 61 y old male with severe coronary artery disease. The ejection fraction (top left) is abnormally low at 0·34. The summed left anterior oblique projections of the end systolic (bottom left) and end diastolic (bottom right) images show markedly reduced wall motion; the computer-generated line representation of ventricular motion (top right) demonstrates global hypokinesis with superimposed areas of focal akinesis.

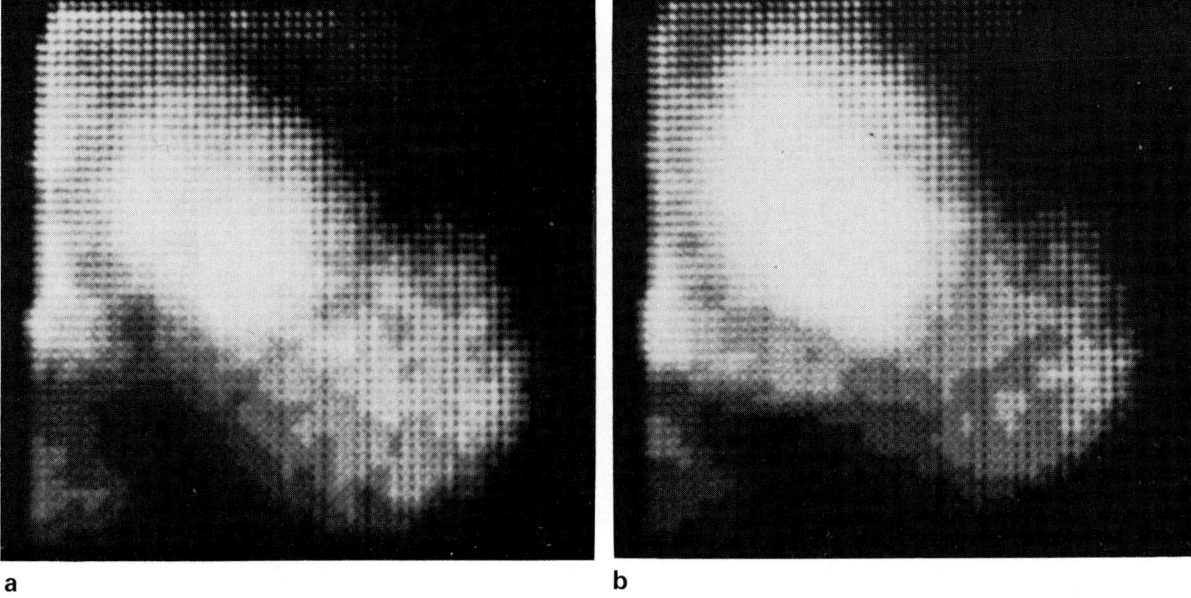

a   b

Fig. 3.19 Gated cardiac blood pool study in the left anterior oblique projection demonstrates huge ventricular aneurysm seen in (a) end systole and (b) end diastole, in a 54 y old male with history of severe myocardial infarction 6 months earlier.

of patients with rapidly changing or unstable ECGs. Both techniques have gained widespread clinical use in the evaluation of ventricular function following myocardial infarction (Fig. 3.17), coronary artery disease and its repair (Fig. 3.18) and in the demonstration of ventricular aneurysms (Fig. 3.19)

Shunt detections

As noted on page 116, intracardiac shunts may be diagnosed with radioisotopic techniques. The procedure is simple and safe for the patient, usually involving no more than intravenous administration of a radiopharmaceutical and frequently eliminating the need for more complex and life-threatening radiographic procedures. An intracardiac shunt may be detected by observing the passage of a bolus of intravenously administered radiopharmaceutical, such as ^{99m}Tc pertechnetate or ^{99m}Tc serum albumin aggregates, using a SFOV or LFOV gamma camera. The location and quantification of the shunt usually require computer analyses. These techniques are also valuable to assess surgical procedures that are used to correct shunts.

Vascular abnormalities

In the evaluation of vascular abnormalities, the bolus injection of the radiopharmaceutical is given in a peripheral vein for both venous and arterial abnormalities. The radiopharmaceutical may be one that is rapidly cleared from the blood such as ^{99m}Tc sulphur colloid or ^{99m}Tc DPTA, so that repeat studies may be performed, or one that is less rapidly cleared such as ^{99m}Tc pertechnetate. The studies are most commonly used to evaluate the presence of thoracic or abdominal vessel aneurysms (Fig. 3.20) or blocks in collateral circulation in both the arterial and venous systems from a variety of causes (Fig. 3.21). These studies are usually conducted with either a SFOV or preferably a LFOV camera system. The changes in blood flow patterns are sometimes evaluated quantitatively using computer processing techniques.[77]

Skeletal

The development of ^{99m}Tc labelled phosphates and diphosphonates in the early 1970s has greatly expanded the role of skeletal imaging into many clinical areas.[103, 104] Currently, the agents of choice include ^{99m}Tc methylene diphosphonate (^{99m}Tc

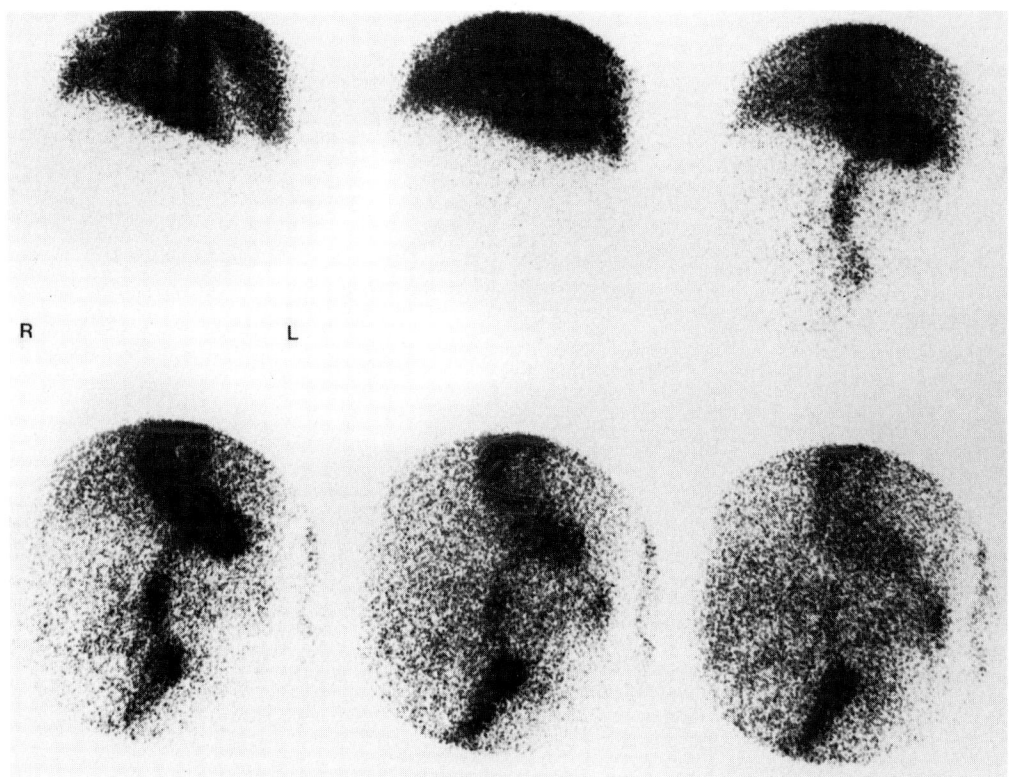

Fig. 3.20 Serial, 2 s images obtained during a radionuclide angiogram demonstrate a large aneurysm of the abdominal aorta with obstruction to the run-off into the left iliac artery.

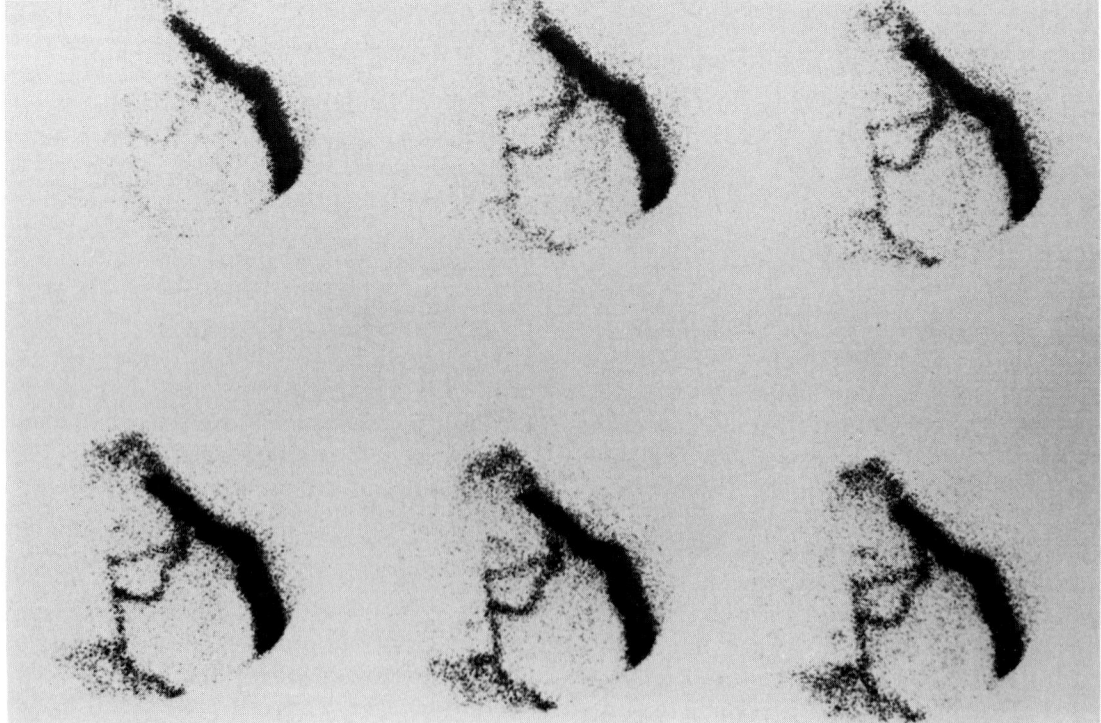

Fig. 3.21 Serial, 1 s images obtained during a radionuclide superior vena cavagram in a 37 y old male with mediastinal lymphoma. These demonstrate a complete obstruction to the superior vena cava and left subclavian vein with marked collateral circulation.

MDP), ^{99m}Tc hydroxyethylidene diphosphonate (^{99m}Tc HEDP) and ^{99m}Tc pyrophosphate (^{99m}Tc PPi).[95, 112] Skeletal imaging studies are most commonly carried out with a LFOV camera system; multiple static views or a combination of a whole body image and selected static views are recorded.

The more important clinical applications of skeletal imaging include the following: (1) The workup of patients for metastatic disease in bone or primary bone tumour (Fig. 3.22). This procedure is the most sensitive diagnostic method for detection of bone neoplasms and is still the most common clinical use of skeletal imaging.[35, 70] In patients with primary bone neoplasms, such as osteosarcoma, the procedure can be used to detect the presence of metastases in other bones and soft tissues.[98] (2) The evaluation of patients with osteomyelitis where the perfusion status of the afflicted bone and the delayed uptake pattern (Fig. 3.23) is studied to allow separation of osteomyelitis from cellulitis or other soft tissue inflammatory conditions, such as septic arthritis.[37] The response of the osteomyelitis to therapeutic regimens may also be assessed by

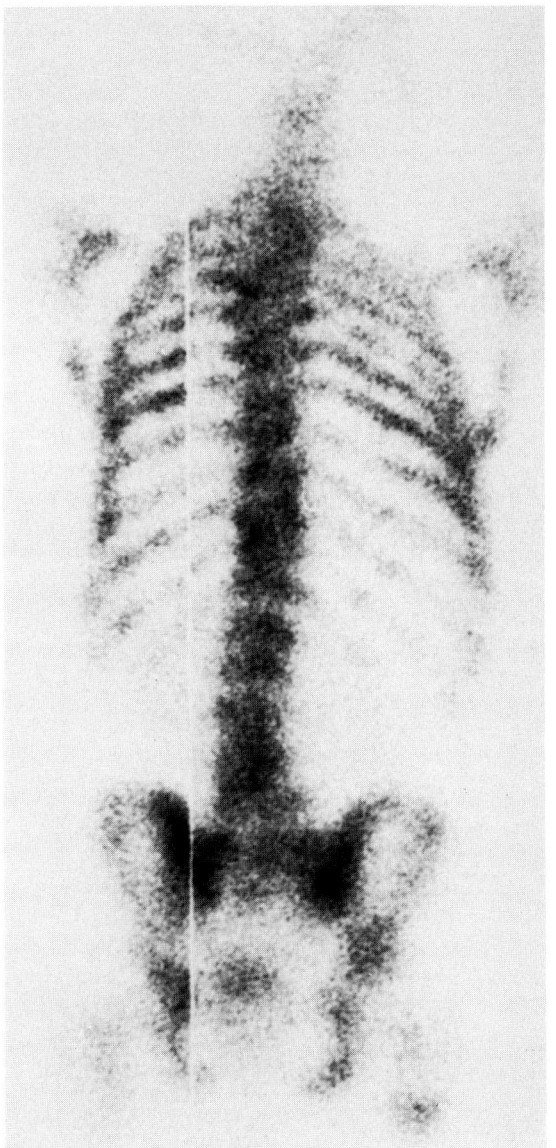

Fig. 3.22 Posterior, total body image performed 2 h after the intravenous injection of 555 MBq of ^{99m}Tc MDP in a 66 y old male with a primary carcinoma of the prostate. Image demonstrates wide-spread osseous metastatic lesions in the spine, rib cage, pelvis and extremities. Note the absence of normal renal uptake frequently associated with widespread diffuse metastatic lesions.

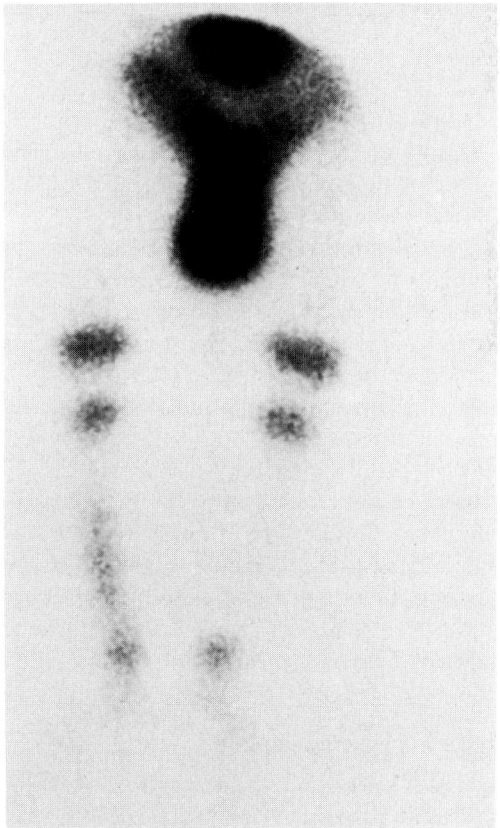

Fig. 3.23 Anterior gamma camera image of the lower limbs of a 2 y old infant with a tender right leg and refusal to move the leg for 3 days. Routine radiographic examination of this leg was normal. The large focus of abnormal activity in the right tibia is consistent with osteomyletis. At surgery, a staphylococcus osteomyelitis was found.

124 SCIENTIFIC BASIS OF MEDICAL IMAGING

skeletal imaging. At times, a ^{67}Ga citrate study may be necessary for full evaluation.[56] (3) The evaluation of patients suffering from stress fractures, or fractures in areas where the radiographic demonstration is difficult, such as in the sternum and scapula.[55] (4) The detection and monitoring of osteonecrosis and other vascular impairment diseases; great care and attention must be placed on the early perfusion images, as well as on later bone deposition.[9, 114] (5) The evaluation of a variety of metabolic conditions; the use of bone imaging techniques in this application is dependent on the quantitative estimates of the uptake and clearance of bone seeking radiopharmaceuticals.[47] (6) The evaluation of the arthritis; bone imaging techniques can detect the location and severity of joint involvement and be used to study the response to therapeutic regimes.

Haematological system

Evaluation of haematological function with imaging techniques involves visualisation of the bone marrow.[36] This is usually accomplished by one of two methods. One method visualises the reticuloendothelial component of the bone marrow using a labelled colloid, such as ^{99m}Tc sulphur colloid. A second method visualises the haemopoietic portion of the marrow with a radiopharmaceutical such as ^{111}In chloride or iron-52 (^{52}Fe) citrate. Both types of study are usually conducted with a LFOV gamma camera with total body imaging capability; adequate studies may be also performed, however, by recording static views using a SFOV or LFOV gamma camera. The procedure is frequently used to demonstrate the site and extent of marrow function within the body (Fig. 3.24), the assay of myeloproliferative states, and to determine the location for marrow biopsy.

Liver and spleen imaging

Evaluation of the liver commonly depends upon the reticuloendothelial component of this organ, and its ability to accumulate colloidal materials. The most widely used radiopharmaceutical is ^{99m}Tc sulphur colloid. The study is usually performed with a gamma camera; both the early perfusion and the later static deposition stages of the intrave-

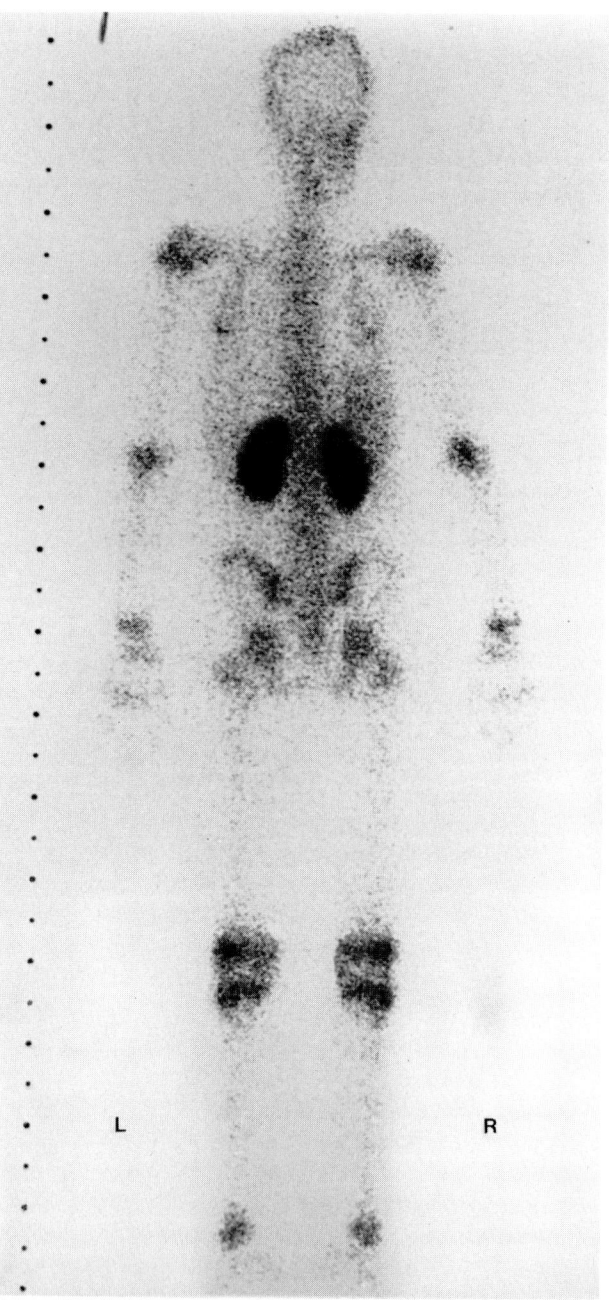

Fig. 3.24 Total body posterior image obtained 48 h after the intravenous administration of 52 MBq of ^{111}In chloride in a 11 y old girl with myelofibrosis. This image demonstrates normal bone marrow distribution in a child of this age.

nously administered ^{99m}Tc sulphur colloid are recorded.

The major clinical applications of this procedure are: (1) evaluation of the liver for space occupying disease, such as tumour, abscess or cyst; (2) evaluation of hepatic trauma; (3) identification for biopsy sites; and (4) evaluation of liver size and its relationship to other organs and masses.

Space occupying lesions are identified as defects within the uniform activity pattern of the liver (Fig. 3.25). Computed tomography and ultrasonic techniques are also used for this clinical application.[86] At present, neither procedure offers significant advantage over the radionuclide liver scan, especially in the search for metastatic disease. As better contrast agents for CT study are developed, this situation may change. Further increases in sophistication of ultrasonic instrumentation may have the same result. Radionuclide liver images and serum liver function studies are conducted frequently in patients with primary tumours known to metastasise to liver. If these tests are normal, no further evaluation is performed. If the findings suggest the present of metastatic disease, again no further tests are generally needed. If the results are equivocal, however, further evaluation with either ultrasound or CT is carried out. With this scheme, angiography and/or biopsy are rarely necessary. In patients with tumours such as lymphoma where the abdomen will be examined by CT and/or ultrasound, the liver is initially studied during the examination. A similar approach is taken with hepatic trauma (Fig. 3.26). The exact interrelationship of the three diagnostic modalities varies greatly from institution to institution, being very dependent upon the equipment available, the expertise of those who perform and interpret the imaging studies and the laboratory's ability to handle emergency cases.

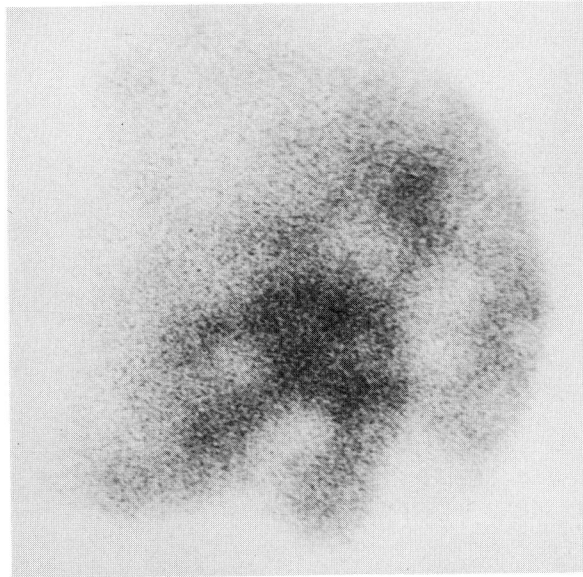

Fig. 3.25 Anterior view image of liver obtained following the intravenous administration of 185 MBq of ^{99m}Tc sulphur colloid. This study demonstrates marked metastatic involvement in the liver for this 41 y old female patient with breast carcinoma.

Hepatobiliary imaging

Radionuclide imaging studies play an important role in the study of the hepatobiliary system. Although ^{131}I rose bengal has been the principal radiopharmaceutical used to study this system for many years, recently ^{123}I rose bengal and several ^{99m}Tc labelled compounds, particularly the ^{99m}Tc labelled derivatives of iminodiacetic acid (IDA) and ^{99m}Tc labelled pyridoxylidene glutonate (PG), have made significant inroads into the study of acute cholecystitis and other hepatobiliary problems. These radiopharmaceuticals offer considerable advantage over the ^{131}I rose bengal in that improved image quality is obtained in the same or less time and the test is accompanied by less radiation dose to the patient. Serial images obtained with the ^{99m}Tc labelled radiopharmaceuticals visualise the extraction of the radiopharmaceutical from the blood by the hepatocytes and its excretion into the bile, accumulation in the gall bladder and final excretion into the gut.[116] Hepatobiliary imaging is particularly useful in the differentiation of surgical from nonsurgical jaundice and for the evaluation of cystic duct patency, offering a dynamic differentiation between chronic colecystitis and cystic duct obstruction. Other indications include the assessment of biliary reflux and postoperative status of the biliary system. The importance of being able to assess the clearance of the radiopharmaceutical makes it essential to conduct this procedure on a camera system which allows the collection of dynamic images.

Splenic imaging

The spleen may be imaged using either a colloidal preparation such as ^{99m}Tc sulphur colloid,

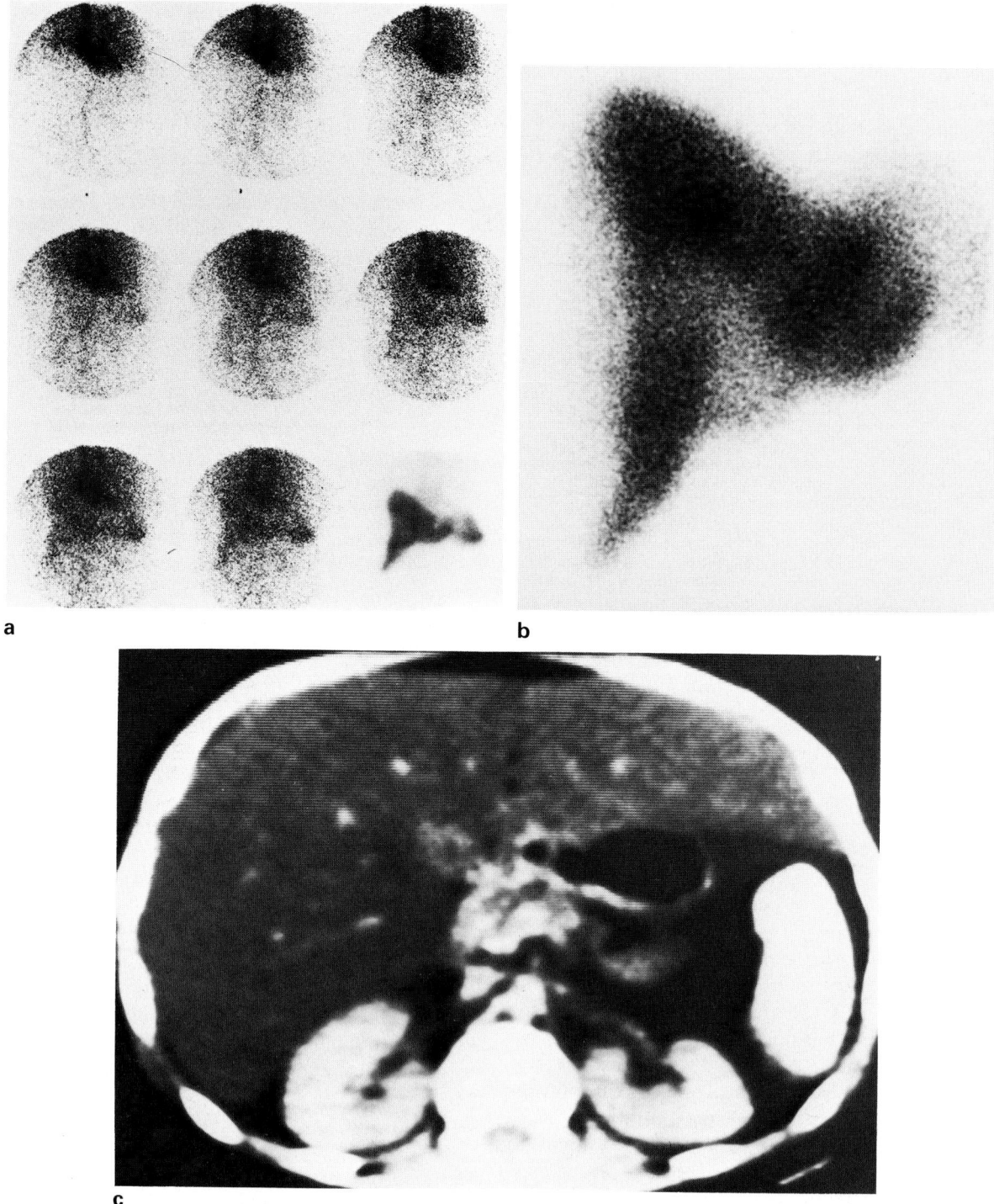

Fig. 3.26 (a) Serial, 3 s images obtained during ^{99m}Tc sulphur colloid perfusion study of the liver demonstrate displacement of the liver medially from the lateral body wall. (b) Right anterior oblique view of the liver demonstrates two filling defects, with the larger along the lateral wall and the smaller, more centrally placed. This 21 y old female complained of abdominal discomfort 2 days after minor trauma to the left upper quadrant of the abdomen. (c) CT section images of the liver were interpreted as normal. At operation, two subcapsular haemotomas were found.

currently the most widely used agent, or ^{99m}Tc labelled damaged red blood cells. The routine spleen imaging procedure is similar to that used for looking at the reticuloendothial component of the liver, namely, performance of a radionuclide angiogram and then multiple static images in a variety of projections. Clinical indications are also similar, including the assessment of involvement by tumour, abscess or trauma. Similarly, the relationship between the radionuclide approach, CT and/or ultrasonography is dependent upon the equipment and expertise available at a given institution.

Renal and genitourinary imaging

The choice of instrumentation and radiopharmaceutical combination is particularly critical in the study of the kidney. The selection must be based on the specific renal function measurements required in individual cases. For example, if it is wished to study the glomerular filtration of the kidney, an agent must be chosen specifically for this purpose. Labelled insulin and para-amino hippurate and ^{99m}Tc DTPA are radiopharmaceuticals which might be considered for this procedure. If the cortical region of the kidney is to be studied, a radiopharmaceutical should be chosen which maintains a significant residual fraction of the activity in the renal cortex following its primary clearance and excretion by the kidney. Mercury-197 (^{197}Hg) labelled chlormerodrin, ^{99m}Tc iron ascorbic acid, ^{99m}Tc DTPA, and ^{99m}Tc dimercaptosuccinic acid (DMSA) are frequently used for this diagnostic problem. Making use of conventional computer processing of camera imaging data, functional estimates of a variety of renal parameters can be determined. These include: gross blood flow, effective renal plasma flow, urinary extraction rates, differential renal function between kidneys or regions within the kidneys, urine flow calculations, bladder emptying capabilities, rate of bladder reflux with urination and residual volume determinations. The more important clinical applications include the study of the following problems.

Obstruction

Here a rapidly cleared agent such as ^{99m}Tc DTPA is used as the radiopharmaceutical of choice. This study is frequently combined with an ultrasound examination of the kidneys although dilated caliceal systems are usually quite easy to visualise on the radionuclide study.

Renal vascular hypertension

Here it is possible to calculate differential renal function, effective renal plasma flow and drainage capability by using either an agent such as ^{99m}Tc DTPA or ^{99m}Tc glucoheptonate. These studies are usually performed early in the workup of patients suspected of having renal vascular hypertension, both as a diagnostic and selective tool before going on to more complex and hazardous diagnostic procedures.[68]

Vascular problems

Agents such as ^{99m}Tc DTPA or glucoheptonate are used most commonly in conjunction with a gamma camera to allow differentiation of major and minor arterial obstructions, frequently avoiding the need for angiography. This approach is helpful also in the diagnosis of renal venous thrombosis.

Trauma

When the kidneys are evaluated for trauma, a radiopharmaceutical which localises in the cortex is most commonly used. ^{99m}Tc DMSA is preferred as it allows for the evaluation of the perfusion of the kidney and, in addition, provides for the determination of renal parenchymal damage from lacerations, contusions or haematoma. Frequently, CT or an ultrasound study is performed separately or in conjunction with this renal radionuclide study.[52] Once again, the initial choice of approach is quite dependent upon the equipment and expertise available within a given medical institution.

Renal transplants

Rapid perfusion imaging is usually the first step in evaluation of renal transplants to assess the patency and the function of the vascular graft. This study generally gives best results when performed with two different agents such as ^{99m}Tc DTPA and ^{123}I or ^{131}I labelled hippuran. It is the combined

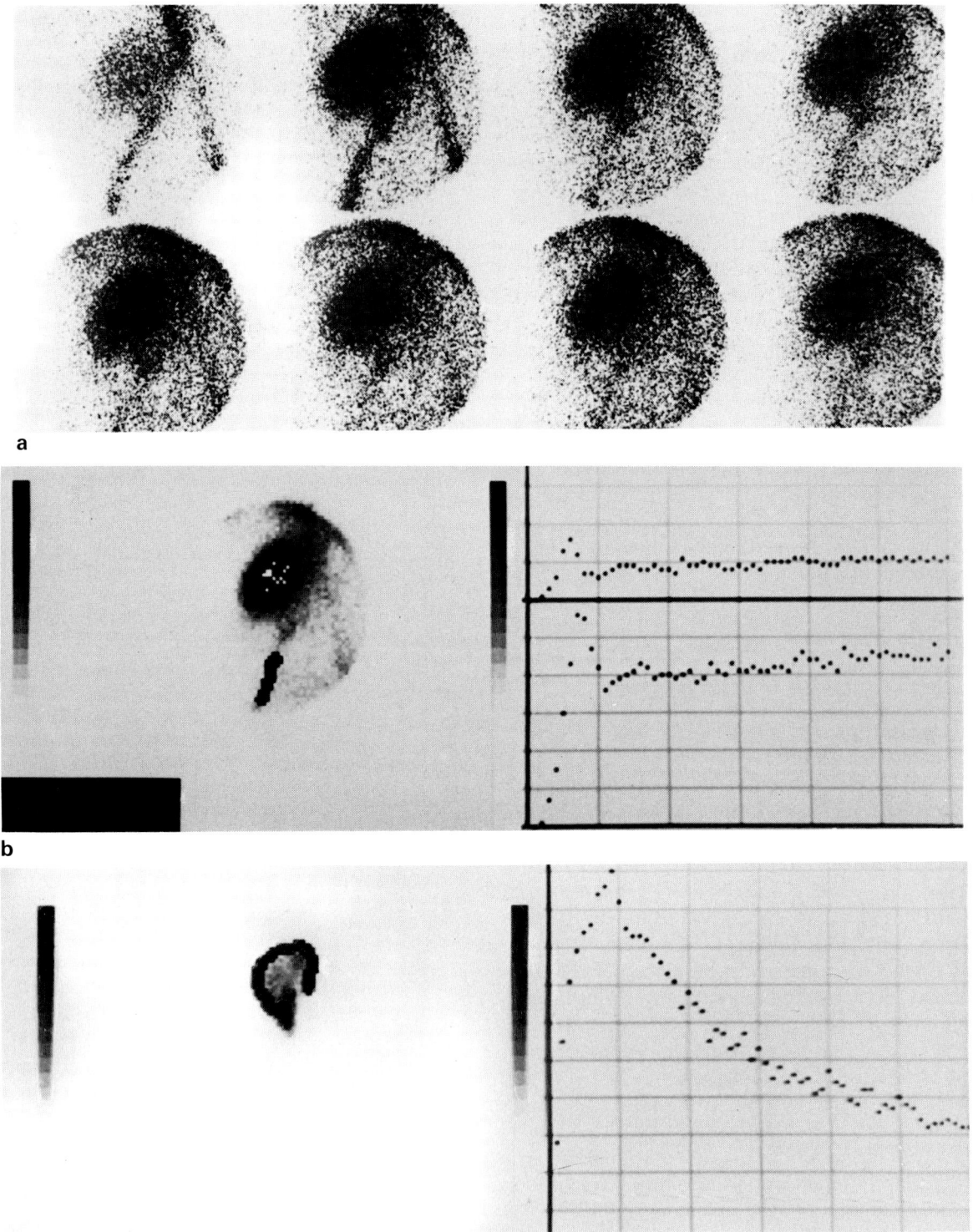

Fig. 3.27 Renal study in 18 y old male who is 3 d post cadaver renal transplant. (a) 3 s serial images obtained during radioisotopic angiogram performed after the bolus intravenous administration of 370 MBq of ^{99m}Tc DTPA. These demonstrate good vascular perfusion of the transplanted kidney. (b) Activity clearance curves obtained from the computer processed images in (a) confirm normal perfusion. (c) The renal activity clearance curve obtained from a subsequent study using 5 MBq of ^{131}I hippuran also demonstrates normal function of the transplanted kidney.

functional parameters which allow differentiation between acute tubular necrosis and acute or chronic rejection (Fig. 3.27).

Testicular pathology

Most cases of severe testicular disease may be readily differentiated on clinical grounds alone. Approximately 5 per cent of such cases need to be studied in order to differentiate testicular torsion from epididymitis, tumour or abscess. A perfusion and subsequent localisation imaging study of the testes, using ^{99m}Tc pertechnetate or ^{99m}Tc DTPA, differentiates testicular torsion from the other processes.[46] Testicular torsion and its lack of perfusion may also be accurately evaluated using Doppler ultrasonic imaging techniques. Such an approach is preferable, if available, since it contributes no radiation dose to the patient.

Radionuclide cystography

The draining capabilities of the bladder may be evaluated by directly instilling an agent, such as ^{99m}Tc pertechnetate, sulphur colloid or aggregates of albumin in sterile water or saline, into a catheterised bladder. Dynamic images of the bladder during micturition are obtained to determine if reflux is present or not. If computer processing capabilities are available, the amount of reflux as well as the residual volume can be determined.[78]

An indirect estimate of these abnormalities may be obtained by imaging the patient in the same manner using a renal agent which is rapidly cleared by the kidney. ^{99m}Tc DTPA has been found to be a suitable tracer for this approach to assessing reflux. This approach is frequently preferred since it provides a good estimate of renal function and bladder emptying dynamics while sparing the patient the discomfort of direct catheterisation of the bladder.

Endocrine imaging

Thyroid

Evaluation of thyroid function and anatomy remains the most common, by far, of all endocrine radionuclide imaging studies. ^{131}I has been the pri-

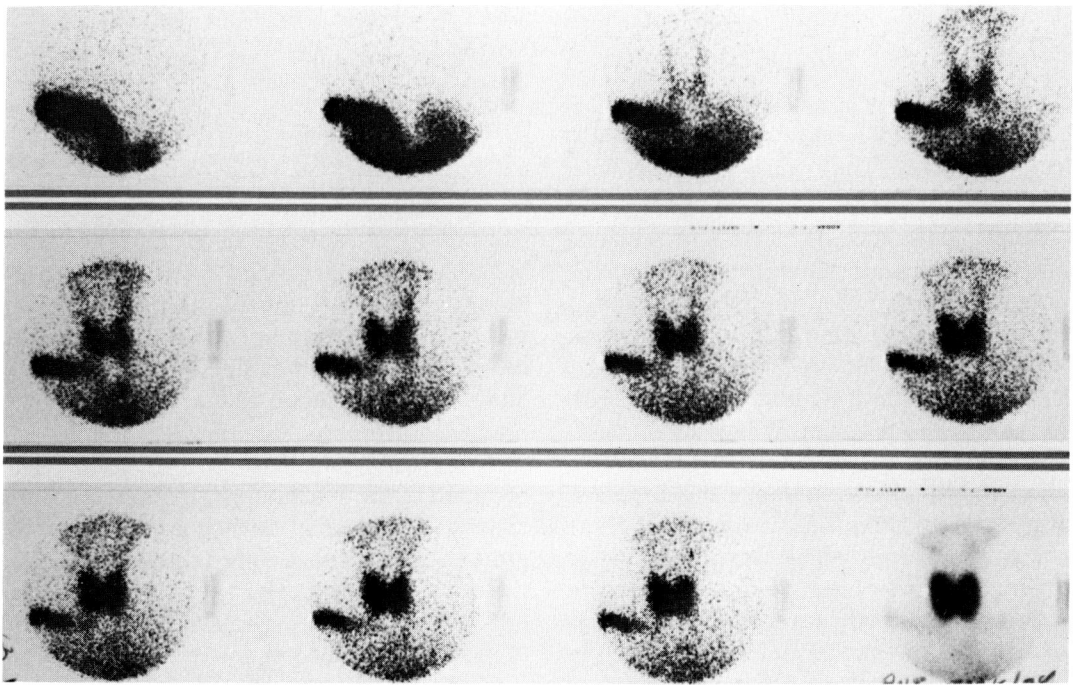

Fig. 3.28 Serial, 2 s images obtained following the intravenous administration of 185 MBq of ^{99m}Tc pertechnetate in a 22 y old female patient with Grave's disease. Note marked increase in vascularity to the thyroid gland, as well as early appearance of blood flow to the gland. A single anterior static image (lower right) shows a marked enlargement of the gland associated with greatly increased uptake of ^{99m}Tc pertechnetate.

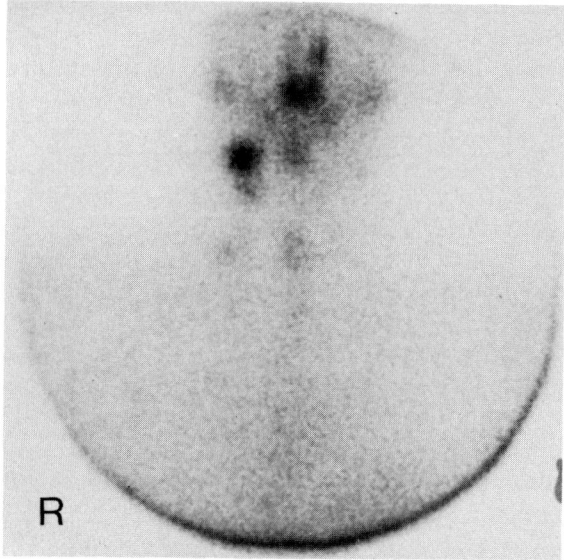

Fig. 3.29 Anterior image of the neck and upper chest performed 48 h after the oral administration of 185 MBq of ^{131}I as sodium iodide in a 23 y old male who had a mixed papillary follicular carcinoma of the thyroid removed 18 months prior to imaging. This study demonstrates abnormal activity in the thyroid bed and functioning metastatic activity in the right anterior cervical lymph node chain. The demonstration of function within the thyroid metastases makes this patient eligible for treatment with large dose ^{131}I therapy.

mary agent for imaging this gland although its use is decreasing in most major centres because of its high radiation dose to the patient and the thyroid gland. Newer agents include ^{99m}Tc pertechnetate (which images only the trapping capability of the gland) and ^{123}I.[65] Imaging of the thyroid gland is usually carried out with an evaluation of vascular perfusion of the gland followed by imaging of the gland morphology. These are best carried out with a SFOV camera, usually with pinhole or converging collimation.

The most widespread utilisation of this approach remains in the evaluation of the functional characteristics and workup of a patient with known or suspect nodular development within the gland to provide differentiation between benign and malignant nodules. It also remains an important step in the evaluation of hyperthyroid patients to assess the size of the gland (Fig. 3.28). Finally, it is an essential step in the determination of function within metastatic thyroid cancer (Fig. 3.29).[10]

Adrenal imaging

Imaging of the adrenal glands is performed following administration of an ^{131}I labelled compound, 6β-^{131}I-iodomethyl-19-nor cholest-5(10)-en-3β-ol (NP-59).[107] Subtraction techniques using ^{99m}Tc sulphur colloid and ^{99m}Tc gluconate are frequently used to enhance the image of the adrenal glands. The study is most commonly performed to allow differentiation of normal visualisation from that associated with adrenal hyperplasia.

Pancreas and hyperparathyroid imaging

These studies have been performed following the administration of ^{75}Se labelled selenomethionine in an attempt to provide differentiation between the presence and absence of neoplasm, cystic changes or hyperplasia in the case of the hyperparathyroid glands. In the area of the pancreas, pancreatic imaging has been replaced in most institutions by either ultrasound or CT procedures. If functional information is desired concerning presence and location of the parathyroid glands, this remains a viable study.

Tumour and inflammation imaging

Tumour imaging is most commonly performed following the administration of ^{67}Ga citrate. Other clinically applicable agents in current use would include ^{111}In chloride and ^{111}In bleomycin. These agents are most commonly visualised using total body imaging capabilities with a LFOV gamma camera system. Tomographic imaging devices enhance the appreciation of the location of abnormal uptake in neoplastic disease (Fig. 3.30).

To date, the most encouraging results have been obtained in the evaluation of lymphomas, lung carcinoma and several of the pediatric age tumour groups. These studies are performed not only in the initial staging workup of the patient as a baseline, but offer the best return in the evaluation of the efficacy of therapeutic regimens (Fig. 3.31).[43]

Gallium-67 citrate has shown itself to be useful in demonstrating the presence of inflammatory disease within the body. Best results are obtained with a total body imaging approach, as already men-

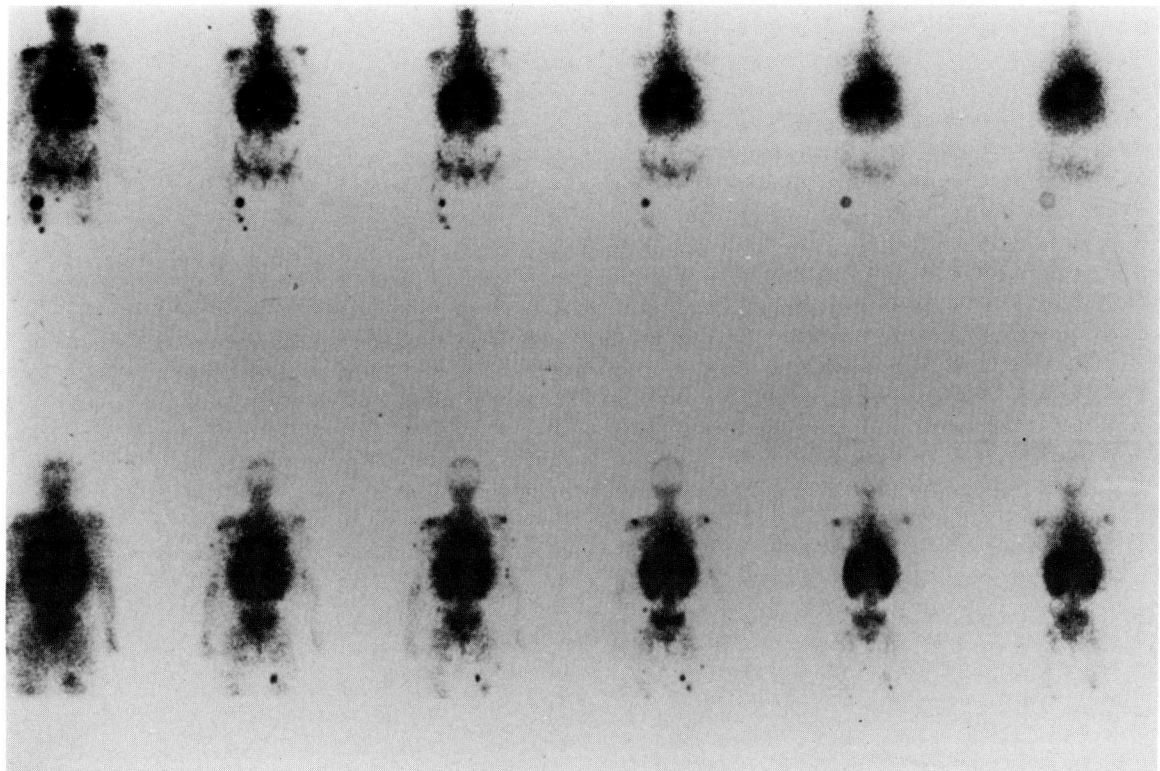

Fig. 3.30 Tomographic images obtained with a longitudinal plane tomographic scanner after the intravenous administration of ^{67}Ga citrate to a patient with lymphoma. The tomographic display begins with the most anterior view (upper left corner) and proceeds through the body in longitudinal fashion to the most posterior view (lower right corner). This study demonstrates abnormal activity in the mediastinal and inguinal nodal regions.

tioned. The uptake of ^{67}Ga is associated with the inflammatory change and not the true lesion mass (Fig. 3.32). As a result, the use of this technique has been best in the evaluation of patients with nonlocalising symptoms, such as fever of unknown origin, which suggests inflammatory disease. If a clinical situation presents where the symptoms of inflammatory disease are in a specific organ or area of the body, the first step should be ultrasonography or CT. The gallium scan may then be performed, if necessary, if no abscess or mass lesion is discovered by the other diagnostic modalities.

More specific radiopharmaceuticals for the detection of inflammatory disease are under investigation. Most promising of these would appear to be the ^{111}In oxine leucocytes. An investigation involving the latter radiopharmaceutical suggest that it may be a useful agent for the study of inflammatory disease.[96]

Miscellaneous

Salivary gland imaging

^{99m}Tc pertechnetate accumulates in the salivary glands and is excreted in the oral cavity. Adequate images of the salivary gland may be carried out with a gamma camera. This is useful in the evaluation of several disease entities affecting the salivary glands including tumour, Sjögren's syndrome and other causes of dry mouth.

Gastric mucosal imaging

^{99m}Tc pertechnetate is heavily concentrated by gastric mucosa, presumably by parietal cells. This property allows for imaging of gastric mucosa in normal and ectopic locations. The most common utilisation of this is in the demonstration of bleeding from Meckel's diverticulum, where serial scin-

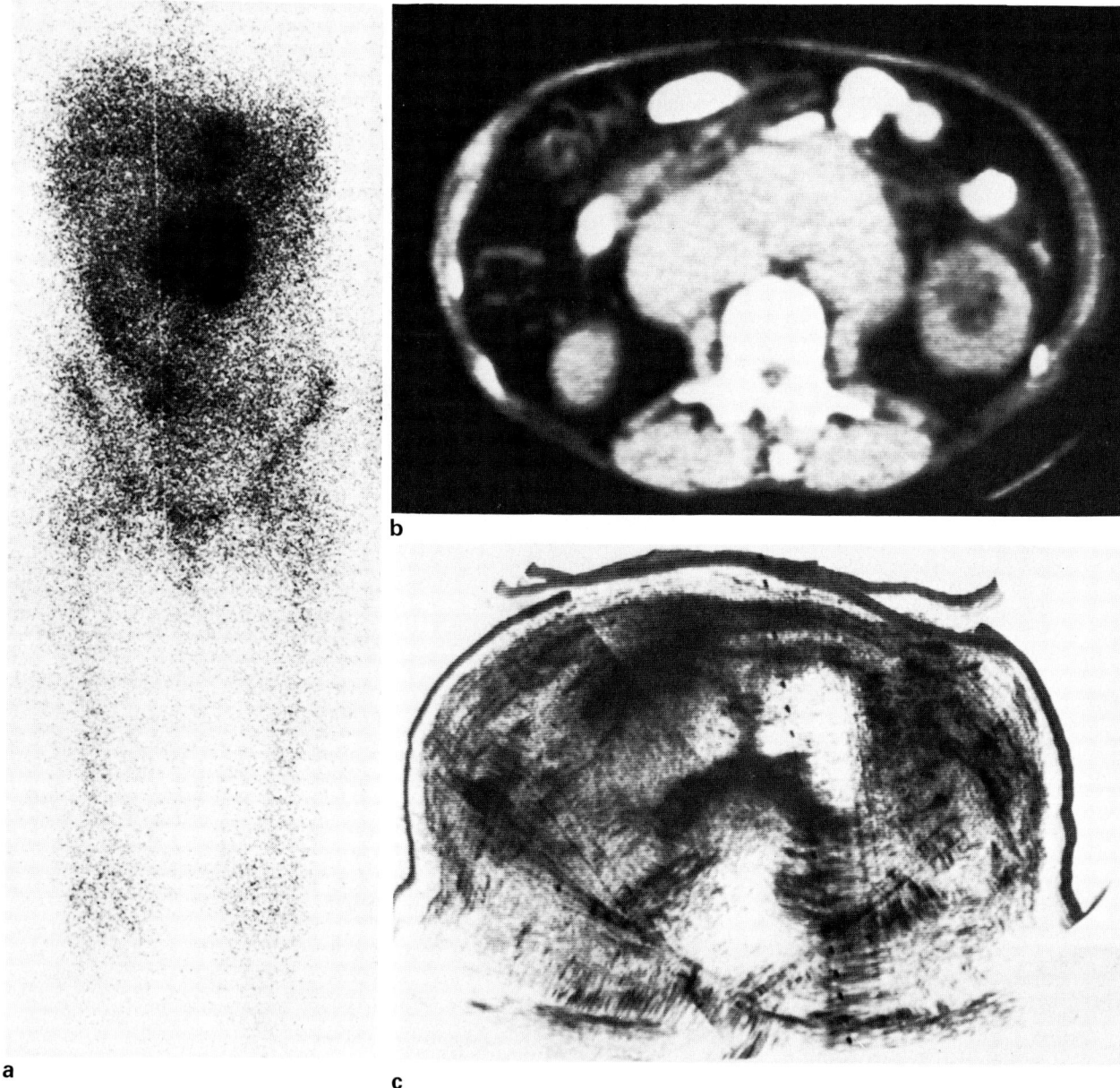

Fig. 3.31 (a) Anterior view of lower half of total body images performed with ^{67}Ga citrate as part of routine follow up evaluation of a 37 y old female with lymphoma. At this time, the patient was felt to be in clinical remission. This study demonstrates markedly abnormal ^{67}Ga accumulation in the paraaortic and abdominal lymph nodes. The (b) CT and (c) ultrasonic images correlate well with the abnormal findings demonstrated initially on the Ga-67 images.

tigrams of the abdomen are obtained following intravenous administration of ^{99m}Tc pertechnetate. In addition, this procedure is useful in the diagnosis of Barrett's œsophagus and in the demonstration of pulmonary and mediastinal cysts that contain gastric mucosa.

Stomach motility

Utilising test meals of liquid radiopharmaceuticals such as ^{99m}Tc sulphur colloid or ^{99m}Tc pertechnetate, it is easy to determine gastric emptying times, gastric absorption times and gastric reflux.

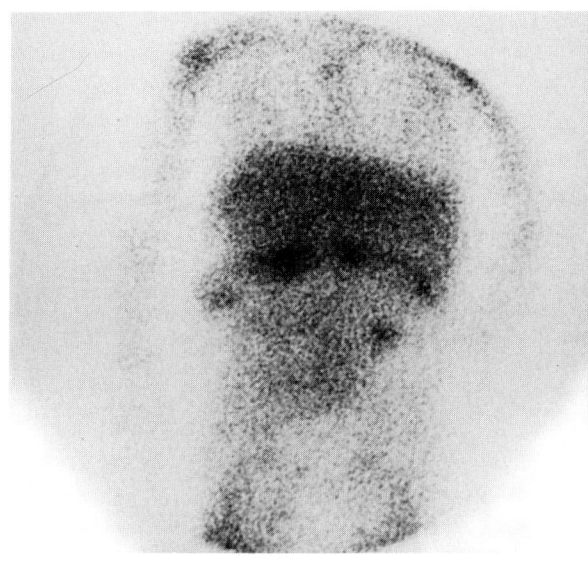

Fig. 3.32 Anterior ^{67}Ga image in a 3 y old male with fever of unknown origin occurring three weeks after surgical exploration of the abdomen for possible tumour. Multiple abnormal collections are seen along the surgical line and in the left lower quadrant. Ultrasonography was felt to be within normal limits. At surgery, these abnormal areas correlated with multiple pockets of inflammatory change and pus formation.

Thrombus detection

A variety of methods are employed for the detection of lower leg thrombophelebitis. These include scintillation probe measurements of ^{125}I fibrinogen and camera assays of radioisotopic venograms of agents such as ^{99m}Tc pertechnetate. ^{99m}Tc macroaggregated albumin is also used to demonstrate the flow venogram as well as the holdup of the particles on thrombi. Other radiopharmaceuticals that have had more limited clinical application include ^{111}In oxine labelled leucocytes and ^{99m}Tc plasmin.

Lacrimal duct imaging

In patients who have excessive lacrimation, the patency of the lacrimal duct may be readily assessed by imaging the clearance of a small volume of ^{99m}Tc pertechnetate which has been placed on the orbit. Serial images are recorded using a gamma camera with pinhole collimation. This provides visualisation of the passage of the radioactive material through the palpebral fissure to the lacrimal sac and into the nasal-lacrimal duct. This study is also useful for evaluating the postoperative efficacy of surgical procedures for restoration of duct flow.

SUMMARY

The direction of the development of radionuclide imaging procedures in nuclear medicine is progressively moving towards the assay of function and metabolism with less emphasis being given to procedures which only offer anatomical or structural information. Most of the newer imaging systems, including several of the ECT systems, offer dynamic as well as static imaging capabilities. A considerable amount of investigative effort is being directed to the development of radiopharmaceuticals which can be used to assess organ function and regional physiology. It is expected that as new procedures are introduced which make use of these developments, radionuclide imaging will play an increasingly significant role in patient care.

Acknowledgements

Figure 3.30 was kindly provided by Ernest Fordham. We are grateful to Technicare Corporation, Solon, Ohio, for Figure 3.4, to General Electric Company, Medical Systems Division, Milwaukee, Wisconsin, for Figures 3.6 and 3.8, and to Siemens Gammasonics, Nuclear Medicine Division, Des Plaines, Illinois, for Figure 3.11.

REFERENCES

1. Alderson, P. O., Gado, M. H. & Siegal, B. A. (1977) Computerized cranial tomography and radionuclide imaging in the detection of intracranial mass lesions. *Sem. nucl. Med.*, 7, 161–73.
2. Allen, H. C. Jr, Risser, J. R. & Green, J. A. (1954) Improvement in outlining of thyroid and localization of brain tumors by the application of sodium iodide gamma-ray spectrometry techniques. In *Proceedings of the 2nd Radioisotope Conference*, vol 1, p. 76. New York: Academic Press.

3. Allison, J. D. (1980) Cadmium telluride matrix gamma camera. *Med. Physics*, **7**, 202–6.
4. Anger, H. O. (1958) Scintillation camera. *Rev. Sci. Instr.*, **29**, 27–33.
5. Anger, H. O. (1968) Tomographic gamma-ray scanner with simultaneous readout of several planes. In *Fundamental Problems in Scanning*, ed. Gottschalk, A. & Beck, R. N., pp. 195–211. Springfield: Thomas.
6. Anger, H. O. (1974) Tomography and other depth-discrimination techniques. In *Instrumentation in Nuclear Medicine*, ed. Hine G. J. & Sorenson, J. A., vol 2, pp. 61–100. New York: Academic Press.
7. Atkins, H. L., Robertson, J. S., Croft, B. Y., Tsui, B., Susskind, H., Ellis, K. J., Loken, M. K. & Treves, S. (1980) MIRD dose estimate report no. 9, estimates of radiation doses from radioxenons in lung imaging. *J. nucl. Med.*, **21**, 459–65.
8. Barrett, H. H., Wilson, D. T. & De Meester, G. D. (1973) Fresnel zone plate imaging in radiology and nuclear medicine. *Opt. Eng.*, **12**, 8–12.
9. Bauer, G., Weber, D. A., Ceder, L., Egund, N, Hansson, L. I. & Stromqvist, B. (1980). Dynamics of Tc-99m methylenediphosphonate imaging of the femoral head following hip fracture. *Clin. Orthop. Rel. Res.* **152**, 85–92.
10. Beierwaltes, W. H. (1978) Treatment of thyroid carcinoma with radioactive iodine. *Sem. nucl. Med.*, **8**, 79–94.
11. Bender, M. A. & Blau, M. (1960) Autofluoroscopy: the use of a non-scanning device for tumor localization with radioisotopes. *J. nucl. Med.*, **1**, 105.
12. Berger, H. J., Gottschalk, A. & Zaret, B. (1978) First-pass radionuclide angiocardiography for evaluation of right and left ventricular performance: computer applications and technical considerations. In *Nuclear Cardiology: Selected Computer Aspects*, pp. 29–44. New York: Society of Nuclear Medicine.
13. Berger, H. J., Matthay, R. A., Pytlik, L. M., Gottschalk, A & Zaret, B. L. (1979) First-pass radionuclide assessment of right and left ventricular performance in patients with cardiac and pulmonary disease. *Sem. nucl. Med.*, **9**, 275–95.
14. Bowley, A. R., Taylor, C. G., Causer, D. A., Barber, D. C., Keyes, W. I., Undrill, P. E., Corfield, J. R. & Mallard, J. R. (1973) A radioisotope scanner for rectilinear, arc, transverse section and longitudinal section scanning: (ASS-the Aberdeen Section Scanner). *Br. J. Radiol.*, **46**, 262–71.
15. Brookeman, V. A. (1980) Performance characteristics of seven-pinhole tomography. *J. nucl. Med.*, **21**, 28.
16. Brookeman, V. A. & Hilson, A. J. W. (1980) The use of seven-pinhole tomography in liver imaging, a phantom and clinical evaluation. *J. nucl. Med.*, **21**, 87–8.
17. Brownell, G. L., Burnham, C. A., Chesler, D. A., Correia, J. A., Correll, J. E., Hoop, B. Jr, Parker, J. A. & Subramanyam, R. (1977) Transverse section imaging of radionuclide distributions in the heart, lung and brain. In *Reconstruction Tomography in Diagnostic Radiology and Nuclear Medicine*, ed. Ter-Pogossian, M. M., Phelps, M. E., Brownell, G. L., Cox Jr, J. R., David, D. O. & Evens, R. G., pp. 293–307. Baltimore: University Park Press.
18. Brownell, G. L., Correia, J. A. & Zamenhof, R. G. (1978) Positron instrumentation. In *Recent Advances in Nuclear Medicine*, ed. Lawrence, J. H. & Budinger T. F., vol 5, pp. 1–49. New York: Grune and Stratton.
19. Budinger, T. F. (1977) Instrumentation trends in nuclear medicine. *Sem. nucl. Med.*, **7**, 285–97.
20. Budinger, T. F., Derengo, S. E., Gullberg, G. T., Greenberg, W. L. & Huesman, R. H. (1977) Emission computer assisted tomography with single-photon and positron annihilation photon emitters. *J. Comput. Assist. Tomog.*, **1**, 131–45.
21. Buell, U, Kazner, E., Rath, M., Steinhoff, H., Kleinhans, E. & Lanksch, W. (1979) Sensitivity of computed tomography in serial scintigraphy and cerebral vascular disease. *Radiology*, **131**, 393–8.
22. Cassen, B., Curtis, L., Reed, C. & Libby, R. (1951) Instrumentation of I-131 used in medical studies. *Nucleonics*, **9**, 46–50.
23. Chio, M. Y., Barrett, R. G., Simpson, C., Arendt, J. W. & Gindi, G. R. (1969) Three-dimensional radiographic imaging with a restricted view angle. *J. opt. Soc. Am.*, **69** (issue no 10).
24. Cho, Z. H., Eriksson, L. & Chan, J. (1977) A circular ring transverse axial positron camera. In *Reconstruction Tomography in Diagnostic Radiology and Nuclear Medicine*, ed. Ter-Pogossian, M. M., Phelps, M. E., Brownell, G. L., Cox Jr, J. R., David, D. O. & Evens, R. G., pp. 393–421. Baltimore: University Park Press.
25. Cho, Z. H. & Farukhi, M. R. (1977) Bismuth germanate as a potential scintillation detector in positron cameras. *J. nucl. Med.*, **18**, 840–4.
26. DeLand, F. H., Kim, E. E., Domstad, P. A. & Magoun, S. L. (1980) Contributions of the seven-pinhole collimator to cisternography. *J. nucl. Med.*, **21**, 88.
27. Dillman, L. T. & Von der Lage, F. C. (1975) Radionuclide decay schemes and nuclear parameters for use in radiation-dose estimation. NM/MIRD Pamphlet no 10. New York: Society of Nuclear Medicine.
28. Ehrhardt, J. C., Oberley, L. W. & Cuevas, J. M. (1978) *Imaging Ability of Collimators in Nuclear Medicine.* Rockville: US Department of Health, Education and Welfare, HEW Publication (FDA) 79–8077.
29. Enzmann, D. R., Norman, D., Price, D. C. & Newton, T. H. (1979) Metrizamide and radionuclide cisternography in communicating hydrocephalus. *Radiology*, **130**, 681–6.
30. Ewins, J. H., Armantrout, G. A., Camp, D. C., Kaufman, L., Hattner, R. S., Price, D. C., Larenz, V. S., Hosier, K. E. & Lee, K. L. (1977) A clinical high purity germanium gamma-camera. In *Proceedings of the International Symposium on Medical Radionuclide Imaging*, vol I, p. 149, IAEA SM-210/62.
31. Folland, E. D., Hamilton, G. W., Steven, M. L., Kennedy, J. W., Williams, D. L. & Ritchie, J. L. (1977) The radionuclide ejection fraction: A comparison of three radionuclide techniques with contrast angiography. *J. nucl. Med.*, **18**, 1159–66.
32. Fordham, E. W. (1977) The complementary role of computerized axial transmission tomography and radionuclide imaging of the brain. *Sem. nucl. Med.*, **7**, 139–59.
33. Francis, J. E., Bell, B. R. & Harris, C. C. (1955) Medical scintillation spectrometry. *Nucleonics*, **13**, 82–8.
34. Freeman, L. M. & Blaufox, M. D. (ed) (1971) Radionuclide studies of the central nervous system. *Sem. nucl. Med.*, **1**, (issue no 1).
35. Front, D., Hardoff, R. & Robinson, E. (1978) Bone

scintigraphy in primary tumors of the head and neck. *Cancer*, **42**, 111–7.
36. Gilbert, E. H., Earle, J. D., Glatstein, E., Gloris, M. L., Kaplan, H. S. & Kriss, J. P. (1976) Indium-111 bone marrow scintigraphy as an aid in selecting marrow biopsy sites for the evaluation of marrow elements in patients with lymphoma. *Cancer*, **38**, 1560–7.
37. Gilday, D. L., Paul, D. J. & Paterson, J. (1975) Diagnosis of osteomyelitis in children by combined blood pool and bone imaging. *Radiology*, **117**, 331–5.
38. Glass, H. I. & Silvester, D. J. (1970) Review article: cyclotrons in nuclear medicine. *Br. J. Radiol.*, **43**, 589–601.
39. Gottschalk, S. C., Smith, K. A., Wake, R. H. (1980) Comparison of seven pinhole and rotating slant tomography of a cardiac phantom. *J. nucl. Med.*, **21**, 27.
40. Graham, L. S. & Perez-Mendez, V. (1977) Special imaging devices. In *Nuclear Medicine Physics, Instrumentation, and Agents*, ed. Rollo, F. D., pp. 271–321. St. Louis: C V Mosby.
41. Hauser, M. F. & Gottschalk, A. (1978) Comparison of the Anger tomographic scanner and the 15-in. scintillation camera for gallium imaging. *J. nucl. Med.*, **19**, 1074–7.
42. Hayes, M. (1980) Lung imaging with radioaerosols for the assessment of airway disease. *Sem. nucl. Med.*, **10**, 243–51.
43. Herman, T. S. & Jones, S. E. (1978) Systematic restaging in patients with Hodgkin's disease: a southwest oncology group study. *Cancer*, **42**, 1976–82.
44. Hine, G. J. & Erickson, J. J. (1974) Advances in scintigraphic instruments. In *Instrumentation in Nuclear Medicine*, ed. Hine, G. J. & Sorenson, J. A., pp. 1–59. New York: Academic Press.
45. Hoffer, P. B., Bekerman, C. & Henkin, R. E. (eds) (1978) *Gallium-67 Imaging*. New York: Wiley.
46. Holder, L. E., Martire, E. R. H. & Wagner, H. N. Jr (1977) Testicular radionuclide angiography and static imaging: Anatomy, scintigraphic interpretation and clinical indications. *Radiology*, **125**, 739–52.
47. Holmes, R. A. (1978) Quantification of skeletal Tc-99m labeled phosphates to detect metabolic bone disease. *J. nucl. Med.*, **19**, 330–1.
48. ICRU Report 32 (1979) *Methods of Assessment of Absorbed Dose in Clinical Use of Radionuclides*, pp. 1–22. Washington: International Commission on Radiation Units and Measurements.
49. Jaszczak, R. J., Murphy, P. H., Huard, D. & Burdine, J. A. (1977) Radionuclide emission computed tomography of the head with Tc-99m and a scintillation camera. *J. nucl. Med.*, **18**, 373–80.
50. Moore, F. E. (1979) Whole-body single-photon emission computed tomography using dual, large-field-of-view scintillation cameras. *Phys. Med. Biol.*, **24**, 1123–43.
51. Johns, H. E. & Cunningham, J. R. (1969) *The Physics of Radiology*, pp. 674–86. Springfield, Illinois: Thomas.
52. Kahn, P. (1979) Renal imaging with radionuclides, ultrasound, and computed tomography. *Sem. nucl. Med.*, **9**, 43–9.
53. Kaufman, L., Camp, D. C., McQuaid, J. H., Armantroul, G. & Lee, K. (1974) Delay line readouts for high purity germanium medical imaging cameras. *IEEE Trans. nucl. Sci.*, **NS-21**, 625.
54. Keyes, J. W., Jr, Orlandea, N., Heetderks, W. J., Leonard, P. F. & Rogers, W. L. (1977) The humongotron-a scintillation-camera transaxial tomograph. *J. nucl. Med.*, **18**, 381–7.
55. Kim, H. R., Thrall, J. H. & Keyes, J. W. Jr (1979) Skeletal scintigraphy following incidental trauma. *Radiology*, **130**, 447–51.
56. Kolvas, E., Rosenthall, L., Ahronheim, G. A., Lisbona, R. & Marks, M. I. (1978) Serial Ga-67 citrate imaging during treatment of acute osteomyelitis in childhood. *Clin. nucl. Med.*, **3**, 461–6.
57. Koral, K. G., Rogers, W. L., Knoll, G. F. (1975) Digital tomographic imaging with time-modulated pseudorandom coded aperture and Anger camera. *J. nucl. Med.*, **16**, 402–13.
58. Kristensen, K. (1979) Quality control analysis at the hospital. In *Radiopharmaceuticals II: Proceedings 2nd International Symposium on Radiopharmaceuticals*, pp. 1–14. New York: Society of Nuclear Medicine.
59. Kuhl, D. E., Chamberlain, R. H., Hale, J. & Gorson, R. P. (1956) A high-contrast photographic recorder scintillation counter scanning. *Radiology*, **66**, 730–9.
60. Kuhl, D. E., Edwards, R. Q., Ricci, A. R., Yacob, R. J., Mich, T. J. & Alavi, A. (1976) The MARK IV system for radionuclide computed tomography of the brain. *Radiology*, **121**, 405–13.
61. Lambrecht, R. M. (1979) Positron-emitting radionuclides-present and future status. In *Radiopharmaceuticals II: Proceedings 2nd International Symposium on Radiopharmaceuticals*, pp. 753–66. New York: Society of Nuclear Medicine.
62. Li, D. K., Treves, S., Heyman, S., Kirkpatrick, J. A., Lambrecht, R. M., Ruth, T. J. & Wolf, A. P. (1979) Krypton-81m: a better radiopharmaceutical for assessment of regional lung function in children. *Radiology*, **130**, 741–7.
63. Lim, C. B., Chu, D., Kaufman, L., Perez-Mendez, V., Hattner, R. & Price, D. C. (1975) Initial characterization of a multi-wire proportional chamber positron camera. *IEEE Trans. nucl. Sci.* **NS-22**, 388–94.
64. Lin, M. S. & Goodwin, D. A. (1976) Pulmonary distribution of inhaled radioaerosol in obstructive pulmonary disease. *Radiology*, **118**, 645–51.
65. Massin, J. P., Planchon, E. & Perez, R. (1977) Comparison of Tc-99m pertechnetate and I-131 in scanning of thyroid nodules. *Clin. nucl. Med.*, **2**, 324–33.
66. Mauderli, W., Luthmann, R. W., Fitzgerald, L. T., Urie, M. M., Williams, C. M., Tosswill, C. H. & Entine, G. (1979) A computerized rotating laminar radionuclide camera. *J. nucl. Med.*, **20**, 341–4.
67. McAfee, J. G. & Subramanian, G. (1975) Radioactive agents for imaging. In *Clinical Scintillation Imaging*, ed. Freeman, L. M. & Johnson, P. M., 2nd ed, pp. 13–114. New York: Grune and Stratton.
68. McAfee, J. G., Thomas, F. D., Grossman, Z., Streeten, D. H. P., Dailey, E. & Gagne, G. (1977) Diagnosis of angiotensinogenic hypertension: the complementary roles of renal scintigraphy and the saralasin infusion test. *J. nucl. Med.*, **18**, 669–75.
69. McNeil, B. (1976) A diagnostic strategy using ventilation-perfusion studies in patients suspect for pulmonary embolism. *J. nucl. Med.*, **17**, 613–6.
70. McNeil, B., Pace, P. D., Gray, E. B., Adelstein, S. J. & Wilson, R. E. (1978) Preoperative and follow-up bone scans in patients with primary carcinoma of the breast. *Surg. Gynec. Obstet.*, **147**, 745–8.

71. MIRD Dose Estimate Report No. 2 (1973) Summary of current radiation dose estimates to humans from Ga-66, Ga-68 and Ga-72 Citrate. *J. nucl. Med.*, **14**, 755–6.
72. MIRD Dose Estimate Report No. 3 (1975) Summary of current radiation dose estimates to humans with various liver conditions from Tc-99m sulfur colloid. *J. nucl. Med.*, **16**, 108A–B.
73. MIRD Dose Estimate Report No. 5 (1975) Summary of current radiation dose estimates to humans from I-123, I-124, I-125, I-126, I-130, I-131 and I-132 as sodium iodide. *J. nucl. Med.*, **16**, 857–60.
74. MIRD Dose Estimate Report No. 8 (1976) Summary of current radiation dose estimates to normal humans from Tc-99m as sodium pertechnetate. *J. nucl. Med.*, **17**, 74–7.
75. Moore, R., Alpert, W., Lazewatsky, J. & Strauss, H. (1980) Variable angle slant hole collimator. *J. nucl. Med.*, **21**, 28–9
76. Muehllehner, G., Atkins, E. & Harper, P. V. (1977) Positron camera with longitudinal and transverse tomographic ability. In *Medical Radionuclide Imaging*, vol I, pp. 291–307. Vienna: IAEA.
77. Muroff, L. R. & Freedman, G. S. (1976) Radionuclide angiography. *Sem. nucl. Med.*, **6**, 217–30.
78. Nasrallah, P. F., Conway, J. J., King, L. R., Gelman, A. B. & Weiss, S. (1978) Quantitative nuclear cystogram: aid in determining spontaneous resolution of vesicoureteral reflux. *Urology*, **12**, 654–8.
79. Newell, R. R., Saunders, W. & Miller, E. (1952) Multichannel collimators for gamma-ray scanning with scintillation counters. *Nucleonics*, **10**, 36–45.
80. Nickles, R. J. & Meyer, H. O. (1978) Design of a three dimensional positron camera for nuclear medicine. *Phys. Med. Biol.*, **23**, 686–95.
81. O'Mara, R. E. & Mozley, J. M. (1971) Current status of brain scanning. *Sem. nucl. Med.*, **1**, 7–30.
82. Oppenheim, B. E., Hoffer, P. B. & Gottschalk, A. (1976) Nuclear imaging: a new dimension. *Radiology*, **118**, 491–4.
83. Ortendahl, D. A., Kaufman, L., Rowan, W., Herfkens, R. & Price, D. (1980) Recent developments in single photon emission computed tomography with a small germanium camera. *J. nucl. Med.*, **21**, 17.
84. Parisi, A. A., Tow, D. E., Felix, W. R. & Sasahara, A. A. (1977) Noninvasive cardiac diagnosis; Parts I, II and III. *New Engl. J. Med.*, **296**, 316–320, 368–74, 427–32.
85. Parkey, R. W., Bonte, F. J., Buja, L. M., Stokely, E. M. & Willerson, J. T. (1977) Myocardial infarct imaging with Tc-99m phosphates. *Sem. nucl. Med.*, **8**, 15–28.
86. Petasnick, J. P., Ram, P, Turner, A. A. & Fordham, E. W. (1979) The relationship of computed tomography, gray-scale ultrasonography and radionuclide imaging in the evaluation of hepatic masses. *Sem. nucl. Med.*, **9**, 8–21.
87. Phelps, M. E. (1977) Emission computed tomography. *Sem. nucl. Med.*, **7**, 337–65.
88. Ramanna, L., Tashkin, D. P., Taplin, G. V., Elam, D., Detels, R., Coulson, A. & Rokaw, S. N. (1975) Radioaerosol lung imaging in chronic obstructive pulmonary disease: comparison with pulmonary function tests and roentgenography. *Chest*, **68**, 634–40.
89. Renaud, L., Joy, M. L. G. & Gilday, D. L. (1979) Fourier multiaperture emission tomography (FMET). *J. nucl. Med.*, **20**, 986–91.
90. Richardson, R. L. (1977) Anger scintillation camera. In *Nuclear Medicine Physics, Instrumentation, and Agents*, ed. Rollo, F. D., pp. 231–70. St. Louis: Mosby.
91. Robertson, J. S., Marr, R. B., Rosenblum, M., Radeka, V. & Yarnamoto, Y. L. (1973) 32-Crystal positron tranverse section detector. In *Tomographic Imaging in Nuclear Medicine*, ed. Freedman, G. S., pp. 142–53. New York: Society of Nuclear Medicine.
92. Rocha, A. F. G. & Harbert, J. C. (1979) *Textbook of Nuclear Medicine: Clinical Applications*, pp. 84–108. Philadelphia: Lea & Febiger.
93. Rogers, W. L., Koral, K. F., Mayans, R., Leonard, P. F., Thrall, J. H., Brady, T. J. & Keyes, J. W. Jr (1980) Coded-aperture imaging of the heart. *J. nucl. Med.*, **21**, 371–8.
94. Rollo, F. D. (1977) Evaluating imaging devices. In *Nuclear Medicine Physics, Instrumentation, and Agents*, ed. Rollo, F. D., pp. 436–52. St Louis: Mosby.
95. Rudd, T. G., Allen, D. R. & Smith, F. D. (1979) Technetium-99m-labeled methylene diphosphonate and hydroxyethylidine diphosphonate-biologic and clinical comparison: concise communication. *J. nucl. Med.*, **20**, 821–6.
96. Segal, A. W., Deteix, P., Garcia, R., Tooth, P., Zanelli, G. D. & Allison, A. C. (1978) Indium-111 labeling of leukocytes: a detrimental effect on neutrophil and lymphocyte function and an improved method of cell labeling. *J. nucl. Med.*, **19**, 1238–44.
97. Shosa, D. W., O'Connell, J. W. & Hattner, R. S. (1980) Motivation for the rotating slant hole approach to scintillation camera tomography. *J. nucl. Med.*, **21**, 27.
98. Siddiqui, A. R., Wellman, H. N., Weetman, R. M. & Smith, W. L. (1979) Bone scanning in management of metastatic osteogenic sarcoma. *Clin. nucl. Med.*, **4**, 6–11.
99. Silvester, D. J. & Waters, S. L. (1979) Radionuclide production. In *Radiopharmaceuticals II: Proceedings 2nd International Symposium on Radiopharmaceuticals*, pp. 727–44. New York: Society of Nuclear Medicine.
100. Stokely, E. M., Sveinsdottir, E., Lassen, N. A. & Rommer, P. (1980) A single photon dynamic computer assisted tomograph (DCAT) for imaging brain function in multiple cross sections. *J. Comput. Assist. Tomog.*, **4**, 230–40.
101. Strauss, H. W. & Pitt, B. (1977) Thallium-201 as a myocardial imaging agent. *Sem. nucl. Med.*, **7**, 49–58.
102. Strauss, H. W., McKusick, K. A., Boucher, C. A., Bingham, J. B. & Pohost, G. M. (1979) Of linens and laces – the eighth anniversary of the gated blood pool scan. *Sem. nucl. Med.*, **9**, 296–309.
103. Subramanian, G. & McAfee, J. G. (1971) A new complex of Tc-99m for skeletal imaging. *Radiology*, **99**, 192–96.
104. Subramanian, G., McAfee, J. G., Blair, R. J., Kallfelz, F. A. & Thomas, F. D. (1975) Technetium-99m-methylene diphosphonate – a superior agent for skeletal imaging: comparison with other complexes. *J. nucl. Med.*, **16**, 744–55.
105. Ter-Pogossian, M. M., Phelps, M. E., Hoffman, E. J. & Mullani, N. A. (1975) A positron-emission transaxial tomograph for nuclear imaging (PETT). *Radiology*, **114**, 89–98.
106. Ter-Pogossian, M. M. (1977) Basic principles of computed axial tomography. *Sem. nucl. Med.*, **7**, 109–28.
107. Thrall, J. H., Freitas, J. E. & Beierwaltes, W. H. (1978) Adrenal scintigraphy. *Sem. nucl. Med.*, **8**, 23–41.
108. Vogel, R. A., Kirch, D., LaFree, M. & Steele, P.

(1978) A new method of multiplanar emission tomography using a seven pinhole collimator and Anger scintillation camera. *J. nucl. Med.*, **18**, 648–54.
109. Vogel, R. A., Kirch, D. L., LeFree, M. T., Rainwater, J. O., Jensen, D. P. & Steele, P. P. (1979) Thallium-201 myocardial perfusion scintigraphy: results of standard and multi-pinhole tomographic techniques. *Am. J. Cardiol.*, **43**, 787–93.
110. Wagner, H. N. Jr & Emmons, H. (1966) Characteristics of an ideal radiopharmaceutical. In *Radioactive Pharmaceuticals*, ed. Andrews, G. A., Kniseley, R. M. & Wagner, H. N. Jr, pp. 1–32. Oak Ridge: USAEC, CONF-651111.
111. Weber, D. A., Keyes, J. W. Jr, Benedetto, W. J. & Wilson, G. A. (1974) Tc-99m pyrophosphate for diagnostic bone imaging. *Radiology*, **113**, 131–7.
112. Weber, D. A., Keyes, J. W. Jr, Wilson, G. A. & Landman, S. (1976) Kinetics and imaging characteristics of ^{99m}Tc labeled complexes used for bone imaging. *Radiology*, **120**, 615–21
113. Weber, D. A. (1978) Computers in nuclear medicine-introductory concepts. *Sem. nucl. Med.*, **8**, 107–12.
114. Weber, D. A., Bauer, G. C. H., Hansson, L. I., Ceder, L., Darte, L., Stigsson, L. & Egund, N. (1980) Tc-99m MDP imaging as an early test for femoral head osteonecrosis. *J. nucl. Med.*, **21**, 19–20.
115. Weber, D. A., Wilson, G. A. & O'Mara, R. E. (In press) Computers in nuclear medicine. In *Handbook of Medical Physics*, ed. Waggener, R. West Palm Beach: CRC Press.
116. Weissman, H. S., Frank, M., Rosenblatt, R., Goldman, M. & Freeman, L. M., (1979) Cholescintigraphy, ultrasonography and computerized tomography in the evaluation of biliary tract disorders. *Sem. nucl. Med.*, **9**, 22–35.
117. Williamson, B. R. J., Teates, C. D., Howard, B. Y., Barczak, R. J. & Mosby, R. (1977) Clinical evaluation of the Cleon Imager. *J. nucl. Med.*, **18**, 1123–7.
118. Winchell, H. S., Sanchez, P. D., Watanake, C. K., Hollander, L., Anger, H. O. & McRae, J., (1970) Visualization of tumors in humans using Ga-67 citrate and the Anger whole-body scanner, scintillation camera and tomographic camera. *J. nucl. Med.*, **11**, 459–66.

4

Ultrasonic imaging

P. N. T. Wells

FUNDAMENTAL PHYSICS OF ULTRASOUND*

Ultrasonic waves

The pitch, or frequency, of the sound which can be heard by normal young people occupies a fairly well-defined section of the spectrum of the frequency of mechanical vibration. Sound frequencies extend from about 20–20 000 Hz. (1 Hz (hertz) = 1 cycle/second. Thus, 1 kHz = 1000 c/s, 1 MHz = 1 000 000 c/s.) For example, the middle C note in music has a frequency of 256 Hz. The term *ultrasound* is used to describe 'sound' the frequency of which is beyond the sonic, or audible, range.

Like sound, ultrasound travels through a medium at a definite *speed*. Everyone is familiar with the delay which occurs between, for example, a distant flash of lighting and the following clap of thunder, due to the sound travelling at much lower speed than the light. Sound travels in the form of a *wave*, and (unlike electromagnetic radiation such as radio waves, light and X-rays) the wave is really a mechanical disturbance of the medium through which the sound energy is being transported. An example of this kind of wave motion can be seen as waves spread out on the surface of water into which a stone has been thrown; meanwhile, other, invisible, pressure waves—called *longitudinal* waves—travel through the water under the surface.

Ultrasonic longitudinal waves are used in medical diagnostic applications. Ultrasonic diagnosis depends upon physical measurements of the ways in which ultrasonic waves interact with biological materials, especially with the soft tissue structures of the body.

Any medium may be considered to be made up of very many tiny particles. Each particle contains many millions of molecules, so that it is continuous with its surroundings, but it is so small that ultrasonic wave variables in the medium (such as pressure) are constant within it. In the absence of an ultrasonic disturbance, the particles are at rest, each in a particular position in the medium. A wave travels through the medium as a result of the transmission of the disturbance between neighbouring particles. The *speed* at which the wave travels depends upon the coupling between particles (the *elasticity* of the medium) and their inertia (which in turn depends on the *density* of the medium, since this controls the acceleration for a given force).†

The speed, measured in metres/second (m s^{-1}) in biological materials are indicated in Figure 4.1. For practical purposes, the speed in any given material is effectively independent of the frequency of the ultrasound.

Wave motion can be represented graphically as illustrated in Figure 4.2. If the wave is moving forward at a speed = c, and the wavelength = λ when the frequency = f, it follows that the speed is equal to the product of the wavelength and the frequency, since the frequency is equal to the number of cycles (each one wavelength long) which pass a fixed point in space in one second. Expressed in symbols.

$$c = f\lambda \qquad (4.1)$$

At a fixed point in space, one cycle of oscillation occurs during a time interval equal to one period of the wave. The frequency is equal to the number of oscillations which occur in 1 second, so that, if

---

*This subject is dealt with in more detail elsewhere.[41]

†The actual relationship is c = $\sqrt{(K/\rho)}$, where K is the elasticity of the material, and ρ is its density.

ULTRASONIC IMAGING

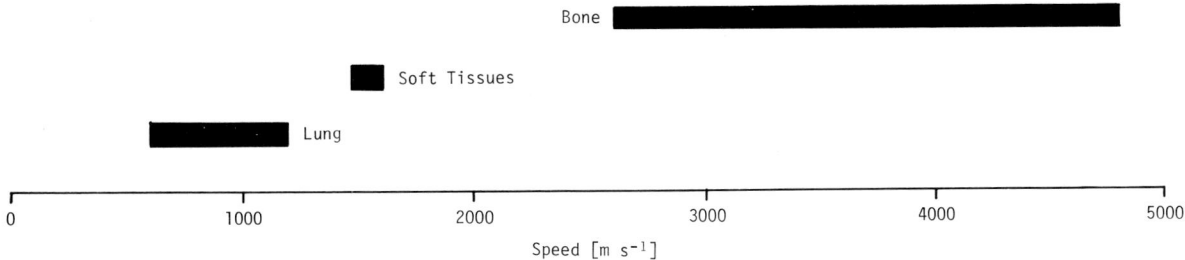

Fig. 4.1 Speeds of ultrasound in biological materials. The horizontal bars correspond to the ranges of the speeds which have been measured experimentally.[40]

the period = τ, it follows that

$$f = 1/\tau \qquad (4.2)$$

The data in Figure 4.1 indicates that the speed of ultrasound in soft tissues is about 1500 m s^{-1}. Substitution of this value in Equation 4.1 relates frequencies to wavelengths, and Table 4.1 gives these results for a range of frequencies, together with the corresponding periods calculated from Equation 4.2.

Table 4.1 Periods and wavelengths of ultrasonic waves at several frequencies, corresponding to a speed of 1500 m s^{-1}.

Frequency, MHz	1	1.5	2.5	3	5	10
Period, μs	1	0.67	0.4	0.33	0.2	0.1
Wavelength, mm	1.5	1	0.6	0.5	0.3	0.15

Behaviour of ultrasonic waves at boundaries

In a uniform homogeneous medium, an ultrasonic wave travels along a straight line, just as light does. Like light, however, ultrasound may be reflected and deviated (*refracted*) when it encounters the boundary separating two media. The behaviour of the wave at such a boundary depends on the different properties of the two media.

A simple situation is illustrated diagrammatically in Figure 4.3. There are two properties of the media on each side of the boundary which are important in determining the behaviour of the wave. The first of these is the speed of ultrasound in each medium. The ratio of the speeds controls the amount of refraction which occurs. The actual relationship is $\sin \theta_i / \sin \theta_t = c_1/c_2$ where θ_i and θ_t

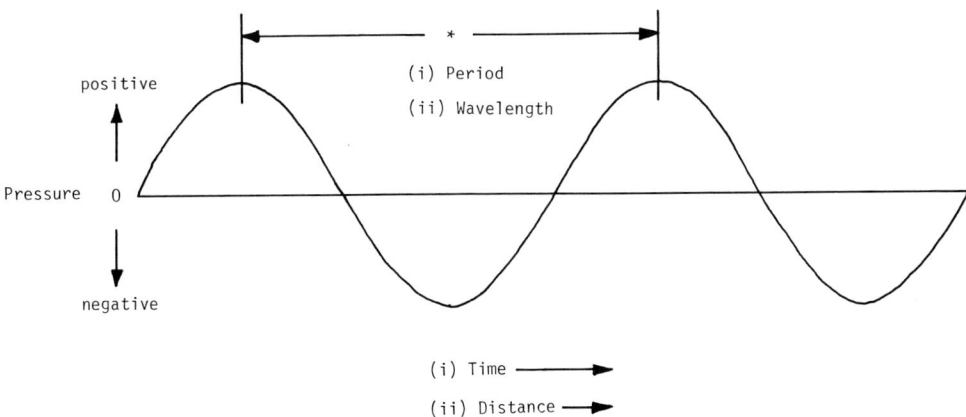

Fig. 4.2 Graphical representation of an ultrasonic wave. This wave has a single fixed value of frequency (the corresponding sound wave would be said to be *monotonic*). The *ordinate* here represents the alternating pressure, but it could equally well represent any other wave variable, e.g. particle displacement from the rest position. Moreover, depending on the choice of the *abscissa* (i) if abscissa represents *time*, the graph then shows how the pressure changes with the time at some fixed point in space, and the time interval * corresponds to the *period* of the wave, equal to the time for the disturbance to complete *one cycle* of oscillation; or (ii) if, the abscissa represents *distance*, it shows distribution of the pressure in space at some fixed instant in time, and the separation * corresponds to the *wavelength* of the wave, equal to the distance between consecutive cycles of the wave.

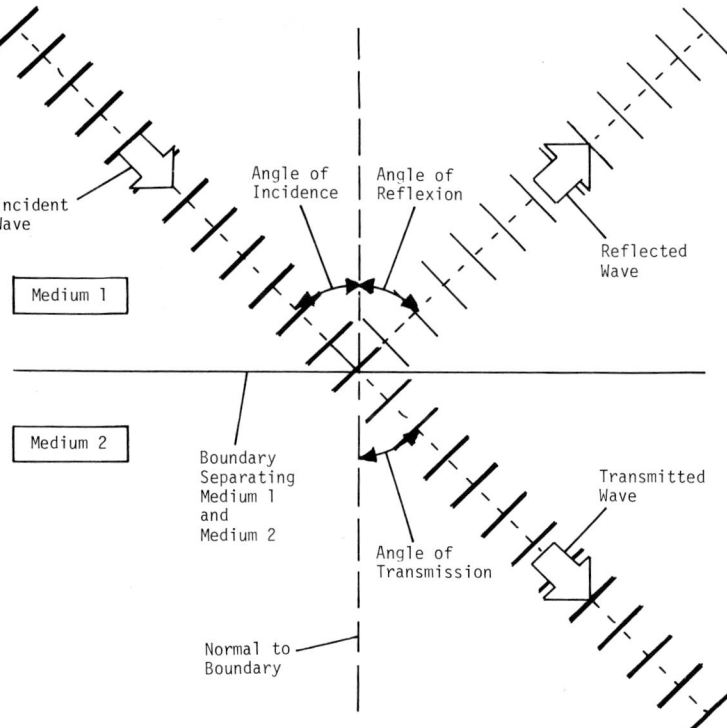

Fig. 4.3 The behaviour of a wave incident on a plane boundary separating two typical media which differ in characteristic impedance.

are the angles of incidence and transmission, and c_1 and c_2 are the speeds in the incident and transmitting media. If the speeds are equal, there is no refraction, the angles of incidence and transmission are equal, and the incident wave is transmitted from the first to the second medium without deviation. Fortunately, the speeds in different soft tissues are all quite similar, and refraction can be neglected when ultrasonic diagnosis is restricted to these tissues. Thus, ultrasound can be assumed to travel in more or less straight lines.

The second important property of the two media is their *characteristic impedances*. The values of the characteristic impedances on each side of the boundary determine how the incident ultrasound is shared between transmission and reflexion. The characteristic impedance Z of a medium is equal to the product of its *density* ρ and the speed of ultrasound within it; in symbols,

$$Z = \rho c \qquad (4.3)$$

If the characteristic impedances of the two media are equal, there is no reflexion, and all of the incident ultrasound is transmitted across the boundary. If the characteristic impedances differ, however, some of the ultrasound is reflected. Just as in optics, the angle of reflexion is equal to the angle of incidence, and the reflexion is said to be *specular*. The energy carried by the incident wave is shared between the transmitted and reflected waves. This sharing process has to satisfy two conditions. Firstly, the two media must remain in contact. Secondly, in each medium the ratio of the particle pressure and the particle velocity (two of the quantities which define the wave) must be equal to the characteristic impedance. The mathematics of the situation is rather complicated; the simplest situation occurs at normal incidence, when

$$R = [\,(Z_2 - Z_1)\,/\,(Z_2 + Z_1)\,]^2 \qquad (4.4)$$

where R is the fraction of the incident energy which is reflected when a wave travelling in a medium of characteristic impedance Z_1 meets the boundary with a medium of characteristic impedance Z_2. As can be seen from Table 4.2, the amount of reflexion depends on the relative values of Z_1 and Z_2, so that almost total reflexion occurs if Z_1 and Z_2 are very different, and only a little reflexion occurs if Z_1 and

Table 4.2 Fraction R of incident energy reflected at the boundary between media with characteristic impedances equal to Z_1 and Z_2.

	\multicolumn{7}{c}{Value of Z_2}
	$\gg Z_1$	$10Z_1$	$1.1Z_1$	Z_1	$0.9Z_1$	$0.1Z_1$	$\ll Z_1$
R	1	0.67	0.002	0	0.003	0.67	1

Z_2 are rather similar. To put this into perspective, refer to Figure 4.4, which gives values of the characteristic impedances of some biological materials. Characteristic impedance is measured in kilograms/square metre/second ($kg\,m^{-2}\,s^{-1}$). The characteristic impedances of the soft tissues are so similar that, for example, the energy carried in the wave reflected back into the liver with normal incidence at a liver-to-kidney boundary is only about 6 per cent of that in the incident wave. On the other hand, in this example about 94 per cent of the incident

which, in any plane perpendicular to the direction of propagation of the wave, every particle always experiences a disturbance identical to that of every other particle. In principle, there is no limitation to the lateral extension of a plane wave, but in practice, plane wave conditions can often be assumed without introducing serious errors.

It is important to realise that the results of calculations of reflexion at a plane boundary may not apply to a similar characteristic impedance discontinuity in the form of a small obstacle, a rough surface, or an ensemble of small obstacles. (In this context, 'small' implies dimensions of around a few wavelengths or less.) The *specular* component of reflexion is replaced, by an amount depending on the geometry, by components of *scattered* energy. As illustrated in Figure 4.5, the distribution of the scattered ultrasound can be explained by consider-

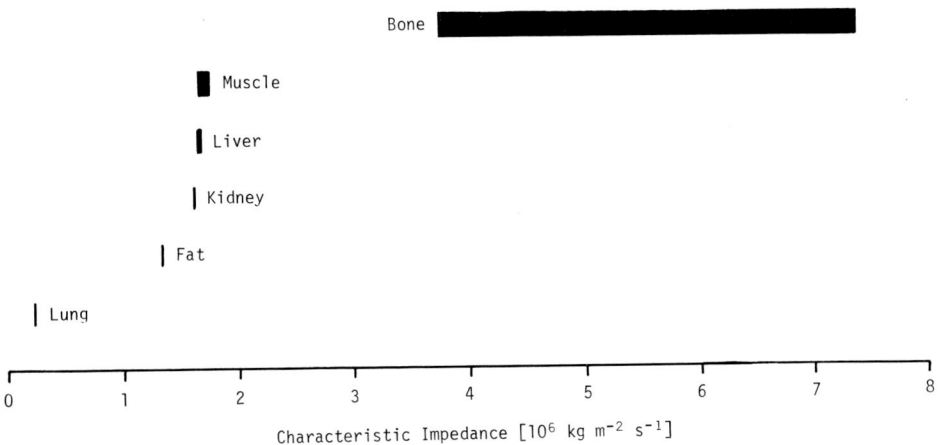

Fig. 4.4 Characteristic impedances of biological materials. The horizontal bars correspond to the ranges of measurements reported in the literature. The soft tissues all have characteristic impedances quite close to $1.5 \times 10^6\ kg\,m^{-2}\,s^{-1}$ because all have densities of around $1000\ kg\,m^{-3}$, and speeds of about $1500\ m\,s^{-1}$. In contrast, the density and speed for lung are both much lower, whilst those for bone are higher.[40]

energy is transmitted beyond the boundary into the kidney. In contrast, about 50 per cent of the incident energy is reflected at a soft-tissue-to-lung boundary, and about 30 per cent at a soft-tissue-to-bone boundary. The situation is even more extreme at a soft-tissue-to-air boundary, where about 99.9 per cent of the incident energy is reflected.

Plane waves, scattered waves and interference

The waves discussed so far in this chapter are what are known as *plane waves*. A plane wave is one in

ing the characteristic impedance discontinuity to be composed of very many tiny areas, each much smaller than the wavelength in size. Each of these areas scatters the incident plane wave as a spherical wavelet.* These separate wavelets combine to form

---

*If the obstacle is extremely small in relation to the wavelength, the intensity (see p. 144) of the wave which returns to the source (for given conditions of characteristic impedance) is directly proportional to the sixth power of the radius of the obstacle, and to the fourth power of the frequency. This means that doubling the radius increases the scattered intensity by a factor of 64, and doubling the frequency increases it by a factor of 16.

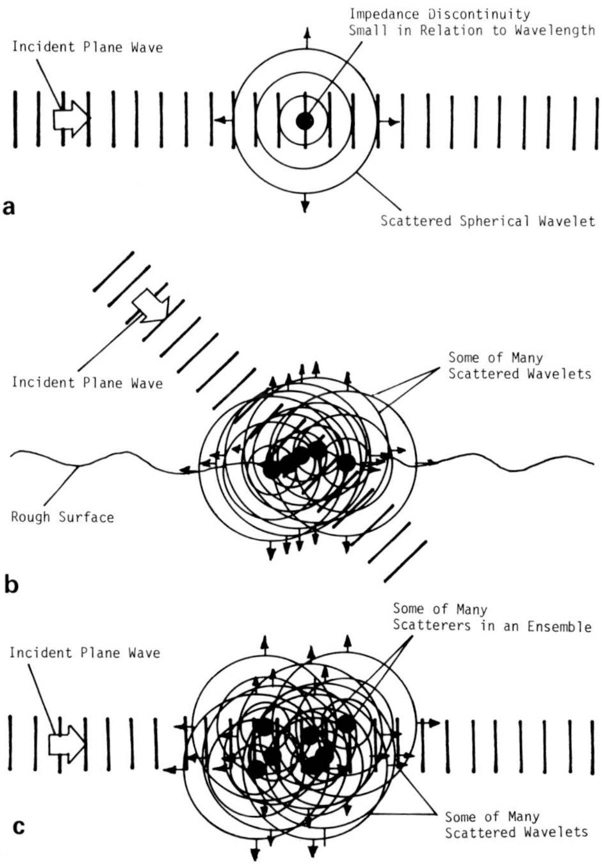

142 SCIENTIFIC BASIS OF MEDICAL IMAGING

Fig. 4.5 Scattering. (a) Spherical scattering by a small isolated discontinuity. (b) Scattering by a rough surface; the scattered field is the resultant of every separate spherical wavelet. (c) Scattering by an ensemble of small discontinuities; again the scattered field is the resultant of the contributing wavelets.

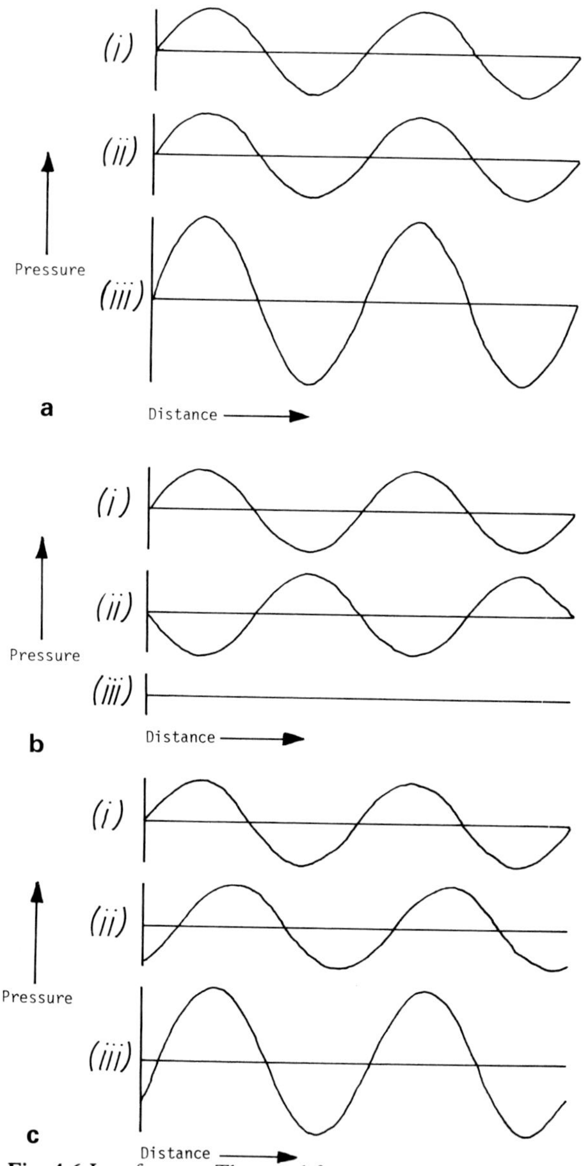

the reradiated ultrasonic distribution. In order to understand the way in which these wavelets combine, it is necessary to introduce the concept of wave *interference*. This is illustrated in Figure 4.6. The effect of the interference between scattered wavelets is rather like that of a light diffuser, such as a ground glass screen, in optics: the scattered ultrasonic radiation is spread over a wider angle than that of the incident wave. Moreover, if the target is not stationary (as, for example, as in the case of blood which is a moving ensemble of scatterers), the amplitude of the reflected ultrasound *fluctuates* with time.

It is often convenient, for example in analysing interference, to consider a parameter of a wave known as its *'phase angle'*. This term arises from the mathematical description of a wave. If the in-

Fig. 4.6 Interference. The equal-frequency waves (i) and (ii) are superimposed to combine to form a resultant wave (iii). (These diagrams illustrate the pressure distribution with distance from the same point along the ultrasonic waves at a fixed instant in time, but they could be used to represent the pressure changing with time at some fixed point in space, simply by labelling the abscissa as 'time' instead of 'distance'.) (a) Positions in space of the maxima, minima and zeroes of (i) and (ii) are identical and (iii) has a pressure amplitude equal to the sum of the separate pressure amplitudes of the two waves. (b) Although the positions in space of the zeroes of (i) and (ii) are identical, the pressure maxima in (i) coincide with the minima in (ii); (i) and (ii) *interfere* so that the combined wave (iii) has an amplitude equal to the difference between the amplitudes of its two contributors (and it is equal to zero if the two waves are of equal amplitude). (c) Somewhere between (a) and (b), the time-positions of the zeroes and maxima and minima of (iii) are shifted from those of (i) and (iii), although the frequency is unchanged.

stantaneous pressure is designated p, and the time as t, then

$$p = p_o \sin(\phi + \omega t) \quad (4.5)$$

where p_o is the value of the maximum pressure, and $(\phi + \omega t)$ has the dimensions of an angle. The quantity ω is called the *angular frequency*. Angular frequency is measured in units of radians/second, (rad s^{-1}) and is given by $\omega = 2\pi f$. When multiplied by time it gives a time-varying angle which is equal to zero when $t = 0$. Because the wave pressure is not necessarily zero when $t = 0$, the angle ϕ is added to ωt to take account of this. The entire angle $(\phi + \omega t)$ is called the *phase angle* of the wave.

It is easy to explain wave interference in mathematical terms. Some examples are illustrated in Figure 4.7.

Doppler effect

In the situation illustrated in Figure 4.8, the frequency of the reflected wave is equal to that of the

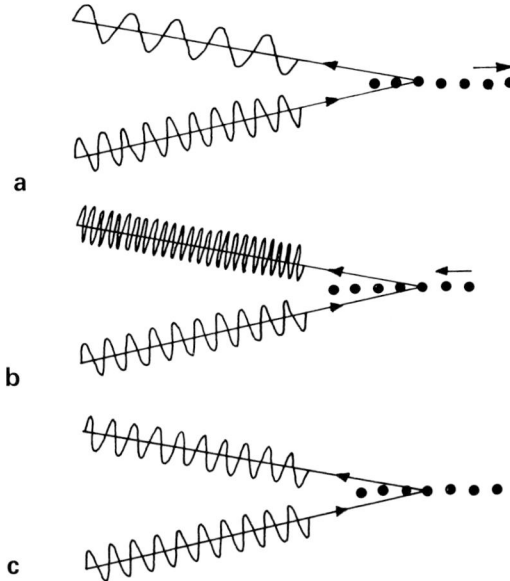

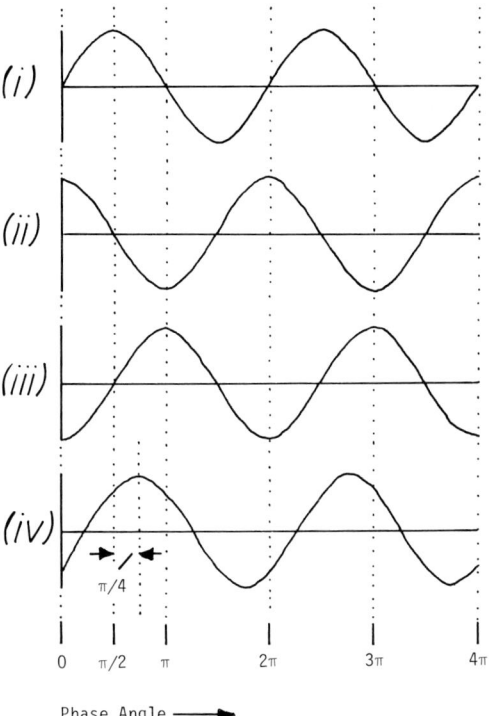

Fig. 4.8 The Doppler shift in the frequency of a wave returned from a moving target. In this example, the target consists of an ensemble of scatters. (a) The target is stationary with respect to the source, and the frequency of the reflected wave is equal to that of the incident wave. (b) The ensemble is moving towards the source of the ultrasound, and the frequency of the reflected wave is shifted upwards. (c) The ensemble is moving away from the source, and the frequency of the reflected wave is shifted downwards.

transmitted wave if the reflecting boundary is stationary (i.e. has no component of velocity along the direction of wave motion). Movement of the reflecting boundary towards the source, however, results in a compression of the wavelength of the reflected ultrasound, and *vice versa*. The speed of ultrasound in the medium in which the ultrasound is travelling has a fixed, constant value. Consequently a change in wavelength must be accompanied by a shift in frequency, so that the relationship expressed in Equation 4.1 remains satisfied. The phenomenon is called the *Doppler effect*.

If the ultrasound strikes the moving reflector at normal incidence, the Doppler shift frequency ($f_D = f' - f$, where f is the frequency of the incident

Fig. 4.7 The phase of a wave. Waveforms shown here all have the same frequency and amplitude. (i) can be represented by: $p = p_o \sin(\omega t)$, where p is the wave variable (such as pressure), and p_o the maximum value of p, and ω the *angular frequency*, equal to $2\pi f$. (ii) can be represented by: $p = p_o \sin(\omega t + \pi/2)$. Thus waveform (ii) *leads* waveform (i) by a *phase angle* of $\pi/2$ radians (180°). Similarly, waveform (iii) *lags* by a phase angle of $\pi/2$ radians, and may be represented by: $p = p_o \sin(\omega t - \pi/2)$. Waveforms (ii) and (iii) differ in phase by π radians, and are said to be exactly *out of phase*, or in *antiphase*. Waveform (iv) is at an intermediate phase angle to waveform (i); in this example, it lags by $\pi/4$ radians (which is equal to 45°).

wave, and f' is the received frequency) is given by

$$f_D = 2\, vf/c \quad (4.6)$$

where v is the velocity of the reflector *towards* the source of ultrasound. Strictly this relationship is only true if $v \ll c$, but this is generally the case in diagnostic applications. (The direction is important: f_D is positive for movement towards the source, and negative for movement away. Determination of this is the basis of the directionally sensitive Doppler system discussed on page 164.)

In diagnostic applications of the Doppler effect, if often happens that the direction of the motion of the reflector (or ensemble of scatterers) is at some particular angle γ to that of the incident wave, although the incident and reflected waves are effectively coincident. Then

$$f_D = 2\, v\, (\cos \gamma)\, f/c \quad (4.7)$$

ATTENUATION OF ULTRASOUND

Power, intensity and the decibel notation

Ultrasonic waves carry energy. *Power* is defined as the rate at which energy is delivered. It is measured in units of watts, abbreviated by W; 1 W = 1 joule/second, (J s^{-1}). 1 J is the amount of heat required to raise the temperature of 1 kg of water through 0·000 24 K. The ultrasonic *intensity* of a wave is equal to the quantity of energy flowing through unit area in unit time. Intensity may be measured in units of watts/square centimetre, abbreviated W cm^{-2}. The SI base unit is the watt/square metre, but this involves an inconveniently large area in relation to practical situations in biomedicine.

The absolute value of the ultrasonic intensity of a wave is an important consideration in relation to the possible occurrence of biological effects and associated hazards (see p. 176). In relation to ultrasonic diagnosis, however, it is frequently very convenient to measure the *ratios* between pairs of intensities, or amplitudes, particularly if the amplitude of one is taken as the reference for the comparison with others. In this way the need for absolute measurement may be avoided, and, because ultrasonic waves are generally both generated and detected electrically, relative wave amplitudes can be expressed as ratios of *voltages*. Rather than expressing the voltages as simple ratios, however, it is usually much more convenient to express these ratios in *decibels*. The decibel is a logarithmic unit, and its use allows even large voltage ratios to be described by quite small numbers, and moreover the arthimetic product of two or more voltage ratios is obtained by the addition of the corresponding decibel levels (and similarly, division is achieved by their subtraction).

If two waves to be compared have powers P_1 and P_2 respectively, and amplitudes A_1 and A_2, then

(relative levels in decibels)
$$= 10 \log_{10} (P_2/P_1) = 20 \log_{10} (A_2/A_1) \quad (4.8)$$

This relationship for amplitudes exists because the power carried in a wave is proportional to the square of (for example) its pressure amplitude, and the logarithm of the square of a number is equal to twice the logarithm of the number. Some values calculated from Equation 4.8 are illustrated in Figure 4.9.

It is important to realise that it is meaningless to express an absolute value of any quantity in terms of decibels, unless a reference level is also stated. Thus, for example, an intensity of -40 dB with respect to 1 W cm^{-2} is equal to 0·0001 W cm^{-2} (i.e. 100 μW cm^{-2}): note that intensities relating to a particular area can be compared in the same way as total powers. Similarly, the amplitude ratio of two waves, one 20dB and the other 40dB below

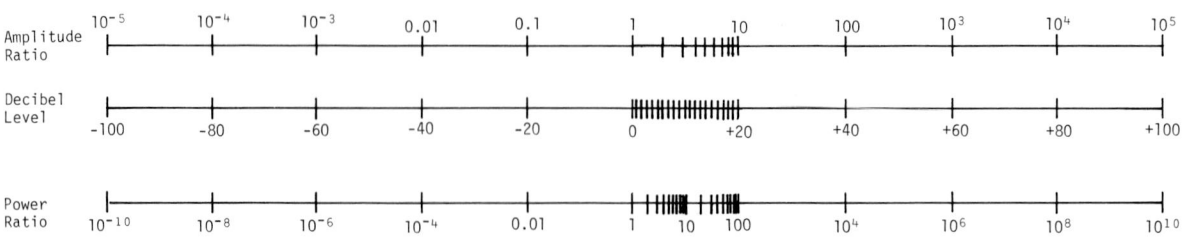

Fig. 4.9 Bar chart showing the decibel levels corresponding to ranges of ultrasonic amplitude and power ratios.

the same reference, is equal to 10 (i.e. the first wave is 20dB greater in amplitude than the second).

Attenuation

In general, the transmission of energy is a process which is accompanied by a reduction in intensity. In practice, the only exception to this occurs when a beam is focused sufficiently strongly so that the gain in intensity due to concentrating the power (so that it flows through a smaller area) more than compensates for the loss due to attenuation. This is, for example, the basis of radiography, in which the image is directly related to the different attenuation rates of X-rays in the various tissue structures under investigation. In ultrasonic diagnostic methods based on the detection of echoes from within the body, however, the principal effect of attenuation is progressively to reduce the amplitudes of echoes from deeper structures, making them more difficult to detect.

There are two processes, illustrated in Figure 4.10, by which the intensity of an ultrasonic wave may be *attenuated* during its propagation. First, the ultrasonic energy flowing through a particular area may be reduced as a result of the re-direction of the wave. There are three mechanisms which may be involved; none results directly in actual loss of ultrasonic energy, but simply change the direction of a proportion of the initial wave energy. Thus, the wave may *diverge* from a parallel beam, so that the ultrasonic power flows through an increased area; beam formation is discussed on page 149. Next, the same result may be due to the *scattering* of some of the wave power by small discontinuities in characteristic impedance (see p. 141). Finally, the wave may be *partially reflected* (as described on p. 139) so that the power of the wave which remains travelling in the initial direction is reduced.

The second attenuation mechanism involves the actual reduction in the total ultrasonic vibrational energy by conversion into heat. This is known as *absorption*. In biological soft tissues, it seems that the most important contribution to absorption is due to *relaxation processes* in the protein constituents of the tissues. Biological macromolecules like proteins have complex arrangements, and their components are not stationary, but vibrate or spin

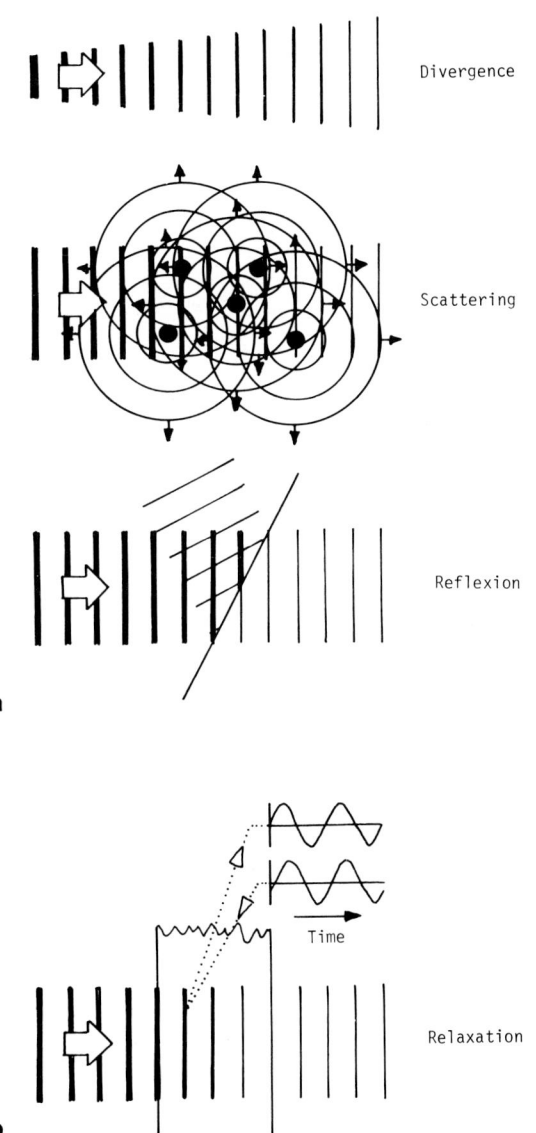

Fig. 4.10 Processes causing attentuation of ultrasonic intensity. (a) Redirection of the wave, by divergence, scattering or reflexion, resulting in a reduction in the ultrasonic energy flowing through a particular area. (b) Return of an out-of-phase fraction of the wave from a relaxation process, resulting in energy loss due to interference.

within the structured lattice. The energy stored in the spins, for example, may be changed by changing the applied pressure. The redistribution of the total energy is a process which occupies a certain period of time, depending on the particular molecular modification which is involved. Pressure is one of the quantities which vary during the passage of an ultrasonic wave. At very low frequency, the time which is required for the energy to be redistributed within the molecule is negligible in relation to the period of the wave, and so the energy which is stored within the molecule moves between the various states without any loss. At very high frequency, on the other hand, the pressure changes so rapidly that there is insufficient time for any energy to be redistributed during a single period of the wave, and again there is no associated energy loss. At some particular intermediate value of frequency, however, the energy which is being redistributed returns to the ultrasonic wave at the time in each cycle when it is out-of-phase (see p. 142). The resultant interference is associated with actual loss of energy. This phenomenon is called a *relaxation process*, because the energy temporarily stored in the molecule *relaxes* back into the ultrasonic wave. Although a given relaxation process has its maximum effect at some particular value of frequency, its influence extends over a fairly wide range of frequencies. Moreover, there is evidence that relaxation processes exist which extend over the whole range of frequencies used in ultrasonic diagnostic techniques.

Figure 4.11 represents the situation in which a wave is attenuated as a result of propagation through a material. In the simplest case, the characteristic impedance of the material and its surroundings may be taken to be equal, so that the reduction in the amplitude of the wave depends only on the distance which it travels through the attenuating medium. It is then very convenient to express the attenuation coefficient of the material in units of decibels per centimetre, abbreviated dB cm^{-1}. Thus, in the example illustrated in Figure 4.11, the amplitude of the transmitted wave is αd dB below that of the incident wave.

The attenuation experieced by a wave in travelling through a given material depends not only on the thickness of material, but also upon the ultrasonic frequency. In biological soft tissues, the attenuation coefficient turns out to be roughly proportional to the frequency, over the whole range of frequency used in ultrasonic diagnostic techniques. For example, in a given thickness of material, doubling the frequency approximately doubles the attenuation.

Because of the approximately linear relationship, in soft tissues, between attenuation and frequency, the attenuation coefficient divided by the frequency, that is, α/f, is roughly constant over the whole range of frequencies used in ultrasonic diagnostic techniques. α/f is conveniently expressed in units of decibels/centimetre/megahertz, abbreviated dB cm^{-1} MHz^{-1}. Typical values of α/f are given in Figure 4.12, for various materials of importance in ultrasonic diagnosis.

GENERATION AND DETECTION OF ULTRASONIC WAVES

Piezoelectricity

At megahertz frequencies such as are employed in diagnostic applications, ultrasound is both generated and detected by the piezoelectric effect. Piezoelectric materials are called *transducers* because they provide a coupling between electrical and mechanical energies. In piezoelectric crystals, the electric charges bound within the crystalline lattice of the material are arranged in such a way that they react on an applied electric field to produce a mechanical effect, and *vice versa*. In the undeformed state, the centre of symmetry of the positive charges coincides with that of the negative charges, and, because the positive and negative charges are equal in magnitude, there is no effective potential across the transducer. If the transducer is compressed, the centres of symmetry no longer coincide, so that a charge difference appears if the transducer is extended. The converse piezoelectric effect occurs because the application of an electric field tends to move the centres of symmetry of the

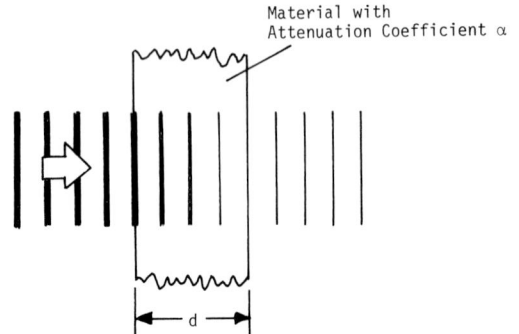

Fig. 4.11 Attenuation of ultrasound as a result of propagation across a distance d in a material with attenuation coefficient α.

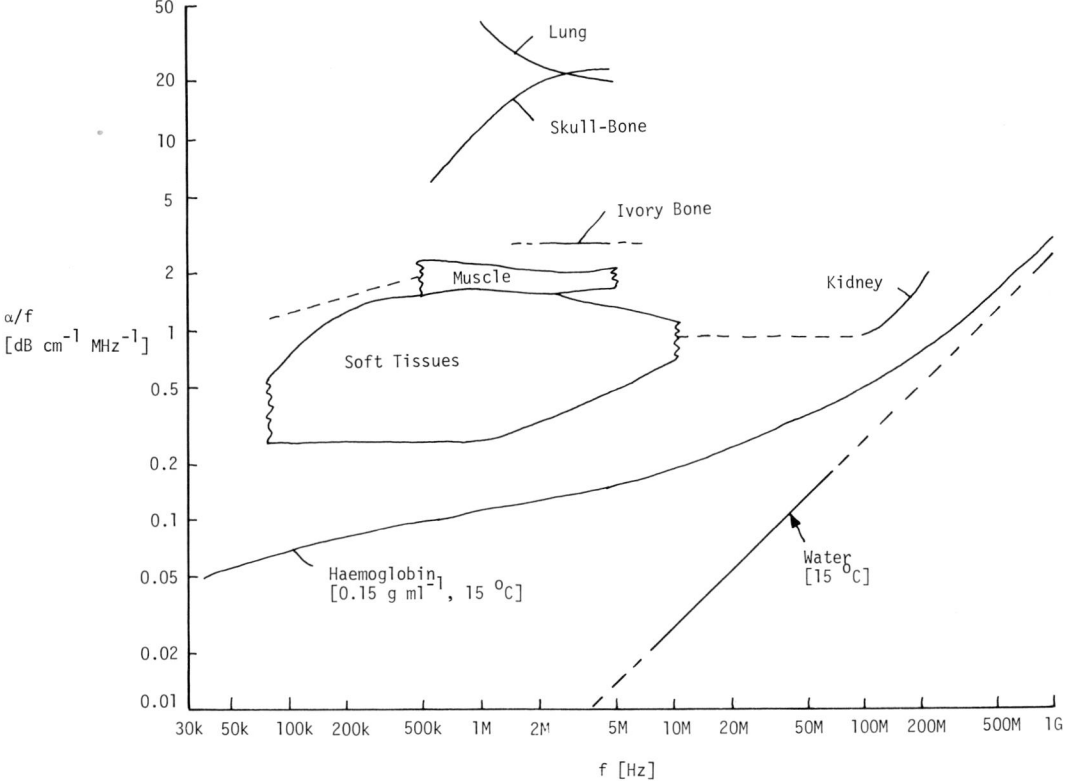

Fig. 4.12 Transmission loss data for biological materials. Note that similar mammalian tissues have been grouped together, regardless of species, and that no account has been taken of temperature or of tissue 'freshness'. Moreover, the distinction has not been made between absorption and attenuation, since this is often not clear in the published literature from which these data were collected.[40]

positive and negative charges in opposite directions, causing the transducer to deform. Thus, piezoelectric transducers can act both as generators and detectors of ultrasonic waves. Moreover, at least up to quite large amplitudes, they are linear devices.

Although there are many natural crystals which are piezoelectric (the best known is quartz), the

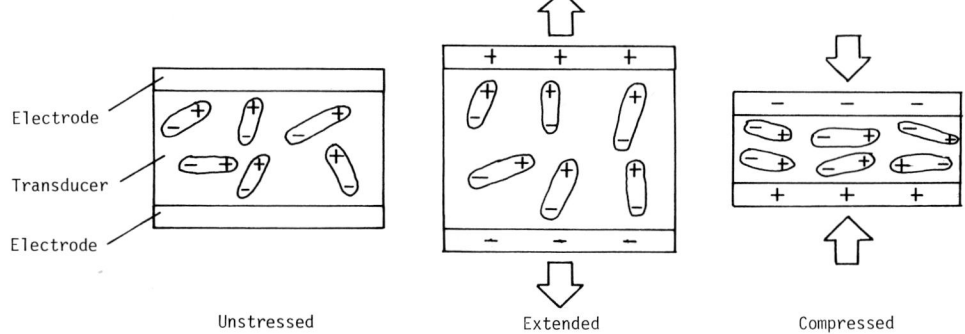

Fig. 4.13 The interaction between force and electric charge distribution is a piezoelectric transducer of the polarised ferroelectric variety. The arrows indicate the directions of the applied stresses, and the resultant surface charges are indicated at the electrodes. The converse effect accounts for the deformation of the transducer in response to an applied voltage.

most commonly used transducer material is the synthetic ceramic lead zirconate titanate. This material is polarised during manufacture to make it strongly piezoelectric. It belongs to the group of materials, called *ferroelectrics*, in which there are many tiny electric charge domains which are preferentially orientated in a particular direction by the polarisation process. This is represented diagrammatically in Figure 4.13; the name 'ferroelectric' is given by analogy to 'ferromagnetic' materials with their preferentially orientated magnetic field domains.

Transducers for diagnostic applications

Most diagnostic applications of ultrasound employ narrow beams of energy. Such a beam is often best generated and detected (see p. 147) by a disc of piezoelectric material electrically excited through two electrodes, one on each parallel surface. The transducer resonates at the frequency at which its thickness is equal to half the wavelength. For example, the ultrasonic speed in lead zirconate titanate is about 4000 m s^{-1}, and the transducer thickness is 1 mm at 2 MHz.

In pulse-echo diagnostic systems (see p. 151), the transducer is required to respond to energy pulses of very short duration. This requires that the transducer response should be *damped* by its mounting. Figure 4.14 shows a typical form of construction of a probe for the generation and detection of short pulses. The mechanical damping is provided by a block of highly absorbent material (for example, fine particles of tungsten, which act as scatterers, suspended in epoxy resin, which absorbs the scattered ultrasound) attached to the rear surface of the transducer. The ultrasonic insulator (for example, rubberised cork) between the case of the probe and the transducer-backing block assembly minimises the coupling of ultrasonic energy into the case. Such coupling is undesirable because the case may be made of low-loss material, such as metal, and is likely to *ring* for some time in response to an ultrasonic transient. Ringing of the case would be detected by the transducer as an *artifact*. The front surface of the transducer is attached to a plastic lens which focuses the ultrasonic beam (see p. 150). For short pulse operation, the plastic layer in front of the transducer should ideally be $\lambda/4$ in thickness, and of characteristic impedance equal to the geometric mean of the characteristic impedances of the transducer and the load in order to achieve maximum efficiency. Because the thickness of the lens changes with the radius, the quarter-wave thickness criterion cannot be satisfied over the whole surface and a compromise is necessary to optimise the performance.

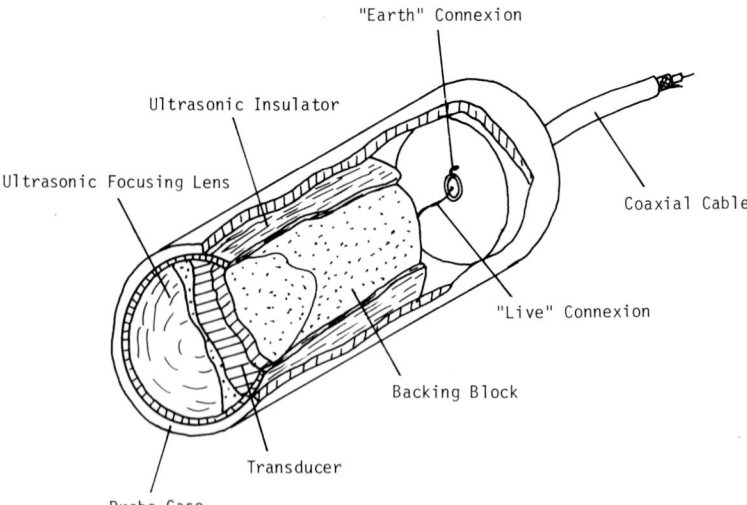

Fig. 4.14 Construction of a typical transducer probe for short pulse operation. The electrical connexions are made to thin metal electrodes bonded to the flat surfaces of the transducer. Usually, the rear electrode is *live*, and the front electrode is connected to the metal case which is *earthed* (or *grounded*).

The pulse response of a typical transducer of this type is shown in Figure 4.15. The pulse shape can be specified in terms of its *zero-crossing frequency*, and the *duration* between specific *threshold* levels below the *peak amplitude*. These are important quantities in the estimation of the *resolution* of a pulse-echo diagnostic system (see p. 152).

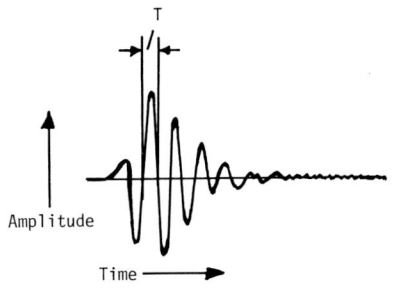

Fig. 4.15 Pulse response of a typical diagnostic ultrasonic transducer. The zero-crossing frequency is equal to $1/T$, and this is twice the 'ultrasonic frequency' of the pulse. The ripple which follows the pulse is due to several effects, including radial resonance of the transducer and the ringing in the probe case.

THE ULTRASONIC FIELD

Steady state conditions

As previously mentioned (p. 148) disc transducers are commonly used in diagnostic applications. The steady state ultrasonic field produced by such a source (and the sensitivity distribution of such a transducer operating as a receiver) may be calculated from the application of Huygen's principle. This principle, well known in optics, states that the surface of a radiating source may be considered to be made up of innumerable small sources, each radiating a uniform spherical wavelet; the wavelets interfere to form the ultrasonic beam. If I_0 is the intensity at the surface of the transducer, and I_z is the intensity at a distance z from the transducer along the central axis, then

$$I_z/I_0 = \sin^2 \{ (\pi/\lambda) [(a^2 + z^2)^{1/2} - z]\} \quad (4.9)$$

where a is the radius of the disc. This relationship is illustrated for a typical example in Figure 4.16. Moving along the central axis towards the source, the intensity increases until a maximum is reached at a distance z'_{max} from the source given by

$$z'_{max} = a^2/\lambda \quad (4.10)$$

provided that $a^2 \gg \lambda^2$. The region between the source and z'_{max} is called the *near field* (or Frésnel zone), and the region beyond this is the *far field* (or Fraunhofer zone). The beam in the near field is roughly cylindrical. Deep in the far field, the

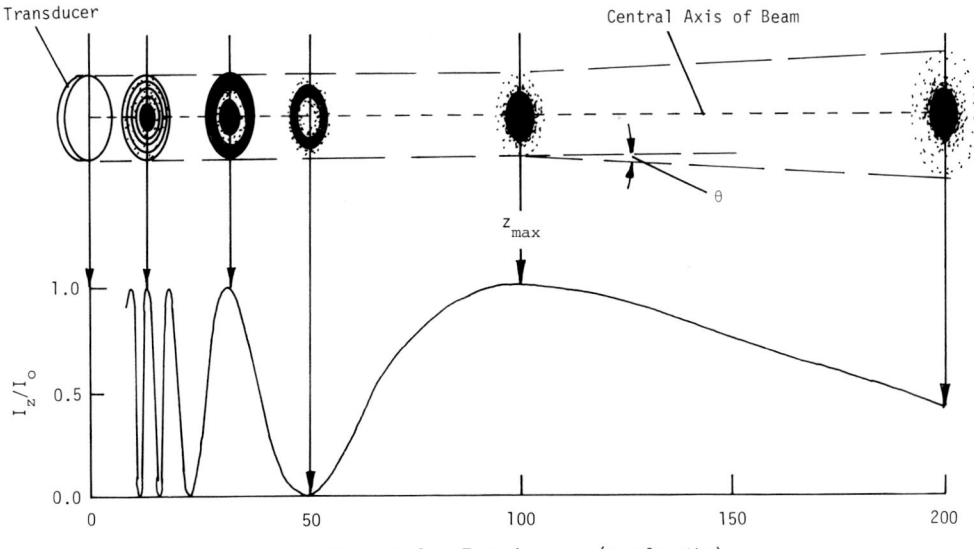

Fig. 4.16 The ultrasonic field of a typical disc transducer; in this example the distribution shown is for a transducer of 20 wavelengths diameter (i.e. 20 mm at 1·5 MHz in water). The ultrasonic beam normal to the central axis is circular in section, and the elliptical diagrams represent oblique views of such sections.

directivity function is given by

$$D_s = \frac{2 \mathcal{J}_1 (ka \sin \theta)}{ka \sin \theta} \quad (4.11)$$

where θ is the angle relating D_s to the central axis of the beam, k is the wave number $= 2\pi/\lambda$, and $\mathcal{J}_1$ is the first order Bessel function. Thus the main lobe of the beam diverges at an angle $\pm \theta$ about the central axis, given by

$$\theta = \sin^{-1} (0.61 \, \lambda/a) \quad (4.12)$$

Thus, when considering the shape of the ultrasonic beam produced by a plane disc transducer, it should be remembered that the length of the near field *increases*, and the divergence in the far field *decreases*, with *increasing* diameter of the transducer and with *increasing* frequency (which is equivalent to *decreasing* wavelength).

In the near field, an ultrasonic beam may be focused over a limited depth of field. This greatly improves the resolution of the system (see p. 152). The materials, such as plastics, from which ultrasonic lenses may be constructed generally have higher propagation speeds than water or soft tissues, so that converging lenses are concave (Figs. 4.14 and 4.17).

In considering the phenomenon of focusing, a useful concept is that focusing occurs at the point in the field at which the contributions from the entire surface of the transducer all arrive together, or 'in phase'. Thus, lenses function by introducing appropriate thicknesses of material in which the speed differs from that in the medium, so that the transit times along ray paths of different lengths to the source are all equal (Fig. 4.17a). Focusing may be achieved by the use of a concave transducer giving equal length ray paths from the transducer surface to the focus (Fig. 4.17b). Figure 4.17c shows how the combined effects of convergence due to a concave transducer, and divergence due to a convex plastic lens, can make it possible for a flat-faced (or even slightly convex) probe to produce a focused ultrasonic beam. This trick is often used in practice, because the alternative concave probe face is difficult to use in skin contact scanning, as it tends to trap air which interferes with the ultrasonic coupling with the patient.

Another method by which focusing can be introduced is by means of appropriate time grading

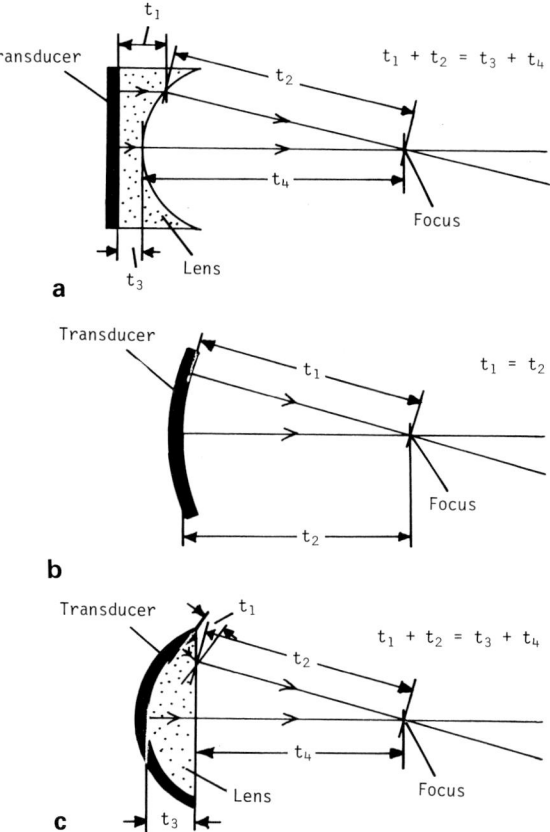

Fig. 4.17 Methods of focusing an ultrasonic beam. In all cases, the time delays are equal along all ray paths between the surface of the transducer and the position of the focus. (a) Plane transducer with concave plastic lens. (b) Concave transducer. (c) Concave transducer with convex lens, producing a focused beam from a probe with a flat (or even slightly convex) surface.

across an array consisting of small transducer elements. This is discussed on page 160.

Transient conditions

If the transducer produces a transient ultrasonic disturbance, as distinct from a steady state continuous wave such as is dealt with on page 149 the ultrasonic field is modified because, at any particular point in the field, the contributions from the different elementary parts of the source surface may not be equal. As a result, the sharply defined near field inhomogeneities of the steady state become increasingly smeared and homogeneous as the pulse length is reduced.

PULSE-ECHO DIAGNOSTIC METHODS

An ultrasonic pulse is reflected when it strikes the boundary between two media of differing characteristic impedances, and the time delay which occurs between the transmission of the pulse and the reception of its echo depends on the propagation speed and the path length. The propagation speeds in different soft tissues are so closely similar (approximately equal to that in water, and around 1500 m s^{-1}; see p. 139) that a constant relationship between time and distance can usually be assumed. Ultrasound travels 10 mm in about 6·7 μs at this speed.

The ultrasonic pulse-echo method depends on the estimations of the ranges and directions of echo-producing targets within the tissue volume interrogated by the ultrasonic beam. Instruments range in complexity from the simple range-finding A-scope with hand-held probe, through the time-position recording system and the static two-dimensional B-scope, to real-time systems gathering data from two-dimensional planes within three-dimensional volumes.

The A-scope

The basic elements of the simplest type of pulse-echo system for medical diagnosis, called an *A-scope*, are illustrated in Figure 4.18. The rate generator (or 'clock') simultaneously triggers the transmitter, the swept gain generator (or 'time gain control', 'tgc', generator), and the timebase generator. The voltages which appear across the transducer in the probe are amplified by the receiver, and the output from the receiver is arranged to deflect the timebase line on the display. Thus, vertical deflexions of the horizontal timebase occur at positions corresponding to echo-producing targets along the ultrasonic beam within the patient. Rapid repetition of the process (typically at least 1000 times/second) results in a flicker-free display.

Swept gain

A substantial improvement in the usefulness of the displayed information is obtained if the echo signals from deeper structures are amplified more than those which originate closer to the probe. This is because deeper echoes are more attenuated by the greater tissue path length; swept gain compensates for this. Ideally, swept gain should lead to similar deflexion amplitudes on the display for sim-

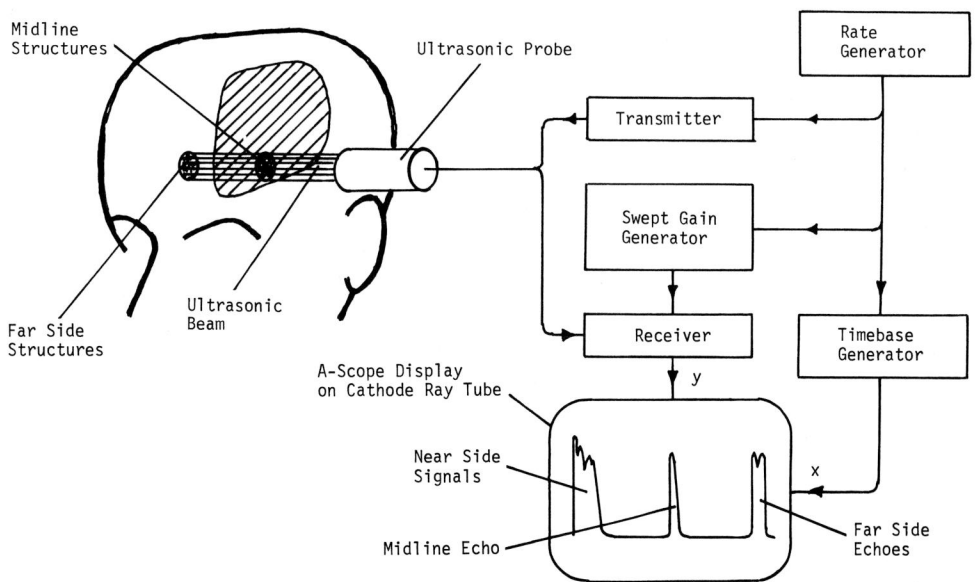

Fig. 4.18 Basic elements of the A-scope. The output from the receiver is connected to the vertical (*y*) deflexion plates of the cathode ray tube, and that from the timebase generator, to the horizontal (*x*) plates.

ilar surfaces, irrespective of their distances from the probe. In practice, however, accurate swept gain is difficult to achieve, for two main reasons.

Firstly, there is a variation in the attenuation rates of different tissues, so that compensating on the basis of 1 dB cm^{-1} MHz^{-1} (for example, setting the swept gain rate at 4 dB cm^{-1} for operation at 2 MHz, taking the go-and-return path length into account) is at best only a compromise. Secondly, the energy in the ultrasonic pulse is distributed over quite a wide frequency spectrum, and the higher frequency components of the pulse are increasingly attenuated with increasing penetration, since the attenuation coefficient in soft tissues is roughly proportional to the frequency. This exacerbates the problem of applying accurate swept gain compensation.

Resolution in pulse-echo systems

Three important concepts have to be introduced into a discussion of the resolution in ultrasonic pulse-echo systems. The first is that of *noise*. This is the term used to describe those signals, ultimately appearing at the display, which are generated within the instrument itself; they do not carry information about the tissues being studied. The satisfactory detection of the information-carrying signals requires that they should be greater in amplitude than the noise signals on which they are superimposed. The second important concept is that there are practical limitations to the *power* which can be transmitted into the patients, due both to the physical limitations of the transducer and to the biological limitations of the hazardous exposure. The other concept is that of *dynamic range*. This term, which is usually expressed in decibels (see p. 144), describes the range over which relevant signal variation occurs (e.g. the range from some threshold level to the maximum which can be accepted by the display).

Within the limitations imposed by noise and the maximum permissible transmitted power, the maximum useful dynamic range of the echoes received in conventional medical diagnostic pulse-echo systems is about 100 dB. This dynamic range is shared between the variations in echo amplitude at particular ranges, and the attenuation of echoes which increases with distance. In practice, at any particular range, an echo amplitude variation of about 30 dB is the maximum which may usefully be employed, since the azimuthal resolution is unlikely to be acceptable with a larger dynamic range. Therefore, around 70 dB is available to provide swept gain compensation for attenuation. An attenuation of 1 dB cm^{-1} MHz^{-1} corresponds to 0·15 dB per wavelength, or to 0·3 dB per wavelength of penetration (taking account of the go-and-return path). With 70 dB of swept gain, a penetration of 233 wavelengths would thus seem to be possible; 200 wavelengths is a more realistic figure.

The resolution of any imaging system may be defined in several different ways. The usual definition is that the resolution is equal to the reciprocal of the minimum distance (in range or in azimuth) between two point targets, at which separate registrations can just be distinguished on the display. An alternative definition, equivalent in concept but usually more convenient in practice in considering ultrasonic pulse-echo systems, is that the resolution is equal to the reciprocal of the distance which appears on the display to be occupied by a point target in the field. Measurements based on this definition avoid problems which arise due to interference between waves scattered by two closely spaced point (or line) targets.

The resolution cell is the volume of material within which the interaction providing the data takes place. Except in simple and idealised situations, the dimensions of the resolution cell depend on its particular position along the axis of ultrasonic beam. As shown in Figure 4.19, the length of the resolution cell depends on the duration of the ultrasonic pulse, and its width, on the diameter of the ultrasonic beam. The effective values of the pulse duration and the beamwidth are determined by the dynamic range lying between the maximum echo amplitude and the detection threshold of the diagnostic system.

In principle, the *range resolution* can be increased by reducing the duration of the ultrasonic pulse. Since little can be done to improve the shape of the pulse, which always resembles that shown in Figure 4.15, the only way in which this can be achieved is by increasing the ultrasonic frequency. Since, as has already been explained in this Section, the penetration is limited to little more than about 200 wavelengths, it is necessary to compromise between range resolution and penetration. Consequently, in practice the minimum achievable pulse duration is often best considered as being equiv-

ULTRASONIC IMAGING   153

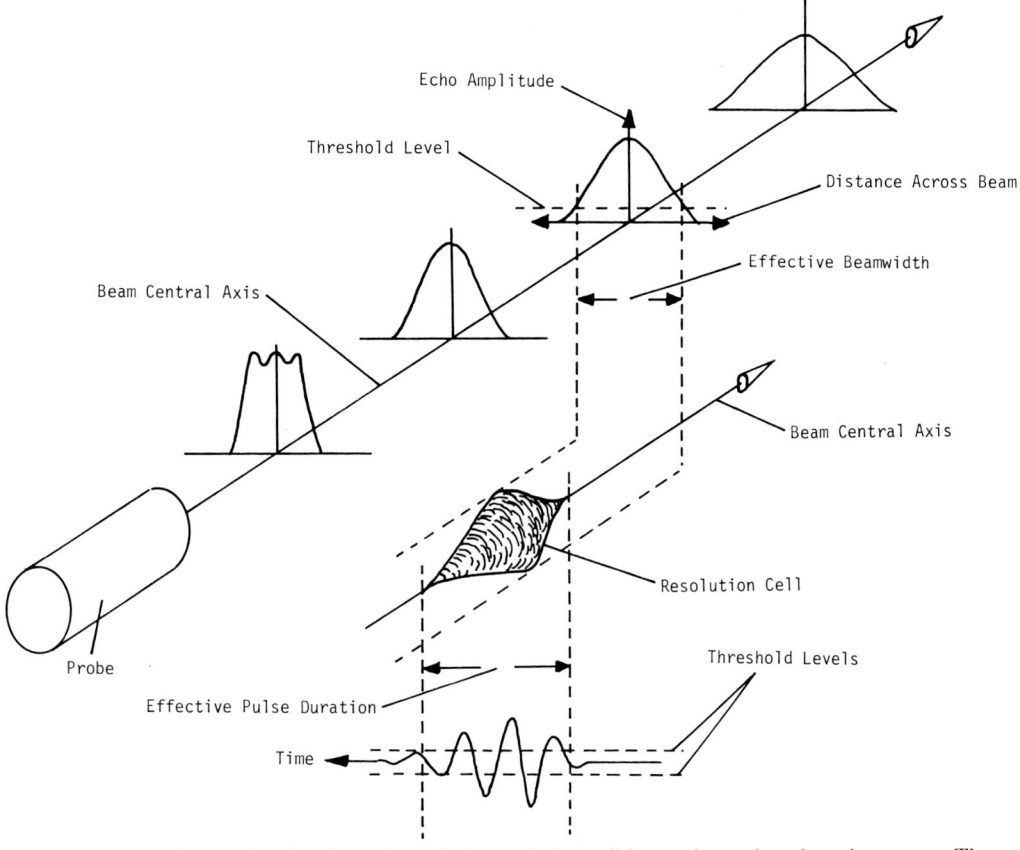

Fig. 4.19 Factors determining the dimensions of the resolution cell in an ultrasonic pulse-echo system. The axial length of the resolution cell corresponds to the duration of the echo pulse envelope which exceeds the threshold level of the system (see bottom of diagram and Fig. 4.15). The diameter of the resolution cell is equal to the effective beamwidth, which is determined by the system threshold (as illustrated in relation to the beam profile) and which depends on the space-position along the central axis and the time-position within the pulse.

alent to about two cycles of ultrasonic 'frequency*' with a dynamic range (between the chosen threshold level and the peak pulse amplitude) of say, 10 dB. The corresponding resolution is approximately equal to the reciprocal of two 'wavelengths'.

Somewhat similar considerations apply to the *lateral resolution*. It follows from the relationships developed on page 149 that increasing the ultrasonic frequency allows a transducer with a smaller diameter to be used whilst maintaining the beam geometry in terms of dimensions (in wavelengths) and angular divergence. An additional point to be remembered is that the beamwidth can be reduced

over a limited depth in the near field by focusing with a lens or a curved transducer. In the absence of focusing (i.e. with a plane disc transducer), the width of the beam extending for about 1·2 times the length of the near field beyond the transducer (the beam may begin to diverge significantly beyond this, unless the transducer is very large: see Equation 4.12) may be taken to be around 10 wavelengths, again with a dynamic range of 10dB. Focusing typically reduces the beamwidth to around two wavelengths.

It is often helpful to consider the wavelength to be the factor which controls the dimensions of the structures which are but examined by any particular instrument. Thus, optimum results are obtained in abdominal, cardiological and neurological investigations at frequencies of 2–4 MHz (corre-

---

*Note that the 'frequency' and and 'wavelength' of such a short pulse is a simplistic concept, since a short pulse has a substantial frequency bandwidth.

sponding to wavelength of about 0·8–0·4 mm, and maximum penetrations of 200–100 mm). For vascular and 'small parts' scanning, frequencies of 3–5 MHz are used (wavelengths, 0·5–0·3 mm; penetrations, 100–50 mm). Ophthalmological scans are made at frequencies of 8–20 MHz (wavelengths, 0·2–0·1 mm; penetrations, 40–20 mm).

Multiple reflexion artifacts

A serious limitation of the pulse-echo method is due to the multiple reflexions, or reverberations, that the ultrasonic pulse may suffer during its propagation. For example, in Figure 4.18 echoes returning to the probe from within the patient are themselves partially re-reflected at the probe surface, and these pulses themselves act as if they were transmitted pulses, relatively small in amplitude and appropriately delayed in time. Echoes of these small pulses produce registrations, if they are large enough to be detected, at positions corresponding to twice the distances at which the true echoes are registered. These 'multiple reflexion' artifacts may often be quite easily recognised because of their regular spacings. Those due to gas and bone are generally inconveniently large, and they are a fundamental limitation in ultrasonic diagnosis. In echocardiography, common sources of multiple reflexion artifacts are the ribs and lung.

The B-scope

The information obtained with a pulse-echo system is a combination of range and amplitude data which can simply be presented as an A-scan (see p. 151). The same information, however, may alternatively be displayed on a brightness-modulated timebase, in such a way that the brightness increases with echo amplitude; this type of display is called a B-scan. The B-scope is the basis of the *time-position recording* technique (the *M-mode* recording technique which is the cornerstone of echocardiography), and of the *two-dimensional scanner* (of which three main types—the *static B-scanner*, the *water-bath coupled scanner*, and the *real-time scanner* are in common clinical use).

Time-position (M-mode) recording

A time-position (M-mode) recording of structure position along the ultrasonic beam may be generated from a B-scan as shown in Figure 4.20. Most

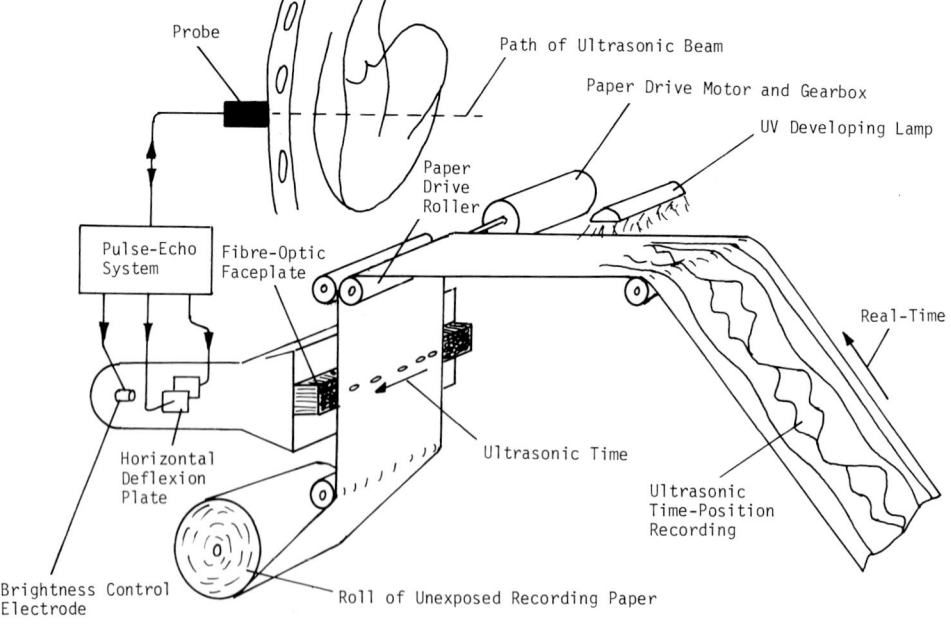

Fig. 4.20 Time-position recording system using a continuous strip of photographic paper sensitive to ultraviolet light. The B-scan is displayed on a cathode ray tube with a fibre-optic faceplate. This display is extremely bright, and a continuous image of the time-position trace is produced (and developed within a few seconds) as the paper is driven at constant speed past the cathode ray tube.

instruments based on this principle generate time and distance (i.e. ultrasonic timebase) markers on the recording to assist in interpretation.

A time-position recording is composed of many separate B-scan lines lying side-by-side. Conventionally, increasing distance into the patient is represented by more downward deflexion on the recording, and earlier time, horizontally towards the right. The time required to form a single B-scan line depends on the depth of penetration; for example, a time of 133 µs corresponds to a depth of 100 mm. Structures within the body do not move a significant distance during so short a time, so that (provided that the pulse repetition rate is fast enough) the movements of structures such as heart valves may be studied.

Two-dimensional B-scanning

The production of an image of a cross-section through soft tissue structures of the body may be accomplished by relating the positions of registrations on the display to the positions of the corresponding echo-producing structures within a defined two-dimensional plane in the patient.

Before about 1975, ultrasonic two-dimensional scanners were generally designed to produce tissue maps with the emphasis on the display of organ boundaries. The best scans were considered to be those in which the anatomy was depicted by thin white lines on a black background, for which purpose a black-and-white display is ideal. It has now become clear, however, that the echo amplitude conveyes useful diagnostic information, and that gray-scale displays are generally greatly superior to those limited to presenting black-and-white images. The gray-scale capability of a display system can be described in terms of the dynamic range of the image. The dynamic range may be expressed

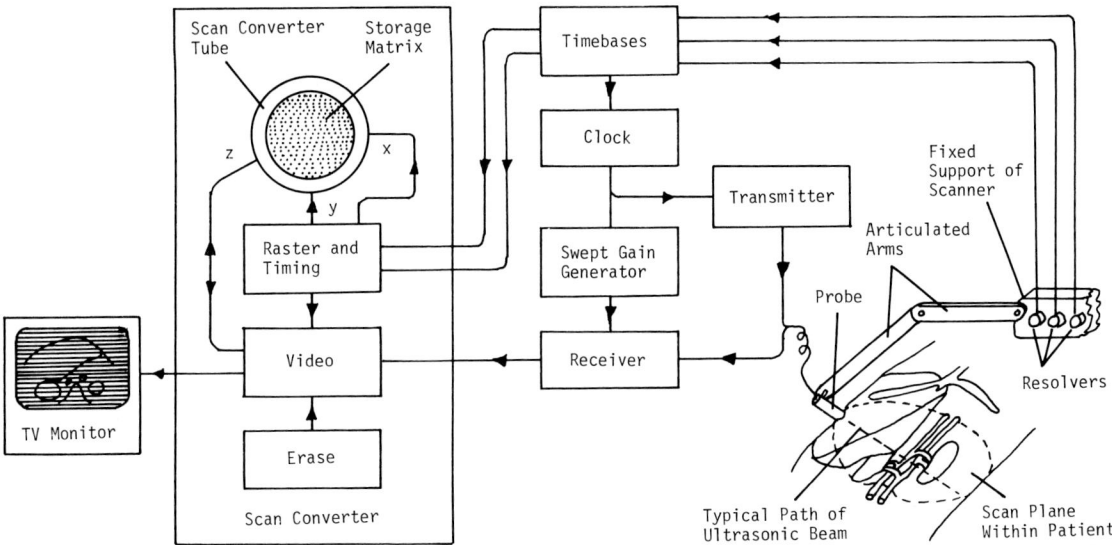

Fig. 4.21 Basic elements of a typical hand-operated two-dimensional static B-scanner. The ultrasonic part produces an intensity-modulated signal written on the storage matrix of the scan converter. (*Digital* image storage (Fig. 4.23) is now commonly used in place of the analogue type shown here, but the latter is easier to understand in an initial explanation of the principles involved.) The positions in which the echo signals are recorded are determined by the two timebase generators, controlled by three resolvers mounted on the fixed support of the scanner. Two articulated arms constrain the probe so that it can be moved only in a defined two-dimensional plane, in contact with the patient (coupling is provided by means of oil or propietary gel smeared on the skin). The resolvers measure the horizontal and vertical positions of the probe and the direction of the ultrasonic beam. This arrangement results in the timebase being driven across the storage matrix from the corresponding position and in the same direction as the ultrasonic beam travels across the patient. Changes in beam orientation are followed by corresponding changes in that of the timebase. Thus, echoes from any particular reflecting point in the patient register at the same position on the storage matrix, independent ultrasonic beam direction. As the probe is scanned across the patient, echo signals produce registrations on the storage matrix creating a charge pattern that is a two-dimensional representation of the anatomical cross-section through the patient. It is displayed as an image on the TV monitor by raster-scanning of the scan converter storage matrix. Time-sharing of the scan converter operation allows the image to be viewed whilst scanning is in progress, and the stored image can subsequently be studied on the monitor, or the image may be photographed, either directly from the monitor or on a multiformat camera.

as the number of decibels separating the minimum and maximum displayed amplitudes between which changes in amplitude produce perceptible changes in brightness.

Static B-scanners

The first type of ultrasonic two-dimensional scanner to come into widespread clinical use was of the so-called static variety. A typical instrument is illustrated in Figure 4.21. This type of scanner is commonly used in ultrasonic visualisation of the pregnant uterus and its contents, and of the relatively static contents of the abdominal cavity.

Water-bath scanners

The second type of two-dimensional scanner employs water coupling between the transducer and the patient. Instruments of this type range from full-scale abdominal and general-purpose scanners, to relatively compact systems designed for visualising superficial small parts such as the thyroid gland, the testis, and the peripheral blood vessels. Eye scanners also are usually in this category.

Some water-bath coupled scanners, particularly the smallers ones, can produce complete images very rapidly. Before describing these instruments, it is necessary to introduce the concept of *real-time* scanning. For the purposes of discussion, a real-time scanner is defined here as being one which produces sequential images at a rate fast enough to follow changes in the spatial relationships within the scan plane. Such changes may be due either to physiological movements within the defined spatial plane, or to movements of the scanner bring different structures into the scan plane, or to a combination of these two types of motion. For example, in studying the movements of the heart valves, a frame rate of, say, 100/second might be necessary to satisfy this definition of real-time, whereas a frame rate of 4/second might be adequate to follow changes as a scanner is moved over the surface of the abdomen.

Some examples of water-bath coupled scanners are illustrated in Figure 4.22. The use of a water-bath allows a relatively larger transducer to be used than would be possible with the transducer in contact with the patient; this allows significant focusing to be applied, with consequently high resolution (see p. 153). Moreover, the mechanical movement causing the scanner action is remote from the patient, so sensitive and soft structures can be examined without discomfort or spatial disturbance.

Real-time scanners

Fast real-time scanners produce images at a rate which is high enough to avoid flicker when they are displayed sequentially. This is true for image frame rates of greater than about 20 s^{-1}. At slower frame rates, the eye is distracted by the transient appearance of the image. This can be avoided by the use of a digital scan converter (Fig. 4.23). Appropriate logic circuitry allows the data stored in the RAM to be read out continuously and displayed in analogue form on a television monitor. Meanwhile, the image data can be refreshed line-by-line. The effect of this is that a flicker-free image appears on the display, and, as the ultrasonic beam slowly scans through the patient, the previous image is wiped out and updated by the new image. Another advantage of this method of storage is that the operator can freeze any image as it appears, if it seems to merit detailed study.

Ultimately the frame rate is limited by the speed of ultrasound in tissue. If, for example, a penetration of 150 mm is required, the time which elapses between the transmission of the ultrasonic pulse and reception of the echo from the maximum range is equal to 200 μs (taking the speed to be 1500 m s^{-1}). The corresponding maximum pulse repetition rate is 5000 s^{-1} (although in practice 2000–3000 s^{-1} would be more likely to be used). Thus the maximum image line rate is 5000 s^{-1}, equal to the product of the number of lines per frame and the number of frames per second. Again, for example, at 40 frames s^{-1}, there are 125 lines per frame.

Some of the many methods of rapid scanning to produce real-time images are illustrated in Figure 4.24. The mechanical method shown is yet another way of directing the ultrasonic beam of a conventional transducer through an appropriate scan pattern. This particular arrangement, using a rotating wheel with several transducers 'looking' in sequence radially through the rim, is a popular one because it avoids the disadvantage of vibration associated with an oscillating transducer in contact with the skin, whilst being relatively easy to construct and simple to maintain.

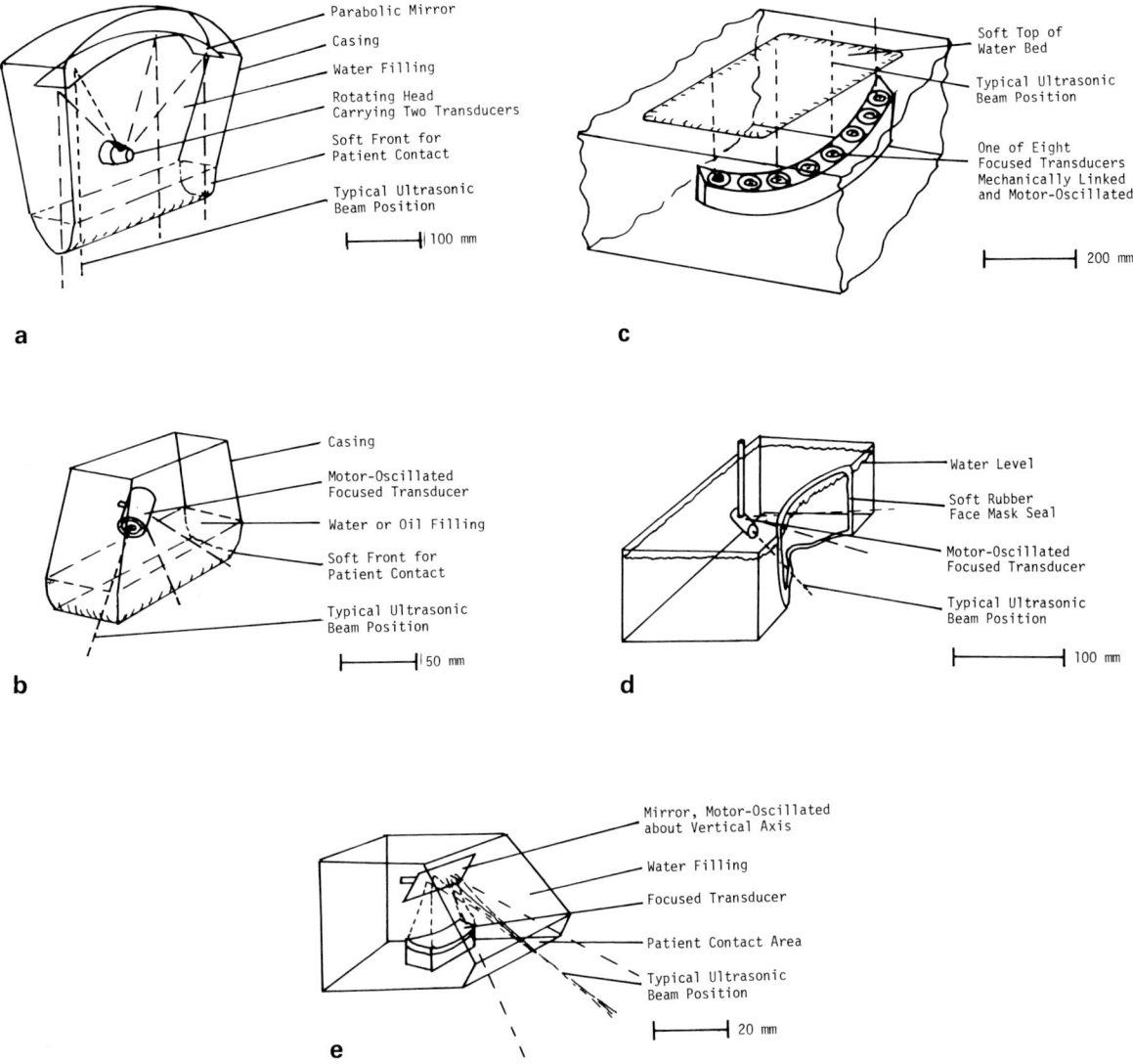

Fig. 4.22 Two-dimensional scanners employing water-bath coupling between the transducer and the patient. Abdominal scanners (a) with rotating transducer mounted at the focus of a parabolic reflector to produce a rectangular scan format, as the ultrasonic scan lines are parallel in the patient, (b) with oscillating transducer mounted some distance from the patient's surface to produce a trapezoidal scan format. (c) General purpose instrument, suitable for scanning the adult abdomen, the neonate and infant (including the brain), and the breast; the transducers are linked together and oscillated mechanically to produce scans with any desired degree of compounding. In a compound scan each volume element of tissue is examined from several different directions. Likelihood of detecting specular reflexions is increased (p. 141) but image may be degraded by variations in propagation speed along different path lengths, or by even quite small inaccuracies in setting up the instrument. (d) Eye scanner, with oscillating transducer producing a trapezoidal scan format. (e) 'Small parts' scanner, with a focused ultrasonic beam reflected by a rotating, off-axis, mirror, to produce a trapezoidal scan format.

Electronic real-time scanning

The other two methods illustrated in Figure 4.24. have no moving parts, and instead the scanning is achieved electronically. The principles of the electronically addressed linear array type of real-time scanner are illustrated in Figure 4.25. In the earliest linear array systems, the transducer elements

158 SCIENTIFIC BASIS OF MEDICAL IMAGING

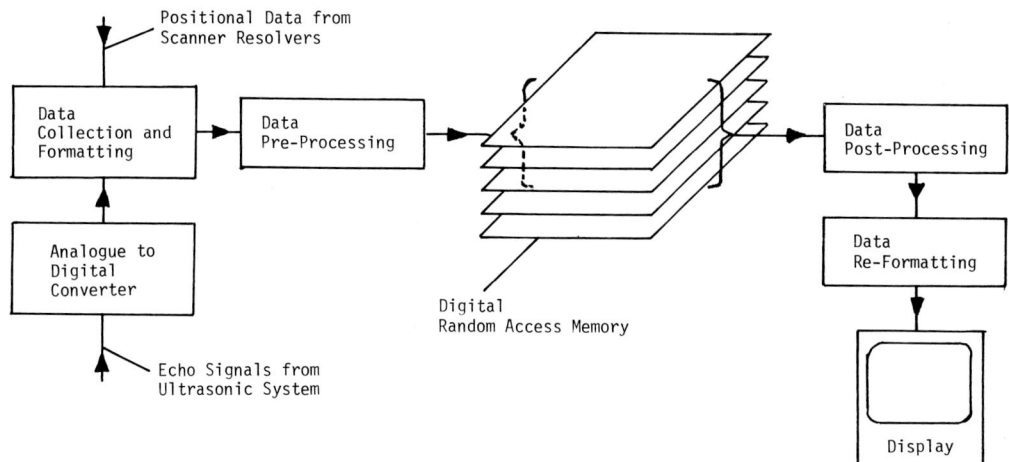

Fig. 4.23 Digital scan converter for two-dimensional image storage. The RAM typically has a capacity of 512 × 512 5-bit words. The analogue echo signals are digitised and stored in the appropriate matrix elements of the RAM addressed by positional data from the scanner. Gray scale capability is limited by digital word length, e.g. a 5-bit word can accommodate a range of input levels from $1-2^5$. In decimals, this is equivalent to 1–32. Thus, 32 discrete gray levels can be stored, corresponding to a dynamic range of about 30 dB. (This may be compared with the 50 dB dynamic range of a well-adjusted analogue scan converter.)

are addressed one at a time. In this situation, a compromise is necessary. On the one hand, it is desirable to have a large number of lines in the image, and this requires a large number of transducers. On the other hand, it is desirable to have good resolution, which depends on having a non-divergent (or even focused) beam of ultrasound. Unfortunately, the beam divergence in the far field increases as the transducer is made more narrow. The difficulty can be circumvented by having an

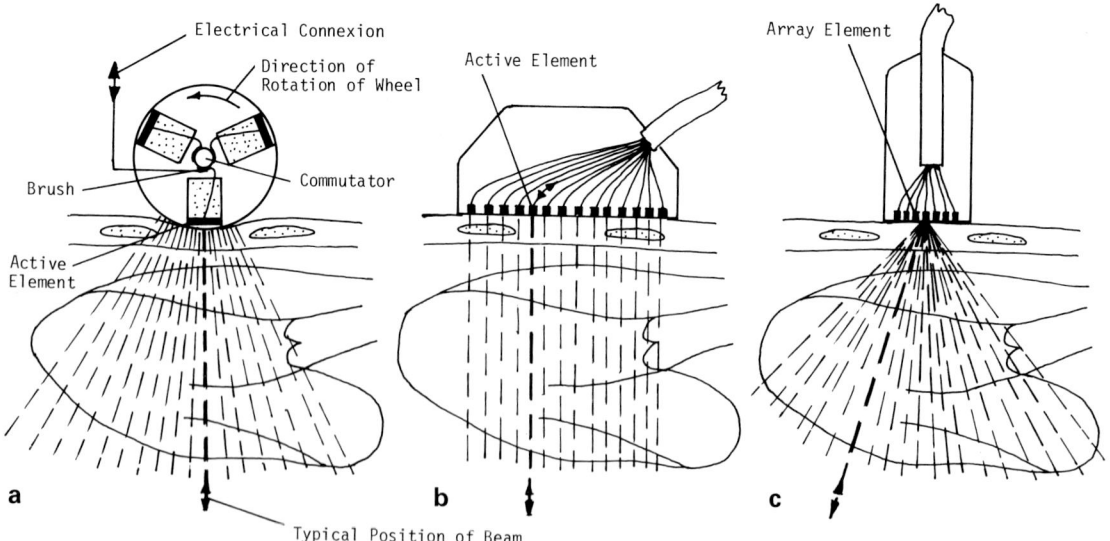

Fig. 4.24 Methods of real-time scanning. (a) Fast mechanical scanner: 3 single-element transducers mounted on a continuously rotating wheel. As each transducer in turn comes into contact with the patient, it sweeps out a new frame made up of an image sector. (b) Electronically scanned linear array transducer array: the transducer elements are addressed sequentially, to sweep out image frames with a rectangular format. (c) Transducer array with electronic beam steering: delays are introduced into the separate signal paths associated with the individual elements in the array, to sweep out image frames with a sector format.

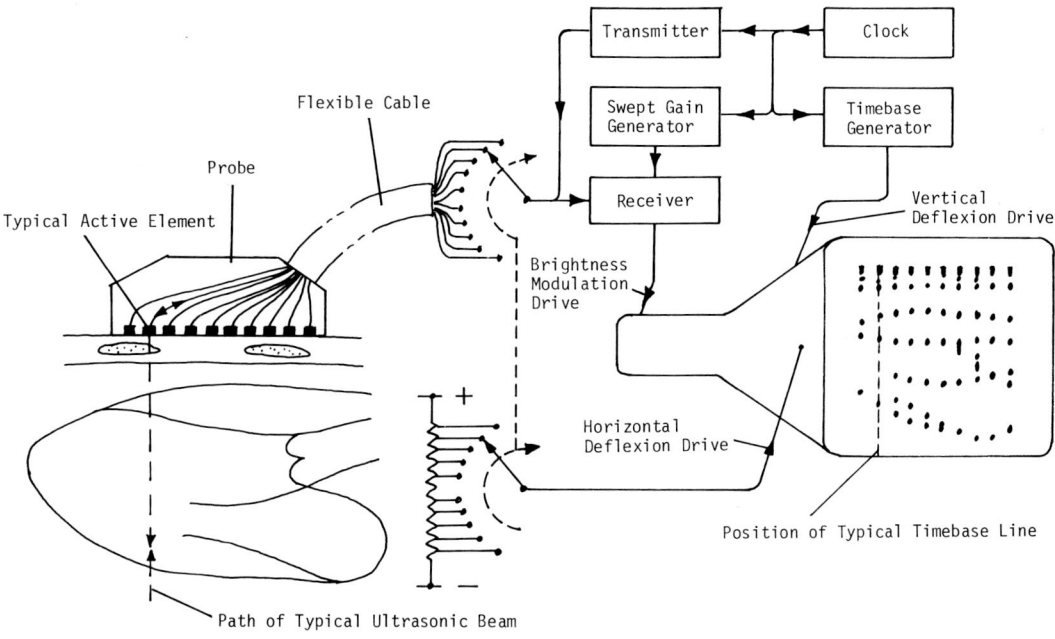

Fig. 4.25 Linear array real-time scanning system. This probe contains 10 separate transducer elements (in a practical system, the number is usually between 20 and 128). The clock, typically operating at a prf of 2000 s^{-1}, triggers the transmitter. Here the transmitter pulse is applied, through a sequencing switch, to one of the transducer elements. (Again, in a practical system, this sequencing switch, and the second switch operating synchronously with it, is usually electronic and not mechanical.) Simultaneously, the clock triggers the timebase generator connected to the vertical deflexion plates of the cathode ray tube display. Echoes returning from within the patient are detected by the transducer element which emitted the original pulse, fed through the sequencing switch, and amplified (under swept gain control, triggered by the clock), to brightness-modulate the display. Each element is rapidly addressed in sequence, and a two-dimensional image is built up by the second sequencing switch applying appropriate horizontal deflexion voltages to the display.

array of many narrow transducers (so that the objective of high line density can be achieved) operated in groups to ensure an adequate aperture (so that the resolution is acceptable). A common arrangement, illustrated in Figure 4.26, is to have 64 elements operated in groups of 4, stepped one element between lines, thus giving 61 lines of ultrasonic information.

An important feature of array operation is illustrated in Figure 4.27. This is the ability to steer and to focus the ultrasonic beam by introducing appropriate time gradings across the array. The effect of this, at least when the beam is directed straight ahead, is equivalent to that of the action of a lens (discussed on p. 150). For transmission, the electronically controlled geometry of the beam is fixed according to the chosen times delays. During reception, however, the position of the focus may be swept continuously (or, at least, the position of the focal zone may be switched in discrete intervals) to coincide with the instantaneous positions of the echo-producing targets along the ultrasonic beam axis.

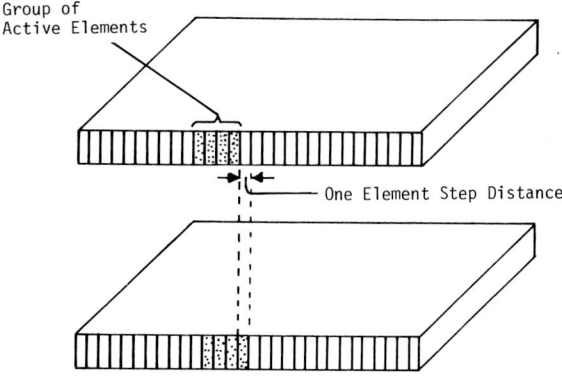

Fig. 4.26 The use of element groups in linear array to provide an adequate aperture whilst allowing the adjacent beam separation to be kept small. A four-element aperture (shown stippled) is stepped along the array, one element at a time.

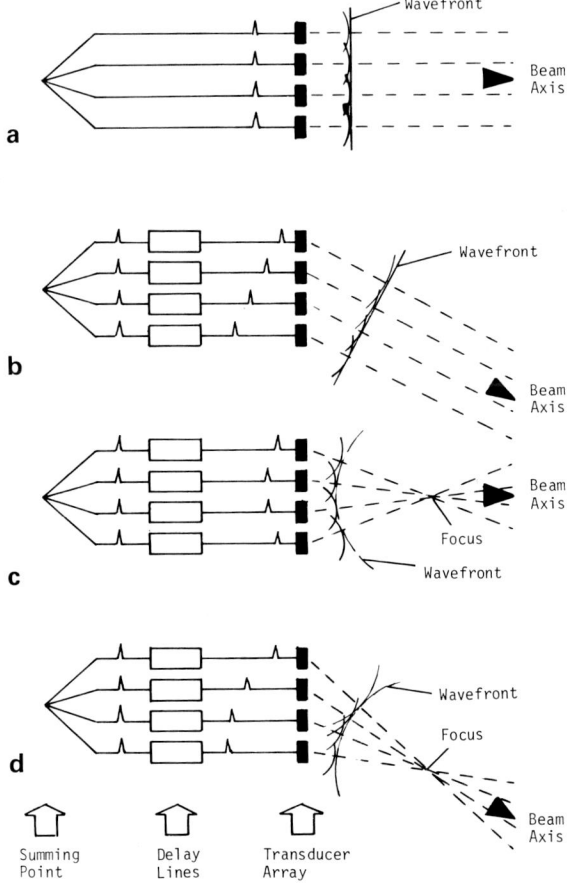

Fig. 4.27 Principles of electronically steered array scanning illustrating the transmission of ultrasound by an array of four long narrow elements; the same principles apply to the reception of ultrasound. The long axes of the elements are normal to the plane of the diagram, and viewed in this direction each element emits a cylindrical wavelet in response to electrical excitation. (a) When the elements are excited simultaneously (as indicated by the simultaneous 'blips' on the connecting wires), the wavelets combine to form a wavefront of which the corresponding beam travels directly away from the array. (b) When the elements are excited in sequence, the beam is deviated off the central axis. (c) When spherical time grading is used, the beam is focused. (d) When the time grading consists of combined linear and spherical distributions, the beam is both deviated and focused.

Figure 4.28 illustrates the improvement in *azimuthal* resolution (i.e. resolution along the length of the array) which can be achieved by applying electronic focusing to a linear transducer array. To gain maximum benefit from this, more elements need to be used in the aperture than are appropriate for an unfocused beam (as in Fig. 4.26).

Although the linear array type of electronic real-time scanner has important clinical applications, especially in examining the abdomen, it does have the disadvantage that flat skin contact has to be maintained over the full length of the imaging aperture. Since the scan format is rectangular, this limits the width of the scan plane through the examined tissue section. In many clinical situations, however, this problem may be avoided by the use of an *electronically steered* array, which, as illustrated in Figure 4.24c, has a trapezoidal scan format and requires only a relatively small contact area with the skin. The term *phased* array is commonly used to describe this system. This term is appropriate in the analogous technique in radar, where the relative frequency bandwidth is so small that within a pulse a particular phase change introduces a time delay which is effectively constant across the pulse frequency spectrum. Strictly speaking, however, the term is inappropriate for diagnostic ultrasound, because the pulse bandwidth is a significant proportion of the centre frequency.

Figure 4.29 is a more detailed diagram showing some of the practical aspects of the operation of a steered array. Typically, electronically steered arrays have around 20 elements, and the external dimensions of the probe are similar to those of a conventional single-element transducer probe.

Of the two main types of real-time scanner, the electronic systems (either linear or steered array) have an advantage which is particularly important in cardiological investigations. This is the ability which they have to allow the selection of one (or more) scan line positions for simultaneous M-mode recording (p. 154) of the movement of a structure identified on the two-dimensional image. The best that can be done with mechanical scanners is first to identify the structure of interest on a two-dimensional scan, and then progressively to decrease the scan angle until there is a single, stationary, line passing through the structure whose motion it is desired to record. The real-time image is presently invariably displayed on a cathode ray tube during the scanning procedure. Except occasionally with electronic linear array systems, the scan format is not TV-raster-compatible, and to make use of standard TV monitors, character generators, and tape recorders, the initial ultrasonic scan dis-

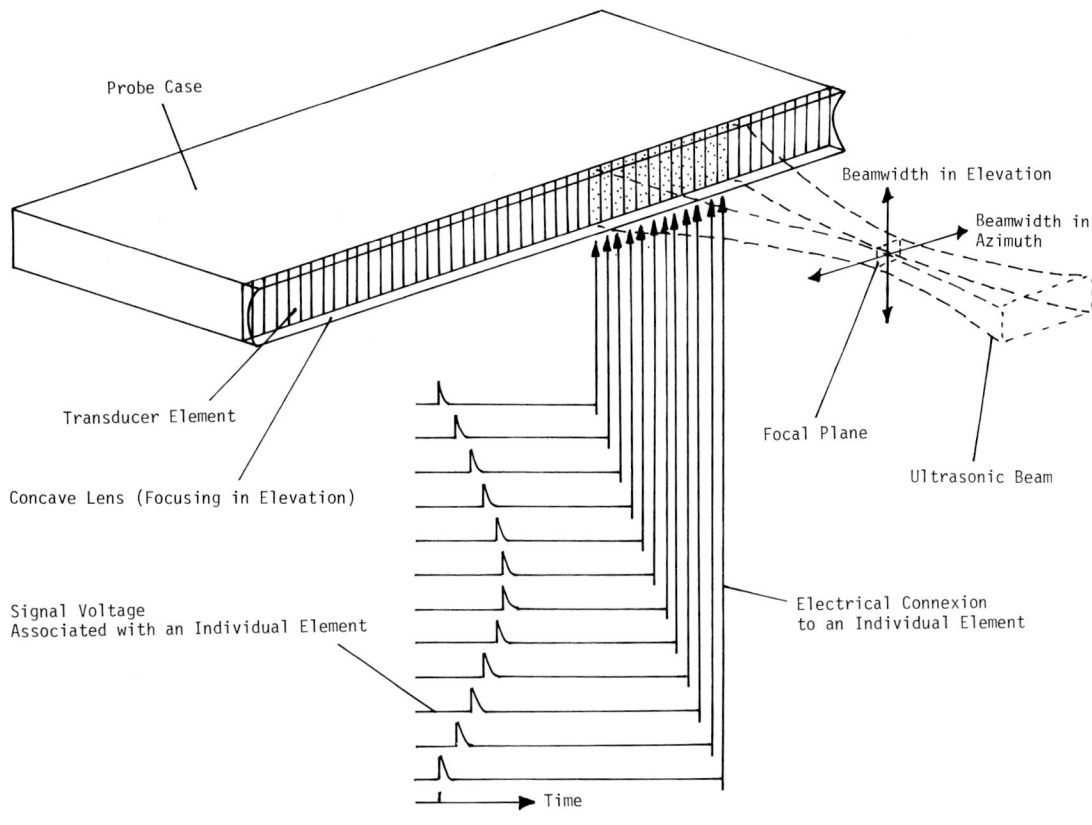

Fig. 4.28 Linear array with electronic focusing in azimuth (this has to be of fixed focal length on transmission, but can be swept on reception), and with lens focusing in elevation. In this example, the elements are used in groups of 12, and there are 51 elements in the array, giving 42 separate lines in the image. The resolution in *elevation* (i.e. the resolution across the width of the array) is improved by focusing with a concave plastic lens.

play tube may be viewed by a closed-circuit TV camera.

It has previously been mentioned in this Section that an image frame rate of at least around 40/s is necessary to follow fast movements such as those of the cardiac valves. It is not possible, however, for the eye of the observer to follow movements presented at this rate. This can only be done if the images are played back from a recording in slow motion; and this is a facility which is available with some video-tape recorders.

In clinical practice, one of the major operational problems in real-time ultrasonic scanning carried out by technicians for subsequent review by doctors is the difficulty of recording the anatomical position of the scan plane. An audio channel for commentary dubbing on the video tape is only a partially successful solution to the problem. A better way is simultaneously to record the ultrasonic scan and a closed circuit TV view of the patient.

Measurements of distance

In many clinical applications, it is important to be able to make measurements of distance from the ultrasonic two-dimensional images. It is not satisfactory to measure directly from the cathode ray tube display, even when the image is stationary for long enough to make this possible, because the image is distorted by non-linearities in the deflexion system. Electronic calipers may be provided to eliminate this problem, and several arrangements have been devised: generally the choice depends on the personal preference of the operator.

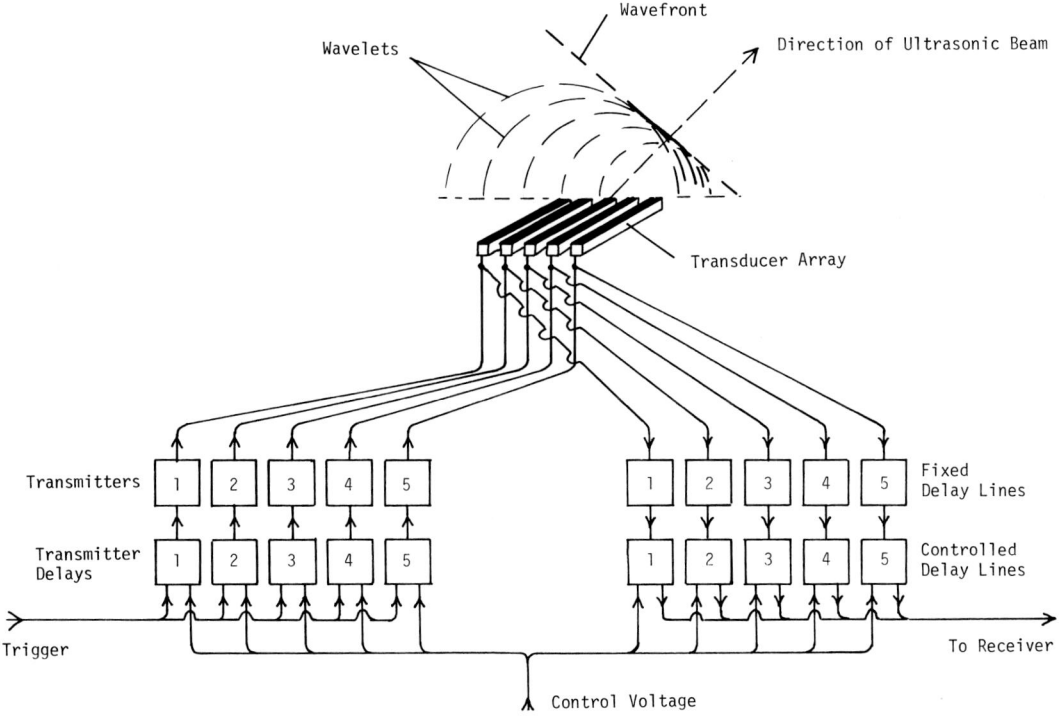

Fig. 4.29 The principles of operation of an electronically steered array for real-time two-dimensional imaging. This type of system produces a sector scan with a radial line scan pattern. Each element in the array is approximately 20 wavelengths long and 1 wavelength in width. Here, transmitter 1 is triggered first, followed in sequence by 2–5. Each transducer element emits a cylindrical wavelet, and the resultant beam is directed perpendicular to the wavefront. The transmitted beam can also be focused, by superimposing a spherical time grading along the array. The same principles apply on reception, but delay lines are required to delay the actual ultrasonic signals detected by each element. Moreover, as negative delay cannot be introduced, each controlled delay line is connected in series with a fixed delay line, chosen so that the beam is steered to the extreme of one edge of the sector when all the controlled delay times are equal.

DOPPLER DIAGNOSTIC METHODS

Ultrasonic Doppler methods are nowadays both widely used and of established value in the study of moving structures in clinical diagnosis. In most applications, the Doppler shift in frequency of a continuous wave ultrasonic beam reflected from a moving structure (or ensemble of scatterers) is used to provide information about the velocity of the structure (or ensemble), either for interpretation by ear, or for analysis by instrument. Two-dimensional Doppler scanning is becoming accepted. Pulsed Doppler systems, which combine the range-measuring capability of the pulse-echo method with the velocity-measuring capability of Doppler, are beginning to demonstrate their potential value in scanning and analysis.

Equation 4.7 relates the Doppler shift frequency to the velocity of the reflector, the angle between the directions of the ultrasonic beam and the motion of the reflector, the ultrasonic frequency and the speed of ultrasound. For example, in the case where no correction for angulation is required (i.e. $\cos \gamma = 1$), a 2 MHz ultrasonic beam is shifted in frequency by about 260 Hz on reflexion from a surface moving at a velocity of 100 mm s^{-1}, if $c = 1500$ m s^{-1} (as is the case in water, blood, and soft tissues). For practical purposes, the Doppler shift frequency may be taken to be proportional both to the ultrasonic frequency and to the reflector velocity. One particularly convenient feature of Doppler methods is immediately apparent: the Doppler shift frequency lies in the audible range and, because the ear is so good at recognising sound patterns, a good deal of useful clinical information can be obtained simply by listening to the signals.

The choice of the ultrasonic frequency depends on the clinical application. A compromise is necessary between the penetration, the variation of Doppler shift frequency for a given variation in target velocity, the sensitivity to small reflectors, and the size and shape of the ultrasonic field. In obstetrics and cardiology, the optimum frequency is generally 2–3 MHz, but in blood flow studies, it may be as high as 10 MHz. The same restrictions and limitations (such as the necessity to maintain good ultrasonic coupling, and the inability to operate successfully through gas) which apply to ultrasonic pulse-echo methods, also apply to ultrasonic Doppler methods. The reflexion (backscattered) ultrasonic Doppler method is used in many types of instrument, simple and complex, for measuring the velocities of structures and flow within the heart and blood vessels. Usually the examination is transcutaneous.

Continuous wave Doppler systems

The block diagram of a continuous wave Doppler system is shown in Figure 4.30. The transmitter operates continuously, providing an output of constant amplitude and frequency. The ultrasonic probe contains separate transmitting and receiving transducers. (These are generally necessary, because it is important to minimise the direct transfer of energy from the transmitter to the radio frequency amplifier*, in order to avoid overloading the receiver.) The output from the rf amplifier consists of a mixture of signals, some of frequency equal to that of the transmitter (these are due to reflexions from stationary structures in the ultrasonic field, and electrical leakage), and some of frequencies shifted by the Doppler effect (due to reflexions from moving structures). These signals are mixed in the demodulator, the output from which contains the difference frequencies between the transmitted ultrasonic wave and the Doppler shifted received waves. The output from the demodulator is filtered to allow these difference frequencies to pass, whilst unwanted (higher) frequencies are stopped. The difference frequencies, which in general fall in the audible range, are amplified, and either an operator listens to them, or they are analysed electronically.

In clinical applications, the Doppler shifted signals do not consist of a single frequency, but they extend over a spectrum of frequencies which changes with time. This is because the beam simultaneously interrogates structures and scatterers moving at different velocities. In some situations, such as in the detection of fetal heart movements, the signal of interest has some strongly distinguish-

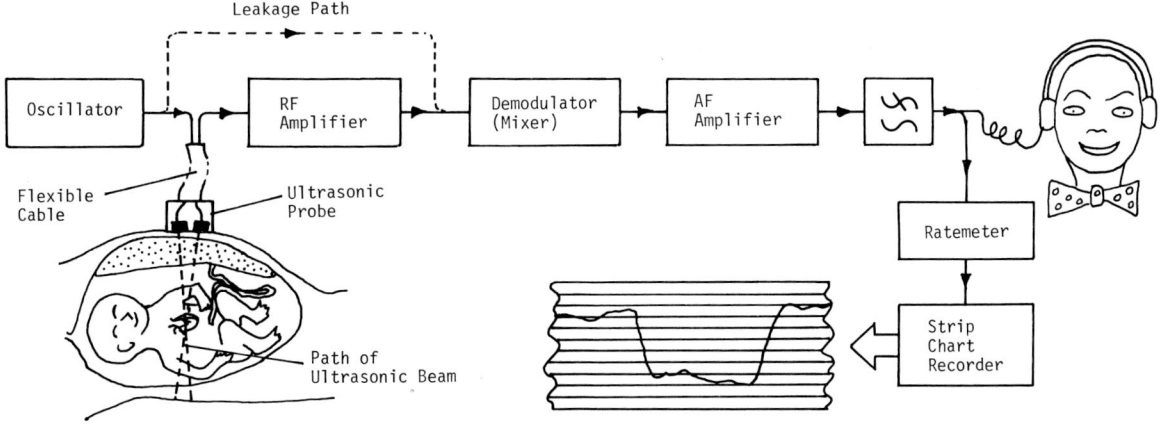

Fig. 4.30 Continuous wave ultrasonic Doppler instrument designed specifically for detecting fetal heart movements, and recording the fetal heart rate. The ultrasonic frequency is typically 2 MHz.

*The term 'radio-frequency' is used because the ultrasonic frequencies used (2–10 MHz) happen to lie within the range of frequencies of electromagnetic waves used for radio transmissions.

ing feature (e.g. loudness), and the information which is clinically relevant may be obtained by means of a simple ratemeter. Most other applications of the Doppler effect are for the investigation of blood flow, and measurements of Doppler shift signals made by ratemeters, such as the zero-crossing frequency meter, need to be interpreted with caution. In most cardiovascular investigations with Doppler techniques, it is generally very much safer to subject the Doppler signals to frequency spectrum analysis; this may be done by on-line or off-line instruments.

Pulsed Doppler systems

The block diagram of a typical pulsed Doppler system is shown in Figure 4.31. This particular arrangement, employing a single receiver channel with an adjustable range-gate, is the simplest possible. More complex instruments, with multiple range gates, can be used to measure velocity simultaneously at several positions along the ultrasonic beam (see p. 169).

In any pulsed Doppler system employing uncoded transmitted signals, there is an upper limit to the frequency which can be detected without ambiguity. This limit is set by the sampling rate, which is equal to the clock frequency. The maximum clock frequency is limited by the ultrasonic transit time to and from the resolution cell, and by the reverberation decay time. It is well known in information theory that if a signal waveform has frequencies in its spectrum extending from zero to an upper frequency f_{max}, it is possible to convey all the information in the signal provided that the sampling frequency is at least 2 f_{max}. This sets an upper limit to the maximum unambiguously measurable velocity vector at any given penetration for a given ultrasonic frequency. For example, the chosen frequency might be 5 MHz, and the necessary penetration, 100 mm. The corresponding maximum pulse repetition rate for this penetration would be 7500 s^{-1}. Theoretically the maximum ultrasonic Doppler shift frequency corresponding to this sampling rate would be 3750 Hz; and substitution in Equation 4.7 reveals that the maximum vector velocity would be about 550 mm s^{-1} (with γ = 0°). It turns out that, at any given frequency and geometry, the product of the maximum vector velocity and the maximum target range is equal to a constant. This is an important consideration which has to be taken into account in designing pulsed Doppler instruments. In the case of blood flow studies, for example, it would otherwise generally be desirable to use a rather higher ultrasonic frequency than is possible in practice. This is because the signal-to-noise ratio would become larger at a higher ultrasonic frequency, but unfortunately the consequential increase in Doppler shift frequency would be beyond the nonambiguous range set by the penetration depth limit in the pulse repetition frequency.

As is hinted earlier in this Section, this range-velocity compromise can be avoided by coding the transmitted pulses, so that several pulses are simultaneously in transit between the transducer and the resolution cell. Coding can, for example, be provided by noise modulation. Although the feasibility of this technique has been demonstrated experimentally, it is not yet widely used.

There is another limitation of the range-gated Doppler method, but one which is more of a theoretical nicety than of practical importance. It arises because the range resolution of the pulse-echo measurement and the velocity resolution of the Doppler measurement are inextricably linked. Conceptually, this arises because it is impossible to measure the velocity of a reflector if its position is exactly measured from the same data. In more precise terms, it becomes increasingly difficult to measure Doppler shift frequency signals superimposed on an ultrasonic pulse, as its duration is shortened (with corresponding increase in frequency spectral bandwidth) to improve the range resolution.

Directionally sensitive Doppler systems

Simple Doppler systems merely measure the magnitude of the frequency difference between the transmitted and received ultrasonic signals, and not the sign of the difference as defined in Equation 4.6. This sign carries the information about the direction of the movement of the target, either towards or away from the probe. This directional information is vital in some diagnostic situations.

If the signal always consists, at any instant in time, of movement (or flow) in only one direction, a detector capable of switching a logic circuit to indicate whether the movement is in the forward or reverse direction would be satisfactory. (This is the method employed in many commercially-manufactured systems, and is explained later in this section.) Almost invariably, however, in practice the Doppler signal consists, at least for some of the time in each periodic cycle, of simultaneous signals from targets moving in opposite directions. Logic circuits are then inadequate, and the forward and

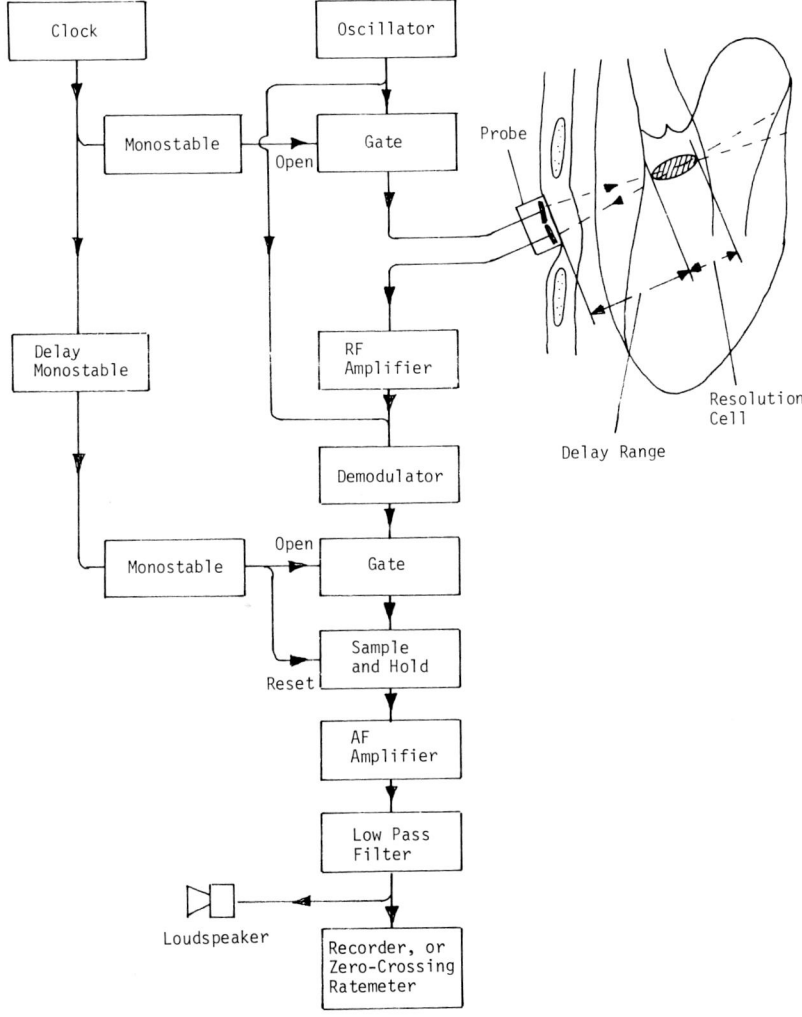

Fig. 4.31 Typical pulsed Doppler system. The pulse repetition rate is controlled by the clock, which triggers the monostable to open the gate to allow the transmitting transducer to be excited for a period corresponding to the width of the target volume which it is desired to study. Echoes returning from within the patient are amplified, and mixed in the demodulator with the signal from the oscillator (equal in frequency to that which was transmitted). The delay monostable triggers the monostable controlling the receiver gate, so that the gate opens to allow a voltage, which is in effect a sample corresponding to the Doppler shift due to motion in the resolution cell, to be stored in the sample-and-hold circuit. The sample-and-hold is reset immediately prior to being updated by a new sample resulting from the following ultrasonic pulse. The output from the sample-and-hold is thus a rectangular wave with a long 'mark' and a short 'space', the envelope of which is an audible signal representing the Doppler shifted information from the resolution cell.

reverse flow signals need to be separated and processed simultaneously and independently. In principle, the simplest way in which this can be done is to use highpass and lowpass filters tuned to the upper and lower sidebands about the transmitted ultrasonic frequency (Fig. 4.32a). The upper sideband consists of signals shifted upwards in frequency by movements towards the ultrasonic probe, and vice versa for the lower sideband. The forward and reverse Doppler-shifted difference signals may then be obtained separately by mixing the outputs from the two filters with a signal at the

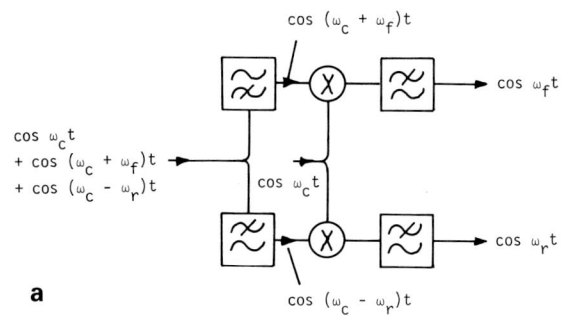

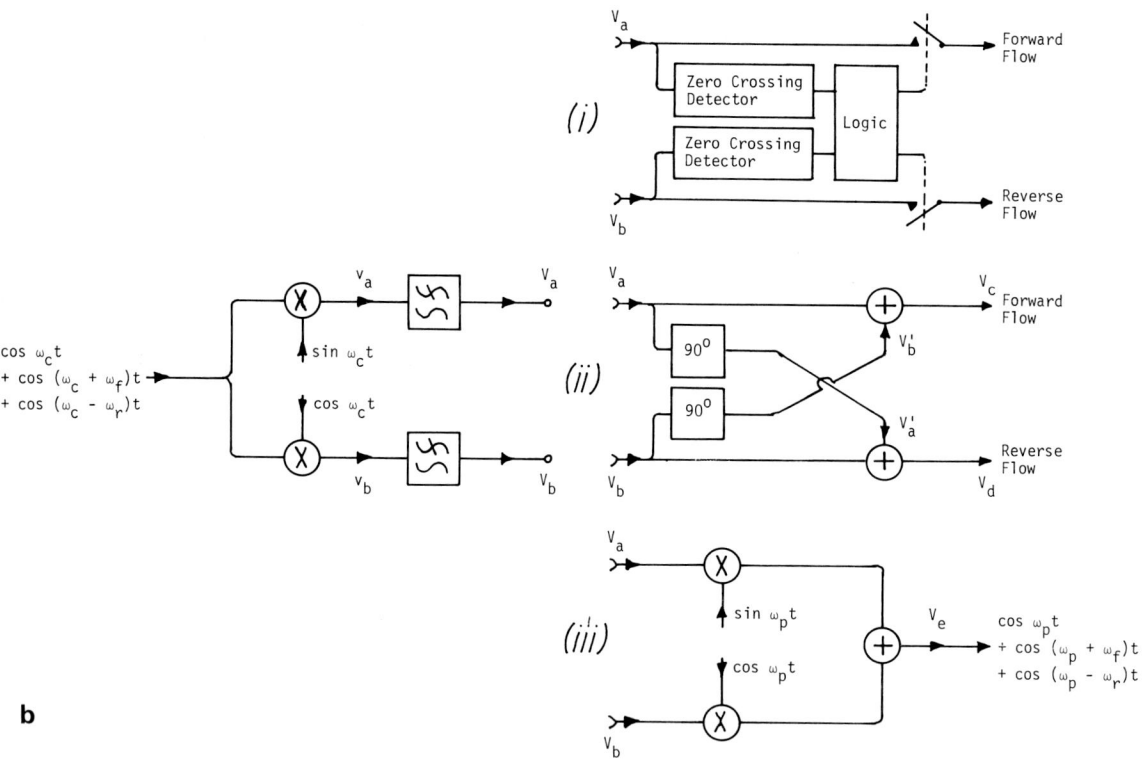

Fig. 4.32 Two techniques for separating Doppler signals according to their directions.[5] The 'raw' Doppler signal can be considered to be made up of three components: $\cos \omega_c t$ represents the component at the transmitted frequency ω_c; $\cos (\omega_c + \omega_f) t$ is the sideband corresponding to forward flow with frequency ω_f; and $\cos (\omega_c - \omega_r) t$ is the sideband with reverse flow frequency ω_r. (a) the highpass and lowpass filters select the upper and lower sidebands respectively, and mixing these signals with a signal at the transmitted frequency ω_c produces, after lowpass filtering, the separate forward and reverse Doppler difference frequency signals. (b) Mixing the 'raw' Doppler signal separately with signals 90° out of phase with each other but both at the transmitted frequency produces two signals V_a and V_b which contain a mixture of both forward and reverse flow signals but which differ in phase by 90°. These signals can be further processed in the following ways: (i) Time domain processing. The zero crossing detectors and logic circuit determine whether V_a leads or lags V_b. If V_a leads, the flow is in the forward direction, and vice versa. (ii) Phase domain processing. The principle of this method is that the reverse flow components are made equal to zero by adding V_a to V_b', V_b' being V_b shifted through 90°, and likewise for the forward flow components. The method depends on the 90° phase shifting networks operating correctly over the whole frequency range of interest. (iii) Frequency domain processing. Mixing V_a and V_b with two signals at the same pilot frequency ω_p but separated by 90°, and adding the results, produces a spectrum with forward and reverse flow signals represented by sidebands above and below the pilot frequency.

transmitted frequency. An advantage of this technique is that the transmitter frequency signal, which may be thought of as the carrier, can be rejected by the sideband filters. The main disadvantage is that the sideband filters, which have to operate at the ultrasonic frequency, are complicated and virtually impossible to adjust. The most commonly used technique of directional separation avoids this disadvantage by making use of the fact that forward flow signals, being higher in frequency than the transmitted signal, lead the transmitted signal in phase, whereas reverse flow signals lag in phase. Three processing systems based on this are illustrated in Figure 4.23b. The first of these is the logic switching system mentioned earlier in this section. The second system gives separate channels for forward and reverse flows, whilst the third equates zero flow to a pilot frequency, with forward and reverse flow signals on the upper and lower sidebands respectively.

Resolution in Doppler systems

The lateral resolution of a Doppler system at any particular distance from the transducer depends on the effective width of the ultrasonic beam. This in turn depends on the beam profile, and the signal processing arrangements including the detector threshold level. The range resolution of a continuous wave Doppler system is, in effect, such that any detectable target gives a signal; the penetration is limited by attenuation. Pulsed Doppler systems have range resolution determined by the effective length of the ultrasonic pulse, and in principle the situation resembles that in a conventional pulse-echo system; the point made at the end of section on pulsed Doppler systems (p. 164) should not be forgotten.

Doppler signal presentation, analysis and display

The simplest method of presenting the Doppler signal is to allow the operator to listen to it. Skilled operators are expert at identifying the signals from various origins, and at separating signals from noise and artifacts. For the solution of some clinical diagnostic problems, such as the confirmation of fetal heart motion, this is perfectly adequate; it may even be the best method. Even allowing for the possibility of later review from a tape recording, however, listening to the signals does not yield quantitative data. The acquisition of quantitative data requires quantitative analysis.

For measuring the rate of approximately periodic and characteristic Doppler signals, such as the regular, loud pulses of sound detected from the fetal heart, a simple ratemeter of the type used in ECG systems is perfectly adequate. The output from such a ratemeter can be recorded on a strip chart (Fig. 4.30).

The analysis of Doppler blood flow signals requires a more sophisticated approach. It has to be admitted, however, that zero crossing counting, which is the approach most commonly used in commercially available instruments, lacks the necessary degree of sophistication. In essence, the *zero crossing counter* consists of a comparator which produces a pulse each time that the signal crosses zero (normally, in one direction), followed by a circuit which converts these pulses into an instantaneous count rate. The method suffers from two main problems. Firstly, it is prone to respond to spurious noise signals superimposed on the Doppler signals. Secondly, at any instant in time, the Doppler signal contains a spectrum of many different frequencies. Although theoretically a zero crossing ratemeter produces an output proportional to the root mean square frequency of such a spectrum, in practice the instrument deserves its reputation for giving unreliable and misleading results.

The class of instrument which has been, and continues to be, traditionally used to avoid the pitfalls of the zero crossing ratemeter is the *frequency spectrum analyser*. The objective of frequency spectrum analysis is to produce a display on which time and frequency are represented on orthogonal axes (usually the x and y axes respectively), and the corresponding signal amplitudes are represented by density or brightness. Figure 4.33 is a typical sound spectrogram. This type of analysis may be performed by recording the signal on a magnetic disc and then replaying it over and over again. The continuously replayed signal is mixed with the output from a stepped frequency oscillator, and this shifts each part of the recorded spectrum in sequence to the passband of a fixed frequency filter. The output from the filter is

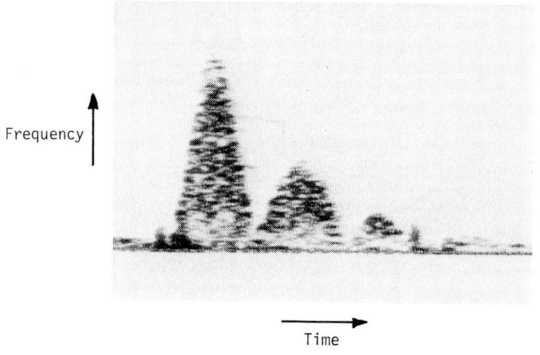

Fig. 4.33 Typical sound spectrogram of an ultrasonic Doppler blood flow signal. This particular spectrogram was made using a system which did not have a directional detector. In considering the spectrum, it is important to realise that the initial blood flow peak, with the highest maximum frequency, is in the forward direction, whereas the second peak actually represents blood flow in the reverse direction.

arranged to control the density of horizontal lines on the recording at vertical positions corresponding to the signal frequency bands.

The sound spectrogram has the great advantage that it allows artifacts to be recognised. Instruments using parallel filter banks, time compression analysers, or fast Fourier transform analysers, can display sound spectrograms in real time. In many clinical applications, however, full frequency analysis is not really necessary and there are three alternative approaches which are more-or-less adequate and which also avoid the hazards of the zero-crossing ratemeter. The first of these is the *time interval histogram analyser*. For each zero crossing event in the Doppler signal, the time period from the previous zero crossing is measured, and a dot is printed on the display at a horizontal position corresponding to the actual time, and at a vertical position which is inversely proportional to the measured time period. The advantage of time interval histogram analysis is that clear recordings (for example, from plug flow in which the signal is practically monotonic) can be safely interpreted, whereas bizarre patterns (for example, from turbulent flow), where caution is necessary, clearly cannot really be interpreted properly. Thus, although the method does not lend itself to quantitative studies, it is a neat way of answering some clinically important questions.

In several applications, the sound spectrogram of the Doppler signals is first obtained, and then the waveform of the maximum frequency envelope is traced by hand around the recording. It is this maximum frequency waveform which is analysed to obtain the diagnostic data. In order to avoid the manual tracing process, a *maximum frequency follower* may be used. Three schemes for implementing this have been reported. The first uses a bank of parallel filters (as in one of the schemes for frequency spectrum analysis) and a logic circuit which identifies which filter in the bank provides, at any instant in time, the signal with the highest frequency in the spectrum above a threshold level. Secondly, a phase lock loop can be arranged to provide a signal proportional to the maximum input frequency. Finally, a servo-controlled loop can automatically maintain the frequency of a local voltage controlled oscillator so that it is at a fixed difference frequency from the maximum input frequency; the controlling voltage is then proportional to the maximum input frequency.

There are some situations, in blood flow studies, in which the mean frequency of the Doppler shift is more relevant information than the maximum frequency. For example, if the blood vessel geometry remains constant, and if the ultrasound beam floods the blood vessel uniformly, the mean Doppler frequency is proportional, at any instant in time, to the average velocity of the blood flowing through the vessel, independent of the flow profile. The instantaneous blood flow volume rate is equal to the product of the average blood flow velocity and the cross-sectional area of the blood vessel. Three different schemes of *average velocity detection* have been reported. The best is probably the mean frequency computer, the output of which is obtained by processing the complete power density spectrum of the Doppler signal. Secondly, the power in each of the outputs from a bank of parallel filters may be summed. Lastly, a phase lock loop with a relatively long time constant can be arranged to give an output proportional to the average input frequency.

Two-dimensional Doppler imaging

In many clinical situations, adequate diagnostic information can be obtained with a hand-held Doppler probe. It is necessary, however, for the investigator to know the anatomy of the structures being studied in order to interpret the results.

In studies of the vascular system it is often useful also to have a two-dimensional map showing the position of blood vessels. The ultrasonic Doppler shifted signals from flowing blood are sufficiently characteristic to allow their presence to be identified by logic circuitry. This capability is exploited in the two-dimensional scanner shown in Figure 4.34.

A two-dimensional scan of a blood vessel made with a continuous-wave Doppler instrument is essentially a plan view, representing the projection of the blood vessel onto the skin surface along the line-of-sight of the ultrasonic beam. The same type of image can be obtained with a pulsed Doppler scanner range-gated to a constant depth (or even to a variable depth, under the control of the operator) within the blood vessel. Because the pulsed-Doppler scanner is capable of measuring range (as well as velocity), and thus of displaying the depth of detected flow, cross-sectional and longitudinal images of the blood vessel lumen can also be produced. Typically a pulsed Doppler scanner has 32 serial gates, each representing flow in a 1 mm increment along the ultrasonic beam, and the system operates at 5 MHz and is directionally-sensitive. Furthermore, in appropriate anatomical situations, it is possible to determine the orientation, lumen cross-sectional area, and flow velocity profile, by means of pulsed-Doppler scanning, and thus to estimate blood flow volume.

A useful refinement of Doppler imaging is

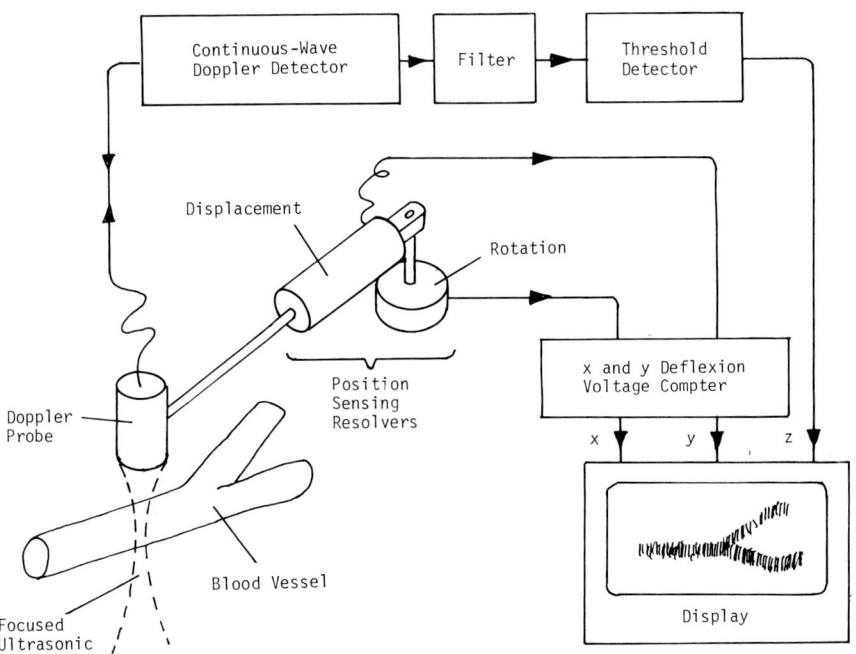

Fig. 4.34 Continuous wave Doppler system for two-dimensional visualisation of blood vessel distribution. The probe is mounted on a two-dimensional co-ordinate measuring scanner, the resolvers of which provide data enabling computation of the x and y voltages that control the deflexion circuits of a direct-view electronic storage tube. The probe is arranged so that the ultrasonic beam is at least slightly inclined to the direction of flow in the vessels to be visualised. When the beam passes through moving blood the Doppler detector generates an output which is filtered (to remove artifacts due to low velocity movements such as those of the probe over the skin) and, provided that the output exceeds a preset threshold level, it switches on the electron beam of the display. A two-dimensional map showing those regions in which flow has been detected is constructed on the display by scanning the probe over the area of skin overlying the vessel. Since arteries and veins often lie close together, a directionally-sensitive circuit is arranged to inhibit the display when flow is detected in the opposite direction to that in the vessel under study.

afforded by colour-coding the display according to the maximum detected frequency. This makes it easier to recognise the presence of turbulence and high velocity jets due to stenosis.

it easier to locate regions of interest quickly, and is virtually essential in studying moving structures such as the heart. A typical duplex scanner is illustrated in Figure 4.35. The two-dimensional im-

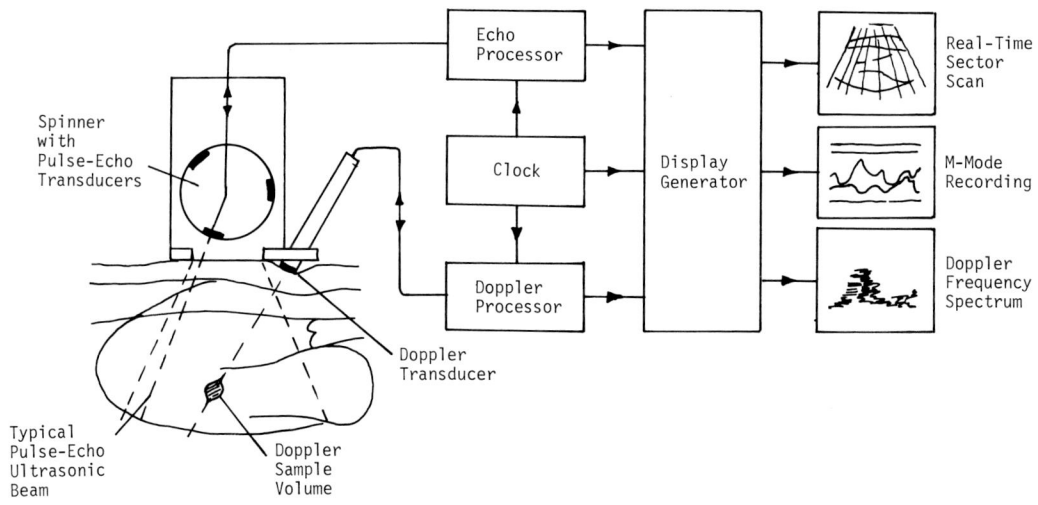

Fig. 4.35 A duplex scanning system, combining real-time two-dimensional pulse-echo imaging (using a rotating wheel, or spinner, with three transducers mounted on its rim to make a trapezoidal scan) with a pulsed Doppler capability. Stopping the rotation of the spinner allows M-mode recordings to be made. This particular instrument employs a separate transducer for Doppler measurements, arranged so that the sample volume can be positioned at any desired position in the image plane.[8] A popular, but less versatile, variant of this arrangement requires the spinner to stop rotation during Doppler studies, and one of the spinner transducers is directed at the region of interest and operated in the pulsed Doppler mode.

Duplex scanning

Although two-dimensional Doppler imaging (discussed on p. 168) is clinically useful because of its ability to display regions and patterns of flowing blood, it has two important limitations. Firstly, the method does not display neighbouring stationary anatomical structures. Secondly, scanning to form an image is a lengthy process, since at least one complete cardiac pulse is necessary to form each element of picture information. Because of these restrictions, the potential of combining two-dimensional pulse-echo imaging with a limited amount of pulsed Doppler information (so-called *duplex-scanning*) is extremely attractive. The pulse-echo image allows regions of interest to be located, and the pulsed Doppler system allows structure motion or blood flow within the regions to be studied rapidly.

Duplex scanning can be based on a static B-scanner (see p. 155), but it is generally more useful with real-time scanning. Real-time scanning makes

age is used to identify structures and to guide the positioning of the sample volume of the pulsed Doppler system.

TRANSMISSION METHODS

Orthographic transmission imaging

The first attempts to use ultrasound for medical diagnosis, in the 1930s and '40s, were based on the expectation that it would be possible to demonstrate tissue masses by the measurement of the attenuation of transmitted ultrasound. (The process is called *orthographic transmission imaging*; the image lies in a plane perpendicular to the direction of wave propagation.) Conventional radiography, after all, produces excellent images of the attenuation of transmitted X-rays.

The early investigators hoped in particular that the method might be used to visualise abnormalities of the brain. Thus they chose one of the least promising organs for their work, since the variations in transmission through the skull mask variations due to changes in the brain.

The attenuation and refraction due to the presence of either gas-containing structures or of bone in the ultrasonic transmission path seem to be insuperable problems preventing satisfactory imaging of overlying regions. Moreover, transmission imaging, even of soft tissues, with conventional ultrasonic beams suffers from serious artifacts due to diffraction and refraction. This particular problem has been solved, however, by the ingenious expedient of transmitting *incoherent* ultrasound through the object.[14] Conventional piezoelectric transducers radiate *coherent* ultrasound, analogous to the coherent light emitted from a laser source, in which there is a smooth in-phase wavefront across the whole extent of the ultrasonic beam. It is the coherent properties of the wave which give rise to many of the problems associated with orthographic transmission imaging. Incoherent ultrasound, which is analogous to light produced by, for example, an electric light bulb, can be obtained from an assembly of numerous small randomly-arranged transducer excited by separate oscillators operating at nominally the same frequency but with no phase-correlating interconnexion.

Figure 4.36 is a diagram showing the arrangement of an orthographic transmission imaging instrument, or *camera*, employing diffuse insonification. The camera provides a real-time image of a depth-of-field typically 10 mm thick and 175 mm in diameter. The signal-to-noise ratio of any ultrasonic system depends, amongst other things, on the intensity of the ultrasound falling on the detector. In this respect transmission imaging is greatly superior to pulse-echo reflexion imaging; the incident ultrasonic intensity is at least an order of magnitude lower to achieve the same signal-to-noise ratio.

Computed tomography

The success of X-ray transmission computed tomo-

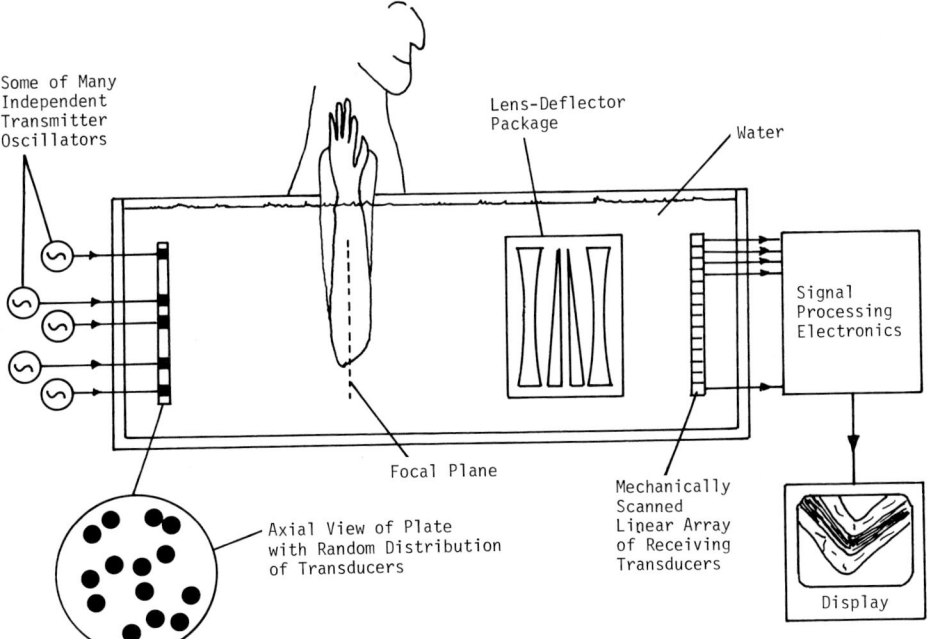

Fig. 4.36 Simplified diagram of an orthographic imaging instrument using incoherent ultrasound.[14] The ultrasonic source is a random array of small transducers excited by independent power oscillators. Having passed through the object, the ultrasonic field is collected and focused by plastic lenses to form an image which is detected by a linear transducer array. This array detects only one picture-line at a time. The complete image is built up in real-time, by repeatedly sweeping the focused ultrasonic image past the linear array. This is done by the two plastic prisms which are continuously rotated in opposite directions.

graphy (Ch. 2) and radioisotope emission computed tomography (Ch. 3) has stimulated efforts to develop the method for ultrasonic imaging.[4] As with orthographic transmission imaging discussed in the previous section, it is necessary for the ultrasonic transmission paths to be free from obstructions by bone and gas. This requirement is more difficult to satisfy in CT scanning, because it is necessary to make measurements of transmission profiles in a complete set of angular orientations (Fig. 4.37) in order to collect the data for image

travelled along the shortest path length, which is the line-of-sight. Time-of-flight profiles can be used to compute maps showing the distribution, pixel-by-pixel, of propagation speed in the tissues in the tomographic plane. (There is no analogue of this in X-ray transmission imaging; radioisotope emission CT using positron annihilation time-of-flight measurement is also essentially different, since the speed of the γ photons is assumed to be constant in that computation process.)

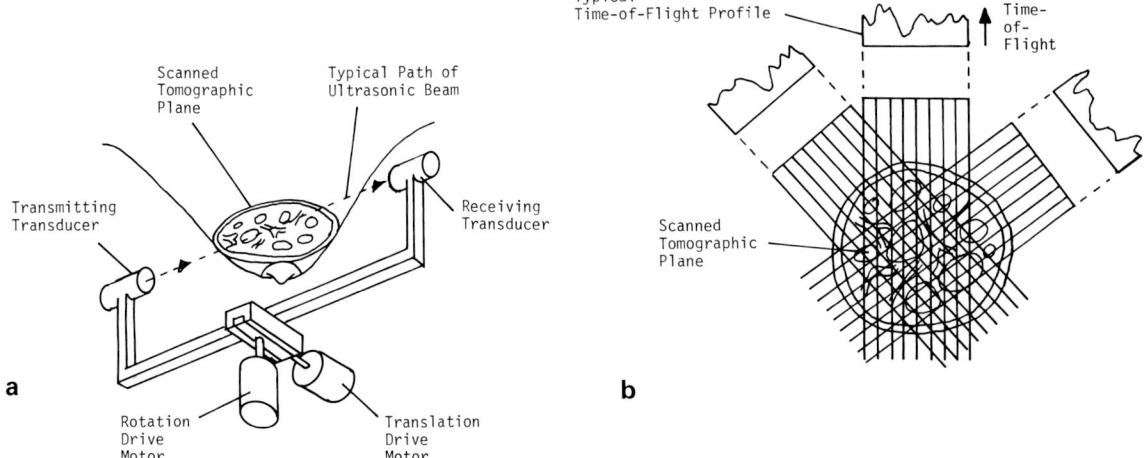

Fig. 4.37 The method of ultrasonic computed tomography. In this example, time-of-flight tomography is being performed by orthodox translate-rotate scanning. (a) Mechanical scanning system. (b) How profiles of time-of-flight are obtained at many angular orientations with respect to the scanned tomographic plane.

reconstruction. Once collected, however, the data are reconstructed by the same algebraic reconstruction or back projection techniques as are used in X-ray CT imaging (see, for example, p. 56).

Computed tomography depends on the validity of the assumption that line-of-sight propagation is maintained across the object being scanned. This assumption is certainly valid for X-rays and γ-rays, and so does not introduce any problem in X-ray transmission or radioisotope emission CT imaging. Unfortunately, however, an ultrasonic beam is deviated by refraction and diffraction in travelling across tissues, so that the attenuation profile in particular may not be a true representation of line-of-sight tissue elements. The problem is less acute for time-of-flight profiles, since the first component of energy to arrive at a receiver set up on the central axis of a transmitter is likely to have

Acoustic microscopy

The use of ultra-high-frequency ultrasound allows images of biological structures to be made with resolutions which are so high that the technique qualifies as *microscopy*. Acoustic (ultrasonic) microscopes operate at frequencies of 10 MHz to 2 GHz[*], and the corresponding wavelengths (in water and soft tissues) range from 150 μm down to 0·75 μm. The wavelengths of visible light range from 0·4–0·7 μm; thus the wavelength of the ultrasound used to form images in the highest frequency acoustic microscopes is comparable with the wavelength of the light used in optical microscopes, and so the resolutions of these two classes

[*]1 GHz = 1000 MHz. The term 'acoustic microscopy' has already become accepted, although a more apt description would be 'ultrasonic' microscopy.

of imaging instruments are similar.

Two different methods of acoustic microscopy have been developed. In principle, the simpler is the *scanning acoustic microscope* (SAM)[24] (Fig. 4.38). The specimen itself is moved in an x-y raster pattern, so that the attenuation of each element of the specimen in turn can be measured while it lies in the focal zone of the highly-focused ultrasonic beam. At gigahertz frequencies, the contribution of viscosity as an absorption mechanism becomes important in relation to relaxation processes (see p. 145). Consequently, it is the viscosity, or elasticity, of the components of the specimen which give rise to contrast in the image; acoustic microscopy makes it possible to study structures in living cells which can only be seen in dead, stained, cells by optical microscopy. A disadvantage of this increase in the importance of viscosity is that the absorption in water is substantial, and it increases with the square of the frequency. In practice, it is the absorption in the coupling liquid which limits the maximum ultrasonic frequency—and hence, the resolution—and lower-absorption alternatives to water for use as coupling liquids are being sought.

The second type of acoustic microscope is the scanning laser acoustic microscope (SLAM)[22] (Fig. 4.39). In principle, the image frame rate of the SLAM is potentially faster than that of the SAM. It cannot be operated at such a high ultrasonic frequency, however, because of attenuation and detection limitations, and so the maximum resolution is not so great. The SLAM is an excellent instrument for studying the physiological function of small organs, such as the hearts of small mammals. Moreover, the phase information in the received signal is retained, and this can be used to generate fringes on the attenuation image, the spacings between which depend on changes in the transit time (due to differences in the speed of ultrasound) through the different materials of which the specimen is composed.

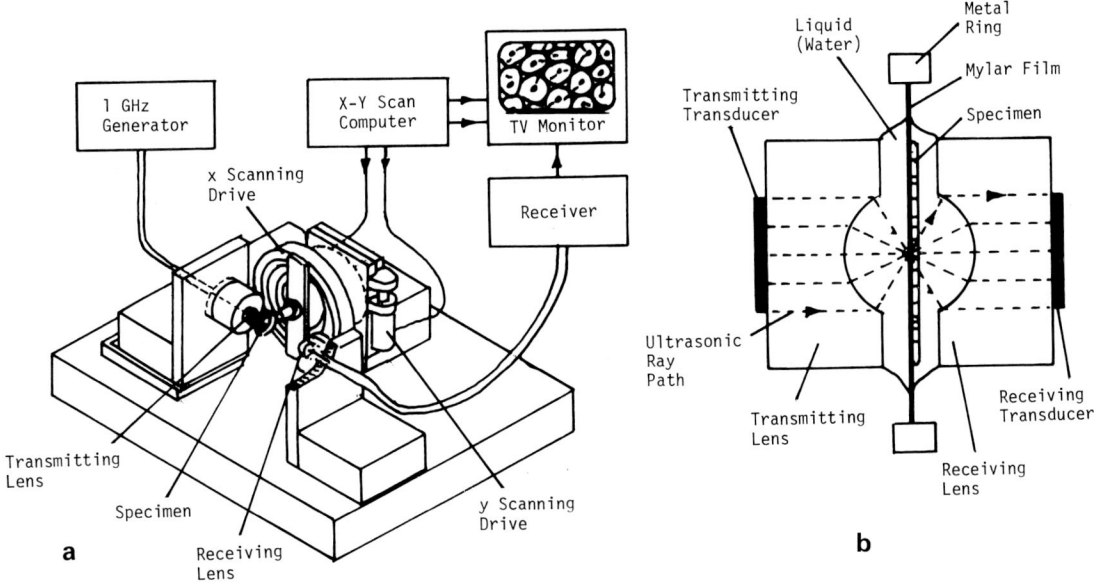

Fig. 4.38 Scanning acoustic microscope designed to operate at frequencies around 1 GHz (1000 MHz).[24] (a) General arrangement. The transmitting and receiving lenses are shown here moved outwards from their operating positions. The specimen is mounted on a Mylar film on a metal ring, and the metal ring is scanned horizontally (x-direction) by a modified audio loudspeaker, whilst the vertical (y-direction) drive translates the specimen in a raster pattern. (b) The relative positions of the acoustic components in the scanning operation. The lenses are made of sapphire, and the thickness of the water film between the outer surfaces of the lenses is about 300 μm. A typical specimen area of 250 μm square is scanned in about 1 s, and the image is made up of 50 000 pixels each corresponding to a 1 μm square of the specimen.

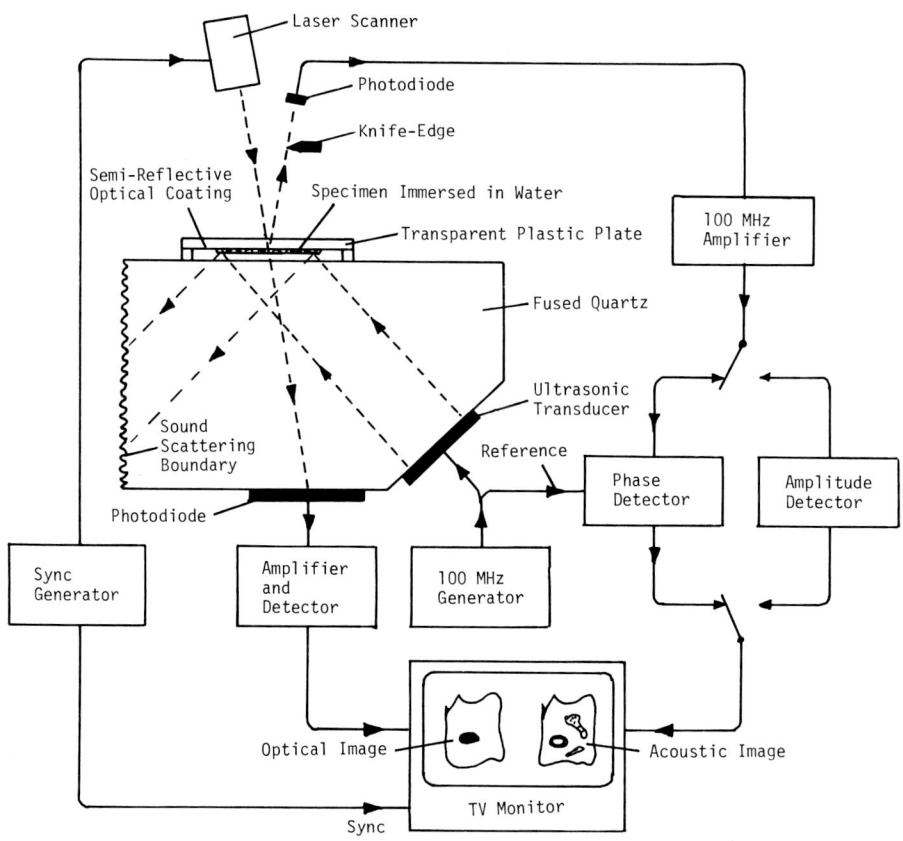

Fig. 4.39 Scanning laser acoustic microscope, designed to operate at frequencies of around 100 MHz.[22] The instrument simultaneously produces acoustic (phase or amplitude) and optical images of the specimen, which can be displayed separately (as represented here) or superimposed. The probing laser beam focused on the semireflective coating of the plastic mirror becomes spatially modulated by the localised surface distortion produced by ultrasound transmitted through the specimen. A fraction of the light is transmitted through the mirror and the specimen to produce the optical image. (In this diagram, the effects of refraction on the ray paths have been neglected.)

ULTRASONIC HOLOGRAPHY

Although the results have been uniformly disappointing—for reasons which are quite easy to understand—no account of ultrasonic medical imaging would be complete without at least a mention of ultrasonic holography.

Ultrasonic holography is analogous to light holography. It is a two-stage process in which the diffraction pattern of an object irradiated by ultrasound is biased by a coherent reference wave and recorded to generate a hologram. A three-dimensional image of the object is created when the hologram is illuminated by a coherent light source.

There are many different arrangements by which ultrasonic holograms may be obtained. One of these arrangements is illustrated in Figure 4.40; it is not the fastest technique, but it is easy to understand, and it really does produce holograms—which is something that some other so-called 'holographic' techniques apparently do not do!

Much effort has been expended in trying to develop ultrasonic holography for medical imaging. At first sight, it has much to offer: if it could be made to work as well as optical holography, it would produce three-dimensional images in real-time. There are, however, several difficult or apparently insuperable problems. The image has a longitudinal distortion of about 2000 to 1, due to the difference between the wavelengths of the ultrasound used to form the hologram (say 1 mm at 1·5 MHz), and the light used for the reconstruction of the image (say 0·5 μm). Specular reflexions, being of large amplitude, mask low-amplitude scattered echoes. There is diffraction in the near fields of the large apertures, of both the transducers and the object. Ultrasonic waves are deviated and distorted as they travel through biological tissues. Perhaps most important and fundamental of all, however, is the fact that phase coherence, on which holography depends, is destroyed by variations in the speed of ultrasound in different kinds of tissue.

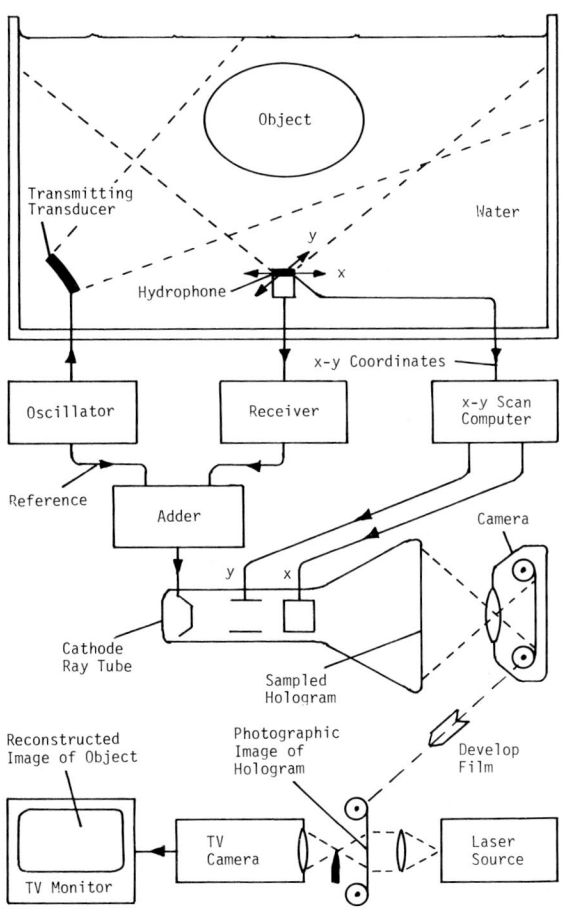

Fig. 4.40 Typical arrangement for ultrasonic holography. The hydrophone receiving transducer is mechanically scanned in an *x-y* raster pattern to generate the hologram by sampling. The reference signal is added electronically. One transmitted pulse is required for each position of the hydrophone; at a pulse repetition rate of 1000 s^{-1}, the scanning time is 1000 s for 10^6 sampling points. The average ultrasonic illuminating intensity required is about 10 mW cm^{-2}.

TISSUE CHARACTERISATION

The objectives of tissue characterisation

In addition to the ability to map structures and to study structure motion, ultrasonic signals allow at least some clues to be gained about the characteristics of the tissues from which they arise. For example, liquid-filled and solid lesions can be distinguished from each other because liquids generally are more *anechoic* (i.e. tend not to give rise to interal echoes of significant amplitude) and are more *transonic* (i.e. transmit ultrasound with low attenuation) than solid tissues. In some situations, there are additional clues; thus, for example, pericardial effusion can be identified not only because it is anechoic and transonic, but also because of its geometry and the free movement of the myocardium within it.

The use of clues of this kind is an elementary—but nevertheless very valuable—form of *tissue characterisation*. Ultrasonic tissue characterisation has been aptly described[16] as ultrasonic *telehistology*—histology at a distance. The objective of tissue characterisation research, in which there is substantial interest, is to move beyond the somewhat subjective methods now being used clinically, and to place the ultrasonic identification of tissues on a quantitative basis.

Tissue characterisation measurements

The first quantitative approach to the interpretation of A-scans seems to have been in connexion with the diagnosis of breast disease.[43] The analysis, based on the measurement of echo amplitude, has been refined and applied to the assessment of ultrasonic liver scans. The echogenicity of the liver is measured in terms of an index representing the sum of the amplitudes of consecutive intrahepatic echoes along the A-scan, divided by the length of the timebase along which the echoes lie. Sufficient A-scans are analysed to give statistical significance to estimates for individuals. The results of one such study[30] are shown in Figure 4.41. The echogenicity of the cirrhotic liver is 6 dB greater than that of the normals. Moreover, if it may be assumed that the distribution of scatterers within the liver is homogeneous, the decrement of echo amplitude with distance reflects the rate of attenuation of

176 SCIENTIFIC BASIS OF MEDICAL IMAGING

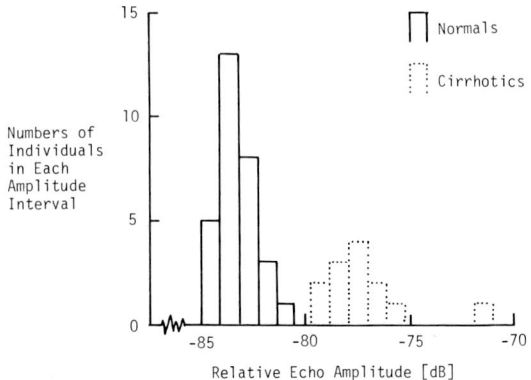

Fig. 4.41 Histogram showing the echogenicity distributions of individuals with normal livers and with cirrhosis.[30] The echo amplitudes are expressed in decibels below the echo amplitude from a perfect reflector at normal incidence in a lossless medium, and the measurements were made using an ultrasonic system with a centre frequency of about 1·7 MHz. The echo amplitude scale is divided into intervals of 0·88 dB.

ultrasound in the liver. The attenuation may be altered in disease. In principle, attenuation can also be measured by ultrasonic CT scanning (see p. 171), but in practice CT scanning of the liver is not possible because of intervening bones and gas-containing structures. CT scanning of the breast is more promising, and, although attenuation measurements are subject to errors, measurements of propagation speed can be used to identify breast carcinoma.

Other approaches to tissue characterisation are based on the measurements of the frequency or angular dependences of the *scattered* echo signals.[17] Most solid biological tissues have loose structure ordering on the scale of the ultrasonic wavelength (in addition to ordering on both smaller and larger scales). Consequently, the scattered echo amplitude and, in particular, the backscattered echo amplitude, are angle dependent. Different specimens of the same type of tissue tend to have similar characteristics in this respect. For example, of three tissues studied at 1 MHz, brain had the highest angular frequency of echo-amplitude fluctuation (~ 40 rad^{-1}), liver had the lowest (~ 10 rad^{-1}), and spleen was intermediate.

Despite the enormous amount of effort which has been expended on tissue scattering studies and the good understanding of the processes involved which has consequently been gained,[28] scattering measurements have not been applied to help solve routine clinical problems. It is, after all, of little clinical relevance to be able to distinguish between the ultrasonic echoes from brain, liver and spleen.

POSSIBLE HAZARDS OF ULTRASONIC DIAGNOSTIC EXPOSURES

Biological effects of ultrasound

The fact that ultrasound can modify biological tissues has been known since before 1920, when the pioneers of sonar (Sound Navigation And Ranging, the underwater analogue of radar) noticed that small fish were killed by their ultrasonic transmitters. Much enthusiasm for the ultrasonic therapy as a cure-all was built up in the 1930s, but the unscientific basis of this work and its indifferent results drove the method into disrepute. Since the beginning of the 1960s, however, there has been steady progress in the understanding of the biological effects of ultrasound.

There are two distinct mechanisms by which ultrasound may produce biological effects. The first of these, the *thermal* mechanism due to heat produced by the absorption of ultrasound, may be discounted as a possible source of hazard in ultrasonic diagnostic investigations, since the average ultrasonic power used is generally around 10 mW cm^{-2}. The corresponding heat can easily be dissipated by convection, conduction (including blood flow) and radiation, without any conceivably significant increase in temperature.

The second mechanism involves *cavitation* which is the term used to describe the behaviour of gas-filled cavities in liquid media supporting ultrasonic waves. *Transient* cavitation is the phenomenon in which voids suddenly grow from nuclei in the supporting liquid, and then collapse, under the influence of the changing pressure in the ultrasonic field. This whole process of growth and collapse occupies less time than the wave period. During the collapse of a bubble, a strong pressure pulse is set up in the liquid and high temperatures occur within the bubble. It is practically certain that the exposure conditions used in diagnostic examinations are too low to cause transient cavitation.

The behaviour of a gas-filled bubble pre-existing in an ultrasonic field of intensity below that necessary to cause transient cavitation is known as *stable* cavitation. A resonant system exists in which the surrounding liquid behaves as a mass set into vibration, the elasticity being provided by the gas in the bubble. A resonant air-filled bubble in water at atmospheric pressure has a diameter of about 0·7 μm at 1 MHz; it is roughly proportionately larger at lower frequencies, whereas, at higher frequencies, the effect of surface tension increasingly modifies this proportionality.

The biological effects of stable cavitation at low megahertz frequencies in liquids of low viscosity are also quite well understood. Stable cavitation is effective at these frequencies if the specimen is rotated to neutralise unidirectional forces. At least about 1000 cycles of oscillation are necessary for stable cavitation to become effective at 1 MHz, and under these conditions DNA is degraded by intensities of a few watts/square centimetre. In solid tissues, however, the bubbles which would be necessary for stable cavitation to occur are likely to be very rare, even if they exist at all.

Not all changes taking place in biological materials as a result of ultrasonic irradiation can be explained simply in terms of thermal or cavitational mechanisms. Some examples of these effects serve to demonstrate this. For instance, blood flow in small blood vessels may be arrested by irradiation with ultrasound of around 0·5 W cm^{-2} at 1 MHz. The phenomenon seems to be due to standing waves. Wound healing may be accelerated, and this effect seems to be marked with 5 min irradiations, on alternate days, using 3·6 MHz with a pulse intensity of 0·5 W cm^{-2}, pulse duration 2 ms, duty cycle 0·2. Heat can almost certainly be excluded as a contributing factor under these conditions. As another example, there is evidence, although not statistically significant, that 5 h irradiation at 40 mW cm^{-2} with 2·25 MHz ultrasound, may be teratogenic in the mouse.

Exposure conditions in ultrasonic diagnosis

Basically, the most direct method of measuring ultrasonic power is by calorimetry. Calorimetry does suffer from a number of difficulties, however, such as slow speed of response and low sensitivity. For the measurement of the ultrasonic power used in diagnostic examinations, it is generally most convenient to make use of the *radiation force* exerted by the ultrasound. An ultrasonic wave exerts a static force on any interface or medium across which there is a decrease in ultrasonic power. This decrease may be due either to attenuation or to reflexion. The physical process which leads to the establishment of the radiation force in an ultrasonic field is not yet fully understood, but it is generally agreed that, in the case of complete absorption of a finite beam of plane waves,[41]

$$F = W/c \qquad (4.13)$$

where F is the radiation force, and W is the incident power. The force F acts in the vector direction of the propagation of the wave. At normal incidence, the force on a perfect reflector is twice the force which would act on a perfect absorber in the same situation; at oblique incidence, the direction of the resultant force may be resolved by taking into account the directions and magnitudes of the forces due to the incident and reflected waves.

Typically, the average intensity used in ultrasonic diagnosis is in the range 10–100 mW cm^{-2}. Substitution in Equation 4.13 shows that an ultrasonic beam with a power of 1 W travelling in water at 20°C produces a force of 6.7×10^{-4} N when it is completely absorbed. This is equal to the force of gravity acting on a weight of about 69 mg. For measuring diagnostic powers, balancing weights of around 1–10 mg is involved. An example of an appropriate balance is shown in Figure 4.42.

In the case of continuous wave Doppler systems, the concept of the average intensity is a simple one. With pulsed ultrasonic beams, however, the average intensity is equal to the intensity of the ultrasonic pulse multiplied by the duty cycle (the ratio of the duration of the pulse to the interval between the emission of consecutive pulses). The duty cycle may be as low as 0·001 (for example, 1 μs pulses at a pulse repetition rate of 1000 s^{-1}), so that the pulse intensity may be as high as 10–100 W cm^{-2}.

Another point is that there are two distinct aspects of ultrasonic irradiation conditions. The first is the *exposure*, which specifies the ultrasonic field parameters, such as intensity, time, frequency, particle displacement amplitude and so on. The second is the *dose*, which specifies the quantity of energy absorbed in the irradiated tissue.

Possibility of hazard

One constructive way of approaching the question

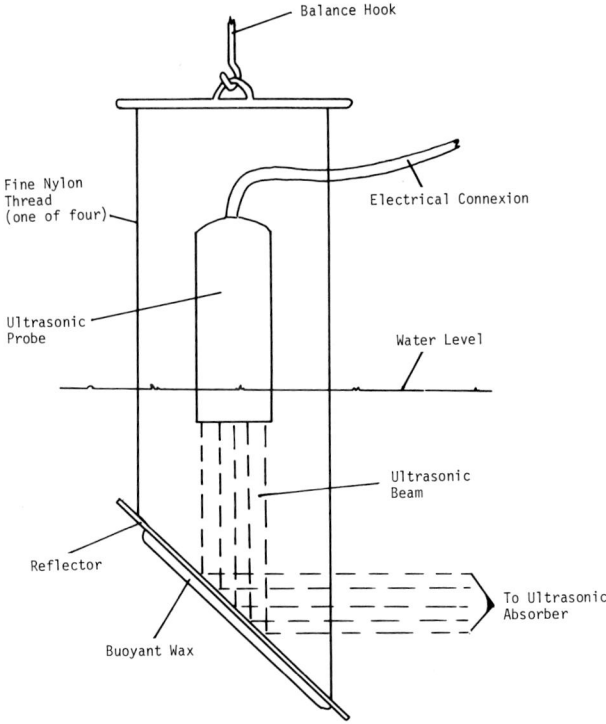

Fig. 4.42 Modified chemical analytical balance for the measurement of the radiation force produced by diagnostic ultrasonic beams.

of whether the ultrasonic exposures used in diagnostic applications may be hazardous is to review the literature on the biological effects of ultrasound. A pair of zones can then be defined on a chart of intensity and time, such that in one zone the conditions have been shown to produce biological effects, and, in the other, they have not. The kinds of biological effects considered include those on chemical systems, macromolecules, isolated cells and cell cultures, tissues and multicellular organs. There is also a small amount of epidemiological data. The results of three literature surveys are indicated in Figure 4.43. Once it has been recognised that a particular irradiation does not fall in the 'safe' region, many considerations need to be taken into account in assessing the 'hazard'. For example, irradiation of an embryo is presumably more 'hazardous' than irradiation, under the same physical conditions, of adult skeletal muscle.

In order to give positive guidance to practising clinicians, the American Institute of Ultrasound in Medicine has issued the following statement:

In the low megahertz frequency range there have been, as of this date, no independently confirmed significant biological effects in mammalian tissues exposed to intensities (spatial peak, temporal average (SPTA) as measured in a free field in water) below 100 mW cm^{-2}. Furthermore, for ultrasonic exposure times (total time; this includes off-time as well as on-time for a repeated-pulse régime) less than 500 s and more than 1 s, such effects have not been demonstrated at higher intensities when the product of intensity and exposure time (as defined above) is less than 50 J cm^{-2}.

The relationship between the conditions specified by the AIUM, and the three literature surveys, is indicated in Figure 4.43. To put these zones into perspective, it is helpful to know that the SPTA intensity used in ultrasonic surgery is typically 100 W cm^{-2}, and in ultrasonic physiotherapy, 1 W cm^{-2}, in comparison with the 0·01 W cm^{-2} typically used in ultrasonic diagnosis. Whilst it would be wrong to be complacent, it is reassuring to observe the most ultrasonic diagnostic techniques employ exposures below the AIUM conditions. Meanwhile, it should be recognised that many unanswered questions remain. For example, do exposure or dosage thresholds exist? Should thresholds—if they do exist—be raised (or lowered) for certain less (or more) sensitive biological systems or organs? Are any effects cumulative and, if so, under what conditions? What are the exposure and dose conditions *in vivo*? To what extent can non-human data be extrapolated to predict effects in man? And can the results be reproduced by other investigators?

PRINCIPAL CLINICAL APPLICATIONS

Applications of pulse-echo techniques

It is impossible, in a short review such as this, to give more than a brief mention even of the most important applications of pulse-echo ultrasonic techniques in clinical practice, to present a few typical results, and to give references to fuller dimensions in the literature.

Angiology

Many of the abdominal vessels, including the aorta, inferior vena cava, portal vein and hepatic, mesenteric and renal vessels, can be visualised.[13] Aneurysms and thrombi can be excellently demonstrated: this may not be possible with X-ray arteriography, since this shows only the lumen of the

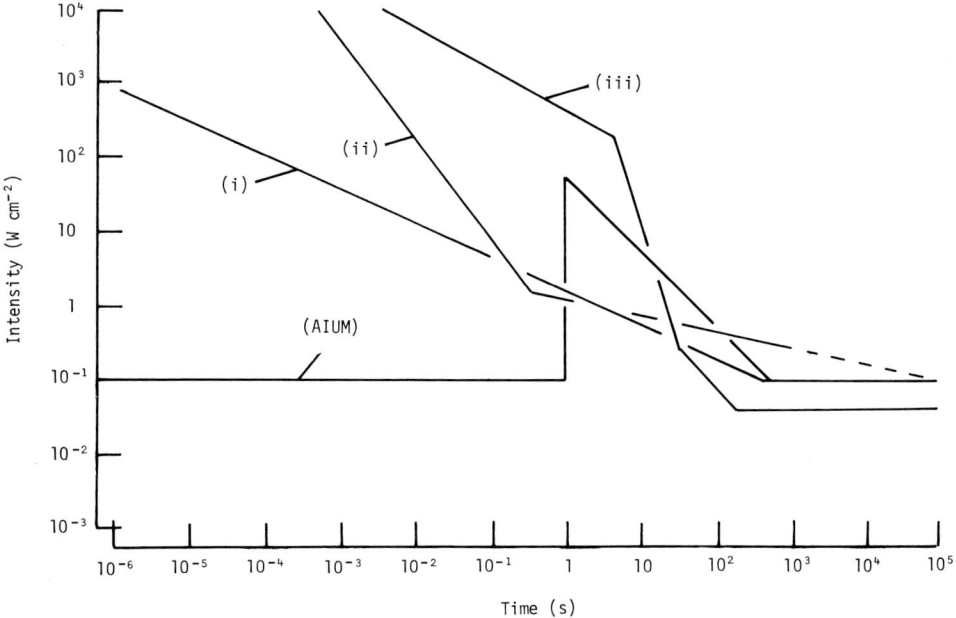

Fig. 4.43 Three pairs of exposure zones, and the AIUM recommendations, showing 'safe' and 'potentially hazardous' conditions, as established from three independent literature surveys. Each line separates one pair of zones, the zone below the line being 'safe'. (i) and (ii) These lines refer to two separate surveys ([37] and [11] respectively) in which the intensity is the time average (TA) value, equal to the product of the on-intensity and the duty cycle, and the time is the total exposure, including intervals between pulses when appropriate. (iii) This line refers to a third survey[39] in which the intensity is the on-intensity (generally the temporal peak, TP) and the time is the on-time. The AIUM conditions relate to SPTA exposures.

vessel. High-resolution images of superficial vessels in the neck and the leg are very good for detecting localised disease.[15] An example of a scan of the carotid artery is shown in Figure 4.44.

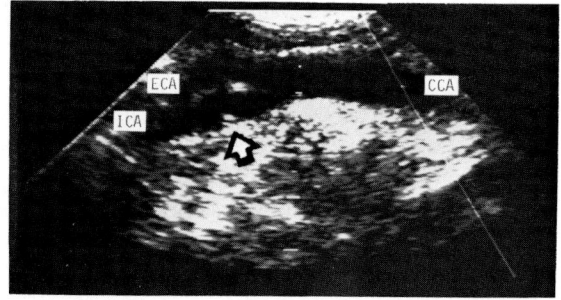

Fig. 4.44 Two-dimensional ultrasonic scan in region of carotid bifurcation, showing common carotid (CCA), internal carotid (ICA) and external carotid (ECA) arteries. The arrow indicates an atheromatous plaque partially obstructing the lumen of the internal carotid artery. This image is a single frame from a study made with a 5 MHz real-time mechanically-scanned pulse-echo scanner.

Cardiology

The possibility that clinically useful information about cardiac structure and function might be obtained was first proposed in 1954,[10] and so echocardiography is historically one of the earliest clinical applications of ultrasound. Nowadays M-mode studies are an essential adjunct in cardiological investigations, and two-dimensional real-time scanning is becoming increasingly indispensible. Traditionally the main application is in cardiac valve studies;[32] the mitral valve is most accessible to ultrasonic examination, the pulmonary valve is most inaccessible, and the aortic and tricuspid valves present intermediate difficulties. Ultrasonic access to the heart is restricted by overlying lung and ribs, and the probe is usually placed in the left parasternal region. Other probe positions, such as at the apex of the heart or in the suprasternal notch, are occasionally used. To examine the valves on the left side of the heart, for example, the ultrasonic beam is directed as illustrated in Figure 4.45. Two examples of M-mode

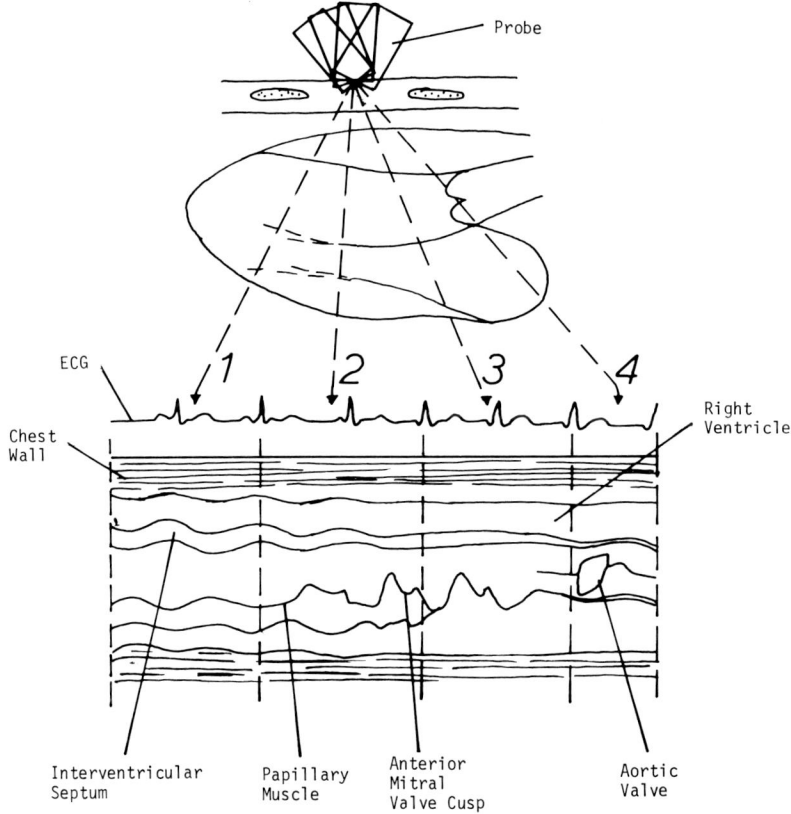

Fig. 4.45 Longitudinal section of the heart shows the structure through which the ultrasonic beam passes as it is aimed in four successive directions through the organ as a time-position scan is made. The time-position scan obtained is shown diagrammatically at the bottom, with the traces from several structures labelled. Position 1 corresponds to the apex of the heart, 4 corresponds to the base of the heart, and 2 and 3 are in between. The time-position scan is shown in relation to a simultaneous recording from an electrocardiograph (ECG).

mitral valve echocardiograms are given in Figure 4.46, showing how the valve movements are modified in disease. Diseases of the valves which can be diagnosed include stenosis, regurgitation, prolapse, calcification, and torn chordae. Moreover, because time and position can be measured, the extent of disease can often be quantitated. Figure 4.47 shows a single frame image from a real-time examination of two-dimensional section of the heart. Other cardiac diseases which can be studied[25] include left atrial myxoma, congenital heart disease, pericardial effusion, torn chordae tendineae, hypertrophic cardiomyopathy, dissecting aortic aneurysm and ventricular and atrial septal defects. Measurements of myocardial motion can be used to estimate stroke volume, and abnormal movements can give clues about the presence of infarcts.

Endocrinology

The thyroid gland is readily accessible to ultrasonic scanning.[36] Not only is it possible to detect, and to distinguish between, cysts and tumours, but also echography is complementary to scintigraphy, which reveals functioning thyroid tissue. The normal adrenal gland is difficult to visualise, being a small structure with little ultrasonic contrast with surrounding tissues and often being obscured by overlying gas-containing structures. In patients with suspected adrenal tumours, however, ultrasonic scanning is a useful preliminary to venography.[9]

Gastroenterology

A considerable amount of detail may be seen in

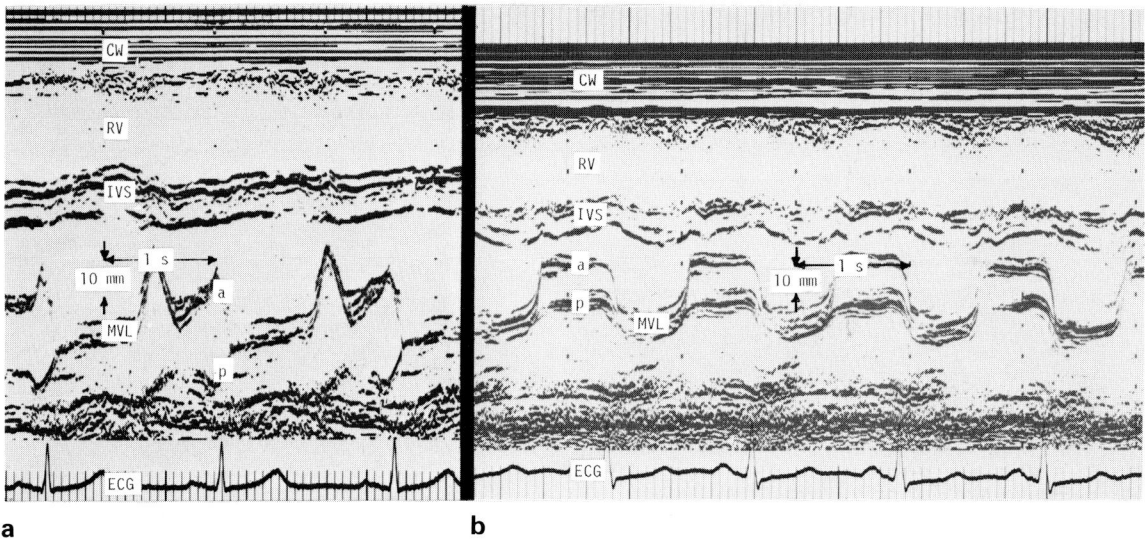

Fig. 4.46 M-mode echocardiograms of the mitral valve. (a) Normal. The ultrasonic probe is in contact with the chest wall (CW), and the ultrasonic beam passes through the right ventricle (RV), interventricular septum (IVS), left ventricular cavity and posterior left ventricular wall. Within the cavity of the left ventricle, the mitral valve leaflets (MVL) are closed during systole, the occurrence of which can be seen by reference to the ECG. During diastole, the anterior cusp (a) and posterior cusp (p) are separated, and move with a characteristic biphasic pattern. (b) Mitral stenosis. The mitral valve cusps are separated by a smaller distance than in the normal during diastole, and the characteristic biphasic pattern of the normal valve is absent because the valve remains as fully open as possible to allow the maximum degree of filling to occur despite the reduced area of the orifice.

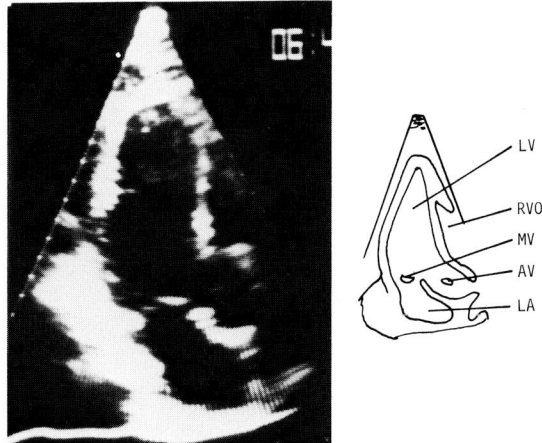

Fig. 4.47 Long axis view of left heart cavities and valves. A mechanical sector scanner with a 60 per cent field of view was placed over the cardiac apex and the plane was positioned to detect the left ventricle (LV), left atrium (LA), right ventricular outflow (RVO), and the base of the aorta. The frame depicts the aortic valve (AV) in its closed position and the mitral valve (MV) as it begins to open. The aortic root passes obliquely through the scan plane producing a non-parallel configuration of its walls. The white dots at the sector margin are spaced at 1 cm intervals.

two-dimensional scans of the liver. It is possible to visualise the gallbladder, the portal vein, the middle and posterior divisions of the right hepatic vein, and the separate vein draining the caudate lobe into the inferior vena cava. Typical scans are shown in Figure 4.48. In the study of liver disease,[35] liquid filled lesions are virtually always detectable, and solid abnormalities, such as metastases, can usually be identified. Generalised liver disease, such as cirrhosis and fatty liver, may be diagnosed by a diffuse increase in the echo amplitude and density in comparison with normal liver. In the case of the jaundiced patient, ultrasonic scanning can help to distinguish between those who require surgery (i.e. those with pancreatic or biliary cancer, strictures or gallstones in the biliary system, or with compression of the biliary system by extrinsic tumour), and those who should be treated medically (i.e. those with obstruction due to metastatic disease, viral hepatitis, cholestasis, cholangitis or cirrhosis). The

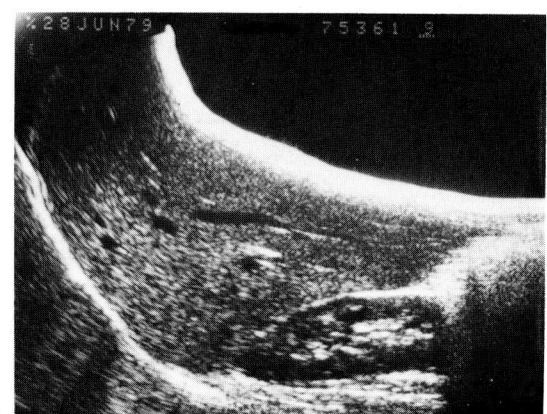
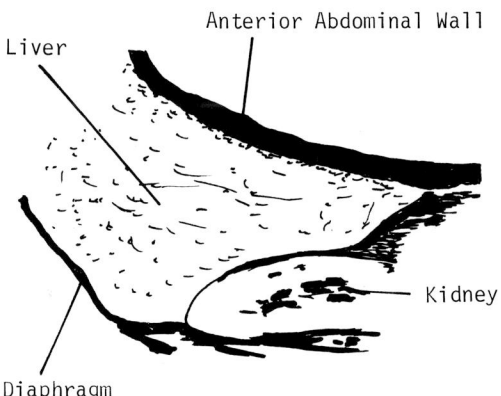

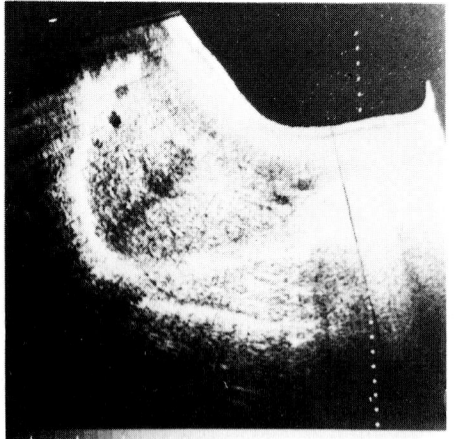
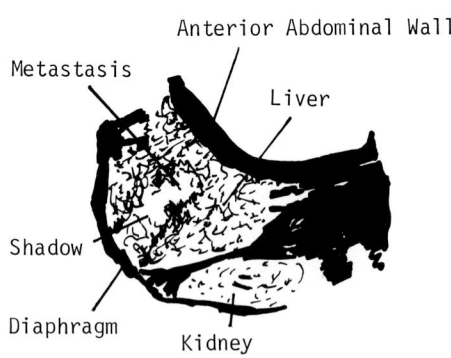

Fig. 4.48 Two-dimensional ultrasonic liver scans. (a) Longitudinal scan of normal liver. Bile ducts and blood vessels are evident as anechoic areas within the liver substance. (b) Longitudinal scan of liver with single metastasis from oat cell carcinoma of lung. (c) Longitudinal section of cirrhotic liver with ascites. (d) Longitudinal section of liver, showing calculus in gallbladder, and inferior vena cava.

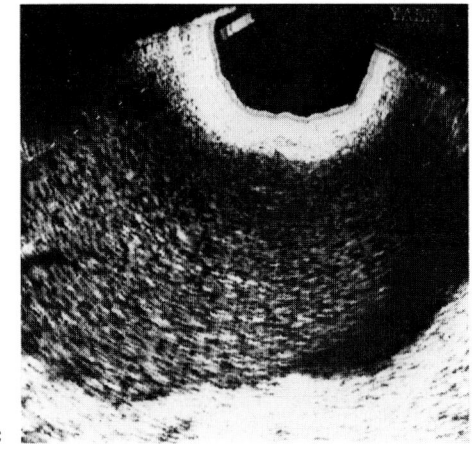
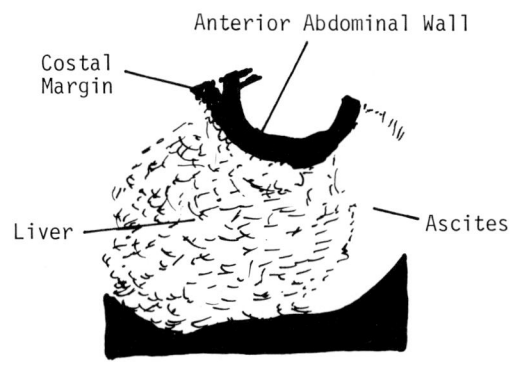

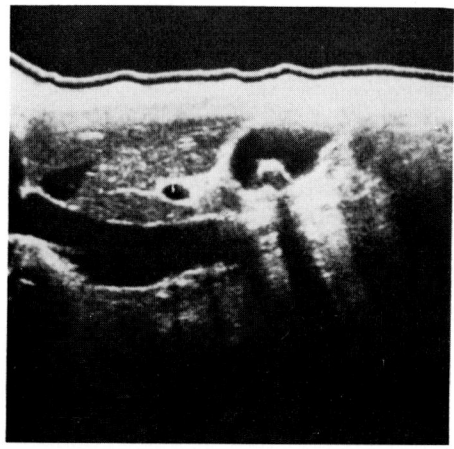
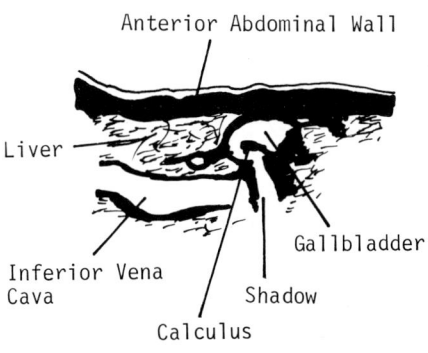

gallbladder is most likely to be visualised in the fasting patient, and gallstones can be identified by their echoes and by the shadows which they cast. Ultrasonic scanning is particularly valuable in patients who cannot tolerate intravenous cholecystography.

The detection of free ascitic fluid in the abdomen suggests the presence of neoplasm, or of liver disease including cirrhosis. Ascites can be visualised as an anechoic, transonic, space between the liver and the abdominal wall.

The spleen is an easy organ for ultrasonic imaging, but, apart from providing evidence about its size, differential diagnosis of splenic diseases on the basis of ultrasonic appearances is difficult.

The pancreas can usually be demonstrated on a slightly oblique scan in a plane just above that containing the mesenteric artery.[33] A typical scan is shown in Figure 4.49. In disease, the pancreas may be enlarged, and its echo texture may be abnormal. The diagnostic accuracies of ultrasonic and CT scanning seem to be similar, and so ultrasound should be the method of choice for the first examination, since it is cheaper, and does not use either contrast medium or ionising radiation.

Ultrasonic localisation is a very useful aid in guiding procedures such as liver biopsy and fine needle aspiration cytology of the pancreas.[19]

Neurology

The use of the A-scope to localise the midline structures of the brain (see Fig. 4.18) was extremely

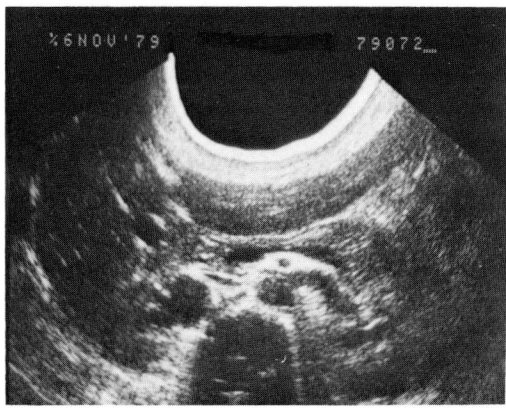 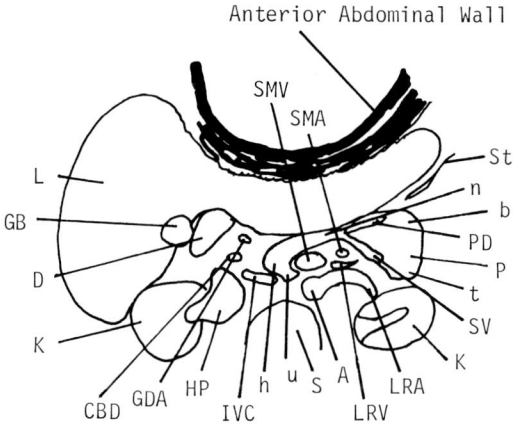

Fig. 4.49 Transverse section through pancreas. The general lie of the pancreas (P) is shown with the head (h) in contact with the duodenum (D), the neck (n) lying across the superior mesenteric artery (SMA) and vein (SMV), while the body (b) and tail (t) extend to the left and posteriorly, in close contact with the splenic vein (SV) and running across the upper pole of the left kidney. The pancreas lies posterior to the liver and stomach. The small uncinate process (u) extends to the left of the head posterior to the superior mesenteric vessels. Detailed structures of importance are the pancreatic (PD) and common bile ducts (CBD) and the gastroduodenal artery (GDA) supplying the head of the pancreas and the duodenum and part of the stomach. Other structures which can be seen in this section are the aorta (A) lying close to the spine and the inferior vena cava (IVC), which in this patient has been lifted anteriorly by a dilated right extrarenal pelvis (hydropelvis, HP) owing to ureteric obstruction. The left renal artery (LRA) and vein (LRV) can be seen. Within the liver, the gallbladder (GB) is in its usual close relationship with the duodenum.

popular in the 1960s. Unfortunately, however, the method is not objective, and its accuracy depends on the skill and clinical acumen of the operator.[42] With the advent of the CT scanner, clinical ultrasonic studies of the brain have virtually ceased. There is some interest, however, in the development of electronically steered array systems specifically for transcranial imaging;[22] the potential advantages of real-time visualisation, with the ability to observe pulsations, are considerable.

Obstetrics and gynaecology

The uterus, whether pregnant or not, is readily accessible to ultrasonic scanning through the anterior abdominal wall. When the uterus is not enlarged, it can be displaced out of the pelvis by allowing the patient's bladder to fill with urine.

Ultrasonic scanning is indispensible in modern obstetric practice.[18] With only a few exceptions, it has replaced radiography. Many obstetricians think that a routine ultrasonic examination should be made of every pregnancy, between weeks 20–24, to establish maturity, to detect multiple pregnancy, and to locate the placenta. Some typical scans are shown in Figure 4.50. The usual way of establishing maturity is by measuring the fetal biparietal diameter. This can be done with an accuracy approaching 1 mm, and the relationships between diameter, growth rate and gestational age are well documented. Most scanners have displays specially designed to facilitate the making of this and other measurements, and electronic calipers of various types are in common use.

As the resolution of scanners—especially real-time scanners—is improved, so it is becoming possible with more certainty to detect fetal abnormalities such as spina bifida. The study of the fetal heart, limb, body and breathing movements is another area of physiological interest.

In gynaecology, ultrasonic scanning is very helpful in identifying carcinomas of the ovary, uterus and cervix. Fibroids are readily visualised, and easily distinguished from ovarian cysts. Ultrasonic scanning is particularly valuable in the very obese patient, where palpation is futile. Surgical strategy can be planned more effectively where the size of the tumour is accurately known, especially when it is desirable to remove a malignant tumour intact to minimise the possibility of neoplastic spread.

Oncology

Ultrasonic visualisation of malignant lesions in many different sites may be of great value in plan-

ULTRASONIC IMAGING 185

ning radiotherapy[3] and in assessing the effects of chemotherapy.[23] Ultrasonic imaging of the breast, however, has so far been rather disappointing. Although very pretty pictures have been produced, as shown in Figure 4.51, the effort needed both to obtain and to interpret them is not negligible and the method can at present only really be used to screen highly selected populations, and possibly to

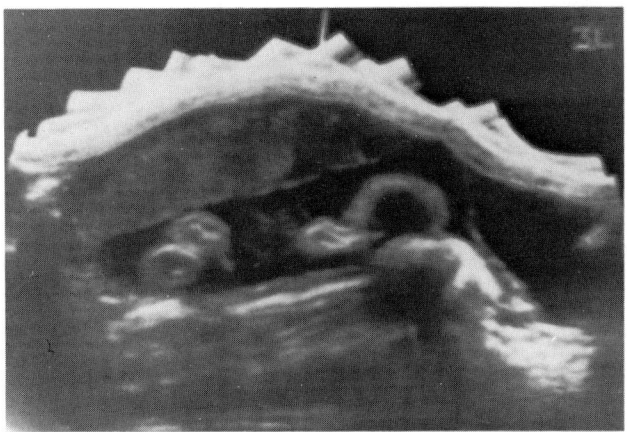
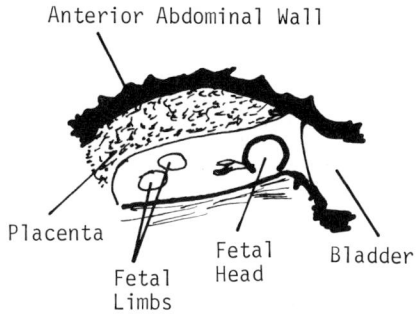

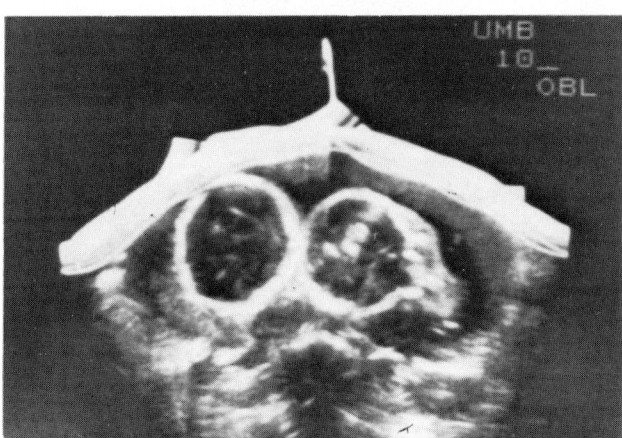
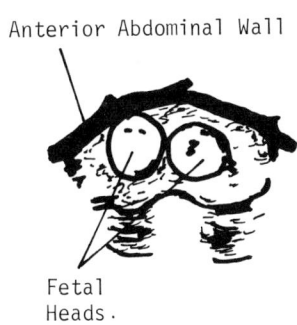

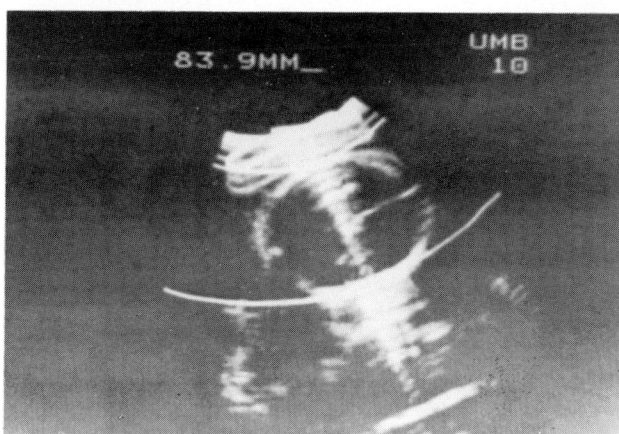
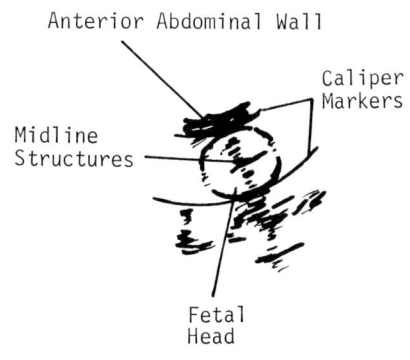

Fig. 4.50 (*Caption overleaf*)

186 SCIENTIFIC BASIS OF MEDICAL IMAGING

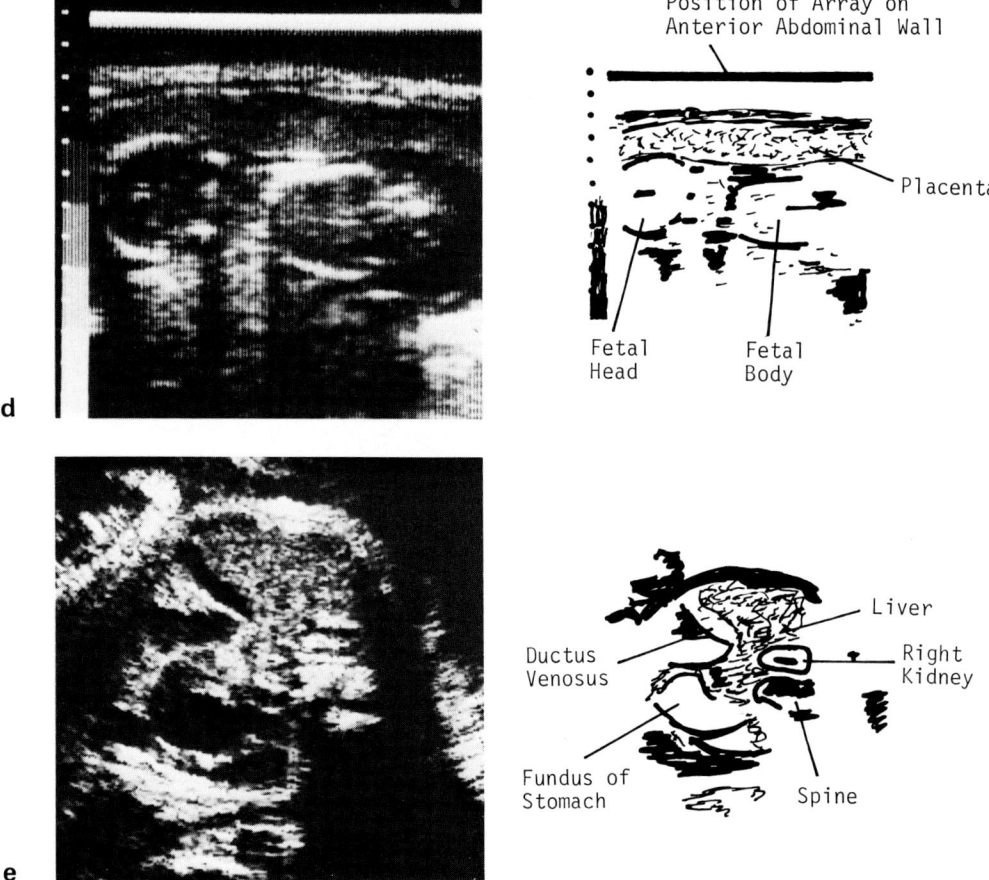

Fig. 4.50 Ultrasonic two-dimensional scans in obstetrics. (a) Longitudinal scan, normal 23-week pregnancy. (b) Twin heads in transverse section, 28 weeks gestation. (c) Fetal head in transverse section, with electronic caliper markers set across the biparietal diameter. The markers indicate a bpd of 83·9 mm, corresponding, in normal pregnancy, to 32 weeks gestation. (d) Longitudinal section of 26 week fetus, made with real-time electronic linear array. (e) Cross-section of fetal trunk *in utero*, showing anatomical details.

compete with X-ray mammography in women with symptoms of breast disease.

Ophthalmology

The eye and orbit are ideal structures for ultrasonic examination, and the application of the method has reached an advanced state.[6] Lesions can be detected and classified, and foreign bodies can be localised. Measurements of the axial lengths of the components of the eye are very useful in optometry.

Urology

The urinary system, with the exception of the ureters and the urethra, can usually be well visualised by ultrasound.[31] Both kidneys can normally be seen in either longitudinal or transverse sections. Some typical scans are shown in Figure 4.52. The ability to distinguish between cystic and solid lesions is very useful, and ultrasonic scanning may be used to determine the best site for cyst puncture or tumour biopsy. It is generally agreed that intravenous pyelography should be the first examination, and that this should be followed by ultrasonic investigation. CT scanning can subsequently settle some of the questions that may remain.

Bladder tumours can be staged by ultrasonic scanning, and this is very important in clinical management.[29] The enlarged prostate can also be

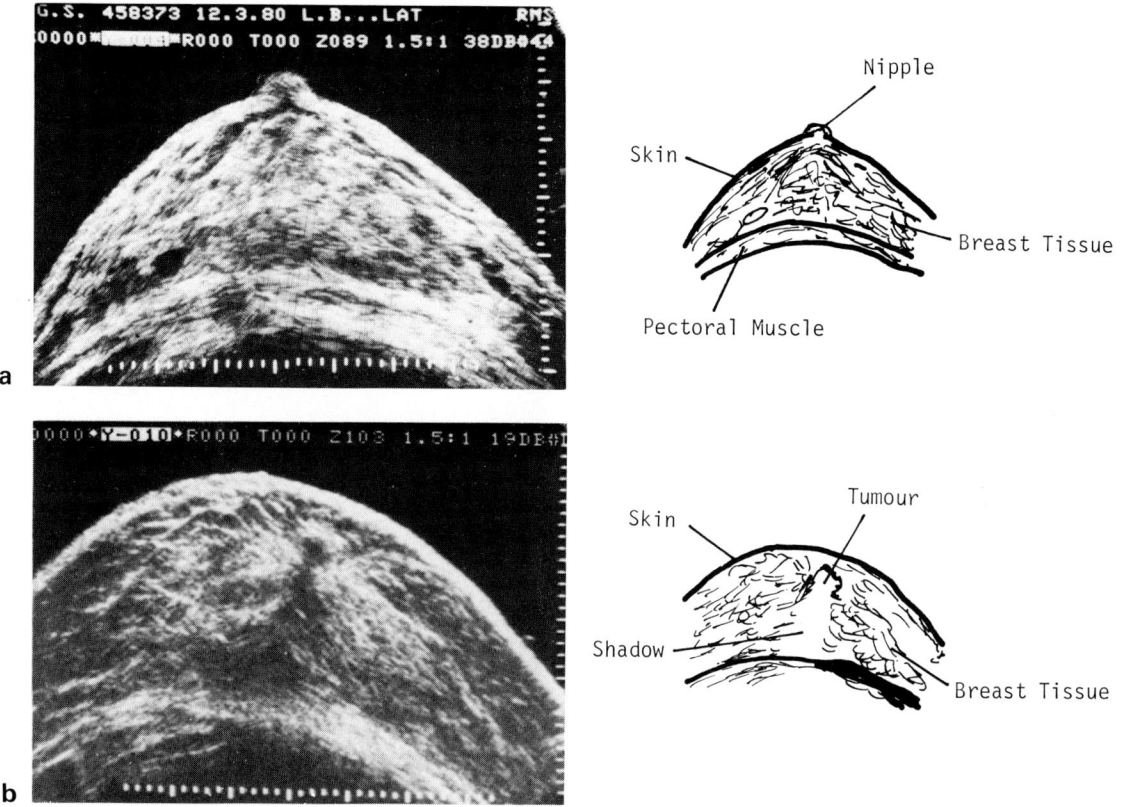

Fig. 4.51 Two-dimensional transverse ultrasonic breast scans, made with a water-immersion scanner. (a) Normal female breast, 28 years old. (b) Female breast with scirrhous carcinoma; note shadowing behind tumour.

seen through the full bladder. Transrectal imaging of the prostate, using a specially designed radial scanner, has the advantage of being able to image the gland without interference by the symphysis.[38]

The testis is quite easy to examine with a small real-time scanner in direct contact with the scrotum.[26] This is a useful aid in dealing with testicular emergencies.

Applications of Doppler techniques

Angiology

In generalised arterial disease, the characteristics of the arteries in the leg may reflect the progress of atherosclerosis throughout the arterial system. Arterial disease may modify the shape of the blood flow pressure pulse at the ankle. This may be determined non-invasively by using the ECG R-wave as a timing reference, and measuring the delays in the arrivals of different parts of the pressure wave beyond a cuff with decreasing pressures, at a Doppler probe positioned over the posterior tibial artery.[20] Another approach to arterial characterisation depends on measurements of the transit times of the arterial pulse past consecutive segments of artery, and from measurements of the pulsatility of the arterial pulse waveforms at the input and output sites of the arterial segments.[44] This is illustrated in Figure 4.53. Measurement of the pulsatility depends on obtaining the waveform of the maximum Doppler shift frequency, and this is usually done manually by tracing from the frequency spectrum, although reliable maximum frequency followers have recently been developed. This approach allows the collateral circulation to be graded into one of four classes, according to its status. More recent studies have introduced the concept of characterising the arterial segment between the heart and measurement site (at the common femoral artery, for example) in terms of the

188 SCIENTIFIC BASIS OF MEDICAL IMAGING

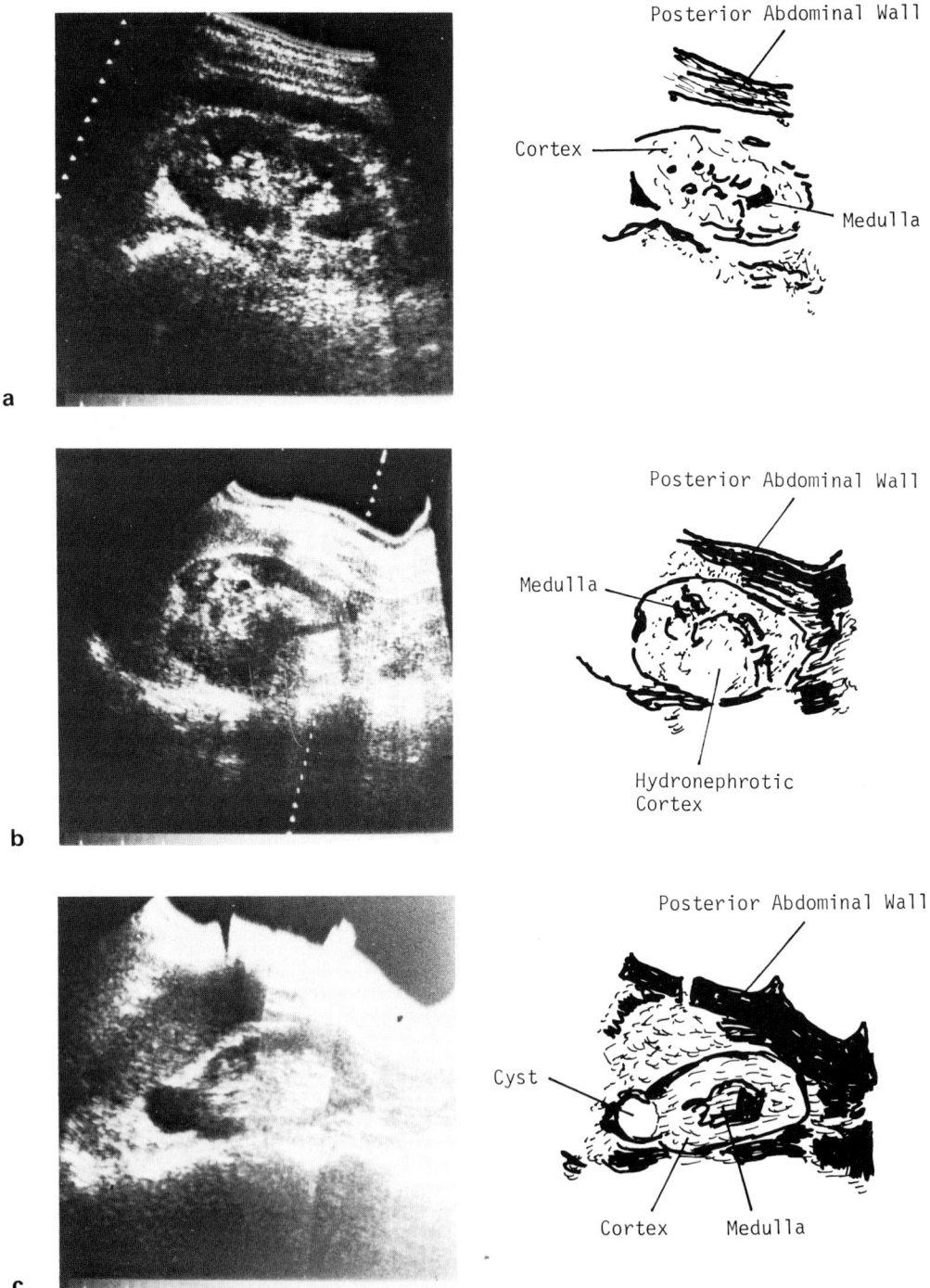

Fig. 4.52 Two-dimensional ultrasonic scans of kidney. These are longitudinal scans through the posterior abdominal wall, at about 40 mm lateral from the midline and slightly oblique to follow the longitudinal axis of the kidney. The patient's head is to the left on each image. (a) Normal kidney. (b) Hydronephrosis. (c) Kidney with upper pole cyst.

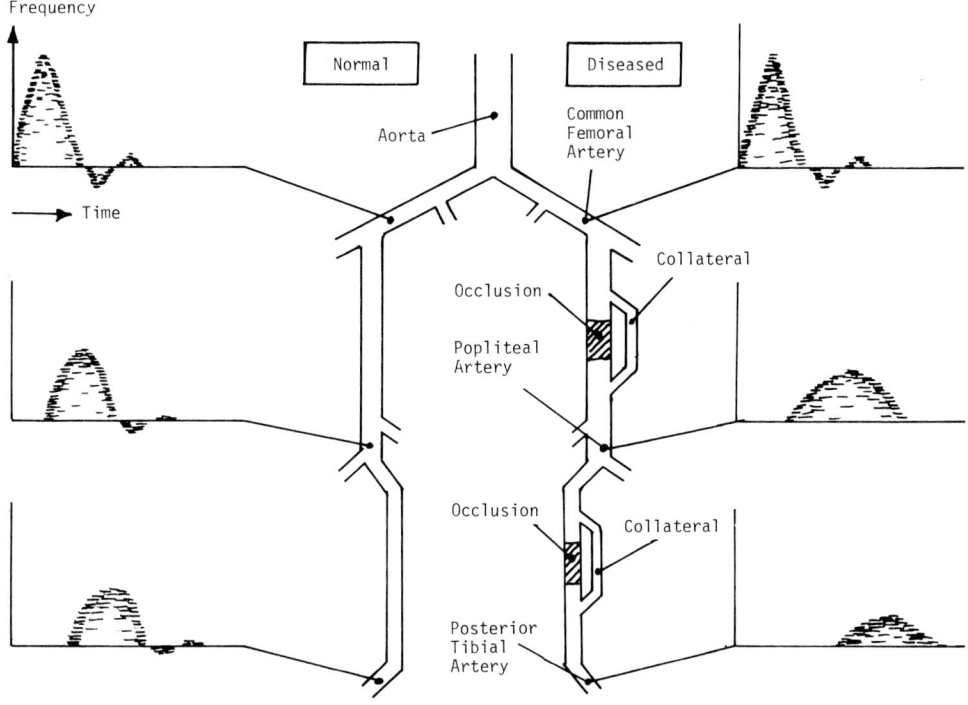

Fig. 4.53 Kinds of ultrasonic Doppler frequency spectra corresponding to blood flow in the arteries of the leg in health and disease. The left-hand side represents a normal arterial tree. The normal transit times between the common femoral site and the popliteal and posterior tibial sites are typically 30–45 ms and 40–55 ms respectively. The other factors which are taken into account are the 'pulsatility index' (defined as the ratio of the peak-to-peak Doppler shift frequencies to the mean Doppler shift frequency) and the 'damping factor' (defined as the ratio of the pulsatility indices at output and input of the arterial segment). Occlusive arterial disease may be classified into four groups, according to whether the collateral has a relatively long or short transit time, and a relatively high or low damping factor.

Laplace transform of the blood flow velocity/time signal. Thus it is possible to obtain numerical indices of arterial stiffness, proximal lumen size, and distal peripheral impedance.[2] These measurements are giving insight into the progression and regression of arterial disease.

Two-dimensional Doppler imaging of blood vessels gives further important data on localised peripheral arterial disease, and is a valuable guide for selecting sites for the monitoring of flow waveforms. The relatively inexpensive continuous wave instruments are only capable of imaging the projection of the blood vessels[7] but pulsed Doppler systems can also make cross-sections and longitudinal-sections, thus increasing the reliability of lesion detection. Examples of such images are shown in Figure 4.54.

Studies of venous flow are limited by the general absence, except in vessels close to the heart, of natural pulsation. Deep vein thrombosis can sometimes be detected by changed flow characteristics in the superficial femoral vein, in response to squeezing the calf or foot.[12] Doppler imaging has a place in assessing the local site of deep vein thrombosis.

These techniques of measuring and visualising blood flow have an important role in monitoring patients in the postoperative period, in addition to their presently better accepted place in diagnosis and preoperative assessment.

Cardiology

In the study of the heart, three main approaches with Doppler techniques have shown some promise. Measurements of flow in the thoracic aorta reflect left heart function.[27] These data can be ob-

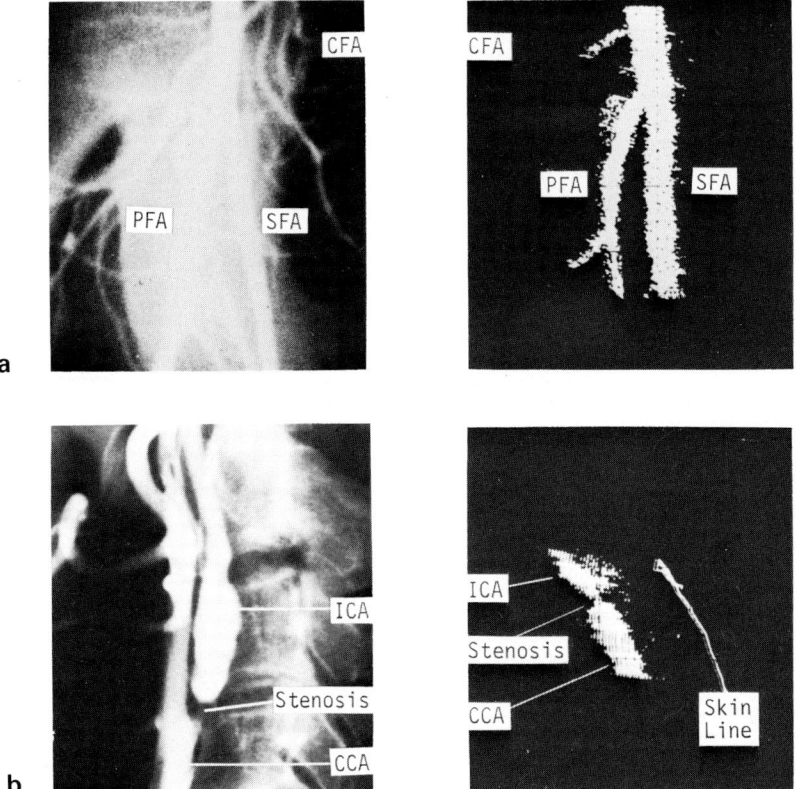

Fig. 4.54 Two-dimensional Doppler images, with corresponding arteriograms. (a) Lateral views of carotid arteries, with stenosis of the internal carotid artery (ICA) close to the bifurcation of the common carotid artery (CCA). (b) Bifurcation of normal common femoral (CFA), superficial femoral (SFA) and profunda femoris (PFA) arteries. These ultrasonic images were made with a 5 MHz pulsed Doppler scanner.

tained with a continuous wave Doppler system operating at a frequency of around 2 MHz, by positioning the probe in the suprasternal notch. The orientation of the aortic arch is such that the ultrasonic beam can, when directed from the suprasternal notch, intersect the direction of blood flow tangentially. Other angles of attack occur, due to the curvature of the vessel, but the highest Doppler shift frequency corresponds to the highest velocity within the beam. The use of real-time sound spectrograph to display directionally-detected Doppler shift signals allows the operator to obtain optimal orientation, and to recognise flow signals from branch arteries which, since they serve the head and neck, are in the opposite direction to the flow in the aortic arch. The spectral display allows turbulence to be identified, and can be interpreted even if the signal-to-noise ratio is poor.

Secondly, the waveforms of blood flow detected with a continuous wave Doppler probe placed transcutaneously over the jugular vein depend on right heart function.[21]

Thirdly, potentially valuable information can be obtained by measuring blood flow within the heart.[1] Thus, the continuous wave Doppler method can be used to measure the instantaneous maximum blood flow velocity within the cardiac chambers, and especially in the region of the valves. Using present techniques, this is not easy to do because of the problems of structure identification in the absence of real-time two-dimensional imaging for guidance. Continuous wave Doppler instruments do not suffer from the range-velocity limitation of pulsed systems, however, and the technique is a sensitive way of detecting regurgitation and turbulence. Generally this disadvantage of pulsed Doppler is not a serious problem at least for qualitative diagnosis, and the great advantage of range selection deserves to be emphasised. The combination of pulsed Doppler flow measurement with real-time two-dimensional visualisation is emerging as an extremely powerful diagnostic tool. The small size of the resolution cell allows turbulent volumes to be detected: in this way, murmurs can be identified which relate to the diastolic rumbles of mitral and tricuspid stenoses, mitral regurgitation, left ventricular outflow obstruction, aortic stenosis, aortic regurgitation, augmented right ventricular filling sound in atrial septal defects, pulmonary stenosis, pulmonary regurgitation, and high velocity flow through the obstruction in coarctation of the aorta. The analyses generally depend on inspection of the frequency spectrum. In many respects, transcutaneous pulsed-Doppler studies can replace intra-cardiac phonocardiography.

FUTURE PROSPECTS

Much research aimed at expanding the horizons of useful applications of diagnostic ultrasound is being carried out in laboratories all over the world. Some of these activities are mentioned earlier in this chapter. Glimpses of others, and the opportunities which they offer for the future, are given in this section.

Portable real-time scanners

Small, hand-held portable self-contained two-dimensional real-time scanners are being developed. These instruments cannot be reduced in size below that set by the display components. At present, there is no alternative to the cathode ray tube; but recent progress with other displays, such as those based on liquid crystals and gas discharge panels, promises to overcome this problem. In the not too distant future, individual cardiologists and obstetricians may expect to have pocket-sized scanners to use in the same way that they use their stethoscopes today. These scanners will be invaluable in the clinic, and will be capable of resolving many diagnostic questions. More difficult and complex clinical conditions will, of course, continue to be investigated by the more quantitative techniques in the laboratory.

High-resolution real-time scanners

The introduction of dynamic electronic focusing has significantly improved the resolution of two-dimensional real-time scanners. Already the resolution of the most advanced instruments is adequate to visualise fetal cardiac structures. Further improvements will certainly make it feasible to screen those at risk of congenital heart disease in early pregnancy, thus giving greater clinical control. The possibility that this type of instrument might also be capable of distinguishing between smooth and ulcerating plaques, and of visualising coronary arteries (although perhaps not in the fetus!) is also very exciting.

Ultrafast scanning

As explained previously in this chapter it is the speed of ultrasound in tissue which ultimately limits the range frame rate in two-dimensional scanning. Basically this must always be true. Contemporary clinical instruments gather picture information in a serial fashion, line-by-line. In principle, however, an array could be used to gather all the received lines simultaneously in parallel, provided that the examined tissue slice could be irradiated uniformly with a suitable pulse of ultrasound. The principal disadvantage would be that the contribution to resolution made by the limited width in azimuth of the transmitted beam in a serial system would be absent, and the principal difficulties would be the practical ones of providing the necessary multitude of electronic receiver channels, and of simultaneously displaying all the resulting timebase lines. Nevertheless, the feasibility of the method has been demonstrated, using optical processing of the ultrasonic signals in order to minimise the complexity.

Two-dimensional arrays

Just as one-dimensional arrays produce two-dimensional images (in real-time), so in principle two-dimensional arrays can be used to examine three-dimensional volumes. Some results have already been published, despite the formidable complexity and high cost of the instrumentation. Another problem, for which a satisfactory solution has yet to be found, is that the data collection time in serial acquisition (i.e. in line-by-line operation) is necessarily a few hundred microseconds per line. The display problem is also difficult. It is not clear that three-dimensional displays which are perceivable by humans are feasible, and it may be necessary to limit the display to a plane or surface selected by the operator. The attraction of three-dimensional scanning is the understanding which it promises to give of the anatomical relationships of abnormally organised structures such as blood vessels.

Intraoperative ultrasonic scanning

Ultrasonic visualisation has a potentially invaluable, but as yet virtually untested, application in surgery. A small, sterilisable, real-time scanner probe and associated display could be used by the surgeon to guide his approach in many operative procedures, for example, in cardiovascular and biliary surgery. The instrument would also provide a method of immediately assessing operative success or technical, probably repairable, failure in the closing stages of intervention. Doppler methods of blood flow detection might be equally valuable in vascular reconstructive surgery.

Acknowledgements

I am grateful to the following colleagues for providing some of the illustrations for this chapter: D. O. Cosgrove (Figs. 4.48a and 4.49); Raymond Gramiak (Fig. 4.47); B. B. Goldberg (Figs. 4.48b, 4.48d and 4.52); Jack Jellins (Fig. 4.51); G. J. Leech (Fig. 4.46); R. J. Lusby (Figs. 4.44 and 4.54a; F. G. M. Ross (Figs. 4.50a, 4.50b and 4.50c); K. J. W. Taylor (Figs. 4.48c and 4.50e); and J. P. Woodcock (Fig. 4.54b).

REFERENCES

1. Baker, D. W., Strandness, D. E. & Johnson, S. L. (1976) Pulsed Doppler techniques. *Ultrasound Med. Biol.*, **2**, 251–62.
2. Bird, D. R., Skidmore, R. & Woodcock, J. P. (1980) The value of Doppler transfer function analysis in the diagnosis of aorto-iliac occlusive arterial disease. In *Diagnosis and Monitoring in Arterial Surgery*, ed. Baird, R. N. & Woodcock, J. P., pp. 121–6. Bristol: John Wright.
3. Brascho, D. J. (1974) Computerized radiation treatment planning with ultrasound. *Am. J. Roentg.*, **120**, 213–23.
4. Carson, P. L. & Scherzinger, A. L. (1980) Ultrasonic computed tomography. In *New Techniques and Instrumentation in Ultrasonography*, ed. Wells, P. N. T. & Ziskin, M. C., pp. 144–65. New York: Churchill Livingstone.
5. Coghlan, B. A. & Taylor, M. G. (1976) Directional Doppler techniques for detection of blood velocities. *Ultrasound Med. Biol.*, **2**, 181–8.
6. Coleman, D. J., Lizzi, F. L. & Jack, R. L. (1977) *Ultrasonography of the Eye and Orbit*. Philadelphia: Lea & Febiger.
7. Curry, G. R. & White, D. N. (1978) Color coded differential velocity arterial scanner (Echoflow). *Ultrasound Med. Biol.*, **4**, 27–35.
8. Daigle, R. E., Rubenstein, S. A. & Baker, D. W. (1977) A duplex scanning system for pediatric cardiology. In *Ultrasound in Medicine*, ed. White, D. & Brown, R. E., vol 3B, pp. 1209–11. New York: Plenum Press.
9. Davidson, J. K., Morley, P., Hurley, G. D. & Holford, N. G. H. (1975) Adrenal venography and ultrasound in the investigation of the adrenal gland. *Br. J. Radiol.*, **48**, 435–50.
10. Edler, I. & Hertz, C. H. (1954) The use of the ultrasonic reflectoscope for the continuous recording of the movements of the heart walls. *K. fysiogr. Sällsk. Lund Föhr.*, **24**, 40–58.
11. Edmonds, P. D. (1972) Interactions of ultrasound with biological structures—a survey of data. In *Interaction of Ultrasound and Biological Tissue*, ed. Reid, J. M. & Sikov, M. R., pp. 299–317. Washington: US Department of Health, Education and Welfare.
12. Evans, D. S. (1971) The early diagnosis of thromboembolism by ultrasound. *Ann. R. Coll. Surg. Engl.*, **49**, 225–49.
13. Filly, R. A. & Goldberg, B. B. (1977) Normal vessels. In *Abdominal Gray Scale Ultrasonography*, ed. Goldberg, B. B., pp. 19–56. New York: Wiley.
14. Green, P. S. (1980) Orthographic transmission imaging. In *New Techniques and Instrumentation in Ultrasonography*, ed. Wells, P. N. T. & Ziskin, M. C., pp. 123–43. New York: Churchill Livingstone.
15. Green, P. S., Taenzer, J. C. & Ramsey, S. D. (1977) A real-time ultrasonic imaging system for carotid arteriography. *Ultrasound Med. Biol.*, **3**, 129–47.
16. Hill, C. R. & Alvisi, C. (eds.) (1980) *Investigative Ultrasonography*, vol 1. Tunbridge Wells: Pitman Medical.
17. Hill, C. R., Nicholas, D. & Bamber, J. C. (1976) Backscattering analysis and ultrasonic imaging. In *Medical Images: Formation, Perception and Measurement*, ed. Hay, G. A., pp. 115–21. London: Wiley.
18. Hobbins, J. C. (ed.) (1979) *Diagnostic Ultrasound in Obstetrics*. New York: Churchill Livingstone.
19. Holm, H. H., Als, O. & Gammelgaard, J. (1979) Percutaneous aspiration and biopsy procedures under ultrasound visualization. In *Diagnostic Ultrasound in Gastrointestinal Disease*, ed. Taylor, K. J. W., pp. 137–49. New York: Churchill Livingstone.
20. Johnston, K. W. & Kakkar, V. V. (1974) Non-invasive measurement of systolic pressure slope. *Archs Surg.*, **108**, 52–6.
21. Kalmanson, D., Veyrat, C., Chiche, P. & Wichitz, S. (1974) Non-invasive diagnosis of right heart diseases and

of left-to-right shunts using directional Doppler ultrasound. In *Cardiovascular Applications of Ultrasound*, ed. Reneman, R. S., pp. 361–70. Amsterdam: North-Holland.
22. Kessler, L. W. (1974) Review of progress and applications in acoustic microscopy. *J. acoust. Soc. Am.*, **55**, 909–18.
23. Kobayashi, T., Takatani, O., Hattori, N and Kimura, K. (1974) Echographic evaluation of abdominal tumor regression during antineoplastic treatment. *J. clin. Ultrasound*, **2**, 131–41.
24. Kompfner, R. (1975) Recent advances in acoustical microscopy. *Br. J. Radiol.*, **48**, 615–27.
25. Lancée, C. T. (ed) (1979) *Echocardiology*. The Hague: Martinus Nijhoff.
26. Leopold, G. R., Woo, V. L., Schieble, W., Nachsheim, D. & Gosink, B. B. (1979) High-resolution ultrasonography of scrotal pathology. *Radiology*, **131**, 719–23.
27. Light, L. H. (1977) Aortic blood velocity measurement by transcutaneous aortovelography and its clinical applications. In *Echocardiology* ed. Bom, N., pp. 233–43. The Hague: Martinus Nijhoff.
28. Linzer, M. (ed) (1979) *Ultrasonic Tissue Characterization II*, NBS Special Publication 525. Washington: US Government Printing Office.
29. Morley, P. (1978). Clinical staging of epithelial bladder tumours by echo-tomography. In *Ultrasound in Tumour Diagnosis*, ed. Hill, C. R., McReady, V. R. & Cosgrove, D. O., pp. 145–61. Tunbridge Wells: Pitman Medical.
30. Mountford, R. A. & Wells, P. N. T. (1972) Ultrasonic liver scanning: the A-scan in the normal and cirrhosis. *Phys. Med. Biol.*, **17**, 261–9.
31. Rosenfield, A. T. (ed) (1977) *Genitourinary Ultrasonography*. New York: Churchill Livingstone.
32. Ross, F. G. M. (1977) Ultrasonic investigation of the heart. In *Ultrasonics in Clinical Diagnosis*, ed. Wells, P. N. T., 2nd edition, pp. 114–41. Edinburgh: Churchill Livingstone.
33. Sample, W. F. & Sarti, D. A. (1979) Diagnosis of pancreatic disease by ultrasound. In *Diagnostic Ultrasound in Gastrointestinal Disease*, ed. Taylor, K. J. W., pp. 85–101. New York: Churchill Livingstone.
34. Smith, S. W., Phillips, D. J., von Ramm, O. T. & Thurstone, F. L. (1976) Real-time B-mode echoencephalography. In *Ultrasound in Medicine*, ed. White, D. N. & Barnes, R., vol 2, pp. 373–82. New York: Plenum Press.
35. Taylor, K. J. W. (1977) Ultrasonic investigation of the hepatobiliary system and the spleen. In *Ultrasonics in Clinical Diagnosis*, ed. Wells, P. N. T., 2nd edition, pp. 97–113. Edinburgh: Churchill Livingstone.
36. Taylor, K. J. W. (1978) The thyroid. In *Atlas of Gray Scale Ultrasonography*, ed. Taylor, K. J. W., pp. 397–403. New York: Churchill Livingstone.
37. Ulrich, W. D. (1974) Ultrasound dosage for non-therapeutic use on human beings—extrapolations from a literature survey. *I.E.E.E. Trans. biomed. Engng.* **BME–21**, 48–51.
38. Watanabe, H. (1978) Prostatic ultrasound. In *Genitourinary Ultrasonography* ed. Rosenfield, A. T., pp. 125–37. New York: Churchill Livingstone.
39. Wells, P. N. T. (1974) The possibility of harmful biological effects in ultrasonic diagnosis. In *Cardiovascular Applications of Ultrasound*, ed. Reneman, R. S., pp. 1–17. Amsterdam: North-Holland.
40. Wells, P. N. T. (1975) Absorption and dispersion of ultrasound in biological tissues. *Ultrasound Med. Biol.*, **1**, 369–76.
41. Wells, P. N. T. (1977) *Biomedical Ultrasonics*. London: Academic Press.
42. White, D. N., Kraus, A. S., Clark, J. M. & Campbell, J. K. (1969) Interpreter error in echoencephalography. *Neurology*, **19**, 775–85.
43. Wild, J. J. & Reid, J. M. (1952) Further pilot echographic studies on the histologic structure of the living intact human breast. *Am. J. Path.*, **28**, 839–61.
44. Woodcock, J. P. (1970) The significance of changes in the velocity/time waveform in occlusive arterial disease in the leg. In *Ultrasonics in Medicine and Biology*, ed., Filipczynski, L., pp. 243–50. Warsaw: Polish Scientific Publishers.

5

Thermographic imaging

C. H. Jones

INTRODUCTION

The normal internal temperature in resting man is maintained within very narrow limits in spite of wide variations in environmental temperature. Under steady state conditions heat flows from production sites in the body to cooler tissues and blood distributes this heat to the body surface from where it is dissipated to the external environment by radiation, convection and evaporation. The importance of deep body temperature as an indicator of disease has been known for centuries; but in recent years attention has also been paid to the significance of skin temperatures. Contact probes such as thermocouples and thermistors are suitable for measuring skin temperatures over relatively small areas but they are tedious to use for mapping temperature distributions over large areas of the body surface. Furthermore, unless the probes are small they can modify the very temperatures they are sensing. Thermography makes use of measuring techniques which portray surface temperature distributions pictorially and this is accomplished either with liquid crystals or infrared scanning equipment.

LIQUID CRYSTAL THERMOGRAPHY

Liquid crystals are a class of compounds which exhibit colour-temperature sensitivity in the cholesteric phase. This phase exists within a specific temperature range and is exhibited by many esters of cholesterol as a state of matter with an ordered molecular arrangement intermediate between a true three dimensional solid and a liquid. The ordered molecular arrangement gives rise to a property which results in maximum scattering of specific wavelengths of light whereas the other light components are transmitted through the material. When the crystals are applied to a blackened surface the transmitted light is absorbed and the scattered light appears as an iridescent colour. A small change in temperature alters the molecular ordering which in turn alters the wavelength of maximal scattering. A given cholesteric liquid crystal always exhibits the same colour at a specific temperature. The disadvantages of this technique are that the skin surface has to be blackened (usually with a water-base paint) and photometric calibration of the liquid crystals is required to determine accurately the colour distribution within a known temperature range. The technique is easy to apply and has been used to detect breast cancer.[8] A record of the liquid crystal image may be obtained by colour photography.

In another method, the liquid crystals are cemented to a pseudo-solid powder (with particle sizes between 10 and 30 μm) and incorporated in thin film supports with a black background. The film (or plate) protects the crystals from chemical and biological contamination and they can be used many times without loss of sensitivity. No painting of the skin surface is required. Liquid crystal plate thermography is used principally for breast investigations[30] but it has also been used where it is not possible to apply liquid crystals directly on to the skin.[20] It is a 'contact method' of temperature measurement and undue pressure between the flexible plate and the body surface can cause a change in the surface temperature distribution: it is not always possible to obtain uniform contact between the plate and the body surface being examined. These difficulties are overcome by infrared temperature measuring systems, and *thermographic imaging* in the following sections refers to infrared thermography and its clinical application.

THERMOGRAPHIC IMAGING

Infrared thermography

Like all other objects, human skin emits infrared radiation as an exponential function of its absolute temperature. The total radiated power per unit area is given by:

$$W_T = \varepsilon \sigma T^4 \qquad (5.1)$$

where W_T expressed in $W\ m^{-2}\ s^{-1}$, ε is the skin's emissitivity, σ is Stefan's constant ($5 \cdot 67 \times 10^{-8}\ W\ m^{-2}\ K^{-4}$), and T is the temperature of the skin in degrees Kelvin.

The emissivity is a wavelength-dependent function which describes the extent to which the surface absorbs and emits radiation like a true *black body*. By definition, a black body is an object which completely absorbs all radiation incident upon it. Obviously human skin does not absorb visible radiation in this way but its emissivity approaches unity throughout the spectral region used in IR thermography. A skin surface whose area is A at uniform temperature T_1 and whose surroundings assumed to be black are at a uniform temperature T_2 loses heat at a rate $W_{\Delta T}$ given by:

$$W_{\Delta T} = A\sigma\ (T_1^4 - T_2^4) \qquad (5.2)$$

If T_1 differs from T_2 by a small quantity ΔT we may write

$$W_{\Delta T} = 4A\sigma T^3 \Delta T \qquad (5.3)$$

This means that for an area of 1 m² which has a temperature 10 K higher than that of its surroundings, the heat loss is about 60 W. The spectral distribution of the emitted radiation depends on the temperature of the surface and can be accurately represented by a theoretical formula first derived by Planck in 1901. This basic law prescribes the radiated power per unit area per unit wavelength interval from a perfect black body radiator as

$$W_\lambda = C_1 \lambda^{-5} (\exp \frac{C_2}{\lambda T} - 1)^{-1} \qquad (5.4)$$

where W_λ = spectral radiant emittance at wavelength λ of a black body at absolute temperature T K, $C_1 = 3 \cdot 74 \times 10^{-16}\ W\ m^2$, and $C_2 = 1 \cdot 438 \times 10^{-2}\ m\ K$.

Radiant energy is emitted in a broad band of wavelengths with a maximum emission occurring at a wavelength dependent upon the surface temperature. It can be shown that the wavelength λ_{max} of the most strongly emitted radiation is inversely proportional to the absolute temperature of the black body radiator, thus

$$\lambda_{max} = (2 \cdot 898 \times 10^3)/T \qquad (5.5)$$

where λ_{max} is expressed in micrometres.

From these equations it is apparent that a skin surface at a temperature of 30° C emits most copiously at a wavelength of about 9·5 μm and significantly over a range of 4–40 μm.

An infrared (IR) temperature measuring device consists basically of a system for collecting radiation from a well-defined field of view, and for focusing it on to a detector which transduces the radiant energy into an electrical signal. There are two categories of detector. These are *thermal detectors* which respond to the heating of the sensor, and *photon detectors* in which the initial absorption of infrared photons results in the freeing of bound electrons.

Photon detectors generally operate within restricted wavelength intervals and the exponent of T in Equation 5.1 varies with the spectral range of the radiation being detected. Temperature differences can still be measured, however, provided that the detecting system is uniformly sensitive throughout the appropriate spectral range.

Thermal detectors

Thermal detectors suitable for clinical use sense radiation by the temperature rise in the absorbing element which affects some temperature-sensitive property. For example, a *bolometer* employs an absorbing element whose electrical resistance is temperature-sensitive. By use of a steady bias current, the change in resistance caused by the temperature change produces a voltage signal which can be amplified electronically. Thermal detectors of this type were used in some of the early types of imaging systems but they are less sensitive and have a lower frequency response than photon detectors.

Pyroelectric thermal detectors are of particular interest.[1] The *pyroelectric effect* is exhibited by certain ferromagnetic crystals, such as barium titanate and triglycine sulphate (TGS). Electrically the sensor behaves as a capacitor on which a charge appears when it is exposed to a change in radiance. A pyroelectric detector presents a spontaneous polarisation in a direction normal to its surface and the magnitude of this polarisation depends upon the temperature of the detector. Absorption of infrared energy by the detector causes a local temperature rise with a consequential change in the polarisation. Pyroelectric detectors have the advantage that they can detect long wavelength radiation without detector cooling which is required for photon detectors. Recently pyroelectric detectors have been incorporated into vidicon type TV tubes and this development is described more fully later.

Photon detectors

A photon detector is usually a semi-conductor type of device in which the initial absorption of an infrared photon results in the freeing of bound electrons or charge carriers. They are designed to function either in a photoconductive mode or in a photovoltaic mode. In the case of a photoconductor, the high electrical resistance of the sensor is decreased on illumination with infrared radiation. A photovoltaic detector employs a junction in which a voltage is produced across a conductor on illumination. Photon detectors are sensitive to infrared radiation within restricted wavelength intervals. So as to reduce thermal excitation of electrons, which would otherwise impair its ultimate sensitivity to infrared, a photon detector is usually cooled. This is commonly achieved by means of liquid nitrogen. The output of a photon detector does not depend on a rise in its temperature and therefore its thermal capacity is of no importance. Its response time constant depends only on the photoelectronic properties of the detector, and is typically a few microseconds.

Indium antimonide (InSb) and cadmium mercury telluride (usually referred to as CMT) are the photon detectors most often used in clinical thermography equipment, but lead tin telluride and germanium detectors have also been used. Typical detector responses are shown in Figure 5.1. Cooled

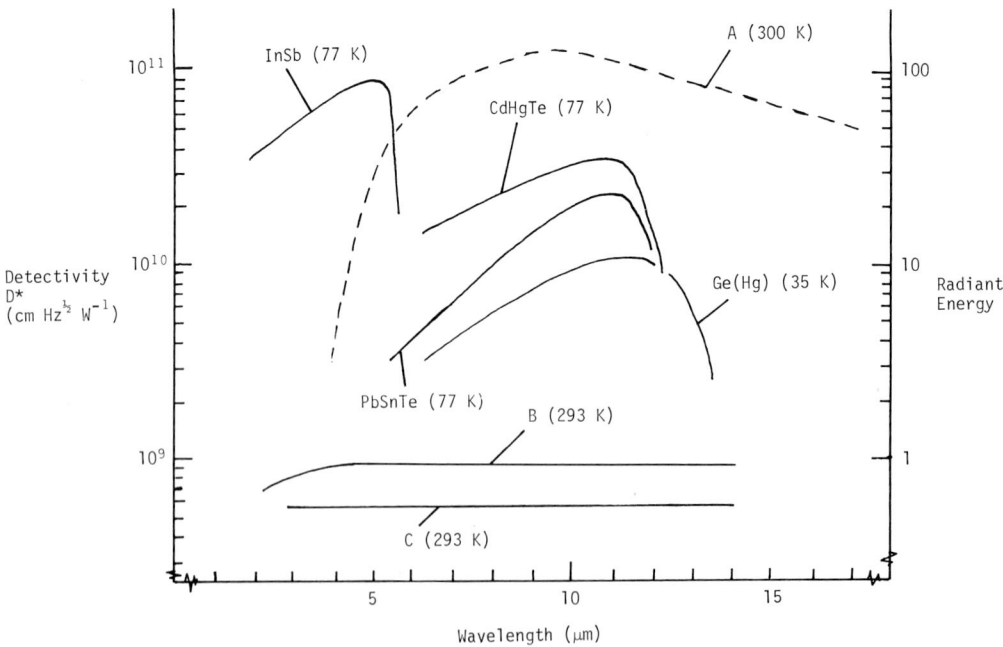

Fig. 5.1 A: spectral distribution of radiant energy from skin at 27 °C (in arbitrary units). The remaining curves represent the detectivities of different types of detectors (InSb: indium antimonide; CdHgTe: cadmium mercury telluride, CMT; PbSnTe: lead tin telluride; Ge(Hg): mercury doped germanium); B: pyroelectric (TGS) detector; and C: thermistor bolometer.

InSb is most sensitive to IR radiation between 2–5·6 μm and CMT to 8–13 μm.

Detector performance

The minimum detectable power W_m of an infrared detector is the incident power which gives a signal-to-noise ratio equal to unity at the output of the detector. Noise is due to thermal and electrical fluctuations both of which are frequency dependent and for this reason the quantity *noise equivalent power* (NEP) is used:

$$\text{NEP} = W_m (\Delta f)^{-1/2} \quad (5.6)$$

where Δf is the frequency bandwidth of the measuring amplifier. For many detectors W_m is proportional to the square root of the area of the detector. A normalised detectivity $D^\star$ describes the detectivity in such a way that the actual area of the detector and the bandwidth used in measuring the detectivity do not affect the result. Thus,

$$D^\star = W_m^{-1} (A \Delta f)^{1/2} \quad (5.7)$$

and

$$D^\star = A^{1/2}/(\text{NEP}) \quad (5.8)$$

When detector systems are to be compared, it is also useful to have some estimate of the temperature resolution of the thermal image. The *noise equivalent temperature difference* (NETD) is a useful parameter for this purpose and is defined as the temperature difference between two black bodies that gives a signal that is equal to the total noise amplitude of the system. An indium antimonide detector working in a wavelength range 2–5·6 μm has a $D^\star$ of about 8×10^{10} cm Hz$^{1/2}$ W^{-1}, and a NETD of about 0·2 K.

Imaging systems

Scanning of the scene in front of the detector can be accomplished in a variety of ways. For example, the Aga Thermovision 680 Medical camera, shown in Figure 5.2, employs a germanium lens to focus the infrared radiation on to a cooled indium antimonide detector through two eight sided rotating prisms. A virtual image is formed by the germanium lens on a plane within the first prism. The image is scanned vertically by rotation of the prism about its horizontal axis, which results in a horizontal virtual line-image being formed within the second scanning prism. The line image is then scanned horizontally in turn by rotation of the second prism about its vertical axis. The indium antimonide detector is used in photovoltaic mode and the sensitive part of the detector is 0·35 mm diameter. This type of imaging system produces an image with 140 lines (210 elements/line) and a scanning frame rate of 16 frames/second, with a temperature resolution of 0·2 K.

Other systems use different methods of scanning, and these include oscillating mirrors and rotating multi-sided mirror drums. Whatever method is employed, the build up of the thermographic picture must be synchronised accurately with the scanning of the patient. The thermal picture is usually displayed on a television image tube. In some instruments avoidance of picture flicker is achieved by electronic storage techniques, but these systems are not ideal for dynamic studies.

Image quality can be improved, and the disadvantage of low frame rates overcome, by using an array of several detectors. Usually the configuration of an array is such that each of the detector elements scans the scene in parallel with a consequential improvement in signal-to-noise ratio. Each line in the picture is scanned by a different detector and therefore channel uniformity must be high otherwise a 'liney' picture results. More recently, serial scan systems have been developed in which each detector in a linear array scans in sequence over every point in the scene, and the signals are appropriately delayed and added to form the image. This method overcomes channel non-uniformity problems but requires very high scanning speeds for the system optics. In practice this difficulty is overcome by a detector array in which elements are grouped in serial rows so that the matrix scan includes a mixture of serial and parallel components.[19] A typical matrix consists of eight linear rows each composed of six elements. Such a system requires fairly complex electronics for connecting the detector output to ensure TV compatibility, but the resulting image is flicker-free and has a temperature sensitivity (NETD) of better than 0·1 K and a high spatial resolution.

Most clinical thermography has made use of single detector systems which provide thermal images

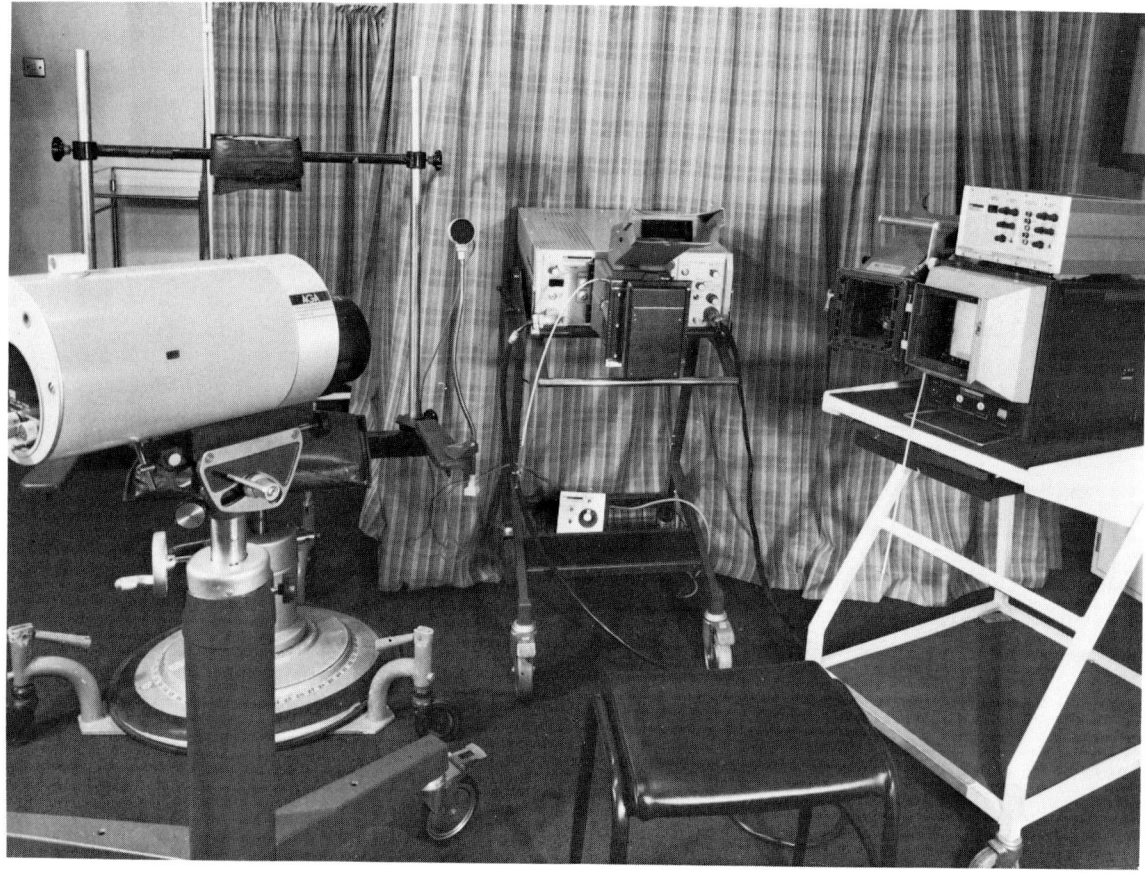

Fig. 5.2 Aga Thermovision 680 medical thermographic system.

with a temperature resolution of about 0·2 K. The angular resolution of an electro-optical imaging system depends largely on the response time of the detector and the characteristics of the scanning optics. This may be defined as the angle in milliradians subtended by an observed object which is small enough to reduce the video signal of the system to half of the maximum signal amplitude obtained for large object angles. Typical values range from 1 milliradian for a CMT detector with a 2 s scan time to 3 milliradians for an InSb detector with a 0·04 s scan time. Table 5.1 lists details of some of the infrared thermography systems which have been used clinically.

Display systems

The signal derived from the detector is amplified and used to modulate the intensity of the electron beam of a TV monitor type picture-tube display unit. The thermal image shows relative temperature differences in a continuous range of gray tones from black to white. The hot area to be displayed may be white or black (inverted mode) depending on the preference of the user. A photographic record of the thermal image is usually required, and this *thermogram* should cover the range of gray tones displayed in the monitor image. Care should be taken not to lose thermal detail by using an inadequate photographic technique.

Some means of quantifying the thermal image is essential. A high quality thermal image which cannot be analysed quantitatively is of little clinical value. Most manufacturers provide a *temperature reference standard* calibrated to an equivalent black body temperature over a temperature range of 28–40 °C. When accurate temperature measurements are required, the temperature standard is placed within the scene being examined. Some standards consist of several temperature sources each of

Table 5.1 Infrared thermography systems: parameter-component descriptions

Parameter-component	Range of values, description	General information
Spatial resolution	0·75–2 milliradians	Close-up lens can be used to improve resolution
Number of horizontal lines (n)	90–625	Large n and e necessary for resolution of vascular components
Elements per line (e)	100–600	10 000–360 000 elements per frame
Field of view	5° × 5° – 40° × 40°	30° × 30° 0·4 × 0·4 m at 0·8 m
Depth of focus (d)	1–30 cm	Large d required for breast thermography
Range of focus (T)	10 cm to infinity	Small T useful for close-up work
Frame rate (f)	0·3 min^{-1} – 60s^{-1}	Low f gives flicker picture, difficult to view and focus, requires long persistence CRT or storage facilities
Noise equivalent temperature difference	0·07 – 0·3°C at 30°C	Governs temperature resolution 0·1 – 0·4°C
Temperature range (t)	25 – 45°C (medical)	2, 5, 10, 15°C ranges useful for medical thermography
Detector	InSb (2 – 5.6 μm, 77 K)	Proven reliability but narrow spectral response
	CdHgTe(2 – 14 , 77 K)	Wide spectral response
	PbSnTe (2 – 14 μm, 77 K)	Wide spectral response
	Ge(Hg) (2 – 14 μm, <30 K)	Used in dual detector systems with InSb: cooling difficult
	Multiple sensor arrays of InSb or CHgTe	Detector matching necessary, high f, good resolution
	TGS pyroelectric vidicon (room temperature)	Inexpensive, inferior resolution, TV compatible
	Thermistor bolometer (room temperature)	Less sensitive than photon detectors
Scanning mechanisms	Scanning mirrors	$f = 0·3$ min^{-1} too slow for dynamic studies
	Rotating silicon prisms	$f = 16$s^{-1}, 25s^{-1} compact, portable system
	Scanning mirror + rotating mirror drum	$f = 4$s^{-1} good spatial resolution
	Rotating mirror drum with offset faces	$f = 46$s^{-1} good for dynamic studies
	Pyroelectric vidicon tube with chopper	Flicker free/real time TV compatible
Display and recording system	Light modulation + film	No display monitor
	Facsimile paper	Slow, poor quality print
	CRT + photography	Good display, isotherms, colour, deflexion, modulation, storage, computer compatible; electronic processing of image

which can be adjusted to a known temperature. In some systems the scanning lines making up the thermal picture can be displayed as temperature profiles, so the temperature magnitude of the profile can be determined relative to that of the temperature standard. The image displays of most commercial systems are equipped with an isotherm function by which a signal is superimposed upon the gray tone picture so that all the surface areas with the same temperature are presented as saturated white. The isotherm can be adjusted as required within the temperature range of the thermogram. The isotherm facility can be used to measure the temperature of an area relative to the known temperature of the reference standard. For example, if in Figure 5.3 the mid-level temperature (indicated by Δ along the lower edge of the image) corresponds to 32 °C, then the isotherm in Figure 5.3b corresponds to 35·7 °C.

Some thermography systems have two isotherm facilities which can be used simultaneously or separately; these are useful for the accurate measurement of temperature differences. One isotherm can be superimposed on the temperature standard, and the other can be adjusted to measure the temperature over a point of interest elsewhere in the image.

A variety of accessories is available for use with commercial equipment. Aga Thermovision provide means by which the average radiant energy emitted

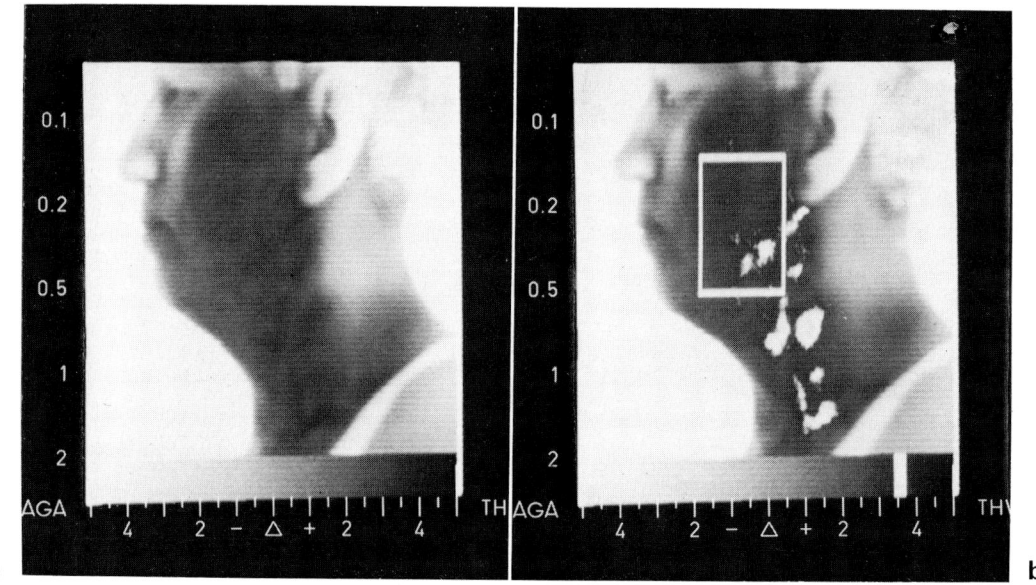

Fig. 5.3 Thermograms of a patient with radiotherapy skin reaction. (a) inverted mode: (white is cold, black is hot). The mid-level temperature Δ is 32 °C, and the temperature range is 10 K. (b) Isotherm showing the hottest area (35·7 °C), and the integrator area.

from one of two selected rectangular areas in the field of view can be measured. The measurement is expressed as a percentage of a preset maximum level. The two areas are presented on the screen of the display unit as outlined boxes whose height, width and position can be selected independently of each other. The maximum and minimum video levels within each box can also be recorded, as illustrated in Figure 5.3b. By means of electronic processing and a colour TV monitor it is possible to display thermal images in colour, each colour representing a predetermined temperature increment. Colour thermograms can be recorded on colour film and these facilitate rapid assessment of temperature differences. Unfortunately colour thermography tends to distort the appearance of the underlying anatomical contours and those heat patterns associated with subcutaneous vasculature.

Some thermography systems provide a digital display option. The gray tone thermogram is supplemented by a raster of digits or symbols each of which represents the measured temperature averaged over a small area. Presentation in this form permits analysis of the thermal image by computer techniques.

It is advisable to check the quality of the displayed image and its photographic record at regular intervals. One method of achieving this is to use a resolution test mask which fits in front of a black body of known temperature such as a temperature standard and record its thermal image and compare with previous thermograms taken in identical conditions. Such an image is shown in Figure 5.4.

PHYSICAL AND PHYSIOLOGICAL FACTORS

General considerations

The measurement of temperature by infrared techniques requires knowledge of the emissivity of the skin, as defined in Equation 5.1. This has been shown to be $0·98 \pm 0·01$ providing the surface is clean and dry and free from cosmetic cream and powder.[29] Subjects being investigated by thermography must have clean dry skin; perspiration on the skin reduces the apparent surface temperature. The temperature distribution over the skin surface depends upon the heat generated in underlying tissues, the thermal properties of the tissues and the skin, and the flow of blood through the subcutaneous vasculature.

Disease or trauma can affect the skin temperature, sometimes causing a temperature increase or in some conditions causing a reduced temperature. Blood vessels which lie within 2 or 3 mm of the surface can be imaged photographically using reflected light and infrared sensitive film, but deeper vessels carrying warm blood also affect the surface temperature distribution.[15] Surface topography also affects the temperature pattern, skin folds and cavities trapping radiant heat. The magnitude of the skin temperature is also influenced by the deep body temperature which is affected by intake of food, physical and hormonal activity and so on. In general, clinical thermography makes use of temperature differences between two similar areas rather than actual temperature magnitudes and many of these difficulties are avoided.

Preparation of the patient

Clinical thermography should be carried out in a draught-free, constant temperature environment. A cool ambient temperature of 19 ± 1 °C is the optimum to ensure reliable standardisation and operation of the imaging equipment. This cools the skin of the patient uniformly and reduces physiological variations associated with ambient changes. If the examination room is air conditioned, the cooler-heater unit must be adequate to balance thermal changes due to heat generated by equipment, personnel and patient as well as any extreme temperature changes due to the disposition of the room. The thermostat controlling the cooler should be sited appropriately within the examination area

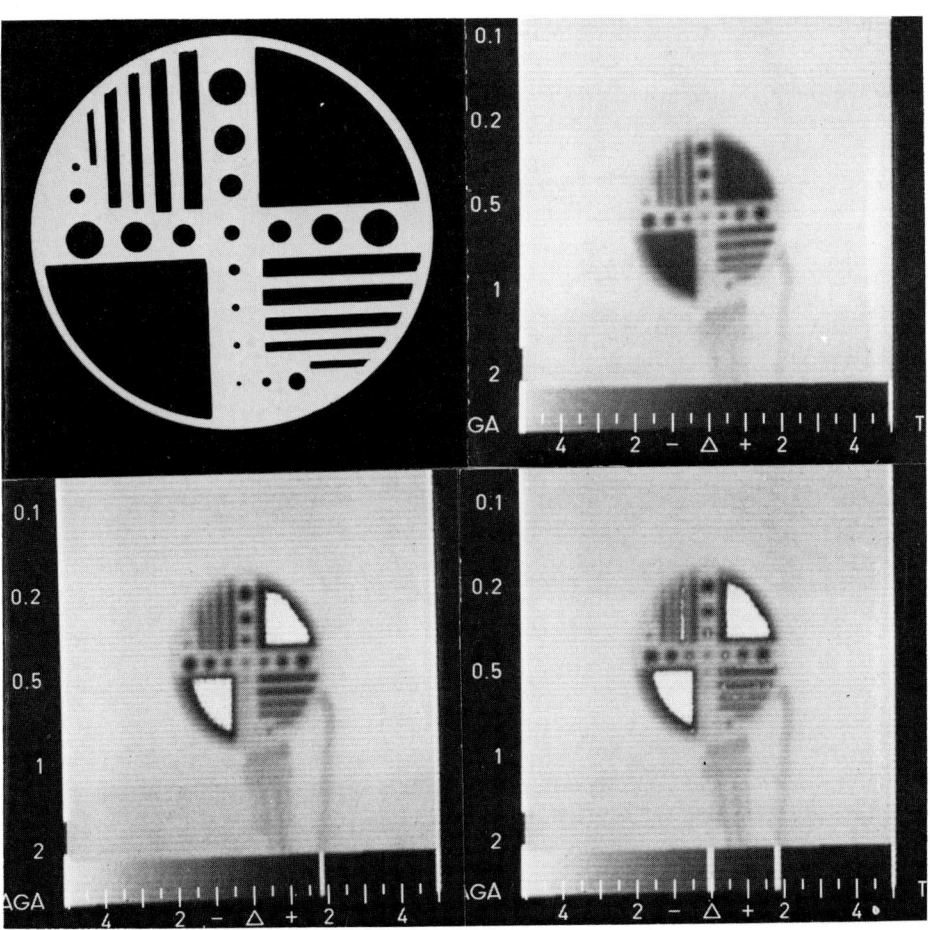

Fig. 5.4 Resolution mask and examples of thermographic images. The mask has a centre hole diameter of 2 mm. The thermograms in the bottom row have single and double isotherms respectively on the left and the right.

and the temperature should be monitored continuously.

Before examination the patient disrobes to expose the area to be examined. It is sometimes necessary for the patient to also remove tight fitting clothing which might affect the blood flow through the area being investigated. The patient should sit or lie restfully for about 12–15 min to equilibrate. Cooling of the patient during this period removes excess heat from the body surface, sharpens up the thermal pattern and helps to stabilise the temperature distribution. It is important that the patient should not be overcooled or uncomfortable during this period of preparation.

Some investigations cannot be carried out in a constant ambient temperature, and patients have to be examined in a ward or clinic. Local cooling of the area or limb can be accomplished by a hand-held cooler fan or by spraying the area with spirit which on evaporation cools the underlying surface. Neither method can be recommended when precise temperature measurements are required but both methods are acceptable for particular investigations such as dynamic studies relating to peripheral vascular disorders or incompetent perforator vein studies.

Thermography is being used to investigate a variety of clinical problems. Most important amongst these are: (1) screening for occult malignant disease; (2) delineation of the extent of known disease; (3) identification of areas with abnormal temperatures which might be the cause of functional impairment of underlying organs or glands; (4) monitoring the effects of various forms of therapy such as reconstructive surgery, radiotherapy or treatment with hormones or drugs; (5) assessing the prognosis of certain diseases; (6) identify functional deficiencies and vascular disorders; (7) studying the effects of acute or chronic trauma; and (8) physiological research such as energy metabolism and peripheral vascular investigations.

It is beyond the scope of this chapter to describe how thermography is used in all these situations, but attention is drawn to a select number of applications which illustrate some of the practical aspects.

Female breast thermography

The development of thermography as a clinical technique has been very closely associated with its use as a diagnostic aid for breast cancer. In 1956 Lawson[18] demonstrated that the skin over malignant tumours in the female breast is often between 1 and 4 K warmer than the surrounding skin.

Although the temperature distribution over the surface of the breast varies considerably from one person to another, each healthy individual has a characteristic pattern (typical examples are shown in Figs. 5.5a and 5.5b) which essentially remains constant over long periods of time. The thermal pattern is closely related to the subcutaneous network of blood vessels and the temperature of blood flowing through those vessels. Neoplasia can alter both the vascular pattern and the blood flow and consequently affect the surface temperature distribution (Fig. 5.5c). In a healthy subject the temperature ranges within 28 and 36.5 °C. There are three areas over which the thermal pattern is frequently prominent: (1) the upper outer aspect of the breast over the lateral thoracic artery which appears as an area of focal thermal activity; (2) an elongated area radiating medially from the areola overlying the subcutaneous mammary vein; and (3) an area circumscribing the areola where subcutaneous blood vessels form deep and superficial plexuses. Vessels which course near the surface of the breast carrying blood from deep within the breast result in prominent thermal profiles over the skin surface with widths at half height of 1–3 cm with gradients of between 1 and 2.5 K cm^{-1} causing temperature increases of up to 4 K.

In order to identify thermal abnormalities more easily, several authors have classified thermograms of healthy women into groups.[9,11] It has been shown that there are at least three types of pattern: (1) patterns with minimal thermal markings which are associated with cold avascular breasts with a mean breast temperature of about 30 ± 2 °C; (2) patterns with prominent thermal markings over both breasts, with a mean breast temperature of about 32 ± 2 °C; and (3) 'patch-type' thermal patterns which cover both breasts and often spread over other areas of the body.

Precise thermal symmetry of both breasts is rare. Even so, most women who do not have breast nodularity or a localised lump tend to have similar surface thermal patterns over both breasts. Each individual has a characteristic thermal pattern

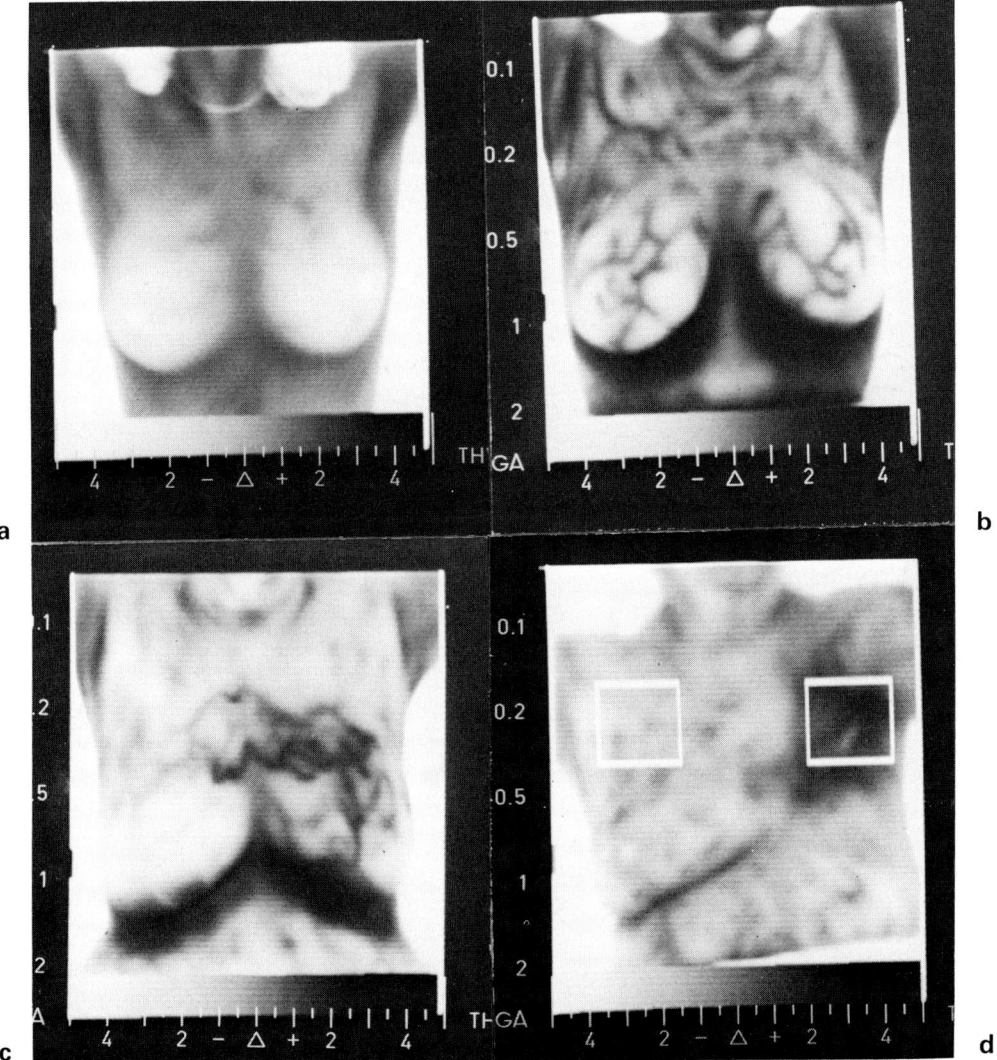

Fig. 5.5 Breast thermograms. (a) Normal avascular breasts. (b) Vascular breasts with benign mammary dysplasia. (c) The left breast has cancer, and has a temperature 3 K higher than the right breast. (d) Patient following left breast mastectomy, with integrator rectangles positioned for monitoring treatment by hormones.

which remains unaltered over a long period of time. The development of a malignant tumour within the breast usually changes the temperature distribution over the surface of the affected breast. The thermographic features considered to be abnormal are: (1) a localised area of temperature increase of about 1·5 K or more; (2) a localised increase in vascularity and its associated thermal pattern (this might be in the form of venous engorgement, dilatation or an increase in the number of superficial blood vessels); (3) unilateral increase in temperature over the areolar area; and (4) a generalised increase in temperature of one breast.

The essential procedure is to compare both breasts using one breast as a control for the other. Similar changes sometimes occur when the tumour is benign, but this is less frequent.

About 70 per cent of breast cancer can be detected by thermography. About 20 per cent of patients with benign disease have abnormal thermograms. In a period of 5 years over 12 000 women have been examined thermographically at the Royal

Marsden Hospital, London.[16] Table 5.2 shows the results for those patients who had biopsies. The correlation of thermography and the stage of the disease for those patients with carcinoma shows that about 60 per cent of early cancers and 80 per cent of late cancers cause abnormal thermal patterns.

Table 5.2 Summary of thermographic and histological results for female breast patients examined at the Royal Marsden Hospital, London.[16] (Note figures in brackets are corresponding percentages.)

Histology	Number of patients	Number of thermograms		
		Abnormal	Equivocal	Normal
Malignant	363(100)	248(68)	47(13)	68(19)
Benign	1101(100)	240(22)	171(15)	690(63)

The results shown in Table 5.2 include women who attended the hospital to be 'screened' for unsuspected cancer. Of the first 5500 women examined at this clinic, 37 carcinomas (0·7 per cent incidence) were found. Sixty-five per cent of these women had abnormal thermograms. Of 5321 women who had complete thermographic examinations, 80 per cent of the thermograms were normal, 8·5 per cent were abnormal, and 11·5 per cent were of doubtful significance. The number of benign conditions producing abnormal thermograms was 75, 23 per cent of the total number of benign lesions in women who had a biopsy for histological verification.

Breast thermography lacks the sensitivity and specificity to be used alone,[14] but some workers find it a useful adjunct to clinical examination and X-ray mammography.[28] It is completely safe and in contrast to mammography it can be used at frequent intervals to monitor patients with chronic benign disease or screen asymptomatic women for occult disease. Patients with abnormal thermograms require further investigation to exclude the possibility of malignant disease. The combination of thermography and ultrasound techniques portends improvement in the overall accuracy of breast disease diagnosis.

Thermography misses at least 30 per cent of very early cancers, but there is evidence that these patients have a better prognosis than those with the same stage of disease who have abnormal thermal patterns. Breast thermography is also used to screen patients for residual disease after radiotherapy[11] and to monitor the response of chest wall recurrences to treatment with hormones or chemotherapy. A typical image is shown in Figure 5.5d.

Scrotal thermography

In man the testes are situated in the scrotum apparently to maintain their temperature a few degrees Kelvin lower than core body temperature. If this normal temperature differential is abolished, spermatogenesis is depressed and may eventually cease. A varicocele caused by reversal of blood flow in the internal spermatic vein interferes with normal circulation of blood in the scrotum and can produce an increase in the temperature of the testes. This condition is not uncommon and affects about 10 per cent of young men and about 20 per cent of subfertile males with a variable degree of impaired spermatogenesis. In some patients it is difficult to be sure clinically whether there is a varicocele or not. In practice it is important to know the extent of the varicocele and to know whether it is unilateral or bilateral. It is also necessary to determine whether any residual veins are of significance after ligation of the varicocele. Scrotal thermography clarifies such situations by providing an objective measurement of the effects of the varicocele on the scrotum.

Thermographic abnormalities correlate well with the presence of internal spermatic vein reflux demonstrated by retrograde caval venography.[5] The non-invasive nature of thermography makes it preferable to phlebography for routine investigation, and because it involves no radiation hazard it can be repeated as often as necessary in sequential studies on an individual patient before and after treatment.

The surface temperature of the normal scrotum after 10 min cooling in an ambient of 19 °C is typically 30 ± 1 °C. The average temperature difference between the testes is less than 0·5 K. A varicocele causes pooling of blood around one or both testicles and increases the scrotal temperature the magnitude and extent of which depend on the size of the varicocele (see Fig. 5.6). A temperature greater than 32 °C is considered to be abnormal especially if this is associated with thermal asymmetry greater than 1 K.

Thermographic examination of the front, under-

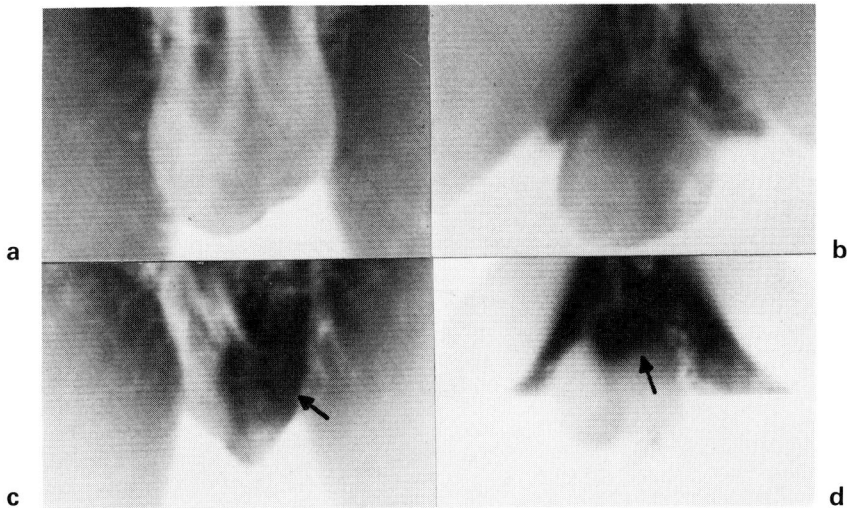

Fig. 5.6 Scrotal thermograms. (a) Anterior; normal, 30 °C. (b) Underview; normal, 31 °C. (c) Anterior; right normal, 30·6 °C; left varicocele, 34·5 °C (as indicated). (d) Underview, small varicocele, 34·4 °C (as indicated).

side and posterior of the scrotum is necessary. The imposition of making the patient assume an uncomfortable position should be avoided. The underside and posterior views are achieved with the aid of a small highly polished aluminium- or front-surface-silvered mirror placed so as to reflect the thermal image of the underside of the scrotum.[17]

Assessment of antirheumatic drug therapy

Thermography has been used to assess the response of rheumatoid arthritis to anti-inflammatory or antirheumatoid drug therapy.[4] Colour isothermograms are taken of the inflamed joint or limb and these are used to determine a *thermographic index* (TI) which has been shown to be a comprehensive measure of the total inflammation recorded in the whole picture. The thermographic index is calculated from the expression

$$\text{TI} = \Sigma \frac{(\Delta t \times a)}{A} \qquad (5.9)$$

where Δt is the difference in K from a base line of 26 °C to each isotherm temperature; a is the area occupied by an individual isotherm area (in square centimetres) and A is the total area of the thermogram (in square centimetres). When the upper isotherm temperature is 32·5 °C and the base line is at 26 °C, the formula gives a TI scale from 1 to 6 which can be read accurately to divisions of 0·1. Reproducible results are achieved when the examination is carried out in a uniform, constant ambient temperature. Serial investigations are carried out at the same time of day to avoid diurnal variations.

The procedure for obtaining coloured isotherms is straightforward, but the generation of the thermographic index from the isotherms is tedious. In practice this difficulty is overcome by computer processing.[23] A rectangular region of interest on the thermal image can be chosen and analysed immediately (Fig. 5.7), by the use of a computer interfaced to the thermography camera. It has been found that, provided examinations are carried out under carefully controlled temperature conditions, the thermographic indices of joints of healthy individuals remain remarkably constant although they have different values for different joints. For example, the normal thermographic index of a joint is about 2·0 for the elbow and about 1·0 for areas of the foot. A value of above 2·0 usually indicates abnormality.

The thermographic index has been used to assess the effect of anti-inflammatory drugs by measuring the rate of fall of the TI caused by the test drug. It has also been used to measure the anti-inflammatory response to intra-articular steroid injec-

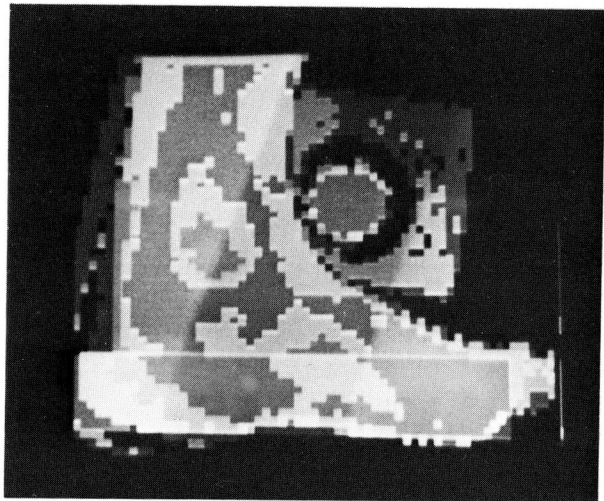 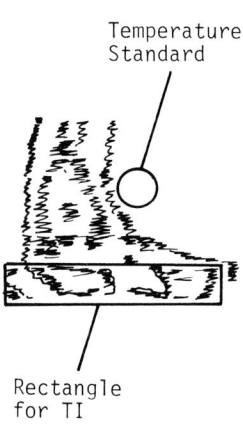

Fig. 5.7 Computer processed thermogram of foot with isotherms at 0·5 K intervals (26·0–32·5 °C), showing rectangle for calculation of thermographic index. (Note that this picture is a black-and-white reproduction of the colour original.)

tions. When the conditions for thermography are rigidly controlled, thermography may be used to follow the patient's response to long term treatment with drugs. The long term changes in TI often occur before other changes in the clinical condition of the patient are observed.

Skin lesions

Mathematical calculations and thermistor probe measurements show that malignant tumours less than 1 cm or so in diameter do not produce sufficient metabolic heat to cause a significant temperature rise in overlying skin, unless the tumour is very superficial. Even when the epidermis is invaded by tumour, the effect on the surface temperature distribution is a result of metabolism and blood flow in the tumour and in surrounding tissue. The effect of metabolism is most marked when the tumour is growing rapidly, such as in the case of malignant melanomas. Temperature increments of 2 or 3 K occur in over 80 per cent of such tumours. Thermography is used in three ways: (1) to detect unsuspected metastatic deposits in a patient with multiple pigmented lesions; (2) to assess tumour activity after treatment by surgery or radiotherapy; and (3) to assess the prognosis of the disease. In this last application, good correlation has been demonstrated between survival and tumour hyperthermia;[12] the more intense the hyperthermia, the poorer is the 5 year survival rate. Temperature increments of at least 2 K have been measured over melanomata on the foot, leg, thigh, abdomen, and face, but other forms of skin cancer can cause similar temperature changes.

Vascular disorders

The temperature of body extremities is largely dependent on blood flow through peripheral vessels, and it is in the study of vascular diseases that thermography has been found to be most useful. Temperature investigations are helpful in the diagnosis and assessment of Raynaud's disease.[13] This is a vascular disturbance caused by spastic contraction of the smaller arteries of the extremities, particularly in a cold environment. Symptoms can be induced by immersion of the hands in iced water. Thermography is used to examine the disturbance under various conditions before and after medication.

Peripheral arterial disease can cause ischaemia necessitating amputation of the affected limb. Selection of the optimum level of amputation in these patients is one of the key factors which determines rehabilitation. Most surgeons depend on a clinical assessment of tissue viability but physical parameters such as skin blood flow, perfusion pressure and ultrasonically derived arterial pressure gradients are also used. Thermography has been shown to be an accurate and reliable method of determining the best site of amputation. The most important factors in the thermographic assessment are the severity of the longitudinal thermal gradient along the limb and the presence or absence of local hypothermia.[27] Typical images are shown in Figure 5.8.

thermograms of a resting subject show the thighs and calves to be cool. In the calf, the subcutaneous border of the tibia and the patella are cooler than the surrounding muscles. Recent calf vein thrombosis produces a diffuse increase in temperature which may involve the whole or greater part of the calf. The temperature increase (of about 2 K) is evident on both supine and prone views. Thermography is able to predict extensive DVT with a

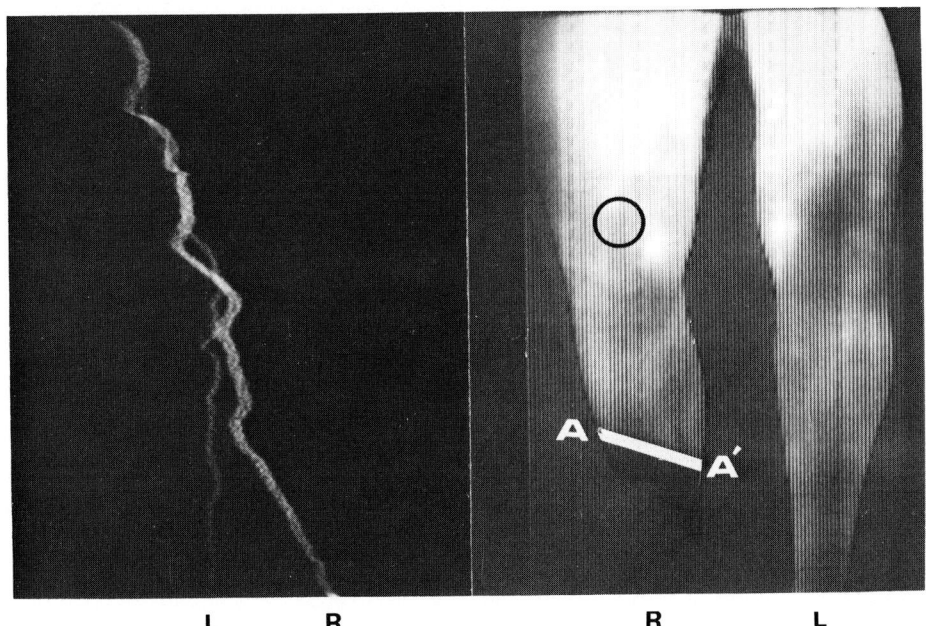

Fig. 5.8 Temperature profiles and lower limb thermogram showing severe ischaemia of right foot. The most distal viable flap level is indicated by A-A'; the patella is ringed. (White is hot, black is cold.)

Deep venous thrombosis complicates major surgery and illnesses such as myocardial infarction and stroke. Confinement, oestrogen therapy and oral contraception also carry some risk. The clinical signs of DVT, calf pain and tenderness, oedema and induration, and an increase in limb temperature, are not always reliable. Phlebography, radioactive iodine fibrinogen uptake, transcutaneous ultrasound, impedance and strain gauge plethysmography can all be used as tests for DVT. Phlebography is perhaps the most accurate means of detecting the presence of a deep venous thrombus and has a high sensitivity and specificity but it is time consuming and requires skilled medical and radiological personnel. Thermography has been used to identify DVT by observing delayed cooling of the affected limb.[6,7] In the absence of DVT, the

high level of accuracy and the innocuous nature of the test enables it to be used daily if required. It is doubtful if thermography is as accurate as phlebography for diagnosis of early limb thrombosis,[24] but there is no doubt about its value when careful attention is paid to the influence of underlying anatomy of the limb.

Thermal pattern changes can be induced physically, and the way in which the temperature distribution alters under controlled stimuli can be used to assess functional aspects of venous disease. Incompetent perforating veins in the leg may be localised in this way.[22] With the patient lying supine, the veins are drained by raising the leg to an angle of about 30°, and the leg temperature is lowered with an ice-cooled wet towel and an electric fan for 5 min. A tourniquet is applied around the upper third of the thigh with just sufficient pressure to occlude the superficial veins, and the patient then stands and exercises the leg. Areas of 'rapid rewarming' below the level of the tourniquet indicate possible sites of incompetent perforating veins. This physiological test gives an objective assessment of a functional derangement and indicates the anatomical sites of incompetent perforators more precisely than subjective clinical methods.

Assessment of trauma

Problems associated with stress to insensitive tissue, such as that arising from limb prostheses, are difficult to resolve and early detection is necessary for effective prevention and control. In the absence of pain, repeated small stresses can prevent healing of the wounded part. Temperature studies in the management of insensitive stumps have been used effectively to aid evaluation of prosthetic devices and to detect irritated tissue prior to frank breakdown.[2]

Thermography is being used to assess trauma caused by a burn or frostbite.[3,21] The treatment of a burn depends upon its severity (the depth of the penetrating injury and the extent on the surface). A first-degree burn shows an erythema on the skin, sometimes accompanied by blisters. A third-degree burn is deeper, shows a complete absence of circulation, the skin is insensitive to pain and has a white colour. It is not always easy to identify a second-degree burn, however, and temperature measurements have been used to assist with this assessment. Third-degree burns have been found to be on the average 3 K colder than surrounding normal skin.

Physiological research

In addition to investigating peripheral vascular physiology, infrared thermography has been used to study body metabolism. Heat emission of the skin of newborn infants over the tissue of the nape of the neck and interscapular region has been measured thermographically as a means of assessing the role played by brown adipose tissue in these areas.[26] It is probable that the special heat production of this tissue (called 'nonshivering thermogenesis') forms an important heat source in human infants during the neonatal period. Thermal imaging allows heat distribution to be studied directly after birth without the hindrance of contact probes.

It has been suggested[25] that the existence of functional brown adipose tissue in man could be identified by local changes in skin temperature during stimulation by a sympathomimetic agent such as ephedrine which increases metabolic rate in man. Ephedrine produces the highest skin temperature in the neck and upper back. These are the areas that correspond to brown adipose tissue locations in the human neonate and adult. Figure 5.9 illustrates how thermography has been used to confirm the existence of these localised areas sensitive to ephedrine. For measurements of this type, instrumentation with a high degree of stability and precise temperature reference standards are required.

RECENT DEVELOPMENTS AND FUTURE PROSPECTS

General considerations

Non-invasive clinical thermography is a safe, fast, uncomplicated technique. It can be carried out by trained technical or paramedical staff, and the nature of the technique is such that it can be repeated frequently without inconvenience or hazard to the patient. It provides a large amount of information about surface temperature patterns which can be of value in the assessment of a variety of clinical problems. Its principal disadvantages are that the origin of an abnormal thermal pattern is not specific and that surface temperatures can be influenced by various physical and physiological factors unrelated to the clinical problem being investigated. The application of infrared technology to clinical problems has resulted in the development of thermographic imaging systems with high spatial and thermal resolutions. Unfortunately, the complexities of this technology are reflected in the high price of commercial thermographic equipment which has restricted the use of clinical thermography to a relatively small number of centres. As a consequence, the development of cheaper imaging systems such as pyroelectric vidicon camera tubes as alternatives to conventional photodetector systems is being pursued by several manufacturers.

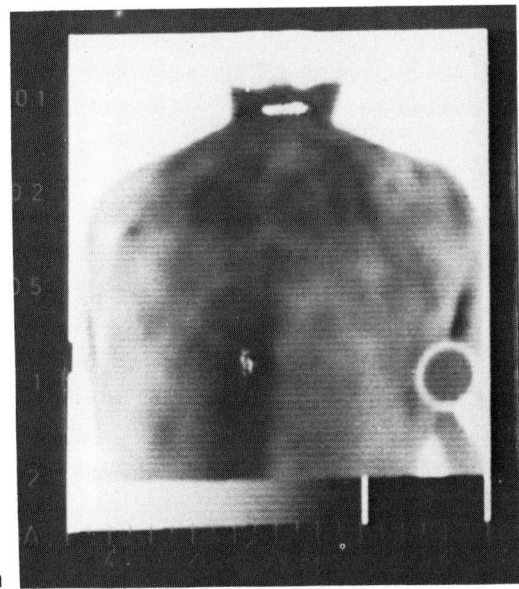 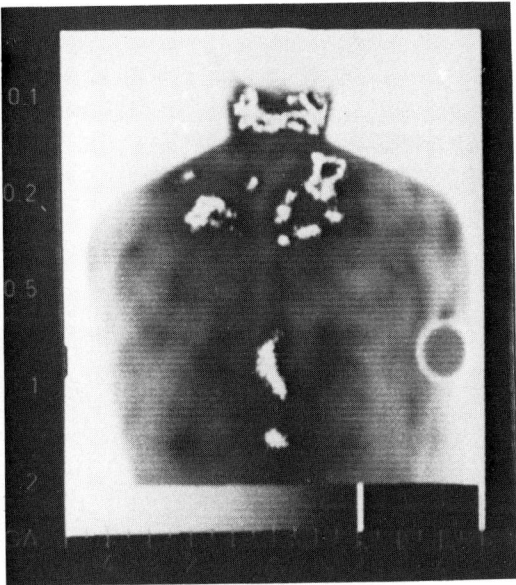

Fig. 5.9 Brown adipose tissue studies. (a) Thermogram of back of male subject showing the location of the hottest area, temperature 32·1 °C. (b) Thermogram showing increase in temperature over probable sites of brown adipose tissue following administration of ephedrine.

Pyroelectric vidicon camera

By means of an infrared lens, the image of the thermal scene is focused onto a pyroelectric target causing temperature differences which induce a charge pattern. This pattern is scanned in a TV raster by the electron beam of the vidicon tube. A signal change is produced only when the target temperature changes so no signal arises from steady incident flux. Modulation of the incident radiation is necessary either by chopping or panning of the thermal scene. The pyroelectric vidicon forms the basis of a simple thermal imaging camera which could be coupled directly to a standard picture monitor and video tape recorder.[31] The focusing lens and faceplate are usually made of germanium to allow transmission of infrared radiation and typical systems are sensitive to 8–12 μm radiation. The whole system is compact and readily portable. Figure 5.10 is a photograph of a typical device.

Pyroelectric vidicons do not require liquid nitrogen cooling and are capable of resolving temperature differences of 0·1 K at low spatial frequencies. At spatial frequencies similar to those encountered in clinical problems the thermal resolution is reduced to about 0·4 K. The basic price of this type of camera is about one quarter that of a single element photodetector system, but improvements in stability and quantification of the thermal image are required before clinical usefulness can be achieved. These technical developments should reduce the cost differences between the systems.

Microwave thermograpy

Infrared thermography records surface temperatures, and any change in subcutaneous temperature is reflected at the surface by convection and conduction of heat through the intervening tissues. Emission of infrared from tissue at 30 °C is most copious at about 10 μm with an intensity about 10^8 greater than radiation with 10 cm wavelength. Detection of such low intensity radiated power, however, is well within the capability of modern microwave radiometers which can readily detect changes in received intensity which correspond to power changes equivalent to temperature differences of 0·1 K. The absorption of microwave radiation by body tissue depends on the frequency and upon the type of tissue. For example, 5 cm of fatty tissue attenuates the incident power by about 35 per cent, whereas, for muscle, the corresponding penetration is only about 1 cm. Since body

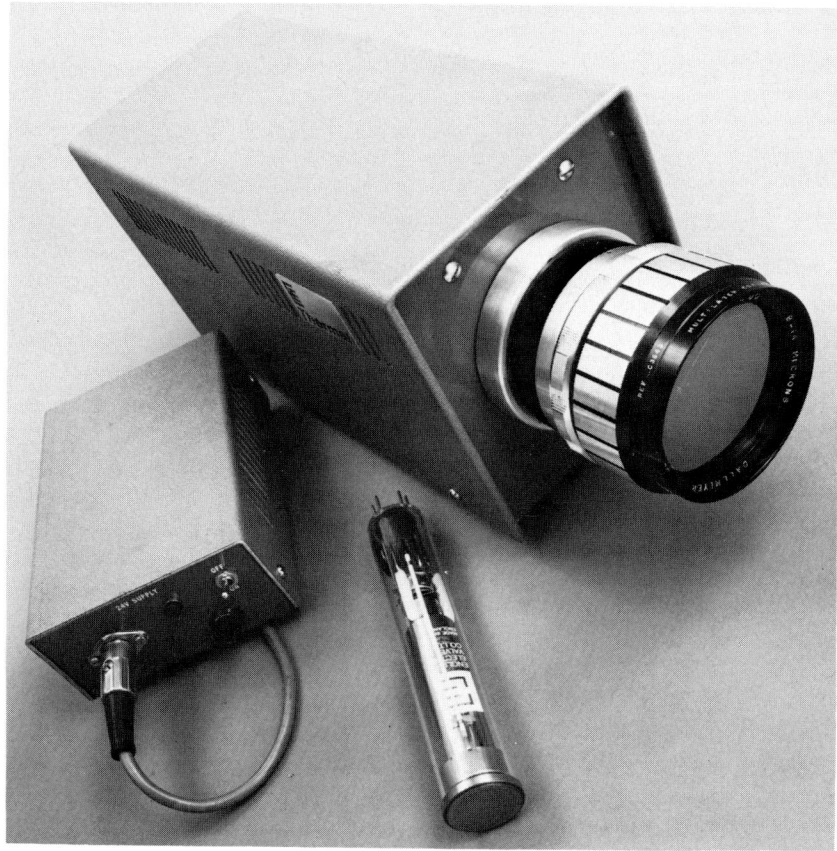

Fig. 5.10 Pyroelectric vidicon infrared camera and tube.

tissue is partially transparent to microwave radiation, the measured temperature corresponds to radiation which originates from a tissue volume extending from the skin surface to a depth of several centimetres. This has been exploited in the development of a microwave scanning system for clinical thermography.[10] Further improvements in this area are anticipated.

In view of the growing interest in cancer treatment by hyperthermia any non-invasive method which gives temperature information about subcutaneous temperatures is likely to be invaluable, even though the spatial resolution of such equipment may be inferior to that achieved on the skin surface by infrared scanning systems.

Acknowledgements

I am indebted to the following for providing some of the illustrations for this chapter, and for allowing them to be reproduced: Polaroid Limited (Fig. 5.2); E. F. J. Ring (Fig. 5.7); V. Spence (Fig. 5.8); N. Rothwell, M. Stock and the Editor of *Nature* (Fig. 5.9); and English Electric Valve Company Limited (Fig. 5.10).

REFERENCES

1. Astheimer, R. W. & Schwarz, F. (1968) Thermal imaging using pyroelectric detectors. *Appl. Opt.*, 7, 1687–95.
2. Bergholdt, H. T. & Brand, P. W. (1973) Thermography: an aid in the management of insensitive feet and stump. In *Proc. Ann. Mtg. Am. Thermographic Soc.*, 211–25.
3. Buwalda, G. (1969) Thermographic assessment of burns and frostbite. In *Medical Thermography*, ed. Heerma van Voss, S. F. C. & Thomas, P., pp. 178–81. Basel: Karger.
4. Collins, A. J., Ring, E. F. J., Cosh, J. A. & Bacon, P. A. (1974) Quantitation of thermography in arthritis using

multi-isothermal analysis. I. The thermographic index. *Ann. rheum. Dis.*, **33**, 113–5.
5. Comhaire, F., Monteyne, R. & Kunnen, M. (1976) The value of scrotal thermography as compared with selective retrograde venography of the internal spermatic vein for the diagnosis of subclinical varicocele. *Fertil. Steril*, **27**, 694–8.
6. Cooke, E. D. & Pilcher, M. F. (1974) Deep vein thrombosis: preclinical diagnosis by thermography. *Br. J. Surg.*, **61**, 971–8.
7. Cooke, E. D. (1978) The fundamentals of thermographic diagnosis of deep vein thrombosis. *Acta thermographica*, suppl. 1.
8. Davison, T. W., Ewing, K. L., Fergason, J., Chapman, M., Can, A. & Voorhis, C. C. (1972) Detection of breast cancer by liquid crystal thermography. *Cancer*, **29**, 1123–32.
9. Draper, J. W. & Jones, C. H. (1969) Thermal patterns of the female breast. *Br. J. Radiol.*, **42**, 401–10.
10. Edrich, J. (1978) Microwave and millimetre wave thermography. *Abstr. 2nd Europ. Congr. Thermography, Barcelona*, abstr. 14.
11. Gautherie, M. & Gros, Ch. M. (1976) Contribution of infrared thermography to early diagnosis, pre-therapeutic prognosis and post-irradiation follow-up of breast carcinomas. *Medicamundi*, **21**, 135–49.
12. Gautherie, M., Grosshans, E. & Juilland, J. (1979) The value of infrared thermography for diagnosis, prognosis and surveillance of malignant melanomas. *Medicamundi*, suppl.
13. Heerma van Voss, S. F. C. (1969) Thermographic differentiation of vascular diseases of the arms. In *Medical Thermography*, ed. Heerma van Voss, S. F. C. & Thomas, P., pp. 142–51. Basel: Karger.
14. Johansson, N. T., Bjurstam, N., Hedberg, K., Hultborn, A. & Johnsen, C. (1976) Thermography of the breast. *Acta chir. scand.*, suppl. 460.
15. Jones, C. H. & Draper, J. W. (1970) A comparison of infrared photography and thermography in the detection of mammary carcinoma. *Br. J. Radiol.*, **43**, 507–16.
16. Jones, C. H., Greening, W. P., Davey, J. B., McKinna, J. A. & Greeves, V. J. (1975) Thermography of the female breast: a five-year study in relation to the detection and prognosis of cancer. *Br. J. Radiol.*, **48**, 532–8.
17. Jones, C. H. & Hendry, W. F. (1979) Thermographic examination of the scrotum. *Acta thermographica*, **4**, 38–43.
18. Lawson, R. N. (1956) Implications of surface temperature in the diagnosis of breast cancer. *Can. med. Ass. J.*, **75**, 309–10.
19. Lawson, W. D. (1979) Thermal imaging. In *Electronic Imaging*, ed. McLean, T. P. & Schagen, P., pp. 325–64. London: Academic Press.
20. Lelik, F., Kezy, G. & Solymossy, O. (1977) The diagnosis of locomotive disorders of domestic animals by contact thermography. *Acta thermographica*, **2**, 13–17.
21. Mladick, R., Georgiade, N. & Thorne, F. (1966) A clinical evaluation of the use of thermography in determining its degree of burn injury. *Plastic reconst. Surg.*, **38**, 512–18.
22. Patil, K. D., Williams, J. R. & Lloyd-Williams, K. (1970) Thermographic localization of incompetent perforating veins in the leg. *Br. med. J.*, **1**, 195–7.
23. Ring, E. F. J. (1975) Thermography and rheumatic diseases. In *Thermography*, ed. Aarts, N. J. M., Gautherie, M. & Ring, E. F. J., pp. 97–106. Basel: Karger.
24. Ritchie, W. G. M., Lapayowker, M. S. & Soulen, R. L. (1979) Thermographic diagnosis of deep vein thrombosis: anatomically based diagnostic criteria. *Radiology*, **132**, 321–9.
25. Rothwell, N. J. & Stock, M. J. (1979) A role for brown adipose tissue in diet-induced thermogenesis. *Nature*, **281**, 31–5.
26. Rylander, E. (1972) Age dependent reactions of rectal and skin temperatures of infants during exposure to cold. *Acta paediat. scand.*, **61**, 1–9.
27. Spence, V. A., Walker, W. F., Troup, I. M. & Murdock, G. (1981) Amputation of the ischaemic limb: selection of the optimum site by thermography. *Angiology*, **32**, 47–63.
28. Stark, A. M. & Way, S. (1974) The screening of well women for the early detection of breast cancer using clinical examination with thermography and mammography. *Cancer*, **33**, 1671–9.
29. Steketee, J. (1973) Spectral emissivity of skin and pericardium. *Phys. Med. Biol.*, **18**, 686–94.
30. Tonegutti, M., Acciarri, L. & Racanelli, A. (1980) Fundamentals of contact thermography in female breast diseases. *Acta thermographica*, suppl. 3.
31. Watton, R., Burgess, D. & Harper, B. (1977) The pyroelectric vidicon: a new technique in thermography and thermal imaging. *J. appl. Sci. Engrg.*, **A 2**, 47–63.

6

Nuclear magnetic resonance imaging

E. R. Andrew

INTRODUCTION

The use of nuclear magnetic resonance as a method of imaging is a relatively recent development which is just beginning to make an impact in medicine. The basic phenomenon of nuclear magnetic resonance (NMR) was discovered at the end of 1945, and gave rise to the subject of NMR spectroscopy, operating in the radio-frequency region of the electromagnetic spectrum. Since its first discovery NMR spectroscopy has become a valuable and versatile technique for analytical, structural and dynamic investigations of all forms of matter in a wide range of disciplines; in its high-resolution form it has become particularly indispensable in chemistry.

As a method of imaging we may note at the outset some of the special advantages that NMR offers, namely that it is non-invasive, penetrates bony structures without attenuation, does not use ionising radiation, and is without known hazard. A variety of names are in use in the literature to describe the subject, and the most common are: *NMR imaging*, *spin mapping*, *zeugmatography*, *NMR tomography*. The reasons for the use of these names will be seen as we go along.

The use of NMR has not been widespread in the medical sciences hitherto, and therefore we begin this chapter with an account of the essential principles, before proceeding to a description of its application to medical imaging.

PRINCIPLES OF NMR

In this section we seek to lay a foundation of the essential concepts of NMR for the benefit of readers with no previous knowledge of the subject. The treatment is necessarily brief and it attempts to convey the basic ideas with the minimum of mathematics. Readers who wish to pursue the fundamentals further are referred to one of the standard textbooks. In an order of increasing difficulty of mathematical treatment books by the following authors may be recommended: Farrar and Becker,[28] Andrew,[3] Carrington and McLachlan,[20] Slichter,[60] Abragam.[1] Of great interest also are the classic papers reporting the discovery of NMR by Bloch and Purcell and their colleagues.[9-12,59]

Atomic nuclei

Our point of departure is the atomic nucleus. We are concerned with ordinary stable nuclei in their normal situation in the atoms and molecules of which all materials, animate and inanimate, are made. In NMR imaging particular attention is focused on the nuclei of hydrogen atoms, namely protons, since from an NMR viewpoint these are particularly favourable nuclei, and since hydrogen is very abundant in all living tissue. Although hydrogen nuclei are especially favourable, there are many other nuclei which are of interest in NMR.

Nuclei which contain an odd number of protons, or an odd number of neutrons, or both, have a spin and a magnetic moment and therefore behave as small spinning magnets. Examples of such nuclei are ^{1}H, ^{2}H, ^{7}Li, ^{13}C, ^{14}N, ^{19}F, ^{23}Na, ^{31}P, ^{35}Cl, ^{63}Cu, ^{127}I. There are in fact over a hundred stable nuclear species with a magnetic moment and spin, and all the chemical elements have at least one naturally occurring magnetic isotope. On the other hand, nuclei which are composed of even numbers of protons and neutrons have no resultant spin and no magnetic moment and cannot be used in NMR. Examples of such even-even non-magnetic nuclei are ^{12}C, ^{16}O, ^{32}S, ^{40}Ca.

The spin or intrinsic angular momentum of a nucleus may be expressed as $I\hbar$, where $\hbar$ is the natural unit of angular momentum given by $h/2\pi$, where h is Planck's constant. The nuclear spin number I is an integer for nuclei of even mass number and a half-integer for nuclei of odd mass number. For even-even non-magnetic nuclei such as ^{12}C, the value of I is zero.

Most work on NMR imaging to date has been carried out on nuclei with $I = \frac{1}{2}$, such as ^{1}H, ^{19}F, ^{31}P and we shall largely restrict our discussion to such nuclei. We should remember however that NMR can be carried out with all nuclei having $I > 0$. Nuclei with $I > \frac{1}{2}$ possess an additional property, namely an electric quadrupole moment, which introduces complications which are avoided by restricting attention to nuclei with $I = \frac{1}{2}$.

Magnetic moments of nuclei are generally expressed in terms of the *nuclear magneton*. This unit is defined as $e\hbar/2M$, where e is the charge on the proton in electromagnetic units, and M is the proton mass; it is defined by analogy with the *Bohr magneton* $e\hbar/2m$, which is the natural unit in which to express the magnetic moment of electrons, atoms and ions; m is the electron mass. Thus the nuclear magneton is much smaller than the Bohr magneton, by the factor m/M, which is close to 1/1836. The proton magnetic moment is 2·79 nuclear magnetons and therefore is 658 times smaller than the magnetic moment of the free electron, which is very close to 1 Bohr magneton.

It is because the magnetic properties of atomic nuclei are so weak that their effects are not apparent in everyday life. The well-known phenomena of ferromagnetism and paramagnetism* have their origins in the magnetic properties of unpaired electrons. Although nuclear magnetism is many orders of magnitude weaker, the magnetic properties of nuclei can nevertheless be measured with great precision by NMR. Moreover the very weakness of nuclear magnets enables them to act as internal probes of their environment in materials of all kinds without significantly influencing their properties, except at extremely low temperatures.

NMR: a classical view

Consider a magnetic nucleus, for example a proton, placed in a magnetic field **B**, as illustrated in Figure 6.1. Its magnetic moment μ experiences a couple

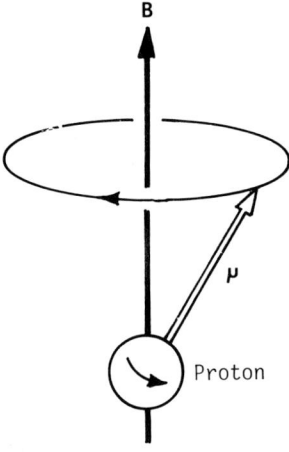

Fig. 6.1 The precession of a proton magentic moment μ in a magnetic field **B**.

tending to turn it parallel to the direction of the field. Since it is spinning, the nucleus responds to this couple in the manner of a gyroscope and its axis precesses around the direction of the field as indicated in the figure. The angular frequency ω of this precessional motion is given by the well-known theorem of Larmor:

$$\omega = \gamma B, \qquad (6.1)$$

where γ is the gyromagnetic ratio of the nucleus, defined as the ratio of its magnetic moment to its angular momentum or spin. We notice that the frequency of precession is directly proportional to the field strength B, and we shall make much use of this proportionality in NMR imaging.

Now let us consider a small glass phial containing 1 ml of water and place it in a magnetic field **B** as in Figure 6.2a. Each water molecule contains two hydrogen nuclei (protons), and therefore the phial contains altogether some 10^{23} protons. We can ignore the oxygen nuclei since ^{16}O has no spin or magnetic moment. We can also ignore the mol-

---

*Substances can be divided into three classes according to their magnetic properties. Ferromagnetic substances have high values of magnetisation. The remaining substances are divided into either paramagnetic or diamagnetic classes, according to whether their magnetisation is in the direction of, or in the opposite direction to, the applied field.

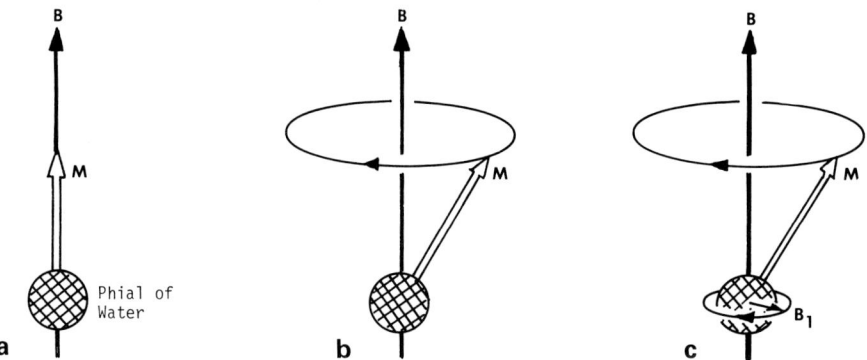

Fig. 6.2 (a) The protons in a phial of water placed in a magnetic field **B** generate a resultant nuclear magnetisation **M** aligned with **B**. (b) The precession of the nuclear magnetisation **M** around the direction of the magnetic field **B**. (c) The application of a synchronously rotating magnetic field B_1 which causes the nuclear magnetisation **M** to move away from alignment with **B**.

ecular electrons since their spins are oppositely paired; indeed apart from the hydrogen nuclei the whole material is diamagnetic. The 10^{23} protons constitute a weak paramagnetic assembly. When the assembly has reached equilibrium in the magnetic field there will be more protons aligned with the field than against, generating a resultant nuclear magnetisation **M** along **B** as indicated in Figure 6.2a.

If we cause this nuclear magnetisation **M** to move away from the direction of **B**, it will precess about **B** as indicated in Figure 6.2b, with just the same Larmor frequency ω given by Equation 6.1, since the precessional motion of **M** is just the precession of the individual protons that make it up.

We can arrange for the nuclear magnetisation **M** to move coherently away from the direction of the magnetic field **B** by applying a small radiofrequency (rf) magnetic field B_1 at right angles to **B**. This rf magnetic field has a component rotating in the same sense as the precession, as shown in Figure 6.2c. The interaction between the nuclear magnetisation **M** and the rotating rf field B_1 produces a small couple tending to turn **M** away from **B**.

It is helpful to visualise the situation in a frame of reference rotating about **B** with angular frequency ω. In this rotating frame the magnetisation **M** is at rest; so too is the rf field B_1 if we have arranged its frequency to be exactly equal to the precessional frequency ω. Therefore, in the rotating frame, **M** experiences a steady couple turning it about an axis normal to both **M** and B_1 and away from **B**. Thus **M** moves away from **B** and precesses coherently with frequency ω.

We notice that it is essential in producing this effect that the applied rf field B_1 should rotate around **B** in the same sense and in exact synchronism with the precessional motion of **M** about **B**. If the rf field has a different frequency **M** and B_1 do not rotate in synchronism; they move in and out of phase and produce no significant effect. Therefore we have a resonance effect when the frequencies of the rf field and the Larmor precession are exactly the same. This is called *nuclear magnetic resonance* (NMR).

This description of NMR in terms of the Larmor precession of the nuclear magnetisation is essentially a classical or 'pre-quantum theory' description. We shall look at the behaviour from a quantum viewpoint in a moment, but we may remark that classical descriptions of NMR phenomena often give good physical insight.

If we surround the phial of water with a coil consisting of several turns of wire, with its axis at right angles to the static magnetic field **B**, the precessing nuclear magnetisation generates an electromotive force (EMF) in the coil, by Faraday's law of electromagnetic induction. This induced EMF, alternating at angular frequency ω, is called a *nuclear induction* signal. It may be amplified and displayed on an oscilloscope and provides a direct way of detecting the NMR phenomenon.

If the rf field B_1 is applied for just a short time,

as a pulse, the nuclear induction signal following the pulse does not last indefinitely but dies away; it is called a *free induction decay* (FID) and its time constant is called the *transverse relaxation time* T_2. For pure water T_2 is a few seconds. The transverse relaxation time is called T_2 to distinguish it from the longitudinal relaxation time T_1 which is discussed later.

From the NMR angular frequency ω we can define an NMR frequency $v = \omega/2\pi$. For protons in a magnetic field B of 1 T (1 tesla = 10^4 gauss) this frequency v is 42·6 MHz. Different species of nuclei have different values of gyromagnetic ratio γ, and consequently their resonance frequencies in a given field strength are all different; for example in a field of 1 T the NMR frequency for ^{13}C nuclei is 10·7 MHz, for ^{19}F it is 40·1 MHz, and for ^{31}P it is 17·2 MHz. Thus there is no problem in distinguishing the resonances from different species of nuclei in a sample; we just tune our receiver in to the correct frequency. In practice in NMR we are always dealing with short-wave radiofrequencies.

NMR: a quantum view

We now look at NMR from the viewpoint of quantum theory. If we place a nucleus of spin ½, such as a proton, in a magnetic field **B**, it may be observed in one of two possible states characterised by magnetic quantum numbers $m = \pm ½$; these states have energy eigenvalues* $\mp\mu B$ as depicted in the energy level diagram in Figure 6.3.

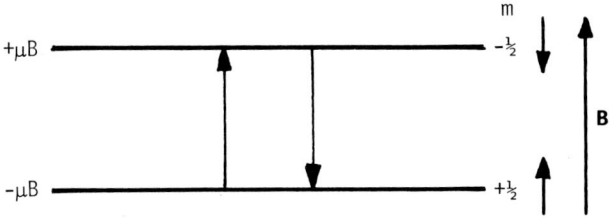

Fig. 6.3 Transitions between the two eigenstates of protons in a magnetic field **B**.

If we now irradiate the proton with electromagnetic radiation of such a frequency v that the quanta or photons have energy hv just exactly equal

*Fixed energy values in which the systems may exist in a steady state.

to the interval between the energy levels so that

$$hv = 2\mu B, \qquad (6.2)$$

a resonant exchange of energy between the proton and the radiation can take place. If the proton is on the lower state it can resonantly absorb a photon and move to the upper state; if it is in the upper state it can be resonantly stimulated to emit a photon and to descend to the lower state. The frequency must exactly satisfy Equation 6.2 if this resonant exchange is to take place, and again we have a NMR phenomenon.

Remembering that the gyromagnetic ratio γ of a nucleus such as the proton is the ratio of its magnetic moment μ to its angular momentum ½ℏ, we may write

$$\mu = ½\gamma\hbar, \qquad (6.3)$$

and upon substituting this in Equation 6.2 we find that the NMR angular frequency obtained from this quantum approach is

$$\omega = 2\pi v = \gamma B, \qquad (6.4)$$

which is identical with the result given in Equation 6.1 from the classical description. This happy agreement between the classical and quantum calculations justifies us in using classical descriptions of NMR behaviour in place of the more rigorous, but often more difficult, quantum descriptions.

The quantum description just given applies to all nuclei with spin ½, such as ^{1}H, ^{13}C, ^{19}F, ^{31}P. The theory may readily be extended to nuclei with spin > ½, for which there are $(2I + 1)$ eigenstates and again the classical and quantum expressions for the NMR frequency are in agreement. Examples of such nuclei are ^{2}H and ^{14}N for which $I = 1$, ^{7}Li and ^{23}Na for which I = 3/2, ^{27}Al, ^{127}I for which $I = 5/2$, ^{43}Ca, ^{133}Cs for which I = 7/2, and ^{209}Bi for which $I = 9/2$.

A simple NMR apparatus

In order to get some 'feel' for the phenomenon and to see what is involved in practice let us consider a very simple apparatus which could be used to detect nuclear magnetic resonance, for example to detect proton NMR in water.

A basic arrangement is illustrated in Figure 6.4. A small sample of water, say 1 millilitre, in a glass

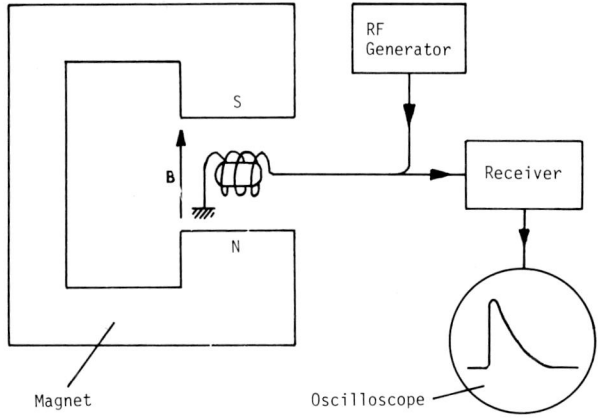

Fig. 6.4 A simple NMR apparatus.

phial, is placed in a coil and mounted between the poles of a magnet. The radiofrequency generator supplies a pulse of rf current at the resonant NMR frequency to the coil, thus producing an alternating magnetic field in the specimen. Strictly we require a rotating magnetic field; however a linearly alternating field along the coil axis of amplitude $2B_1$ may be regarded as the sum of two counter-rotating magnetic fields, each of amplitude B_1. One of these rotating fields is the one required for our NMR experiment; the other is rotating in the opposite sense and is redundant.

After excitation by the resonant pulse of rf radiation the precessing nuclear magnetisation generates a nuclear induction signal in the coil which is then amplified and detected by the tuned receiver and presented as a free induction decay on the oscilloscope. Note that if a Fourier transform (FT) of the FID is taken, the NMR spectrum of the protons is obtained, and for pure water this is an exceedingly narrow response about 0·1 Hz wide. NMR is thus a sharply resonant property, and this is especially so for liquids such as water.

Although NMR spectrometers are in practice much more sophisticated than the diagram of Figure 6.4 might indicate, nevertheless in essentials they all have this basic structure: a magnet, a specimen in an rf probe coil, an rf source, an rf receiver and a display. An NMR system of advanced design may also include a dedicated computer to control its operation, to handle and to store the NMR data and to perform calculations, such as Fourier transformation, on the data.

With such an equipment proton NMR signals may be obtained from any material containing hydrogen atoms. Thus we can get a proton NMR response from water or ice, from gaseous, liquid or solid hydrogen, from polythene and other polymers, from proteins whether solid or in solution, from most organic liquids and solids, from living tissue and, indeed, from any material whatsoever containing hydrogen atoms. In the same way ^{31}P NMR signals may be obtained from any material containing phosphorus atoms. The NMR signal strength is proportional to the number of nuclei which contribute, and therefore is weak if the chemical concentration of the element is dilute, or if the abundance of the isotope studied is low.

Nuclear relaxation

We now consider in more detail the precession of the proton magnetisation **M** in a magnetic field **B**. Let us apply a short resonant rf pulse B_1 for just long enough to turn the magnetisation through 90°, as illustrated in Figure 6.5. Such a pulse is called

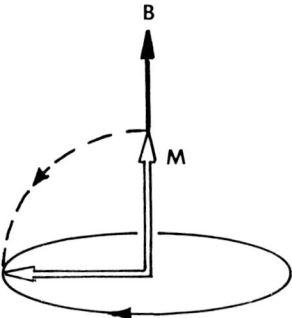

Fig. 6.5 A 90° rf pulse turns the nuclear magnetisation **M** into a plane normal to **B**.

a 90° pulse. After the pulse is completed, the magnetisation **M** precesses as indicated in a plane perpendicular to the field **B**, with angular frequency ω given by Equation 6.1. The nuclear magnetisation is now no longer in equilibrium with the field **B** nor with its surroundings. The protons in the specimen are buffeted by their neighbours and slowly return to the direction of the field **B**. Those that remain precessing in the perpendicular plane get out of phase with each other because they experience slightly differing fields both from within the sample and from outside. For both these reasons the precessing transverse magnetisation decreases and the nuclear induction signal decays to zero. This is the free induction decay (FID) mentioned earlier (p. 215). For water and other simple fluids this decay is exponential, characterised by the time constant T_2, the transverse relaxation time.

Whenever we encounter a damped oscillation in physics, decaying exponentially with time constant t_o say, this corresponds to a response of the system in the frequency domain of Lorentzian form with a width $(1/\pi t_o)$ between half-maximum points. In fact the longer the vibration persists, the more monochromatic it is, and vice versa. Therefore it follows that NMR free induction decay with time constant T_2 corresponds to a frequency response of width $(1/\pi T_2)$. Thus narrow NMR responses correspond to long values of T_2 and vice versa, while broad NMR responses correspond to short values of T_2. Consequently for a sample of water with an intrinsic proton resonance width of 0·1 Hz the corresponding value of T_2 is 3 s.

Now let us consider the effect of applying a 180° rf pulse to the water sample; that is to say a pulse twice as long as the previous pulse. As illustrated in Figure 6.6 the nuclear magnetisation **M** is now

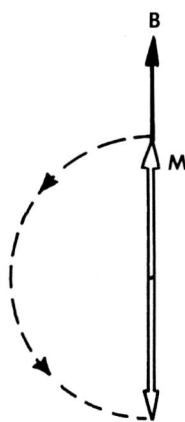

Fig. 6.6 A 180° rf pulse inverts the direction of the nuclear magnetisation **M**.

turned through 180°, and when the pulse cuts off the magnetisation is left pointing in the opposite direction to **B**. It is clearly not now in equilibrium. The fluctuating magnetic fields generated by the molecular motions gradually turn some of the protons round. As they reverse themselves the nuclear magnetisation decreases to zero and then grows along **B** to its full equilibrium length. This return to equilibrium is exponential for most homogeneous materials, and its time constant is sometimes called the *longitudinal relaxation time* T_1; it is however more often called the *spin-lattice relaxation time* T_1. This term spin-lattice relaxation time was originally introduced to describe the return to equilibrium of a nuclear spin system in a crystal lattice. Its use has now become generalised to characterise the return to equilibrium of the nuclear spin system in all forms of matter including fluids, even though in such cases there is no 'lattice' in the ordinary sense.

NMR in liquids and solids

One of the most remarkable characteristics of NMR is the substantial difference in behaviour between the NMR responses of liquids and solids. The most striking feature is that for fluids the resonances are sharp whereas for solids they are usually very much broader. We have seen that for pure water the intrinsic proton resonance width is about 0·1 Hz, whereas for ice at 93 K it is 70 kHz, some 10^6 times broader;[58] the corresponding values of T_2 are 3 s for water and 5 μs for ice.[12]

Another substantial difference lies in the values of T_1 for liquids and solids. For water and other simple fluids $T_1 = T_2$; so in our water example $T_1 = 3$ s. But for ice at 93 K the value of T_1 is 360 s.[58] Not only is this value much longer than for water, but we see that in the solid state $T_1 \gg T_2$.

These significant differences in NMR behaviour between liquids and solids are of particular importance when later on we consider the NMR imaging of structures which contain liquid-like and solid-like regions. For an understanding of these differences we need to consider the underlying mechanisms of relaxation, and of these the most important is that generated by the magnetic interactions between the nuclei.

Each proton in a water molecule experiences a local magnetic field of a few ten-thousandths of a tesla generated by its neighbour proton in the same molecule. In liquid water the molecules tumble and diffuse in a rapid, random and isotropic manner. At 20°C this motion is characterised by a continuous spectrum of frequencies up to about 10^{11} Hz. Therefore the local field experienced by each proton is a rapidly fluctuating field. The spectral components of this fluctuating field at the NMR frequency, which is always less than 10^{11} Hz, are efficient in bringing about spin-lattice relaxation. The fluctuating field is equally efficient in bringing about transverse relaxation; consequently $T_1 = T_2$. A quantitative analysis accounts very satisfactorily for the observed values of T_1 and T_2 in water.[12] On the other hand in solids generally, and in ice at 93 K in particular, the molecules are relatively static. The internal local magnetic fields fluctuate only slowly and have a very weak spectral intensity at the NMR frequency. Consequently the spin-lattice relaxation mechanism is weak and T_1 in solids can often be very long, of the order of minutes or even hours at low temperatures.

On the other hand, just because the local fields are relatively static in solids, there is a wide distribution of precessional frequencies which interfere to give a short FID with a short T_2. It is these static internal magnetic fields in solids which give rise to the broad NMR responses, with consequently very short values of T_2. In fluids, by contrast, the rapid isotropic motion of the molecules averages these internal magnetic fields to very small mean values, and leads to very sharp resonance lines.

The tumbling frequency of a molecule in a liquid is very dependent on the size of the molecule and on the viscosity of the liquid. Consequently, values of T_1 can vary considerably from one liquid to another. Moreover since the viscosity of a liquid is strongly dependent on temperature we are not surprised to find that T_1 varies strongly with temperature. The solution of molecules both large and small in water reduces T_1 for the water protons and the effects encountered are sometimes complex. The cytoplasm of living cells provides an example of reduced relaxation times T_1, in the range of 0·1–1 s, varying from one type of cell to another.[48] The presence of paramagnetic ions and molecules in solution promotes spin-lattice relaxation of the protons; T_1 decreases with increasing concentration of the solution.

High-resolution NMR spectroscopy

We have seen that the proton NMR response from liquid water is a very sharp line at the NMR frequency. If we examine carefully the proton NMR response from ethyl alcohol, CH_3CH_2OH, however, we find that it consists of three separate responses close together as shown in Figure 6.7a.

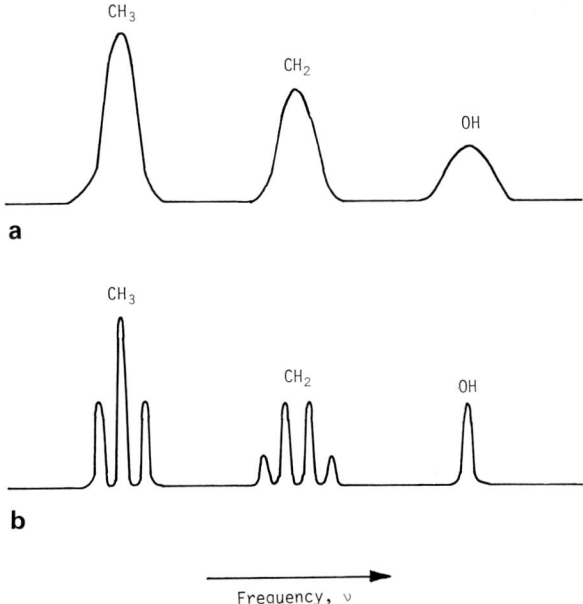

Fig. 6.7 High-resolution NMR spectroscopy. (a) The proton NMR spectrum of ethyl alcohol under resolution sufficient to separate the three chemically-shifted lines. (b) Shows the spin multiplets seen under higher resolution.

The separation between the three lines is proportional to the magnetic field B and is a few parts per million. The lines are only resolved if the field B is very uniform, to better than one part in 10^6. The intensities of the lines are in the ratio 3:2:1 indicating that they originate from the CH_3, CH_2 and OH groups respectively.

This fine structure has its origin in the diamagnetic screening effect of the molecular electrons, whose effects we have so far ignored. Instead of experiencing the magnetic field B, the nuclei actually experience a slightly smaller field $(1 - \sigma)B$, where σ is called the *screening constant*. In practice $\sigma \ll 1$ and for protons $\sigma \sim 10^{-5}$. Therefore we must amend Equation 6.2 to

$$h\nu = 2\mu(1 - \sigma)B. \quad (6.5)$$

The resonance frequency is thus slightly shifted. The exact value of σ depends on the precise electronic environment of the nucleus and therefore differs from one chemical compound to another, and from one chemical group to another. Therefore relative values of σ are called the *chemical shift*. Although for hydrogen atoms differences in σ are only a few parts per million, for other atoms with more electrons σ can be considerably larger.

Further improvement in resolution reveals new fine structure. If the uniformity of magnetic field over the specimen is improved to one part in 10^8, two of the peaks in the alcohol spectrum break into a finer multiplet structure as shown in Figure 6.7b. These *spin multiplets* arise from the magnetic interaction between protons in one group with protons in the neighbouring group via the molecular electrons. It may be shown that for a group with n protons this splits the resonance of its neighbouring group into $(n + 1)$ equally-spaced components with a binomial distribution of intensities. Thus the CH_3 group resonance is split into a triplet with intensities 1:2:1, and the CH_2 group resonance is split into a quartet with intensities 1:3:3:1. Thus this high-resolution NMR spectrum is a 'fingerprint', characteristic of this particular liquid and its molecular structure.

Such high-resolution NMR spectra are of immense value for molecular structure analysis, and most organic chemistry laboratories have high-resolution NMR spectrometers for this purpose. In biochemistry, molecules of biological interest can be investigated by NMR in solutions similar to their normal environment. This rich spectral structure from liquids is not ordinarily obtained with solid specimens because the static internal magnetic fields discussed on page 218 broaden the spectra and obscure the structure.

The resolved structures revealed in high-resolution NMR spectroscopy have not played a central role in the initial development of NMR imaging. Nevertheless recent developments suggest that they may become more important in the future in the imaging of individual chemical species in living systems, and we refer to these developments on page 234.

NMR IMAGING METHODS

One-dimensional projections

In conventional NMR spectroscopy as practised in physics and chemistry, a small specimen, typically less than 1 ml, is placed in the spectrometer coil (p. 216), and its NMR spectra, relaxation times and other parameters are recorded. The specimen is usually homogeneous, the magnetic field is highly uniform, and the NMR spectrum is generated by the whole specimen. In NMR imaging the reverse is the case. The object of interest, for example human anatomy, is heterogeneous and its structure is to be determined and displayed. The magnetic field is deliberately non-uniform; different parts of the specimen are labelled or coded by the particular magnetic field strength they experience, and the NMR spectrum records the spatial distribution of the NMR signal from the specimen. Because the spatial defining magnetic field is coupled to the rf electromagnetic field by the magnetic nuclei in the object, Lauterbur[45] was led to call the subject *zeugmatography* from the Greek word zeugma 'that which joins together'.

Biological systems provide strong proton NMR signals, particularly from water, fat and other fluid or soft components. The intrinsic NMR resonance width of these strongly responding biological components is narrow, typically a few Hz. Therefore, if a linear magnetic field gradient of order 10^{-2} T m^{-1} is superimposed on the usual highly uniform magnetic field, different parts of the specimen experience different field strengths, and remembering the direct proportionality between NMR frequency and field strength (Equations 6.1 and 6.2), we see that the NMR spectrum is a one-dimensional (1D) projection of proton density along the direction of the gradient. This is illustrated in Figure 6.8 for two tubes of water and for a general irregularly-shaped object with an arbitrary internal distribution of mobile protons.

NMR 1D projections were first investigated some years ago with simple glass and liquid structures by Gabillard[29,30] (see also[3]), who also studied their dynamic response. Field gradients are also an essential feature of the study of molecular diffusion in liquids by the NMR spin echo method,[32] in the study of phase separation in ^{3}He–^{4}He solutions,[62] in methods of information storage[2,8] and in the investigation of periodic structures by the NMR 'diffraction' method.[56,57]

One-dimensional projections give some structural information, but for an image we require at least a two-dimensional (2D) representation of

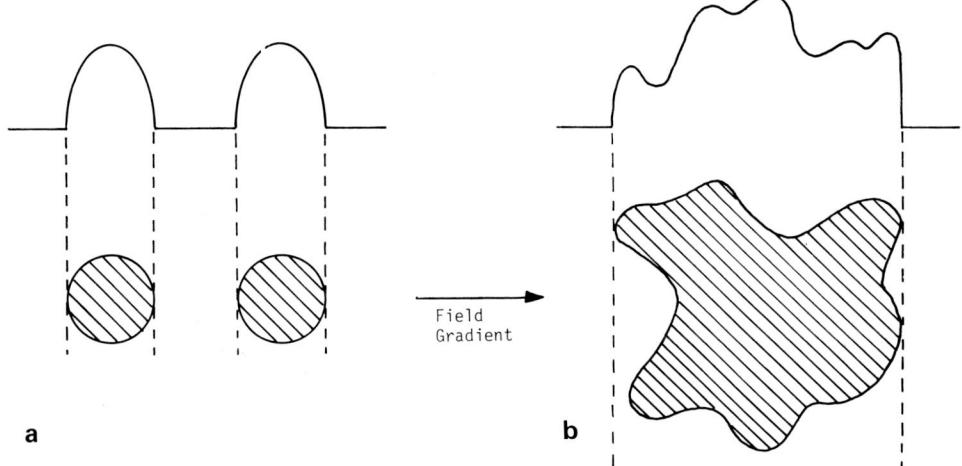

Fig. 6.8 The application of a linear magnetic field gradient generates an NMR spectrum which is a one-dimensional projection of mobile proton density along the gradient direction. (a) Two tubes of water. (b) A general irregularly-shaped object.

nuclear density. Better still we would like to have a 2D image of a thin defined slice in the object; a stack or set of such images of coplanar slices in the object then provides a complete 3D representation of the object.

A number of methods have been devised for proceeding from 1D NMR projections to 2D and 3D NMR images, and these are considered in the following sections. Most of these methods recognise that a field gradient is essentially a 1D probe of investigation, and in order to yield 2D or 3D information a time-dependence must be introduced either by modulating, switching or rotating the gradient.

NMR spectra of the type displayed in Figure 6.8 may be recorded in several ways. We may apply a 90° pulse and record the FID; this may then be Fourier-transformed to yield the NMR spectrum as discussed on page 216. This is *pulsed NMR spectroscopy*. Alternatively we may apply a smaller rf voltage continuously to the coil, and the nuclear induction signal may be continuously received. The frequency of this rf voltage is slowly traversed through the range of interest and the spectrum recorded. This is *continuous wave (CW) NMR spectroscopy*. In the earlier development of NMR the use of CW procedures was widespread, but they have now largely been replaced by pulse methods which have two advantages. First they allow the nuclear system to evolve and relax freely in the absence of a perturbing transmitter signal, so enabling NMR parameters to be measured more directly, and secondly pulse methods enjoy the 'Fourier transform advantage' which results in a great saving of time. The rf pulse excites the nuclear system over the whole frequency spectrum at once, and not at one frequency only; a pulsed NMR spectrometer may thus be regarded as equivalent to many CW NMR spectrometers operating simultaneously in parallel.

Very often the signal/noise ratio in a single recording of an FID is not adequate; in this case the pulses are repeated and the FIDs are accumulated and signal-averaged until the signal/noise ratio is adequate. In order to allow the nuclear magnetisation to relax fully before the next pulse is applied a time of order $5T_1$ is often allowed to elapse between pulses. Alternatively the pulses may be applied more frequently at intervals less than T_1, the nuclear system reaching a state of dynamic equilibrium. Such a procedure is called a driven-equilibrium pulse method. One such method, called the *steady-state free precession* technique (SFP), is referred to later (p. 222).

Projection-reconstruction method

If the magnetic field gradient is applied successively along a number of directions around an axis defined in the object, a series of NMR 1D projections may be recorded. These 1D projections may then be combined by computer to give a 2D projection image of the object, projected on a plane normal to the axis. The method is closely similar to the projection-reconstruction procedures used in computed tomography X-ray scanning pioneered by Cormack[22] and Hounsfield,[42] and described in Chapter 2 of this book. This was the method used by Lauterbur[45] to obtain the first 2D NMR image. In Lauterbur's case, the object consisted of two parallel tubes of water 1 mm diameter, 3 mm apart, and the axis about which the gradient was rotated was parallel to the tube axes.

In general, we can divide our object and its 2D image into an $n \times n$ matrix of picture elements (pixels), and we need to find the NMR response a_{pq} from each of the n^2 matrix elements. If each 1D projection consists of n data values, each of which is a sum Σa_{pq} of n elements, and if n different projections are obtained, we have n^2 simultaneous equations in the n^2 unknown quantities a_{pq}. By computer these may be solved by iterative procedures, by back projection, or other methods, to generate a 2D image of $n \times n$ picture elements.

We should notice one important difference from CT X-ray scanning. In CT X-ray scanning the narrow pencil beams of X-rays define a thin imaging slice. In NMR imaging the whole object within the NMR probe coil is irradiated, and as so far described the method does not provide a thin imaging plane. Therefore the resulting image is a 2D projection image. For an object structured in all three dimensions such 2D projection images do not suffice. Structure in the third dimension is lost, and in the other two dimensions it is blurred. In this situation, the projection-reconstruction approach may be extended to three dimensions by dividing the object into $n \times n \times n$ cuboidal volume elements (voxels); the gradient must now be applied isotropically from n^2 directions, to yield n^3 equations in n^3 unknowns. There is now a very large computing problem. Nevertheless 3D NMR images of a coconut and a pig heart have been obtained by this method with $n = 33$.[44]

It is possible to circumvent this large 3D computing exercise by methods which define a thin imaging slice in the object (Fig. 6.9). In one method, described in more detail later, the field gradient g_z is caused to alternate at a low angular

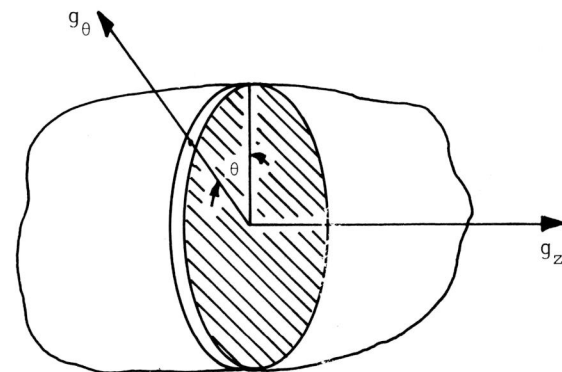

Fig. 6.9 Defining an imaging slice in an object.

frequency Ω_z, so defining a zero field plane of approximate thickness $2\Omega_z$ in terms of angular frequency, or $2\Omega_z/\gamma g_z$ in terms of length. A second, static, gradient g_θ is applied in the plane so defined and a 1D projection is recorded of the protons in the defined slice in the direction of g_θ. This static gradient is applied in successive azimuth directions θ in the plane, and the resulting set of 1D projections is reconstructed to give a 2D NMR image of the defined slice of the object.[17] Another method of defining a slice in the object (see page 223) consists of applying a static field gradient g_z and selectively exciting the protons in the slice by irradiation on a narrow band of wavelengths whose frequencies correspond precisely to the band of resonance frequencies across the slice. A static gradient g_θ is applied in the selected slice, and reconstruction procedures are applied to the resulting 1D projections to obtain a 2D image of the defined slice.[46]

Spin mapping

In the simplest form of this method, conceived and developed by Hinshaw,[33-35] the idea is to define a particular small volume element in the object and record its NMR signal, and then move on to the next element, sequentially scanning all the volume elements of which the object is composed. The image is built up uniquely in 3D without recourse to complex reconstruction computations, mapping out directly the nuclear spin density in the object (hence the name *spin mapping*).

Axes X, Y, Z are defined in the object, with the field **B** along Z. Field gradients are applied along the three mutually perpendicular directions alternating at three asynchronous low frequencies. The field gradient $g_X = \partial B_z/\partial x$ along X, alternating at angular frequency Ω_X defines a zero field, or null, plane parallel to YZ of thickness approximately $2\Omega_X/\gamma g_X$; the field gradients g_Y, g_Z along Y and Z respectively similarly define null planes parallel to ZX and XY of thickness $2\Omega_Y/\gamma g_Y$ and $2\Omega_Z/\gamma g_Z$ respectively. The NMR signal is modulated by these alternating gradients except for the small volume element at the intersection of the three null planes. The output from the NMR spectrometer is taken through a low-pass filter, cutting off below the three modulation frequencies, so that only the signal from the small sensitive volume element is recorded. By varying the relative currents in the coils supplying the alternating gradients, the sensitive point may be scanned television-wise sequentially through a defined imaging plane, and the signal presented synchronously as an image on the oscilloscope. A stack of such 2D images of coplanar slices provides a complete 3D representation of the object.

This is the *single sensitive point* (SSP) method of NMR imaging, and was used by Hinshaw to obtain the first 3D NMR images.[34,35] It is simple and direct, requiring no calculations or computerised reconstructions. Because it is sequential, however, it is a slow method of imaging. On the other hand it should be noted that using this technique it is possible to study NMR at a particular point in a structured object.

The sensitive point method may be greatly accelerated by replacing the alternating gradient along, say, the Y direction (Fig. 6.10) with a static gradient. The NMR spectrum obtained after filtration of the modulated NMR signals is then a 1D projection of the proton density along the sensitive line. This spectrum is obtained by Fourier transformation of the FID following a resonant rf pulse (see p. 220). This has been applied with particular success in the technique[6,7,36-39] in which the n picture elements in one line of the image are obtained in the same time as for one element in the SSP method, and typically represents a hundred-fold improvement in speed. This is the *multiple sensitive point* (MSP) method of NMR imaging.

After recording the NMR signal from one line of n elements, the sensitive line is advanced to the adjacent line of elements. Meantime the Fourier transform of the signal from the previous line is computed and displayed. As the line is scanned progressively through the imaging plane the image is built up line by line.

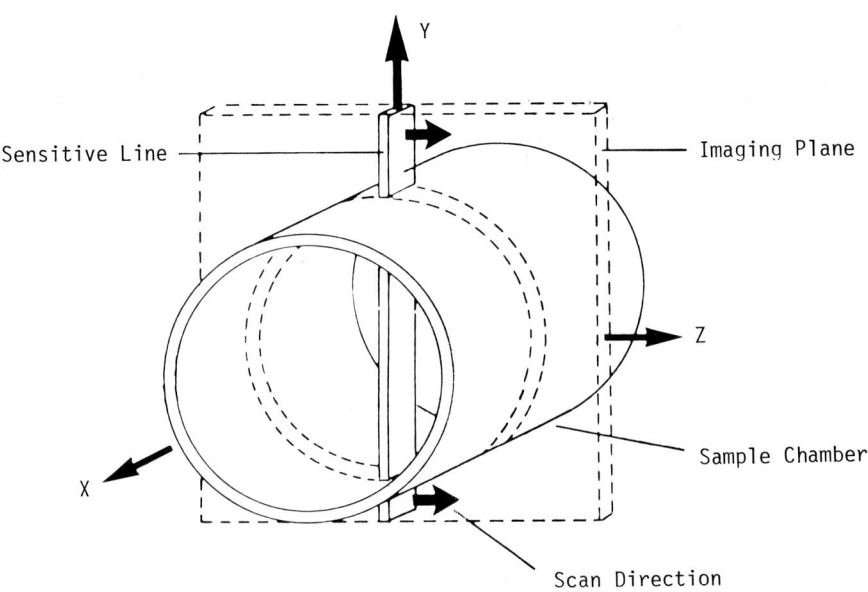

Fig. 6.10 The geometrical arrangement of the sample chamber in the MSP method of spin mapping. The chamber is mounted transversely in the magnetic field **B** which is along the Z direction.

Selective irradiation methods

This method also avoids reconstruction computations by selecting specific planes and lines in the object. Devised by Mansfield and co-workers,[31,51] the idea is to arrange that only the desired elements are excited by the electromagnetic radiation, and is achieved by the use of tailored rf pulse sequences whose rf spectrum covers a carefully selected band of frequencies.

First a field gradient $g_X = \partial B_z / \partial X$ is applied along X (Fig. 6.11) and an rf pulse sequence is

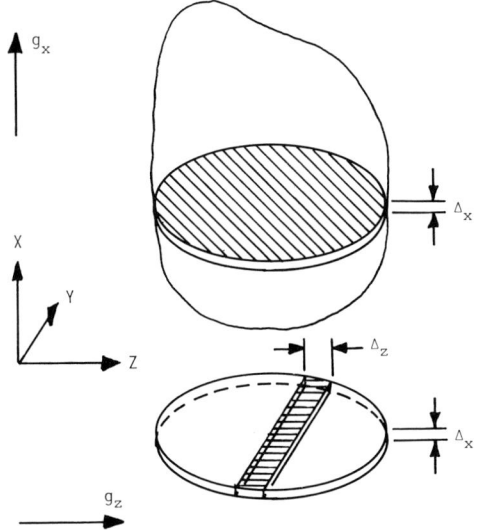

Fig. 6.11 Illustration of the plane and strip defined by selective irradiation.

applied whose spectrum covers with equal intensity all frequencies corresponding to the spread of B_z across the specimen except for those in a narrow band Δx. This sequence is applied for such time as turns all the excited nuclei through 90°. After a brief FID these nuclei remain effectively inert for a time of order T_1. On the other hand the slice of thickness Δx remains untouched. The field gradient along X is now switched off and a field gradient g_Z is applied along Z. Another tailored pulse sequence is now applied which provides a 90° excitation only to nuclei in an elementary strip of width Δz, as indicated in Figure 6.11. At the end of this excitation the gradient g_Z is switched off and a third gradient is applied along Y and the FID is recorded. The Fourier transform of this FID gives the 1D projection of proton density

along this line of elements. A dedicated computer prescribes the tailored pulse sequences, controls the switching of the gradients, moves the line progressively through the plane, and calculates the Fourier transform for each line. Like the MSP method of spin mapping this method is a *line scan* technique of NMR imaging, and traverses a line of elements through a defined imaging plane of the object.

A development of this method is to irradiate a grid of many thin strips simultaneously in the defined slice, instead of a single strip of width Δz. Then by applying a small additional gradient along Y all the strips are examined obliquely and the FID reads the nuclear induction signal from the irradiated strips in the plane. This method is called *planar imaging*.[52] Because the strips must be thin only a small proportion of the nuclei in the object are used in this method. It led to a further refinement, however, in which all the nuclei in the defined slice are used. A spatial periodicity is imposed in the Z direction by periodic reversal of the gradient g_Z. This regular reversal brings the precessing nuclei periodically back into phase as 'spin echoes' which are Fourier transformed to provide a periodicity along Z. Again, adding a small gradient along Y the FID from all the protons in the defined slice is read to give an image of the whole plane. This is called the *echo planar method*.[49] Since it collects signals from the whole defined slice it should be faster than line scan methods, and since the image is obtained from one FID it should take less time than the projection-reconstruction method for which a minimum of n FIDs are required. Preliminary results of the echo planar method have been reported with small annular phantoms[55] and it will be of great interest to see how well the method works with larger biological objects and the human body.

Fourier zeugmatography

In this method devised by Ernst and co-workers[43] a magnetic field gradient is applied along the X direction for a time t_x, is then switched along Y for a time t_y and finally along Z for a time t_z. The FID of all the protons in the specimen is read as a function of t_z. The procedure is repeated for a series of values of both t_x and t_y. The analysis of the method shows that the proton density distribution in the object is the 3D Fourier transform of the family of FIDs; here the spatial co-ordinates (x,y,z) in the specimen and the three times (t_x,t_y,t_z) are conjugate variables.

If the specimen is to be described by an array of $n \times n \times n$ voxels it is necessary to record n^2 FIDs for n different values of both t_x and t_y, reading each FID as n discrete points during t_z. This calls for considerable data storage and handling. For this reason the method has so far only been applied in two dimensions to give a 2D projection image of two tubes of water.

Fourier zeugmatography in 3D makes similar demands on computer capacity to the 3D projection-reconstruction method (p. 220), and as in that case the problems may be substantially eased by selecting a slice in the object and carrying out a 2D Fourier transform in the defined slice.[18] This is *selective Fourier zeugmatography*.

Although Fourier zeugmatography is a sound method of NMR imaging, only recently has its potential been exploited in a modified form by Edelstein, Hutchison *et al*.[63]

Rotating frame zeugmatography

Several of the previous methods of NMR imaging require a magnetic field gradient to be switched rapidly on and off or from one direction to another. In large magnet systems for human NMR imaging this may present substantial technical problems and the rapidly switched gradients may have undesirable physiological effects.[19] In order to avoid field gradient switching, Hoult[41] enlists a gradient of the radiofrequency field B_1 (p. 214).

The main magnetic field **B** is arranged to have a linear gradient in the Z direction, applied all the time and not switched. The rf field B_1 is arranged to have a gradient in the X direction. The rf pulse is applied for a time t_x following which the FID is recorded as a function of time t_z. A set of FIDs is recorded for a series of times t_x. The accumulated FIDs are then subjected to double Fourier transformation in which x, z and t_x, t_y are the conjugate variables, to give the distribution of nuclear density in the XZ plane. The image which results is thus a 2D projection image of the whole object projected along the Y direction. Preliminary 2D projection images have been reported by this method using simple phantoms.

In order to extend the method to 3D a slice in the object must be defined by a method which does not require a switched gradient. An alternating gradient (p. 222) or a carefully profiled field have been suggested, but at the time of writing extension to 3D has not been reported.

Focused nuclear resonance: FONAR

In this method, developed by Damadian et al[24] the object is placed in a static inhomogeneous field, which is very carefully contoured in such a way that only a small volume element in the object, in a saddle-shaped region of the field distribution, is at the proton resonance frequency. The NMR signal from this selected small volume is recorded and the volume element is traversed through a plane in the object, mapping out an image of the NMR signal. FONAR is thus a sequential scanning method; therefore it is simple and direct, but slow. Rather little detail of the technique has been published, but the first human whole-body NMR images were obtained by this method.[26]

NMR IMAGING SYSTEMS

All NMR imaging systems consist of a magnet, an NMR spectrometer and an image display. In this respect the systems are essentially similar to the basic arrangement discussed on page 216 and illustrated in Figure 6.4. Whichever method of NMR imaging is employed the main features of the system are the same, though there are significant differences in detail and sophistication.

Operating frequency

The choice of radiofrequency is determined by several factors which include: (1) considerations of signal/noise ratio; (2) attenuation and phase distortion of the electromagnetic radiation in the object to be imaged; (3) considerations of possible hazard; and (4) the availability of a magnet to provide the magnetic field strength which corresponds to the desired radiofrequency.

In NMR spectroscopy the signal/noise ratio improves with increasing radiofrequency v, typically as $v^{3/2}$.[1,3] Therefore, from this point of view it is desirable to operate at the highest practicable frequency consistent with other constraints.

Biological tissues are moderate electrical conductors. In order to avoid excessive attenuation and phase distortion for human whole body imaging one estimate is that the frequency should not exceed 10 MHz.[14] For smaller objects, such as the human hand and arm and small animals up to say 10 cm in size, the frequency can be increased to 100 MHz without serious trouble. For protons 10 MHz corresponds to a magnetic field of 0·24 T, and 100 MHz to 2·4 T. For other nuclei of lower gyromagnetic ratio γ the corresponding fields are of course higher.

It is not thought that a static magnetic field presents a human hazard (p. 233). Nevertheless codes of practice at accelerator laboratories have limited the exposure of the head and body to 0·2 T and the limbs to 2 T.[4] These limits are conveniently consistent with those cited in the previous paragraph from considerations of rf attenuation and phase shift.

Magnets

The type of magnet selected depends very much on the size of the object to be imaged. For objects not larger than 10 cm in extent, such as fruit and vegetables, small animals, human hands and arms, a water-cooled iron-core electromagnet may be used, similar to those used in conventional NMR spectroscopy, but with a larger gap. A typical magnet of this kind might have a gap of order 12 cm between circular plane parallel polefaces some 40 cm diameter. Powered by a 15 kW supply a field of 0·7 T may be generated, corresponding to a proton NMR frequency of 30 MHz. With the aid of ring shims a uniformity of field of a part in 10^5 may be achieved over the sample dimensions. Field gradients, whether static, alternating or switched, may be generated with the aid of coils mounted on the poles and fed from auxiliary supplies. Magnets of this kind have overall linear dimensions of order 1 m and a mass of order 10^3 kg.

For NMR imaging of the human head or body magnets with a much larger working volume are required. A common configuration is depicted in Figure 6.12. It consists of four air-core water-cooled resistive coils approximating to a 'spherical' geometry. The overall dimensions are of order 2 m, the mass 2×10^3 kg; it has an access of 60 cm diameter through the end coils to take a horizontal patient. Such magnets typically generate a field of 0·1 T with about 20 kW of power.

Large superconducting magnets are now available for wholebody NMR imaging.[5] They have the merit of consuming negligible power, they have excellent constancy of field strength, and can provide much higher fields in magnets of large bore. They are, however, more expensive and require a supply of liquid helium to maintain the magnet windings in their superconducting state at 4 K.

Iron-core electromagnets could in principle be used for wholebody imaging, but it seems doubtful if they offer any advantage. Spare magnets capable of modification for human imaging stand idle in particle physics laboratories, but they tend to be extremely massive with large appetites for power and water.

Spectrometer and image display

The object to be imaged is placed in the magnet inside an insulating cylinder on which is wound an rf coil which generates an rf field $\mathbf{B}_1$ transverse to the field $\mathbf{B}$ of the magnet. This coil is the focal point of the NMR spectrometer. It is supplied with rf current as the NMR frequency, usually in the form of rf pulses, from a crystal oscillator followed by rf gates and a power amplifier. The NMR signals may be picked up by the same coil, or by a separate receiver coil. A pre-amplifier mounted close to the coil takes the NMR signal on to the main amplifiers, where it is followed by analogue-to-digital conversion and signal averaging.

A dedicated minicomputer is usually an integral part of any NMR imaging system. Instructions typed into a visual display unit (VDU) enable the computer to set up the parameters of the spectrometer for the measurement in hand. The computer receives the NMR data from the signal averager and performs whatever calculations are necessary on the data, for example Fourier transformation or projection-reconstruction algorithms. The signals are then passed to the image display

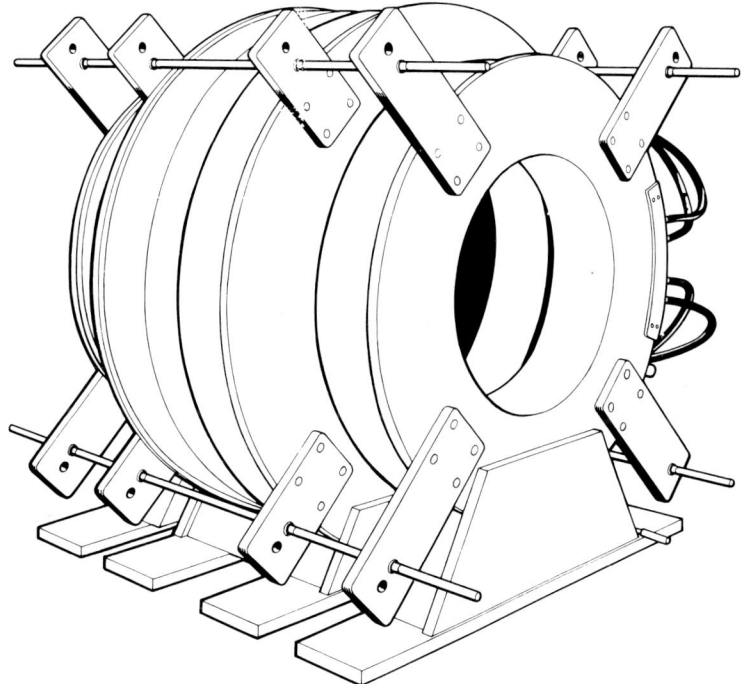

Fig. 6.12 A magnet for human whole-body NMR imaging.

whose parameters may also be set through instructions on the VDU. It is in this area of the NMR imaging system that the greatest variations in detail are found, according to the particular imaging technique adopted and the technical preferences of the design engineer. Typical memory provision is 32k. Permanent storage of image data may be made on disk, diskette, cassette tape or paper tape.

As with other methods of imaging, the digitised output representing an array of $n \times n$ pixels of an NMR image, must be presented on a suitable display. A common form of display is in black and white on an oscilloscope screen. The NMR signal modulates the beam intensity to present a digitised monotonic scale of grays, and a raster scans the beam over the image area. Colour TV monitors are also used to present images in colour with a predetermined colour attribution scheme. When using oscilloscope displays in black and white or in colour, hard copy may be obtained by photography. Images may also be recorded directly in permanent form using electrostatic or heat-sensitive recording instruments, typewriter devices, or computer-driven photoscanners.[15] The whole range of NMR signal from zero to the maximum recorded signal may be displayed. Alternatively a threshold and a ceiling may be interposed to enable a 'window' of arbitrary range to be displayed in order to enhance the discrimination of information in a particular intensity range.

PERFORMANCE OF NMR IMAGING SYSTEMS

Some NMR images

A selection of NMR images obtained by several of the methods described on pages 219–224 is shown in Figures 6.13 to 6.18. Many other images have been published and the reader is referred to the original papers for further examples. Not all the methods described have yet been developed to the point where biological and medical examples can be presented.

In Figure 6.13 is shown a thin proton NMR cross-section image of an intact lemon obtained by the MSP method of spin mapping (p. 222[5,7]). Strong NMR intensity is recorded from the mobile protons in the interior segments of the lemon and weaker signals from the skin and the resolved septum lines. The intensity is presented as 16 gray levels. There is no accepted convention as to

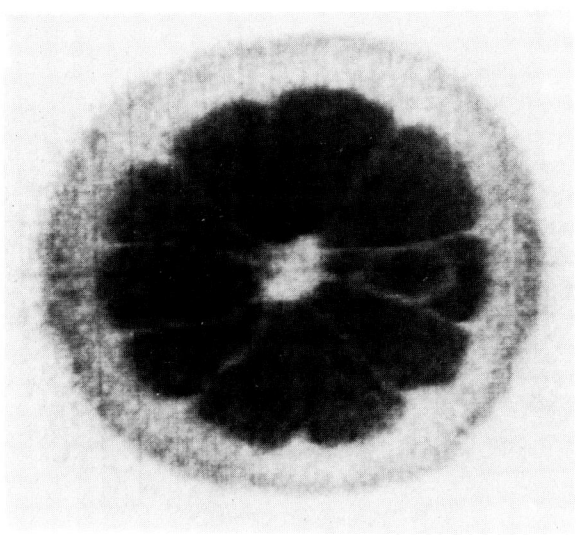

Fig. 6.13 Thin transverse section proton NMR image of an intact lemon.[5, 7]

whether the highest proton signal should be shown black or white. Here the highest intensity is clearly black and the region of zero intensity outside the lemon is shown white. The image was recorded on a 128 × 128 pixel array and is presented on a 256 × 256 point display. Resolution in the image is about 0·5 mm. The thickness of the imaging plane was about 3 mm and the imaging time was 6 minutes.

The NMR image in Figure 6.14 is a cross-section through the mid-phalanx of a live human finger obtained using the selective irradiation line scan method (see p. 223[50]). The diagram alongside the image illustrates the anatomical features which are visible in the image. This image is presented on a 64 × 64 point array using a 16 gray level scale of intensity. The imaging time was 23 min. The convention adopted in Figure 6.14 is white for the highest NMR intensity and black for zero intensity, and therefore is opposite to the convention adopted in Figure 6.13.

The NMR image shown in Figure 6.15 is a thin cross-section image of a live human wrist obtained by the MSP method of spin mapping (see p. 222[36, 38]). The Figure also shows a photograph of a corresponding cadaver cross-section and an anatomical diagram. Dark areas in the image indicate regions that contain high concentrations of mobile protons such as the marrow in the carpal bones and the subcutaneous fat. On the other hand the light areas indicate tissue with few mobile protons such as tendons and the cortical bone. Blood in arteries and veins is light due to its motion through the section during the imaging process. Various tissue types are discriminated and there is clearly a good correspondence between the image and the actual anatomy. A series of such transverse sections has been taken of a live hand and fore-arm and compared with corresponding cadaver sections.[39] The image in Figure 6.15 was recorded on a 128 × 128

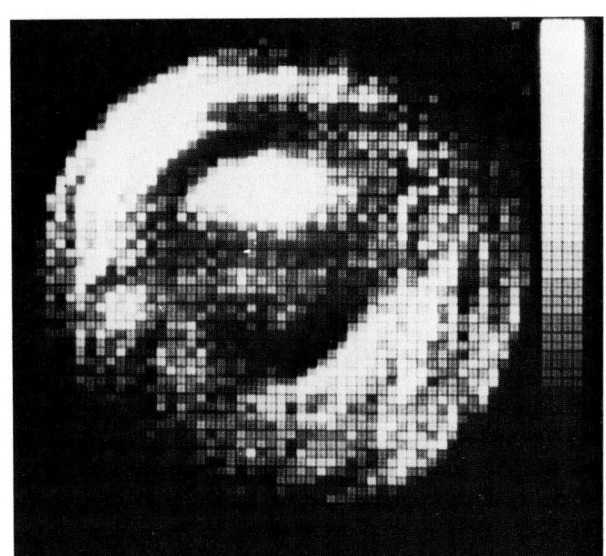
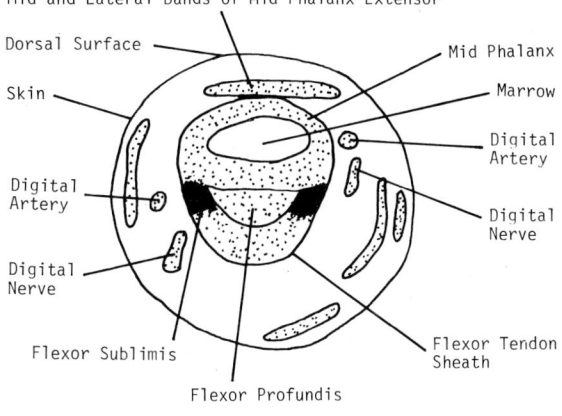

Fig. 6.14 Cross-section proton NMR image of a live human finger.[50]

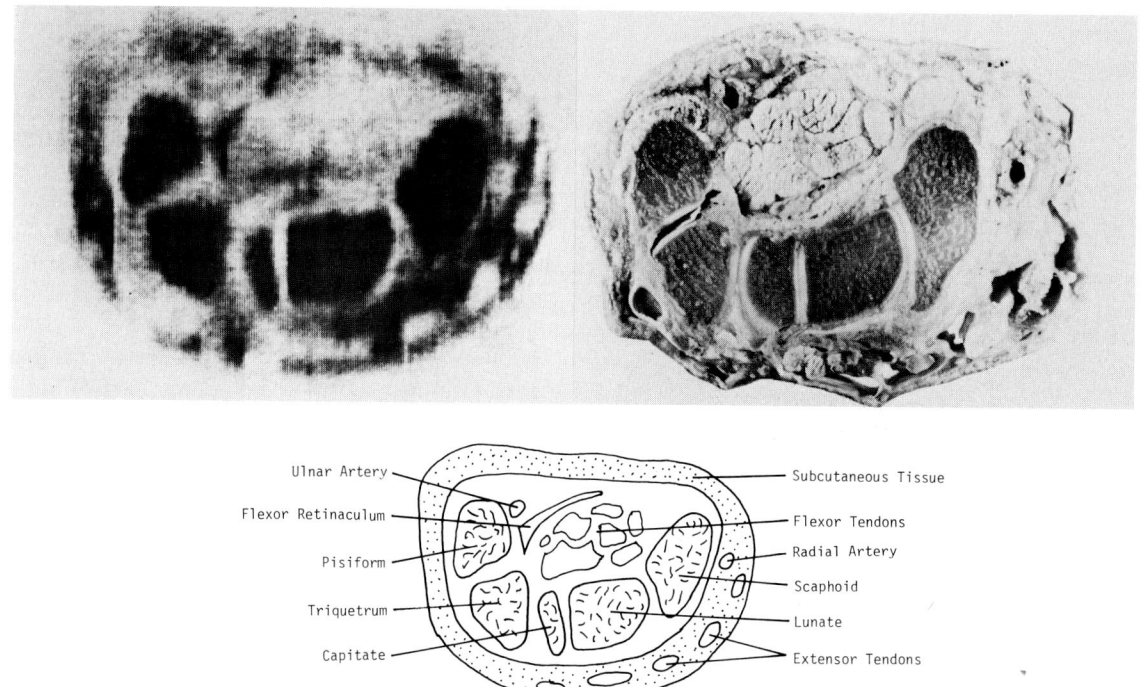

Fig. 6.15 Thin cross-section proton NMR image of a live human wrist. Also shown is a photograph of a corresponding cadaver section and an anatomical diagram.[36,38]

pixel array and presented on a 256 × 256 point display. Resolution in the image is about 0·5 mm. The thickness of the imaging plane is about 3 mm and the imaging time was about 9 min.

The first whole-body NMR image ever made is shown in Figure 6.16. It is a cross-section proton image of a live human chest, and was obtained by the FONAR method (see p. 224[26,27]). The cross-section was taken at the level of the eighth thoracic veterbra. The image is displayed on a 16 level intensity scale. The top of the image is the anterior boundary of the chest wall and the left of the image

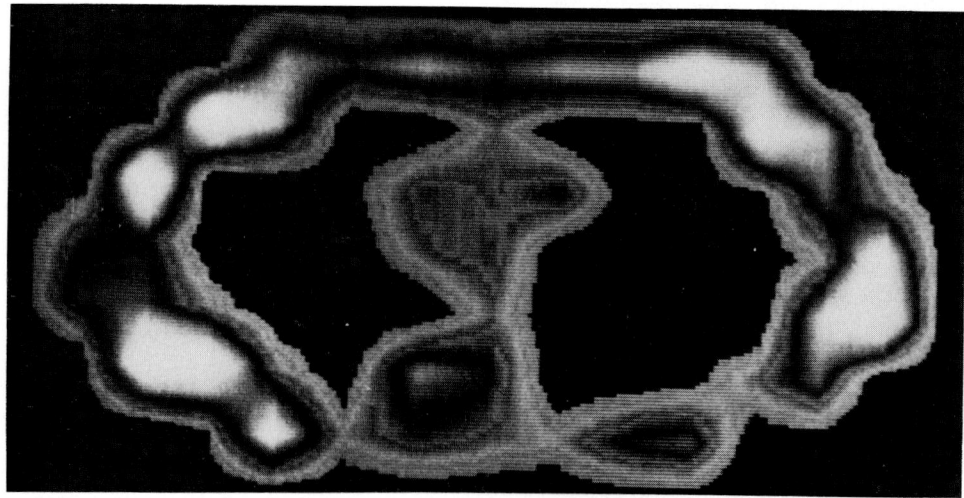

Fig. 6.16 Cross-section proton NMR image of a live human chest.[26,27]

is the left side of the chest. In the body wall there is an alternation of density attributed to intercostal muscle and ribs. The interior dark regions are the two lung cavities. Along the midline the principal structure is the heart; more posteriorly is the aorta. The authors estimate resolution in the image as 6 mm. The imaging time was 4½ hours. Several chest images of patients with cancer of the lung have also been recorded by the FONAR method, in which the tumours are clearly visible.[25] Chest images have also been recorded using a selective irradiation method.[48,61]

Figure 6.17 shows the first NMR cross-section image of the abdomen of a live human subject; the figure also shows an annotated version of the image illustrating the main recognisable features. The image was obtained by the selective irradiation line scan method (see p. 223[53,55]). The subject was placed in a magnet of the type illustrated in Figure 6.12 operating at 0·094 T; the corresponding proton NMR frequency was 4·0 MHz. The imaging slice is 4 cm thick and the image is presented as a 75 × 90 pixel array. The imaging time was 40 min.

An NMR image of a live human head is shown in Figure 6.18 (left). It is a 1 cm thick low ventricular slice obtained in 4 min using the projection-reconstruction method in a defined plane (p. 220) with a more developed system of the type which gave the first NMR head images 6.[21] A CT X-ray image of the same section is shown alongside, Figure 6.18 (right). The striking feature of the NMR image is the strong discrimination between the grey and white matter in the brain, barely perceptible in the X-ray image, due to T_1 differences.

Nature of the image and tissue discrimination

After seeing examples of practical NMR images it is natural to ask what is actually being displayed in the image. The image is not just a 2D representation of proton density $\rho(x,y,z)$ at each point x,y,z in the defined slice of the object. Rather it is a spatial representation of the NMR signal. The NMR signal is certainly proportional to the proton density at each point, since the nuclear magnetisation M at each point is proportional to the proton density. It is also a function, however, of the relaxation times T_1 and T_2 at each point in the section. Furthermore the NMR signal depends critically on the methods of NMR detection and the parameters of the measurement such as the pulse repetition rate. In general the NMR signal at each point, x,y,z may be written as

$$\rho f(T_1, T_2, \ldots)_{xyz}, \quad (6.6)$$

where the function f depends on the details of the method of measurement.

For NMR systems adjusted to the optimum signal-to-noise ratio the function f is generally dependent on the ratio T_2/T_1. For fluids and soft tissues T_1 and T_2 are almost equal as we saw on page 217, and the ratio T_2/T_1 has its highest values. On the other hand, for solid-like materials such as cortical bone and teeth $T_2 \ll T_1$, so that f is small and the NMR signal is weak, even though ρ is not small. This provides an explanation of the tissue discrimination observed in animal and human images. Strong signals are obtained from fluids, fats and soft tissues, intermediate signals from tendon and muscle and other tissues dependent on their 'hardness', weak signals from teeth, cortical bone and voids. Particular parameters such as T_1 may be studied or imaged by examination of the dynamic response of the NMR signal. Relaxation discrimination may be extremely valuable in distinguishing tissues of similar proton density, and in providing spatial information of physiological differences additional to the morphology.

Resolution and the imaging time

The resolution in an image is dependent on a number of factors the first of which is the matrix size $n \times n$. Although the eye interpolates what is presented to it, and images can be interpolated or smoothed by computer, the transverse or planar resolution can never be substantially better than the size of one pixel, or $1/n$ of the linear dimensions of the object. Even this cannot be achieved if the structure of the object varies significantly through the thickness of the slice scanned. Thick slices inevitably degrade resolution.

Although the resolution in an image may in principle be as good as the size of one pixel, and therefore be determined by the size of n which is chosen, in practice it may well not be as good as this. The

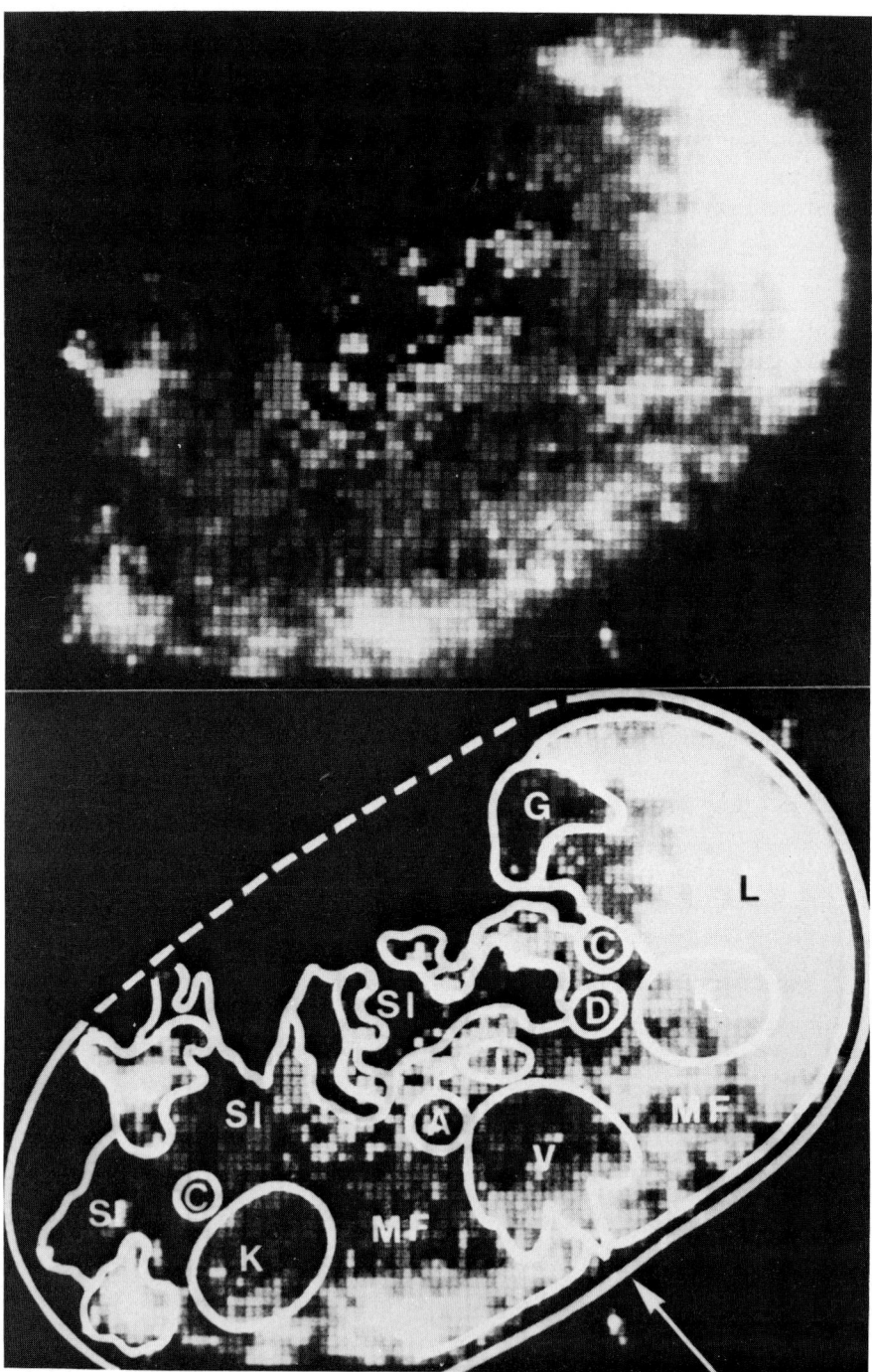

Fig. 6.17 Cross-section line-scan proton NMR image through a live human abdomen at L2–3. The arrow indicates midline posterior. Left side of patient lies to left of the illustration. Bright zones correspond, in general, to high mobile proton content. On the labelled image, A = aorta; C = colon; D = duodenum; G = gallbladder; I = inferior vena cava; K = kidney; L = liver; P = pancreas; S = spleen; SI = stomach and intestines; V = vertebra. Abdominal muscles and retroperitoneal fat (MF) are seen adjacent to the vertebra.[53,55]

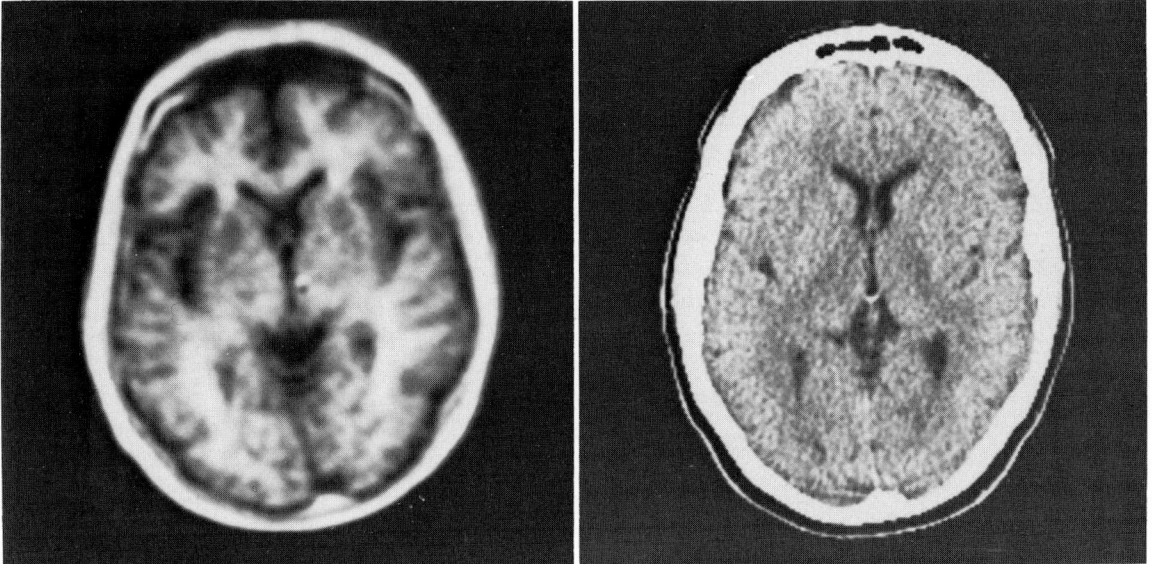

Fig. 6.18: Thin transverse section images through a live human head at low ventricular level: *Left* Proton NMR image, *Right* CT X-ray image.

first reason for failing to achieve the ideal resolution arises from the intrinsic width of the NMR signal. We saw on p. 217 that this is of order $(\pi T_2)^{-1}$ in terms of frequency, and therefore of order $(2/\gamma T_2)$ in terms of magnetic field, using Equation 6.1. Therefore, if the NMR response from one pixel is not to overlap that of the next, the magnetic field gradient must be large enough to ensure that the difference in magnetic field B between two adjacent elements exceeds the intrinsic resonance width. If the linear dimension of the object is d, the size of one pixel is (d/n), and therefore the field gradient must exceed $(2n/d\gamma T_2)$ approximately. For fluids and soft tissues with $T_2 > 0.1$ s this criterion is readily achieved. On the other hand for the more solid-like components with values of T_2 several orders of magnitude shorter the gradient may not suffice to resolve the NMR signals, which in any case are much weaker.

There are many other ways in which resolution may be degraded and distortions or artifacts introduced. They may originate from irregularities in the main field B, or in the rf field B_1, from non-linearity of the gradients, from phase errors, or from movements of the subject or parts of the subject.

It is important to note that there is a close relationship, for any imaging method, between the resolution in an image and the time taken to acquire the image. If it is desired to improve the resolution by say a factor of two in all three dimensions, each voxel is reduced in volume by a factor of eight. If all other parameters are kept constant, it follows that the time required to obtain an NMR signal of the same signal/noise ratio is increased by a factor of 64. In fact, the imaging time increases as n^6. If it is merely desired to improve the resolution in the imaging plane, while retaining the same slice thickness, the picture time increases only as n^4. In either case – for much improved resolution there is a great increase in acquisition time.

Comparison of imaging methods

Since NMR imaging is still in its early years, with many of the methods still at their first stages of development, it would be premature to come to firm conclusions about the relative merits of the methods (p. 219). Nevertheless certain comments may perhaps be made at this stage.

First of all let us ask the strictly practical question, which is of medical significance: which methods at the time of writing have actually produced recognisable proton NMR images of parts of the human anatomy in a time less than, say, 10 min?

The answer is four methods: (1) projection-reconstruction in a defined slice; (2) the multiple sensitive point (MSP) method of spin mapping; (3) the selective irradiation line-scan method; and (4) the spin-warp variation of the Fourier zeugmatography method.[63] Of course some of the other methods may meet this criterion before long, and may indeed do better, but actual achievement is important.

The SSP and FONAR approaches have the merit of extreme simplicity; they require no data processing and enable NMR to be carried out at a specific point in a structured object. As methods of imaging, however, they are of the sequential point type and therefore should take longer to acquire images than methods which scan the slice line by line such as the MSP and selective line scan methods, and this does seem to be borne out in practice. These latter two methods produce proton NMR images with n around 100 in times of minutes. Methods which receive NMR signals from the whole defined slice simultaneously, such as the projection-reconstruction method, should in principle have greater advantages. Data from many projections must be acquired and processed, however, and the times reported so far for this method are not substantially shorter. The method of echo-planar imaging (p. 223), which acquires data from the whole slice in a single FID should in principle be faster and it will be of great interest to watch its development.

In two recent papers attempts have been made to compare the various imaging methods in an objective manner. One approach[18] is strictly theoretical and makes a comparison of the relative times expected for the different methods to acquire an image from a formalised object making certain assumptions about its relaxation properties. The other approach[13] is strictly empirical and makes a comparison by listing the imaging times reported by different workers and adjusting them to common conditions. Both approaches are helpful, though it may perhaps be said of the first that it inevitably takes a simplified model of the object and takes insufficient account of practical problems of implementation, while of the second that it uses published imaging times which may not be equally optimised implementations of the different methods. Nevertheless the conclusions drawn in both papers are broadly consistent with the comments made in the earlier paragraphs of this section.

Potential clinical applications

Although NMR imaging has been carried out on healthy human volunteers, clinical trials are only just beginning. Therefore it is not yet possible to make any assessment of actual clinical applications. Nevertheless we may look ahead and consider how NMR tomography may begin to take its place alongside the more established imaging techniques, and the possible advantages it may offer.

First as a means of human morphological investigation it may be said that the best human NMR images now stand comparison with X-ray CT images so far as the resolution of anatomical detail and geometrical faithfulness are concerned, and are superior to images obtained by radioisotopic imaging or thermographic imaging. In comparison with X-ray CT scanning, at present NMR imaging is slower; whereas the former takes a few seconds, the latter currently takes a few minutes, though this gap may be reduced before long. On the other hand for some parts of the anatomy, for example the head, an imaging time of a few minutes is probably acceptable.

Against the possible disadvantages of being slower may be set a number of positive advantages which NMR imaging can offer: (1) it is non-invasive; (2) it does not involve the use of ionising radiations; (3) it is believed to be without hazard (see p. 233); (4) the electromagnetic radiation penetrates bony structures such as the skull and the spine and into the marrow of bones without significant attenuation; and (5) the method measures the density distribution of hydrogen, the most abundant chemical element in the body, and does so with useful tissue discrimination.

The avoidance of ionising radiation makes the method potentially valuable in examining certain diseases of babies and small children such as hydrocephalus, and for the examination of the fetus in the uterus. The absence of radiation dose will be advantageous also in examinations which require regular, repeated, scans, as in breast cancer screening.

It should be emphasised, however, that NMR imaging is not just a morphological technique, and that it measures not only the spatial distribution of proton density, but also other NMR parameters such as the relaxation times T_1 and T_2 at selected regions in the object. In this way NMR offers the possibility of discriminating tissues of similar density through these additional parameters, and in particular may assist in the discrimination of diseased tissue from adjacent normal tissue.

Experiments by Damadian[23] have shown that values of T_1 and T_2 are generally longer, by a factor of about two, in neoplastic tissue compared with the host tissue. These experiments have been repeated by many other workers in view of their importance, on a variety of tissues. Although there are differences in the experimental results, the general consensus is that T_1 and T_2 are indeed longer for neoplastic tissue than the corresponding normal tissue, though the ratio is not always as large as two. The increased values of T_1 and T_2 for the neoplastic tissues are partly attributed to their higher water content, but other factors very probably contribute. Although these relaxation differences are not fully understood, the empirical difference can be exploited to discriminate pathological tissue. We noted earlier that tumours had been imaged in the human lung, and they have been located in mastectomy specimens.[16,54]

We saw earlier that the rapid transit of blood in the arteries and veins through the imaging plane reduces its effectiveness in producing an NMR signal. Measurements of fluid flow in tubes have been made by NMR using conventional NMR spectrometers and measurements of blood flow have also been made. Therefore, it should be possible to carry out direct measurements of blood flow in specific vessels resolved in the NMR image.

Possibility of hazard

There appear to be three conceivable sources of hazard in human NMR tomography which demand attention, namely the effects of: (1) static magnetic fields; (2) time-varying magnetic fields; and (3) radiofrequency fields.*

*Interim guidance on the risks and on procedures for safe application of NMR in clinical imaging was issued by the UK National Radiological Protection Board in June 1980. This advice is available to those with a practical interest on request to: The Secretary, NRPB, Harwell, Didcot, Oxfordshire OX11 0RQ, UK.

There is substantial literature on biological effects of magnetic fields. Scientific workers have been exposed to fields up to 2 T and have inserted their heads into energised cyclotron magnets. There have been no noticeable ill effects, other than sensations in the mouth, attributed to EMFs generated in metal fillings in the teeth when the head is moved in a magnetic field. So far no volunteer who has been imaged by NMR, whether of the head, chest, abdomen, arms or hands has reported any significant effects. Nevertheless this is not a well charted area, and is one in which we should surely proceed with caution on human subjects. A recent survey of biomagnetic evidence[19] has concluded that health hazards are not likely to be important to the human body in static magnetic fields less than 0·3 T.

As we have seen some imaging systems use alternating or rapidly switched magnetic field gradients. Here again no ill effects have been reported, but there is less evidence and more reason to be careful on account of possible effects on the nervous system, the brain and the heart. Budinger[19] has estimated that temporal variation of fields less than 3 T s^{-1} are not likely to present a health hazard. Therefore low frequency alternating fields below 100 Hz are unlikely to present any hazard, while switched field gradients should be designed with care.

We now turn to the effect of the radiofrequency electromagnetic field, which is essentially a heating effect. Many years of application of short-wave diathermy treatment to various parts of the body including the back, neck and head, have revealed no important hazard in the proper application of the electromagnetic radiation to the parts of the body treated. Although peak power levels in NMR imaging may be at the kilowatt level, typical mean power levels are only a few watts, two orders of magnitude lower than those used in diathermy. In the UK a 'Government Code of Practice' restricts mean radiofrequency exposure of personnel to 100 W m^{-2} continuously and to 500 W m^{-2} for short periods. Budinger[19] reaches a similar conclusion. Exposures during NMR imaging are expected to be below these recommended levels.

Therefore, we conclude on the basis of present evidence, that provided the operating parameters are within the limits stated in the interim guidance,

NMR imaging should present no health hazard.

FUTURE PROSPECTS

Undoubtedly the most important future developments in NMR tomography are concerned with clinical trials, which, as discussed on page 232, are just beginning. NMR imaging has already proved itself as a useful method of interior imaging in a wide variety of systems, both animate and inanimate, and clearly offers considerable promise in medicine, but its evaluation as a practical medical imaging technique in actual clinical situations awaits assessment. Only if clinicians actually do find NMR tomography to be useful, and to have practical advantages over other methods, will it find its way into routine hospital practice. It is likely that the first answers to this important question will begin to appear in the early 1980s, as the clinical trials get under way.

At the same time we may expect further developments in technique to take place. In principle the whole armoury of NMR measurements and methods with all its variations and refinements as practised conventionally on small homogeneous specimens may now be extended and applied in NMR imaging, enabling them to be carried out at a selected region of a structured heterogeneous system, and mapped in 2D and 3D to give images of all NMR properties and parameters.

One example is the possibility of combining NMR imaging with high-resolution NMR spectroscopy (p. 218) to map the spatial distribution of particular chemical species in an object. In the proton NMR images considered so far the chemical shift differences and spin multiplets of the protons in their various different molecular environments have been ignored. The field gradients applied for imaging purposes have so broadened the NMR response as to obliterate the rich fine structure. Lauterbur[47] has shown, however, that with ^{31}P high-resolution NMR spectra obtained in a high magnetic field of 8·5 T it is possible separately to map 2D images of individual phosphorus metabolites, namely creatine phosphate, ATP and inorganic phosphate. If it proves possible to extend this to the human body, it offers the possibility of following the metabolism of specific organs and parts of organs.

While protons are likely to remain the favourite nuclei for NMR imaging on account of their very favourable characteristics coupled with the high concentration of hydrogen in biological systems, nevertheless other nuclei are of interest. In addition to ^{31}P, just discussed, some NMR imaging has been done with ^{19}F,[40] and may have importance in conjunction with fluorinated pharmaceuticals and with fluorocarbon blood substitutes. Other nuclei that may in due course be of interest are ^{2}H, ^{13}C, ^{14}N, ^{15}N, ^{23}Na.

As with all physical techniques used in medicine the future prospects of NMR tomography must inevitably have some relationship with equipment costs. In comparison with other established methods of medical imaging, such as CT X-ray scanning, will NMR tomography be cheaper? For whole-body human imaging the answer to this question is not at all clear. The hardware and software are comparable. On the other hand, smaller equipment for specific applications on hands and arms and breasts could well be substantially cheaper.

Summarising this Section, and indeed this whole Chapter, we see that the prospects for NMR tomography are very exciting and that the future is likely to be full of interest.

Note added in proof

Since completion of the manuscript of this Chapter there have been striking advances in the quality of NMR images reported and the first clinical evaluations are appearing. Examples are to be found in references 64–68.

Acknowledgements

I am indebted to the following for providing some of the illustrations for this chapter, and for allowing them to be reproduced: R. Damadian and the Editor of *Naturwissenschaften* (Fig. 6.16); P. Mansfield and the Editor of the *British Journal of Radiology* (Figs. 6.14 and 6.17); the Editor of *Nature* (Fig. 6.13); the Editor of *Neuroradiology* (Fig. 6.15); the Editor of the *Philosophical Transactions of the Royal Society* (Fig. 6.12); and Thorn-EMI Ltd Central Research Laboratories and the Royal Postgraduate Medical School, Hammersmith, London (Fig. 6.18).

REFERENCES

1. Abragam, A. (1961) *Principes of Nuclear Magnetism*. Oxford: Oxford University Press.
2. Anderson, A. G., Garvin, R. L., Hahn, E. L., Horton, J. W., Tucker, G. L. & Walker, R. M. (1955) Spin echo serial storage memory. *J. appl. Phys.*, **26**, 1324–38.
3. Andrew, E. R. (1969) *Nuclear Magnetic Resonance*. Cambridge: Cambridge University Press.
4. Andrew, E. R. (1977) Zeugmatography. In *Proc. 4th Ampere International Summer School, Pula, 1976* (ed. Blinc, R. & Lahajnar, G., pp. 1–39. Ljubljana: University of Ljubljana.
5. Andrew, E. R. (1980) N.m.r. imaging of intact biological systems. *Phil. Trans. R. Soc. Lond. B.*, **289**, 471–81.
6. Andrew, E. R., Bottomley, P. A., Hinshaw, W. S., Holland, G. N., Moore, W. S. & Simaroj, C. (1977) NMR images by the multiple sensitive point method: application to larger biological systems. *Phys. Med. Biol.*, **22**, 971–4 and 1291.
7. Andrew, E. R., Bottomley, P. A., Hinshaw, W. S., Holland, G. N., Moore, W. S., Simaroj, C. & Worthington, B. S. (1979) NMR imaging in medicine and biology. In *Proc. 20th Congress AMPERE, Tallinn 1978* (ed. Kundla, E., Lippmaa, E. & Saluvere, T.), pp. 53–6. Berlin: Springer.
8. Andrew, E. R., Finney, A. & Mansfield P. (1970) Investigation of pulse storage by nuclear magnetic resonance. *Radar Research Establishment Res. Rep.*, PD/24/026/AT.
9. Bloch, F. (1946) Nuclear induction. *Phys. Rev.*, **70**, 460–74.
10. Bloch, F., Hansen, W. W. & Packard, M. (1946) Nuclear induction. *Phys. Rev.*, **69**, 127.
11. Bloch, F., Hansen, W. W. & Packard, M. (1946) The nuclear induction experiment. *Phys. Rev.*, **70**, 474–85.
12. Bloembergen, N., Purcell, E. M. & Pound, R. V. (1948) Relaxation effects in nuclear magnetic resonance absorption. *Phys. Rev.*, **73**, 679–712.
13. Bottomley, P. A. (1979) A comparative evaluation of proton NMR imaging results. *J. mag. Res.*, **36**, 121–7.
14. Bottomley, P. A. & Andrew, E. R. (1978) RF magnetic field penetration, phase shift and power dissipation in biological tissue: implications for NMR imaging. *Phys. Med. Biol.*, **23**, 630–43.
15. Bottomley, P. A., Hinshaw, W. S. & Holland, G. N. (1978) A computer driven photoscanner for medical imaging. *Phys. Med. Biol.*, **23**, 309–17.
16. Bovée, W. M. M. J., Creyghton, J. H. N., Getreuer, K. W., Korbee, D., Lobregt, S., Smidt, J., Wind, R. A., Lindeman, J., Smid, L. and Posthuma, H. (1980) NMR relaxation and images of human breast tumours *in vitro*. *Phil. Trans. Roy. Soc. B*, **289**, 535–6.
17. Brooker, H. R. & Hinshaw, W. S. (1978). Thin-section NMR imaging. *J. mag. Res.*, **30**, 129–31.
18. Brunner, P. & Ernst, R. R. (1979) Sensitivity and performance time in NMR imaging. *J. mag. Res.*, **33**, 83–106.
19. Budinger, T. F. (1979) Thresholds for physiological effects due to RF and magnetic fields used in NMR imaging. *I.E.E.E. Trans. nucl. Sci.*, **NS-26**, 2821–5.
20. Carrington, A. & McLachlan, A. D. (1967) *Introduction to Magnetic Resonance*. New York: Harper and Row.
21. Clow, H. & Young, I. (1978) Head scans by NMR techniques. *New Scientist*, **80**, 588.
22. Cormack, A. M. (1973) Reconstruction of densities from their projections, with applications to radiological physics. *Phys. Med. Biol.*, **18**, 195–207.
23. Damadian, R. (1971) Tumor detection by nuclear magnetic resonance. *Science*, **171**, 1151–3.
24. Damadian, R., Minkoff, L., Goldsmith, M., Stanford, M. & Koutcher, J. (1976) Field focussing nuclear magnetic resonance (FONAR): visualization of a tumor in a live animal, *Science*, **194**, 1430–2.
25. Damadian, R. (1980) Field focusing N.m.r. (FONAR) and the formation of chemical images in man. *Phil. Trans. Roy. Soc. B*, **289**, 489–500.
26. Damadian, R., Goldsmith, M. & Minkoff, L. (1977) NMR in cancer: XVI. FONAR image of the live human body. *Physiol. Chem. Phys.*, **9**, 97–108.
27. Damadian, R., Minkoff, L., Goldsmith, M. & Koutcher, J. A. (1978) Field-focussing nuclear magnetic resonance (FONAR). *Naturwissenschaften*, **65**, 250–2.
28. Farrar, T. C. & Becker, E. D. (1971) *Pulse and Fourier Transform NMR*. New York: Academic Press.
29. Gabillard, R. (1951) Measurement of relaxation time T_2 in the presence of an inhomogeneous magnetic field. *CR Acad. Sci. (Paris)*, **232**, 1551–3.
30. Gabillard, R. (1952) A steady state transient technique in nuclear resonance. *Phys. Rev.*, **85**, 694–5.
31. Garroway, A. N., Grannell, P. K. & Mansfield, P. (1974) Image formation in NMR by a selective irradiation process. *J. Phys. C: Solid State Phys.*, **7**, L457–62.
32. Hahn, E. L. (1950) Spin echoes. *Phys. Rev.*, **80**, 580–94.
33. Hinshaw, W. S. (1974) Spin mapping. *Phys. Letters*, **A48**, 87–8.
34. Hinshaw, W. S. (1974) The application of time dependent field gradients to NMR spin mapping. In *Proc. 18th AMPERE Congress, Nottingham*, ed. Allen, P. S., Andrew, E. R. & Bates, C. A., pp. 433–4. Amsterdam: North-Holland.
35. Hinshaw, W. S. (1976) Image formation by nuclear magnetic resonance: the sensitive point method. *J. appl. Phys.*, **47**, 3709–21.
36. Hinshaw, W. S., Bottomley, P. A. & Holland, G. N. (1977) Radiographic thin section image of the human wrist by nuclear magnetic resonance. *Nature*, **270**, 722–3.
37. Hinshaw, W. S., Andrew, E. R., Bottomley, P. A., Holland, G. N., Moore, W. S. & Worthington, B. S. (1978) Display of cross-sectional anatomy by nuclear magnetic resonance imaging. *Br. J. Radiol.*, **51**, 273–80.
38. Hinshaw, W. S., Andrew, E. R., Bottomley, P. A., Holland, G. N., Moore, W. S. & Worthington, B. S. (1978) Internal structure mapping by nuclear magnetic resonance. *Neuroradiology*, **16**, 607–9.
39. Hinshaw, W. S., Andrew, E. R., Bottomley, P. A., Holland, G. N., Moore, W. S. & Worthington, B. S. (1979) An *in vivo* study of the forearm and hand by thin section NMR imaging. *Br. J. Radiol.*, **52**, 36–43.
40. Holland, G. N., Bottomley, P. A. & Hinshaw, W. S. (1977) ^{19}F magnetic resonance imaging. *J. mag. Res.*, **28**, 133–6.
41. Hoult, D. I. (1979) Rotating frame zeugmatography. *J. mag. Res.*, **33**, 183–97.
42. Hounsfield, G. N., (1973) Computerised transverse axial scanning (tomography). *Br. J. Radiol.*, **46**, 1016–22.
43. Kumar, A., Welti, D. & Ernst, R. R. (1975) Imaging of macroscopic objects by NMR Fourier zeugmatography. *J. mag. Res.*, **18**, 69–83.
44. Lai, C. M. & Lauterbur, P. C. (1980) True three-

dimensional image reconstruction by nuclear magnetic resonance zeugmatography, (in course of publication).
45. Lauterbur, P. C. (1973) Image formation by induced local interactions: examples employing nuclear magnetic resonance. *Nature*, **242**, 190–1.
46. Lauterbur, P. C., Dulcey, C. S., Lai, C. M., Feiler, M. A., House, W. V., Kramer, D. M., Chen, C. N. & Dias, R. (1974) Magnetic resonance zeugmatography. In *Proc. 18th AMPERE Congress, Nottingham*, ed. Allen, P. S., Andrew, E. R. & Bates, C. A., pp. 27–9. Amsterdam: North-Holland.
47. Lauterbur, P. C. (1980) Progress in N.M.R. zeugmatographic imaging. *Phil. Trans. Roy. Soc. B*, **289**, 483–7.
48. Mallard, J., Hutchison, J. M. S., Edelstein, W. A., Ling, C. R., Foster, M. A. & Johnson, G. (1980) *In vivo* N.M.R. imaging in medicine: the Aberdeen approach, both physical and biological. *Phil. Trans. Roy. Soc. B*, **289**, 519–33.
49. Mansfield, P. (1977) Multiplanar image formation using NMR spin echoes. *J. Phys. C: Solid State Phys.*, **10**, L55–8.
50. Mansfield, P. & Maudsley, A. A. (1977) Medical imaging by NMR. *Br. J. Radiol.*, **50**, 188–94.
51. Mansfield, P., Maudsley, A. A. & Baines, T. (1976) Fast scan proton density imaging by NMR. *J. Phys. E: J. sci. Instr.*, **9**, 271–8.
52. Mansfield, P. & Maudsley, A. A. (1976). Planar spin imaging by NMR. *J. Phys. C: Solid State Phys.*, **9**, L409–12.
53. Mansfield, P., Pykett, I. L., Morris, P. G. & Coupland, R. E. (1978) Human whole-body line-scan imaging by NMR. *Br. J. Radiol.*, **51**, 921–2.
54. Mansfield, P., Morris, P. G., Ordidge, R. J., Coupland, R. E., Bishop, H. M. & Blamey, R. W. (1979) Carcinoma of the breast imaged by nuclear magnetic resonance. *Br. J. Radiol.*, **52**, 242–3.
55. Mansfield, P., Morris, P. G., Ordidge, R. J., Pykett, I. L., Bangert, V. & Coupland, R. E. (1980) Human whole body imaging and detection of breast tumours by N.M.R. *Phil. Trans. Roy. Soc. B*, **289**, 503–10.
56. Mansfield, P. & Grannell, P. K. (1973) NMR 'diffraction' in solids? *J. Phys. C: Solid State Phys.*, **6**, L422–6.
57. Mansfield, P. & Grannell, P. K. (1975) 'Diffraction' and microscopy in solids and liquids by NMR. *Phys. Rev. B*, **12**, 3618–34.
58. Pake, G. E. & Gutowsky, H. S. (1948) Nuclear relaxation in ice at $-180°C$. *Phys. Rev.*, **74**, 979–80.
59. Purcell, E. M., Torrey, H. C. & Pound, R. V. (1946) Resonance absorption by nuclear magnetic moments in a solid. *Phys. Rev.*, **69**, 37–8.
60. Slichter, C. P. (1978) *Principles of Magnetic Resonance.* Berlin: Springer.
61. Sutherland, R. J. & Hutchison, J. M. S. (1978) NMR imaging: image recovery under magnetic fields with large non-uniformities. *J. Phys. E: J. Sci. Instr.*, **11**, 79–83.
62. Walters, G. K. & Fairbank, W. M. (1956) Phase separation in He^3–He^4 solutions. *Phys. Rev.*, **103**, 262–3.
63. Edelstein, W. A., Hutchison, J. M. S., Johnson, G. & Redpath, T. (1980) Spin warp NMR imaging and applications to human and whole-body imaging. *Phys. Med. Biol..*, **25**, 751–6.
64. Doyle, F. A., Pennock, J. M., Orr, J. S., Gore, J. C., Bydder, G. M., Steiner, R. E., Young, I. R., Clow, H., Bailes, D. R., Burl, M., Gilderdale, D. J. & Walters, P. E. (1981) Imaging of the brain by nuclear magnetic resonance. *Lancet*, 11 July, 53–7.
65. Edelstein, W. A., Hutchison, J. M. S., Smith F. W., Mallard, J., Johnson, G. & Redpath, T. W. (1981) Human whole-body NMR tomographic imaging: normal sections. *Br. J. Radiol.*, **54**, 149–51.
66. Hawkes, R. C., Holland, G. N., Moore, W. S. & Worthington, B. S. (1980) Nuclear magnetic resonance tomography of the brain: a preliminary clinical assessment with demonstration of pathology. *J. comput. asst Tomography*, **4**, 577–86.
67. Holland, G. N., Hawkes, R. C. & Moore, W. S. (1980) Nuclear magnetic resonance tomography of the brain: coronal and sogittal sections. *J. comput. asst Tomography*, **4**, 429–33.
68. Smith, F. W., Malland, J. R., Reid, A. & Hutchison, J. M. S. (1981) Nuclear magnetic resonance tomographic imaging in liver disease. *Lancet*, 2 May, 963–6.

Perception and evaluation of images

M. Susan Chesters

INTRODUCTION

The usual reason for forming an image of some part of the body is to decide whether or not an abnormality is present. The task of the observer is two-fold: to detect the abnormality and to recognise it as such. Very little reference is made in this chapter to the mechanism of pattern recognition partly because very little is known about the subject. Since detection must occur for recognition to take place, however, it seems reasonable that considerations of detectability should take precedence over those of recognisability. It is an open question whether, once detection has occurred, recognition can be aided by improving the quality of the image.

Following this reasoning, it appears that the quality of the image should be evaluated initially in terms of its detectability. Since most medical images are at present viewed by a human observer, only detection by such an observer is considered. Furthermore, the imaging device should be designed to facilitate detection by the human observer. To be able to make generalisations about the desirable properties of the image it would be necessary to understand the mechanism of visual detection. Unfortunately relatively little is known about the mechanism at present.

The quality of a given imaging system could be measured by purely objective methods only if the effect of a measured characteristic on detectability were understood. In the absence of a comprehensive theory of detectability such knowledge is lacking and more direct subjective methods of assessment are preferable. The quality of an image is often limited, for example by the dose of radiation that can be given to the patient. The question then arises: is it possible to process a given image to produce one of higher quality? The processing of images is a rapidly evolving technique and new methods are being tried. The use of computers in the production of images has greatly increased the scope of the technique.

PHYSIOLOGY OF THE EYE AND BRAIN

Anatomy of the visual system

Light enters the eye through an aperture known as the pupil. The size of the pupil can be varied by the iris (Fig. 7.1) which surrounds it: the size varies from about 2 mm diameter in very bright light to 8 mm in darkness. The light is then focused by the lens on the retina which forms the rear surface of the eye. The focusing power of the eye is variable by the action of the ciliary muscle. When viewing distant objects the muscles are relaxed but in order to bring nearby objects into focus the eye accommodates, i.e. the eye muscles contract increasing the power of the lens.

The retina is a complex structure containing cells of many types (Fig. 7.2). Although the anatomy of the retina is well-documented,[72,24] the functions of many types of cell remain obscure. Three main categories, however, can be distinguished: (1) the initial receptors called *rods* or *cones*; (2) *bipolar* cells; and (3) *ganglion* cells.

The rods and cones contain photosensitive pigments which are bleached by light. The cells respond to light by passing an electrical potential to the bipolar cells. The cones appear not to respond at low luminances, below approximately 10^{-2} cd m^{-2}, whereas a rod can respond to as few as four to six incident photons.[38] The maximum sensitivity of the rod response, however, is attained only after a

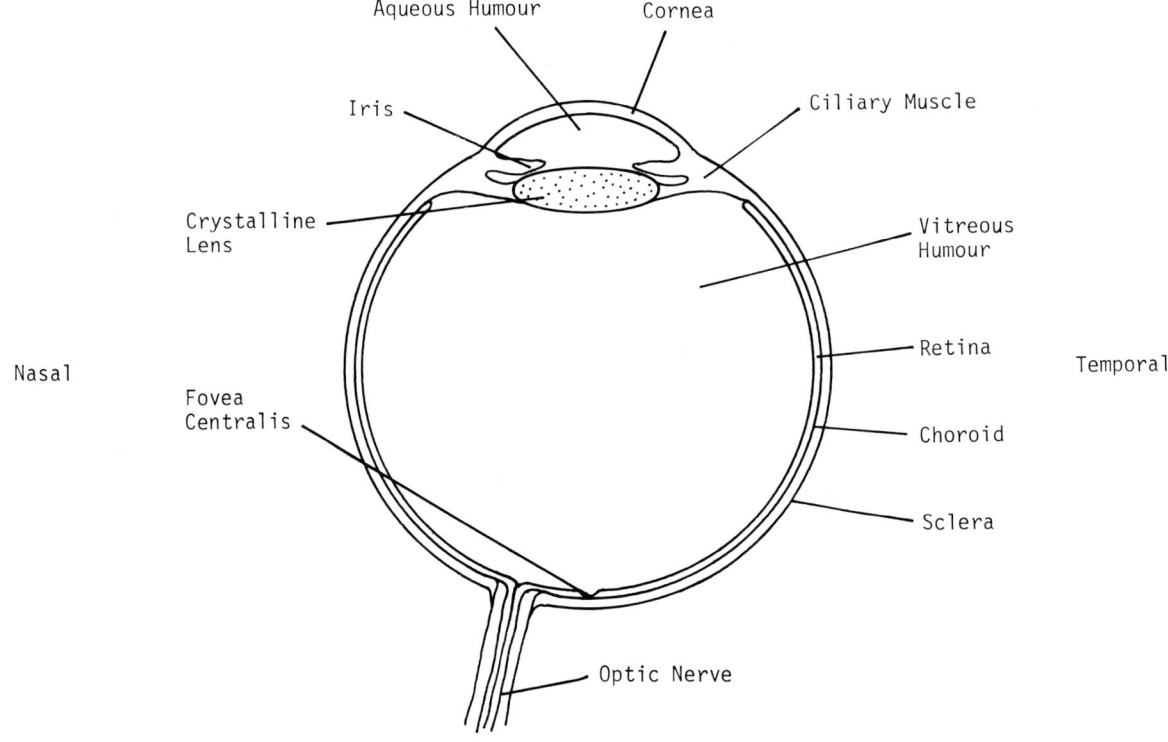

Fig. 7.1 Horizontal section of the human right eye.[56]

period of dark adaptation (of the order of 45 min after the transition from a high mean luminance to complete darkness) to allow for regeneration of the pigment. The rods are less sensitive than the cones over those luminance levels at which the cones are sensitive. The cones are capable of distinguishing colours, but the rods are not.

The sensitivity of the eye to colour (that is, to light of different wavelengths) can be explained by the Young-Helmholtz theory of colour vision. Young (1773–1829) performed experiments in which he showed that any colour in the visible spectrum of light can be matched by the sum of certain proportions of three principal colours, red, green and violet. He suggested that at each sensitive small region of the retina there are three kinds of receptor responding selectively to red, green and violet light. It is now known that in the normal eye each cone contains just one of three kinds of photosensitive pigment that is maximally sensitive in either the red, green or blue region of the spectrum.[12] In about 10 per cent of men and rarely in women, one or more of the three kinds of receptor is either completely absent or is markedly less sensitive than in normal men and women. This minority lacks the normal ability to distinguish colours: commonly, red is confused with green but some people cannot distinguish green and blue. In the complete absence of one type of cone, colour blindness exists. Other less extreme deficiencies resulting in anomalous colour vision can be revealed by colour mixing and matching experiments.

The distribution of the rods and cones across the surface of the retina is not uniform. There is one region called the *fovea centralis* (Fig. 7.1) in which only cones are present. Moving across the retina away from the fovea to the periphery the cone density falls rapidly and is soon far exceeded by the rod density. An image is normally focused on the fovea and within the fovea the diameter of a cone reaches its minimum value. The cones are tightly packed with a spacing, centre to centre, of $0.12 - 0.15$ mrad.[68] The fovea is capable of the best resolution of an image: in fact the cone spacing can be shown to be well-matched to the highest resolv-

PERCEPTION AND EVALUATION OF IMAGES 239

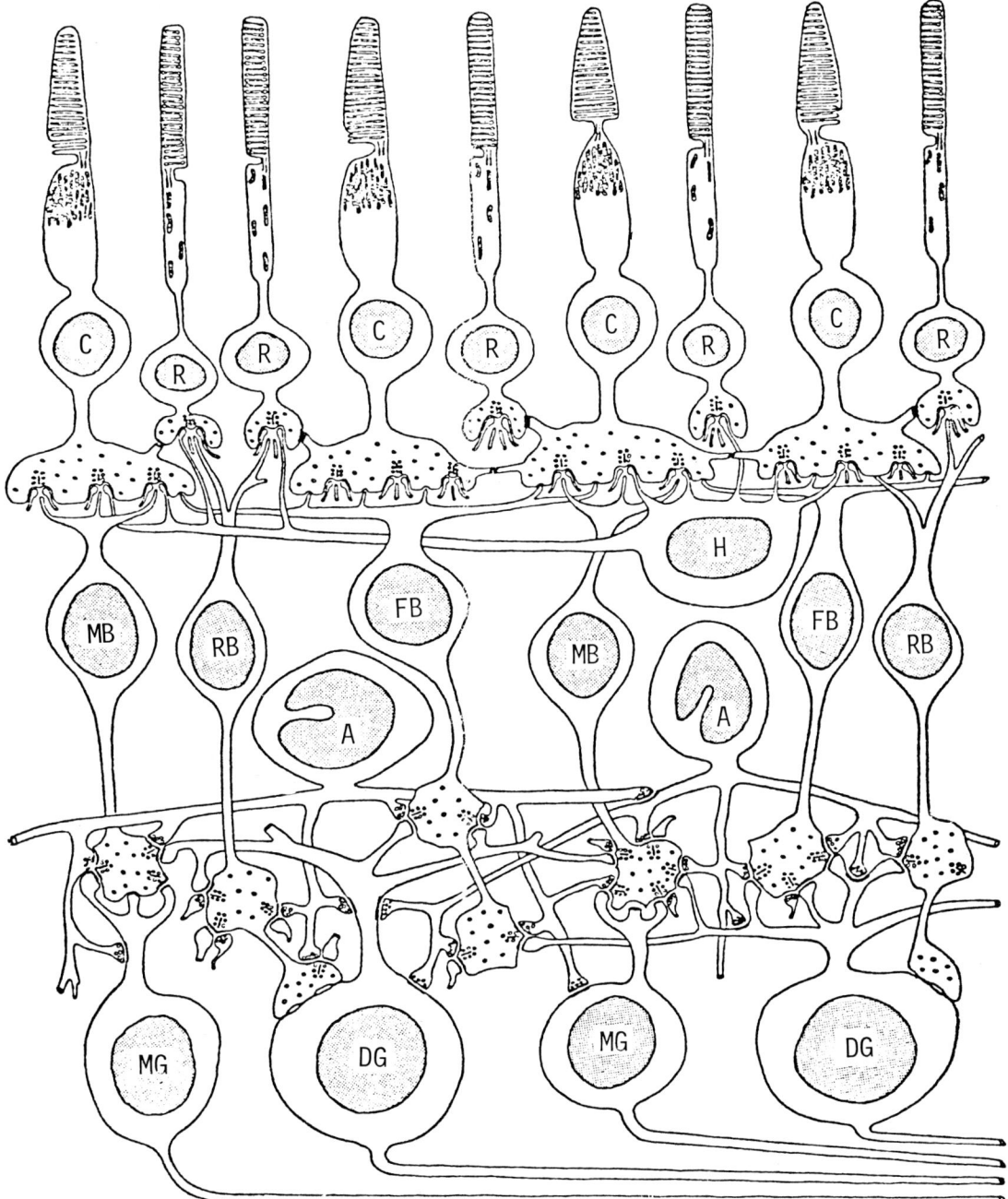

Fig. 7.2 Schematic drawing of the primate retina. The types of cell represented are: R, rod; C, cone; MB, midget bipolar; RB, rod bipolar; FB, flat bipolar; H, horizontal cell; A, amacrine cell; MG, midget ganglion; DG, diffuse ganglion.[24]

able spatial frequency for high mean luminances.[81]

The bipolar cells are more than mere relay stations for the electrical signal. Anatomically there are many interconnexions between them, mediated perhaps by horizontal and amacrine cells, and these connexions could well be used to modify the signal leaving a bipolar cell. Indeed it has been shown that activity in one cell can inhibit the response rate from a neighbouring cell. This kind of interaction has been called lateral inhibition. The inhibitory action of the response of a given cell has been shown to extend not merely to its immediate neighbours but also to quite distant cells.

The bipolar cells transmit electrical signals to ganglion cells. Again there are interconnexions between ganglion cells providing the means for positive and negative interaction between them. Two main types of ganglion cell, classified as X- and Y-types, have been identified in the cat[25] depending on the nature of their response. Similar types of cell have been discovered also in the monkey. In the fovea most cones have a one-to-one connexion with a midget ganglion cell via a midget bipolar (Fig. 7.2). Clearly, this arrangement is capable of preserving the high resolution of the densely packed cones.

Output signals from the ganglion cells are transmitted to the cerebral cortex via the optic nerve (Fig. 7.3). Before reaching the cortex, however,

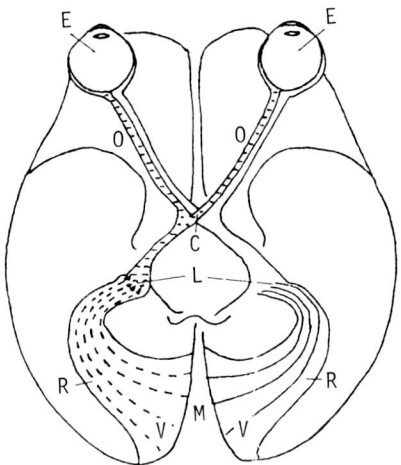

Fig. 7.3 Schematic view from underneath the brain of the primate visual system. E, eyes; O, optic nerve fibres; C, optic chiasma; L, lateral geniculate bodies; R, visual radiation (or geniculo-calcarine tract); V, visual cortex; M, mid-line between the two halves of the brain.[76]

the optic nerve fibres from the inner half of each retina cross at the optic chiasma and are connected to the opposite side of the cortex: those from the outer half are connected to the same side. Thus, the left hemisphere receives input from the left half of the retina of each eye and similarly for the right hemisphere. Therefore it is possible for the brain to compare the messages received from both eyes.

This information could be used in the perception of depth. Input from the optic nerve is received initially by cells of the lateral geniculate nucleus (LGN) situated in the thalamus. Since each cell of the LGN receives input from only one or a very small number of ganglion cells it is not surprising that the response is similar to that of a ganglion cell. LGN cells with X- or Y-type responses have been identified.

Finally, input from the LGN is received by cells of the visual cortex (that part of the cerebral cortex apparently concerned with the analysis of visual information). Overall there is a conformal mapping of the retina on to the visual cortex so that spatial relations are preserved. Cells of the visual cortex are arranged in six layers but more significantly they appear to be connected in columns at right angles to the layers. Cells in a given column are found to respond to stimuli that have certain features in common (p. 241).

Although different classes of *nerve cell* or *neurone* differ considerably in morphology they share certain basic features. The cell body contains the nucleus and extending from the body are branching structures called *dendrites*. Also extending from the cell body in some classes of neurone is a cylindrically-shaped axon which carries the afferent electrical signal from the neurone. The dendrites receive electrical signals from the axons of many other neurones. The point of contact of an axon terminal with a dendrite is called the *synapse*. Transmission of the electrical signal across the synapse is achieved usually by chemical neurotransmitters or more rarely by direct electrical contact. Electrical potentials within the body of the neurone and adjacent to it can be recorded directly by microelectrodes. Neurones in the distal retina respond to electrical stimulation with slow, graded, hyperpolarising potentials (i.e., potentials more negative than the resting potential). This type of response is characteristic of the rods and cones and the horizontal and bipolar cells.[95] In the proximal retina, however, neurones such as amacrine and ganglion cells respond with transient, depolarising potentials (i.e. potentials more positive than the resting potential). If the stimulation received is strong enough these classes of neurone respond by emitting voltage pulses along the axon. The size of the pulse leaving the neurone along the axon is approximately constant: it is the frequency with which pulses are emitted that is determined by the strength of the stimulus received by the neurone. Excitatory stimuli increase the pulse rate initially, although the rate may subsequently decrease even while the stimulus is maintained. Inhibitory stimuli decrease the pulse rate, sometimes to zero, but on removing the stimulus the cell responds vigorously for a time. The X-type of ganglion cell differs from the Y-type in giving a more sustained response. Even in the absence of any stimulus there is considerable activity among neurones belonging to the visual system. This random activity could be an important source of neural noise within the system (p. 243): the term *noise* is used to denote any random activity or possibly an unwanted signal.

The receptive field

The *receptive field* of a neurone[35] is that area of the retina within which visual stimuli provoke a response in the neurone. The stimulus can be either a positive or negative increment of luminance and its effect can be either excitatory or inhibitory. The characteristics of the response of the receptive field can usually be ascertained by moving a point of light across the retina and by recording the electrical activity of the neurone by means of a microelectrode. The receptive field can be regarded as the sampling aperture of the given neurone.

The receptive fields of the neurones that link the cones to the visual cortex directly (the bipolar, ganglion and LGN neurones) are characterised by a centre-surround configuration that is approximately circularly symmetrical. The ganglion cells of the cat are of two distinct kinds.[51] Some cells respond, perhaps only transiently, by increasing their discharge frequency when a spot of light at the centre of their receptive field is switched on: this is called an 'on' response (Fig. 7.4). The discharge frequency of others, conversely, is reduced by switching on the spot of light and increased only when the light is switched off: this is called an 'off' response. The surrounding regions of the receptive fields of both types of cell are antagonistic to their centres. Thus on-centre cells have off-response surrounds, and vice versa. In ganglion cells of the central fovea studied in the monkey the diameters of the centres of the receptive fields are about 1 mrad, but towards the periphery the diameters increase. Maximum response is obtained for a visual stimulus that matches in extent the area

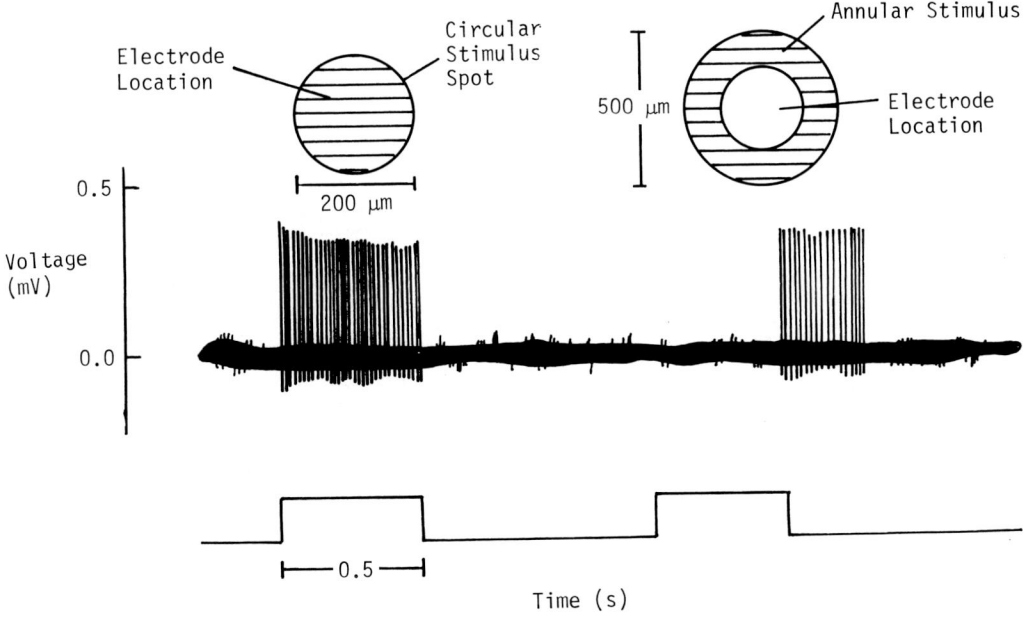

Fig. 7.4 Response potentials recorded from a retinal ganglion cell. The cell responds at the onset of illumination by a central light spot ('on' response) and at the cessation of illumination by a surround annulus ('off' response). The period of stimulation is marked by an upward shift of the time baseline.[76]

of the receptive field centre. If the whole receptive field (both centre and surround) is uniformly illuminated, however, no response is recorded from the cell.

Receptive fields of cells in the visual cortex show more diversity of form. By recording from cells in the visual cortex, four classes of cell – 'circularly symmetric', 'simple', 'complex' and 'hypercomplex'—have been identified according to the characteristics of their receptive fields.[46] The circularly symmetric cells have receptive fields very similar to cells of the LGN. Simple cells are sensitive, however, to bar-shaped stimuli or edges of specific orientations and at a well-defined position in the field of vision (relative to the centre of attention which is focused on the centre of the fovea). Complex cells are equally specific for orientation but respond to correctly-oriented stimuli over a much more extensive part of the field of vision (Fig. 7.5).

increasing the width from its optimal value diminishes the response and zero response is obtained if the receptive field is uniformly illuminated. The stimuli that evoke responses in hypercomplex cells differ in just one respect from those that cause complex cells to respond. If the length of the bar is extended beyond a certain size the response is reduced or even abolished, whereas in complex cells it remains at a constant value. Many cortical neurones that are specific for orientation can be stimulated through either eye although the response through one eye (the dominant eye) can be much greater than that through the other. The receptive fields are very similar whichever eye is used. Cortical neurones with circularly symmetrical fields, on the other hand, appear to respond through only one eye.

Inevitably most of the investigations into the anatomy and physiology of the visual system have

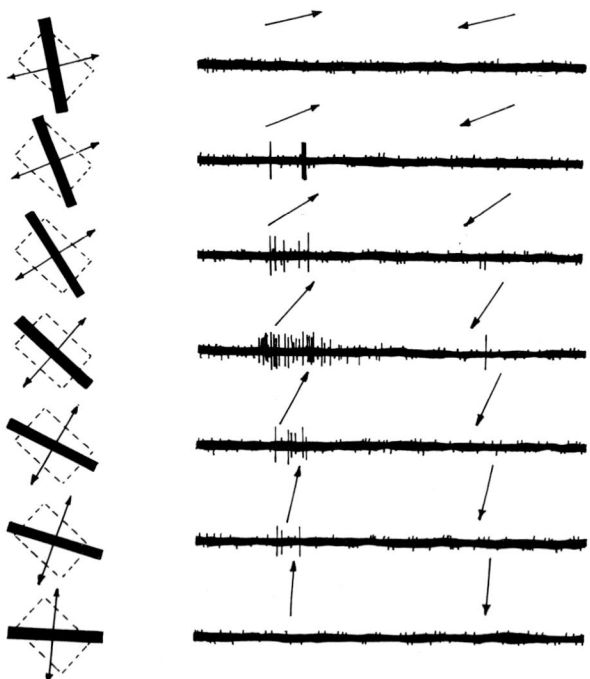

Fig. 7.5 Responses of a complex cell in the visual cortex to various orientations of a moving dark bar. The arrows indicate the direction of movement. The receptive field in the left eye is indicated by the broken lines; it was approximately 6.5×6.5 mrad^2 in size and was situated 70 mrad below and to the left of the point of fixation. The duration of each record was 2 s. The intensity of the background was 20 cd m^{-2} and that of the dark bar 1 cd m^{-2}.[46]

They are usually particularly sensitive to the movement of a bar or edge in one direction at right angles to its orientation. Those cells that respond to bars are also specific for the width of the bar;

been performed on non-human animals. It is always questionable whether the findings in lower animals can be extrapolated to man. Certainly, species differences exist. For example, the stimuli that provoke responses in the ganglion cells of the frog show far greater diversity than those of the cat or monkey. A very few microelectrode recordings have been made on the human visual cortex.[61] Of the 20 cells sampled, all had circularly symmetric receptive fields. The human visual system is likely to resemble most closely that of the monkey. There is certainly clear evidence that the visual cortex of the monkey is capable of considerable analysis of the field of vision.

Visual noise

The absorption of photons by the initial receptors (rods and cones) of the retina is a random process. On average, approximately 55 per cent of incident photons are absorbed by the visual pigment of the rods[98] and of the cones.[49] Of these perhaps 60 per cent cause isomerisation and hence excitation.[4] The number of photons absorbed follows a Poisson distribution. Retinal absorption is certainly one source of noise within the visual system.

There are, however, other possible sources. One is thermal isomerisation of pigment molecules causing responses indistinguishable from those evoked by light. In the absence of light, electrical activity called the dark current can be observed in the retina.[52] It is of a very low amplitude, however, and makes only a minimal contribution to the total noise power except in complete darkness. The dark current among cones is some 3000 times greater than among rods.[2] A correspondingly higher rate of thermal isomerisation of the cone pigments could account for it. The higher noise level among cones could well explain the greater sensitivity of rods at low luminances (see pp. 237 and 244).

Noise could be generated at a synapse if the electrical signal was not reliably transmitted. Thus noise could be introduced at each level of the visual system from the ganglion cell layer to the visual cortex. The noise introduced would not have been processed by the more distal cells. Thus, for example, any lateral inhibitory action occurring among bipolar cells would not affect the noise arising more proximally in, say, the ganglion cells.

Imperfections in the central detecting mechanisms themselves can be responsible for introducing further statistical uncertainty. One attempt to measure the efficiency of these mechanisms has been described.[4] A random-dot pattern is presented to the eye and the dots are of such a high intensity that individually they cannot fail to be detected. The strategy is the same as that employed in the intensification of X-ray images (see p. 265). The result is that just as the principal source of noise in the intensified X-ray image is the random arrival of the quanta, so, in the dot image, variation in the spatial distribution of the dots far exceeds any variation in absorption of the photons that comprise the dots. The observer is required to detect the presence of a signal composed of an area in which the dot density is greater than the surround. It can be shown that the slope of the *frequency-of-seeing curve* of the signal depends on the standard deviation of the number of dots comprising the signal, i.e. on the square root of the mean number of dots within the signal. The observed slope, however, is consistent with the participation in the detection process of only 50 per cent of the dots. The relative noise appears to be greater than can be accounted for by fluctuation in the total number of dots. An additional source of noise between the retina and the threshold decision site would also explain this finding.

Under normal viewing conditions the statistical fluctuations in the visual signal received by the brain are not perceived. When an additional source of fluctuation is introduced into the light entering the eye, however, as for example when the light is generated by X-ray quanta falling on a fluorescent screen, the noise can often be clearly seen (pp. 254 and 265).

Linearity of the visual system

It is important to establish, if possible, whether or not the visual system is linear. Theoretical analysis is considerably simplified if linearity can be assumed, since, for example, Fourier techniques can be applied. It has been accepted for many years, however, that nonlinearity obtains. It has been postulated that a just noticeable difference in luminance, ΔI, corresponds to a fixed unit of sensation.[26] Since, according to Weber's law ΔI is proportional to the mean luminance, I, over a wide range of luminances, it may then be deduced that the eye responds logarithmically to light. Suppose that the visual sensation, S, is some function, $f(I)$, of the luminance I. Then $\Delta S \simeq f'(I)\Delta I$ and if $\Delta S = c$ and $\Delta I = kI$, where c and k are constants, $f'(I) = c/kI$, whence $f(I) = (c/k) \ln I$. More recently, by comparing different signal modalities, it has been suggested that a power law with an exponent of one-third is obeyed.[83]

Nevertheless, if the mean luminance is kept approximately constant, there is some evidence that small increments of luminance can evoke responses that are linearly related to the amplitude of the increment. Some of the evidence is neurophysiological and some psychophysical.

It has been shown that X-type ganglion cells of the cat respond linearly to the contrast of a grating pattern of low contrast.[25] The response tends to a constant level as the contrast is increased. The cells also exhibit linear spatial summation over their receptive fields. X-type cells predominate in the central retina. Y-type cells appear to respond nonlinearly at all contrasts. At the level of the LGN in the cat, linearity of response to the contrast of gratings in X-type cells has also been found.[60] In the simple cells of the cortex, however, the response amplitude is apparently proportional to log contrast.

Some psychophysical evidence also suggests that under certain conditions linearity can obtain. Rectangular waves with duty cycles of 0·5, 0·33 and 0·25 can be synthesised when their first two harmonics are presented monoptically, one eye viewing the fundamental and the other the next higher harmonic.[59] These experiments suggest that no significant nonlinear distortion of the signal takes place at least prior to binocular fusion. Since the simple cells of the cortex are the most distal to receive input from both eyes it seems that the visual system is approximately linear up to this level. Contrast matching and contrast estimating experiments[31] have also shown a linear relationship between estimated contrast and objective contrast.

Although the evidence in favour of linearity is far from conclusive there is probably sufficient to justify the assumption for relatively small contrasts. Fortunately, at least when no noise external to the visual system is present, all the contrasts necessary for threshold detectability are small at the retina. Even though, for small signals, input threshold contrasts increase in inverse proportion to the square of the diameter of the input signal, it can be shown that the maximum contrast at the retina is less than approximately 0·3. This contrast is well within the range found to be processed linearly.

There is one important kind of investigation, the discrimination of signals from noise, in which non-linearity can sometimes be ignored. Suppose the signal and the noise are responsible for two probability distributions of a decision variable, x. It has been shown in connexion with signal detection theory[34] (and see p. 259) that an optimum strategy for discriminating a signal from noise is to accept as a signal all $x > x_C$, where x_C is a chosen criterion value, and to reject as noise all $x < x_C$. If the signal and the noise are transformed by any one-to-one (linear or nonlinear) transformation, the probabilities of the transformed signal and noise lying respectively above and below the transform of x_C are the same as before the transformation. An alternative way of expressing this result is that the *ROC curve* (p. 261) is invariant under the specified transformation. The condition that the signal and the noise are subject to the same transformation, however, is essential. To fulfill this condition in the visual system, one necessary requirement is that the principle source of noise must arise distal to the nonlinearity.

The evidence just reviewed is probably sufficient to justify the assumption of linearity in the analysis of the response of the visual system to signals of low contrast when the mean luminance is kept constant. In the absence of external noise, at the threshold of detectability all signals are of sufficiently low contrast at the retina to be processed linearly by the eye. Furthermore, even for high contrast signals detectability is unaffected by nonlinearity if both the signals and the noise are subject to the same nonlinearity, as when noise external to the visual system is present.

SIGNAL-SPECIFIC, NOISE-LIMITED MODELS OF DETECTION

Historical development

In a classic paper, Hecht, Schlaer and Pirenne[38] demonstrated that fluctuation in the stimulus could be a major factor governing the response of the organism. These results were obtained with a background of zero luminance. Rose[74,75] and de Vries,[23] however, proposed that fluctuation in the absorption of quanta could account for the threshold of detectability of an incremental signal on a background of any luminance. These were perhaps the first suggestions that noise internal to the visual system could influence or even determine detectability. In detecting a disc-shaped signal, the difference between the number of quanta absorbed from the signal and from a corresponding area of the background must exceed the standard deviation of the number of absorbed quanta from the background by a certain constant, k, which is the signal-to-noise ratio (Fig. 7.6). For a signal of di-

contrasts agreed with those observed but for a very limited range of disc diameters. Considerable divergence was found for both large and small discs.

In fact neither Rose nor de Vries attempted to account for the inevitable distortion of the image in its passage through the visual system. It is very unlikely that detection occurs in the retina. Adapting to a grating of high contrast presented to one eye elevates the contrast threshold of a similar grating presented to the other eye[28] suggesting that detection occurs after comparison of the inputs from both eyes becomes possible. Therefore, the image received has been modified in passing through the ocular media of the eye and also pos-

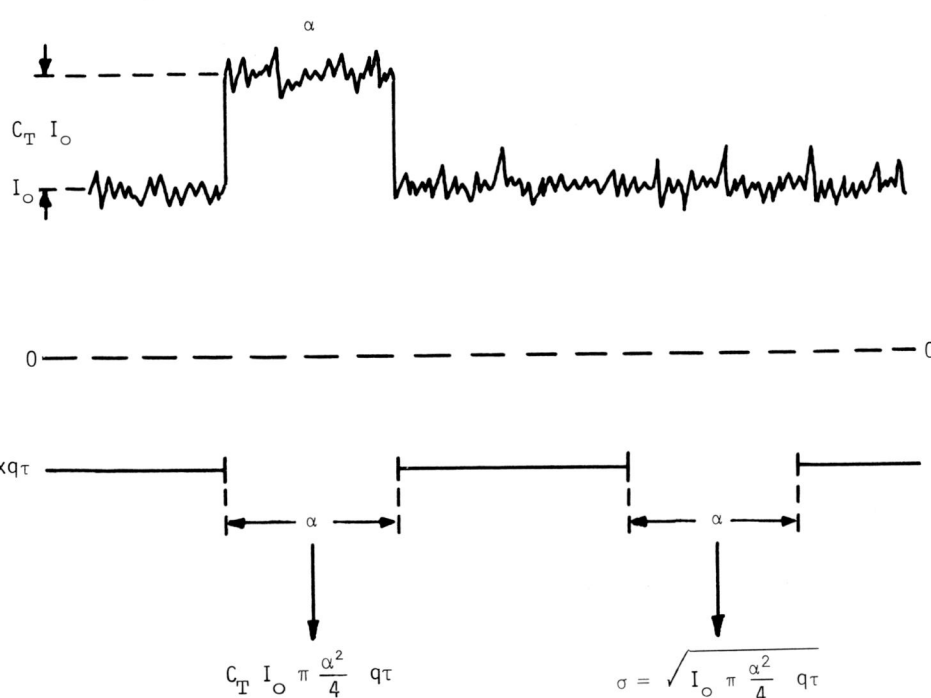

Fig. 7.6 Rose-de Vries model. The intensity within an incremental disc-shaped signal of diameter α and of contrast C_T above a background of luminance I_0 is integrated and compared with samples of equal area of the fluctuation in the background luminance, I_0: τ is the temporal sampling aperture and q is the fraction absorbed of the incident quanta.

ameter α and threshold contrast, C_T, above a background of luminance I_0, $C_T = 2k/\alpha\sqrt{(I_0 q \tau \pi)}$, where τ is the temporal sampling aperture and q is the fraction absorbed of the incident quanta. Rose calculated the threshold contrasts for discs of a range of diameters and for several background luminances. Assuming that $\tau = 200$ ms, $k = 5$ and q is in the range 0·5–5 per cent, his calculated threshold

sibly by neural processing. The modified image is, of course, what the observer 'sees': he or she is unaware of the luminance distribution from which that image derives. The simple concept of signal-to-noise ratio found in the Rose and de Vries models has also been elaborated and extended in signal detection theory.[34] Some of these ideas have been incorporated into a model for the detection of disc-shaped incremental signals which also allows for the modification of the signals and the noise by the unsharpness of the visual system.[17,37,79] These models are outlined after considering the effect of the unsharpness of the visual system on visual signals and noise and the application of signal detection theory to the detection of visual, disc-shaped signals.

A Rose-de Vries model has been applied to the detectability of signals where the principal source of noise arises external to the visual system.[85] It was postulated that X-ray quantum fluctuations limit the detectability of X-ray images. The extended version of the Rose-de Vries model, to be described later, has also been applied to the detectability of images limited by such external sources of noise.

Modification of the object by the visual system

The visual signal received at the retina after passing through the ocular media is relayed through the various layers of the retina and then via the optic nerve to the visual cortex where detection is most likely to occur (p. 244). The anatomy and physiology of the visual system is such as to suggest that considerable processing of the neural signal could take place. The image reaching the retina, however, is already unsharp after passing through the ocular media. The distribution of light from a point source (the point spread function (PSF)) has been measured after a double transit through the ocular media and diffuse reflexion from the retina.[15] The measurement has been repeated for different pupil diameters, giving for each one the point spread function of the ocular media and scattering within the retina. For small pupil diameters, the spread function approaches the diffraction limit, but, for larger diameters, aberrations significantly degrade the image. The most important aberration is the chromatic difference of focus.[92]

Measurement of the effect of additional processing of the signal by the neural system is more difficult. A straightforward approach is to measure the apparent loss of contrast of sinusoidal distributions of light of a range of spatial frequencies thus obtaining directly the modulation transfer function (MTF) of the complete visual system. It can be shown[55] that the MTF is the Fourier transform of the PSF of a linear system. Thus, determination of the MTF is equivalent to measuring the PSF. The measurement of the loss of contrast, however, presents theoretical and practical difficulties. The usual method is to determine the contrast sensitivity (the reciprocal of the threshold contrast) for a range of spatial frequencies. To interpret the contrast sensitivity as proportional to the MTF for all frequencies requires the assumption that the decision criterion (i.e. the level that must be reached by the signal at the detection site for detection to occur, as discussed on p. 248) is constant for all frequencies. This assumption does not necessarily hold in principle. Indeed, if the decision criterion is proportional to the standard deviation, SD, of the noise that limits detectability (i.e., the effective noise) and the effective noise is different for different spatial frequencies (p. 247), the assumption is false. Nevertheless, the contrast sensitivity curve depends on the MTF of the visual system and if due allowance could be made for changes in the decision criterion the MTF could be derived. To obtain reliable information for the low spatial frequencies a large field of vision is required.[45] It has been suggested[45] that sinusoids are detected area by area, where both the height and width of an area are proportional to the wavelength. In this case the noise that limits detectability is sampled over an area proportional to the square of the wavelength of the sinusoid. If the noise power spectrum were uniform, the contrast sensitivity curve could be corrected for changes in the decision criterion by multiplying by the spatial frequency. If the principal source of noise is external to the eye or arises in the retinal receptors, however, the noise power spectrum is proportional to the square of the MTF. Multiplying by the spatial frequency then overcorrects the contrast sensitivity curve at low frequencies although the correction should be reasonably accurate for the higher frequencies. Nevertheless the resulting curve is probably the best estimate available of the shape of the MTF of the visual system: Figure 7.7a shows the normalised and corrected MTF for 10 cd m^{-2}.[91]

The shape of the MTF differs markedly from that of the MTF of the ocular media alone, for a pupil diameter of 3·8 mm corresponding to 10 cd m^{-2},[15] also shown in Figure 7.7a. The MTF of the visual system has been normalised to fit the MTF of the ocular media at high frequencies. At low frequencies the MTF of the visual system increases progressively and is asymptotic to a square law.

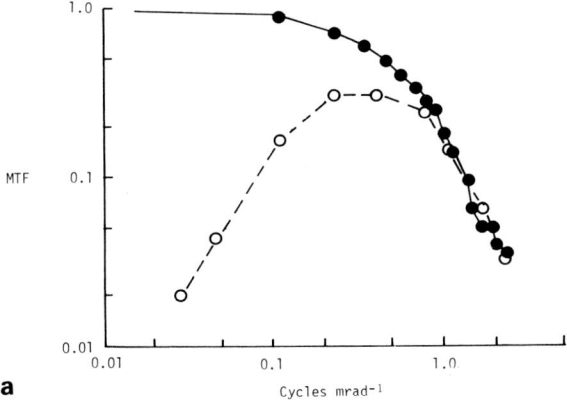

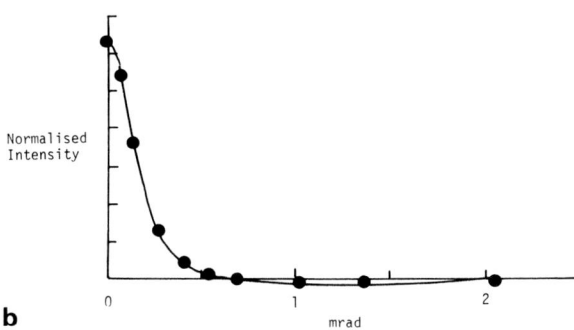

Fig. 7.7 (a) MTF of the ocular media (●) at a mean luminance of 10 cd m^{-2},[15] shown on double logarithmic scales. The MTF of the complete visual system (o) for 10 cd m^{-2} is shown normalised to fit the MTF of the ocular media at high frequencies. (From [91] but corrected for hypothesised changes in the decision criteria.) (b) PSF corresponding to the MTF of the complete visual system shown in (a). Linear scales: the vertical scale is arbitrary. The amplitude of the negative lobe of the PSF has been amplified for clarity of representation.

This characteristic is equivalent to double differentiation in space.[10] The point spread function, PSF, corresponding to this MTF is shown in Figure 7.7b. It has a narrow central core of half-width 0·4 mrad and a much wider negative surround extending to a diameter of about 30 mrad. The effect of convoluting input signals of a range of diameters and of unit intensity with the PSF is shown in Figure 7.8. The profiles of both large and small signals are changed considerably. The central contrast of large signals is reduced almost to zero and the edges are relatively enhanced. Signals that are small compared with the central core of the PSF take on the shape of the PSF although their maximum contrast is proportional to the area of the input signal.

Another possible technique for measuring the MTF of the visual system is subjective matching.[30] The observers adjust the objective contrast of a sinusoidal grating of a certain spatial frequency to match subjectively that of a standard grating of 5 cycles deg^{-1}. The results are somewhat surprising. The most important finding is that if the objective contrast of the standard grating is set at a high level (e.g. two decades above threshold) the same objective contrast is required for gratings of other spatial frequencies to achieve a subjective match. This phenomenon is called *contrast constancy*. As the contrast of the standard is increased above the threshold contrast there is a progressive change in shape from that of the contrast sensitivity curve to a nearly horizontal line. This phenomenon may be the result of a compensatory mechanism in the visual cortex that counteracts the effect on the signal of the initial optical and neural unsharpnesses;[30] the compensating mechanism applies only after the signal has been detected, i.e. after the threshold decision site. Consequently, the compensatory mechanism does not apply either to the signal or to the noise prior to the threshold decision site. Unfortunately, the method of contrast matching gives no information about the MTF that affects the signal and the noise prior to detection.

The signal-specific effect of noise

An important consequence of the Rose-de Vries type of model[36] is the specificity of the interaction between the signal and the noise. The signal is compared with noise sampled over an area of the same size as the signal. The spatial frequencies in the noise spectrum that are of negligibly small amplitude in the transform of the signal make a negligible contribution to the total noise effective for that signal. A practical consequence is that detectability would not be improved by reducing those frequencies in the noise that are not represented in the signal (see p. 273).

A model that leads to a different conclusion has

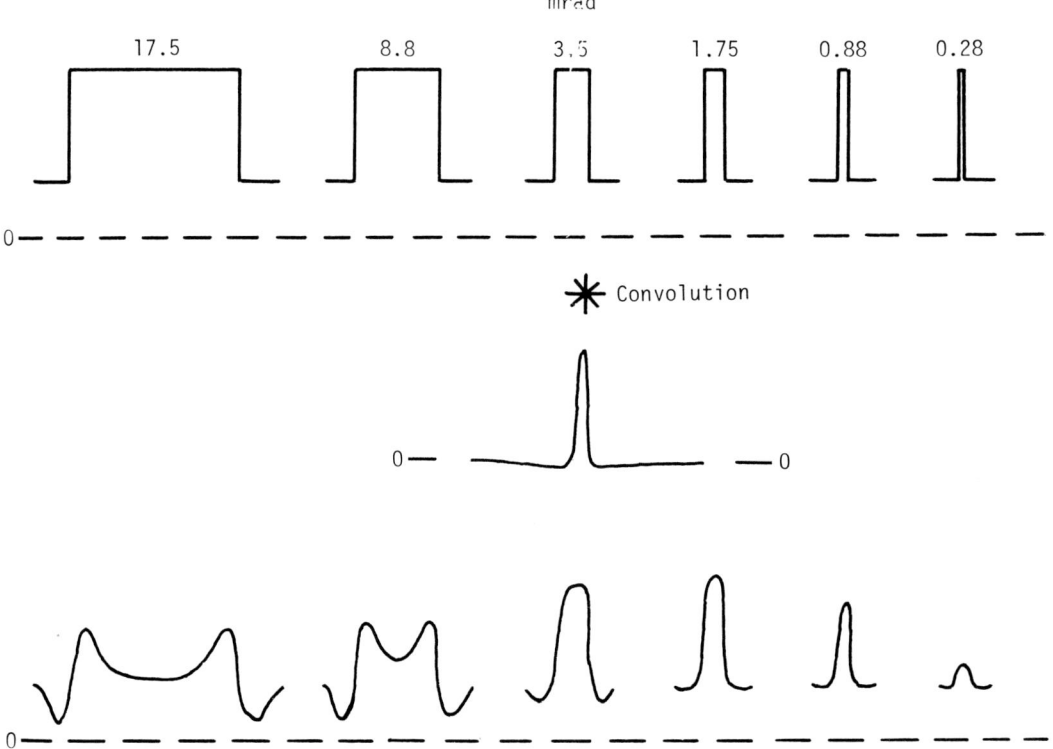

Fig. 7.8 Convolution of disc-shaped incremental signals, ranging in diameter from 17·5–0·28 mrad, with the point spread-function of the visual system.

been proposed.[66] Implicitly, a very small aperture of constant size is used in sampling any signal and the noise. The power of the noise that limits the detectability of any size of signal is constant and the maximum available. The signal is detected if its peak contrast exceeds the coefficient of variation of the noise by a factor k. The variation in threshold contrast of disc-shaped signals with their diameter is then explained solely by the loss of contrast of the signal before reaching the site of detection.

There is direct experimental evidence, however, that changes in the spectrum of noise do not affect all signals equally. If the noise spectrum is changed, e.g. by introducing additional unsharpness into the noise background, there is a decrease in the threshold contrasts of only those signals comparable in extent to and smaller than the unsharpness. Figure 7.9 shows the threshold contrasts for disc-shaped signals displayed on a noise background consisting of the magnified image of photographic granularity. On defocusing the noise, thereby introducing additional unsharpness of diameter 4 mrad, the threshold contrasts of those discs of diameters approximately 10 mrad and less are decreased, whereas the threshold contrasts of the large discs remain virtually unchanged.[17]

Application of signal detection theory to the noise-integration signal-specific model

Further understanding of the detection mechanism has come from *signal detection theory* (SDT) (p. 259). According to this theory the sensory responses, x, evoked by successive samples of a given signal are variable and can be described by a probability distribution, $f(x|s)$, as shown in Figure 7.10. The responses to samples of the background are described by the probability distribution, $f(x|n)$, and are indistinguishable from those evoked by the signal except by their amplitude. One possible strategy that could be adopted by an observer to detect the presence of a signal would be to choose a level of response, D, the decision criterion, and

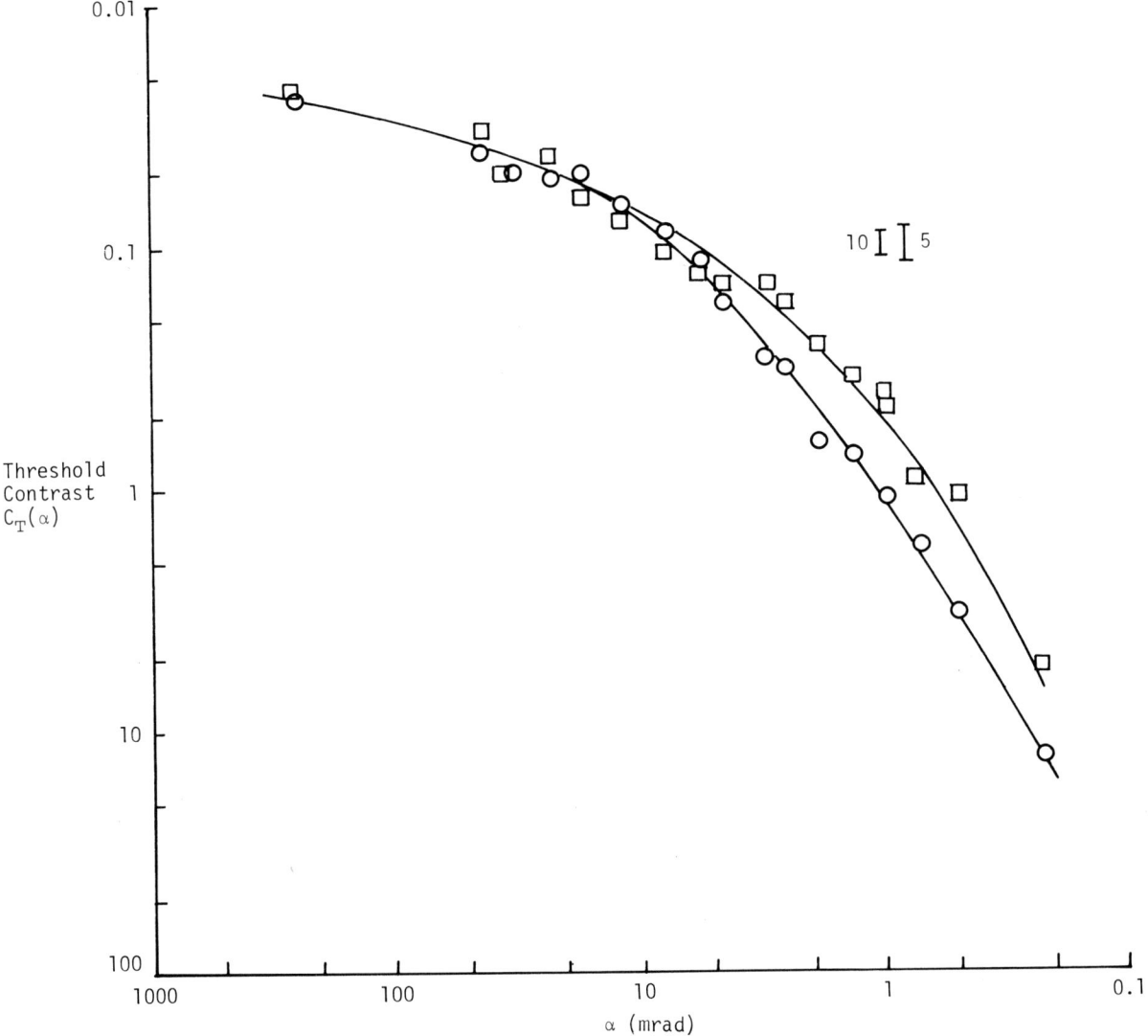

Fig. 7.9 Threshold contrasts, $C_T(\alpha)$, for incremental disc-shaped signals, of initial diameter α mrad, displayed on noise backgrounds of mean luminance 7 cd m^{-2}: focused noise and signals (○); defocused noise and focused signals (□): log scales. Points labelled 'о' and '□' are the means of 10 and 5 observations, respectively. The error bars labelled '10' and '5' are 2 × SE of the means of 10 and 5 observations, respectively.

accept only those responses greater than D as evoked by a signal. The absolute value of D can be expressed in units of the SD, σ, of the responses, x, evoked by the background, i.e. $D = k\sigma$, where k is a multiplying factor. According to SDT the choice of D depends on the costs and benefits of making false and true decisions about the presence or absence of the signal.

When the contrast of the signal is variable and an observer determines its threshold value, he or she adopts a value of D consistent with an acceptably low probability, p, of false positive detection.[37] This probability determines the value of k irrespective of σ: e.g. if p is 0.01, k is the order of two. The sensory response corresponding to the mean threshold contrast of the signal will then be equal to D. It can be inferred from the experimentally observed constancy of the threshold contrast[17] that under constant experimental conditions the observer can maintain D at a constant level for quite

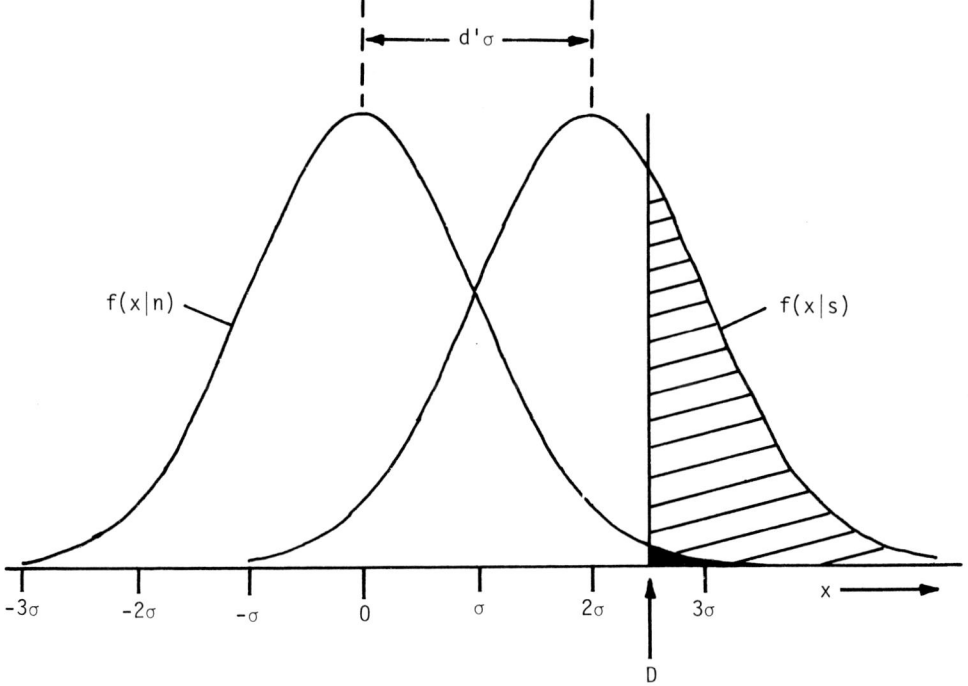

Fig. 7.10 Hypothetical probability distributions of sensory events, x, for samples of noise only, $f(x|n)$, and for samples of signal plus noise, $f(x|s)$. The scale of the abscissa is expressed in units of the standard deviation of the noise, σ. Adopting a decision criterion, D, the true and false positive rates of detection are represented by the shaded and blackened areas, respectively. The distance between the means of $f(x|s)$ and $f(x|n)$ is $d'\sigma$ assuming that the standard deviation of $f(x|s)$ is σ.

lengthy periods. It has further been implied that as long as the costs remain the same, the observer maintains a constant value of p irrespective of variations in σ.[37] The value of σ can be expected to vary widely, for example according to the extent of the signal, the power of the noise in the background, and so on.

The constancy of k and therefore of p can be inferred from the experimental result that changing the value of σ produces a proportionate change in the value of the threshold contrast for a given signal. In Figure 7.11 threshold contrasts for disc-shaped signals displayed on a noise background consisting of the magnified image of photographic granularity can be compared with those for the same signals displayed on a uniformly illuminated background of the same mean luminance, 7 cd m^{-2}. Also shown are the threshold contrasts with backgrounds of a quarter and a sixteenth of the full power of the noise but the same mean luminance: for each signal the threshold contrasts are approximately a half and a quarter, respectively, of those for full power noise.[17] The fact that the mean threshold contrast is found to be proportional to the SD of the threshold contrast for a wide range of signal sizes, background luminances, etc.[21,6] called *Crozier's law*,[41] can also be interpreted as evidence of the constancy of k and p.[37] Implicit in this interpretation, however, are the assumptions that the visual system is linear and that the standard deviations of the responses to the signal and to the background are equal. To infer the constancy of p from the above evidence depends on the adoption of a particular model of visual detection. Direct evidence for the constancy of the value of p could be obtained by direct measurement. Since the values of p normally adopted by observers are very small, however, accurate measurements would require many thousands of presentations of the background.

The temporal sampling aperture

If the noise that limits detectability is dynamic, the

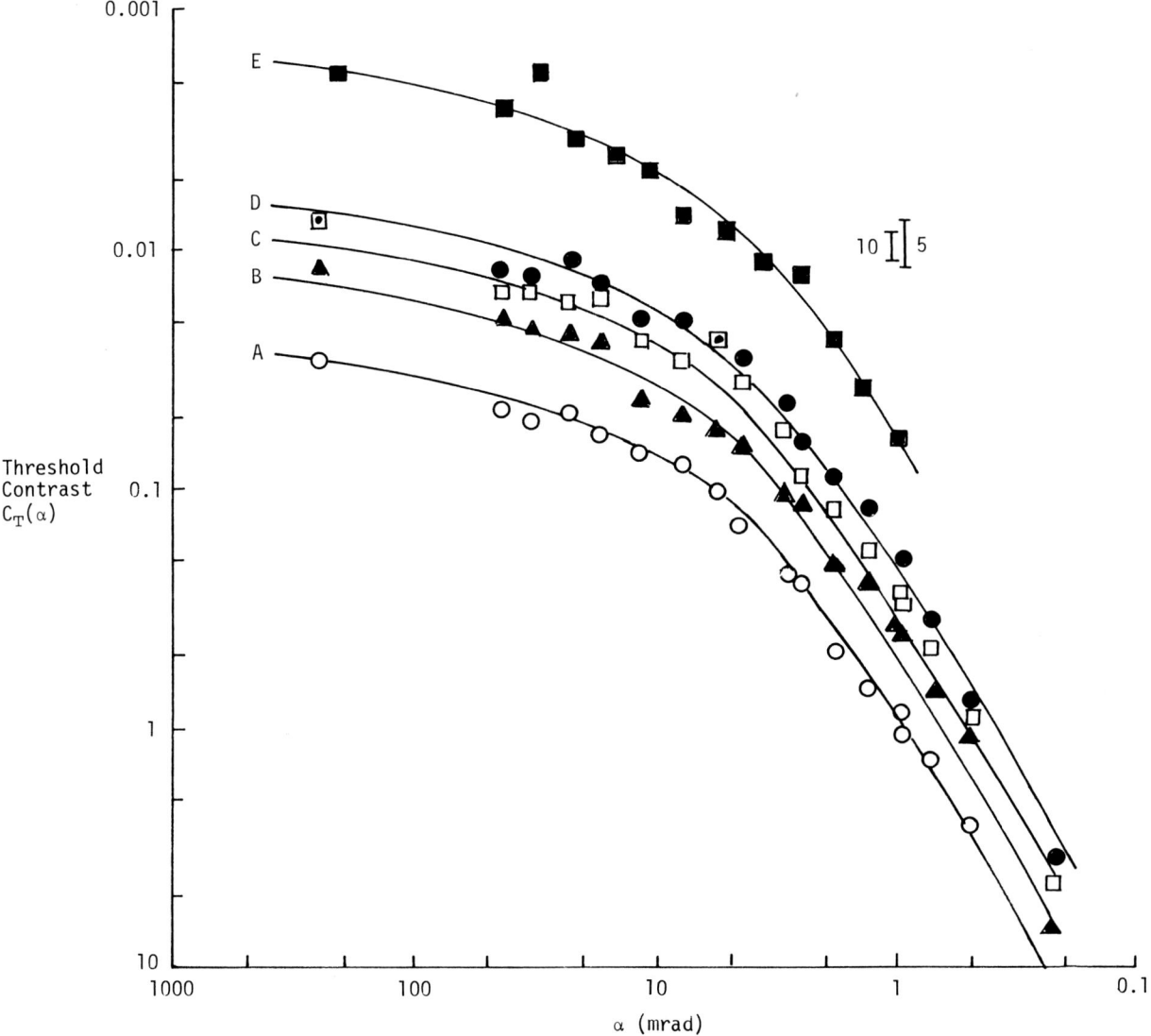

Fig. 7.11 Threshold contrasts, $C_T(\alpha)$, for incremental disc-shaped signals of diameter α displayed on backgrounds of: A, full (○); B, quarter (▲); C, sixteenth (□); D, zero (●) power static noise; and E, dynamic noise (■): all of mean luminance 7 cd m^{-2}: log scales. Contrasts for dynamic noise are reduced 10-fold for clarity. The curve has no theoretical significance and is the same shape, but displaced, for conditions A to E. Points of A and D are the means of 10 observations: points of B, C and E are the means of 5 observations. The error bars labelled '10' and '5' are $2 \times$ SE of the means of 10 and 5 observations, respectively.

temporal as well as the spatial aperture with which the signal and the noise are sampled determines the detectability of the signal. It has been suggested[79] that the temporal impulse response function takes the form $(1/\tau)\exp(-t/\tau)$, for all times $t > 0$, where τ is a relaxation time characteristic of a given mean luminance. It is tacitly assumed that the sampling aperture is small compared with τ. This model can be fitted satisfactorily to observations of contrast sensitivity for signals of limited duration and τ is found to range from 68–220 ms. The relaxation time, τ, however, is to some extent equivalent to a sampling aperture. Since for longer times of presentation it seems that detectability can be improved by multiple separate glimpses of the signal, the interpretation of τ as equivalent to a sampling aperture is not implausible.

There is some evidence that the relaxation time (or sampling aperture) is not constant for different sizes of signal, although it may not be relevant when unlimited time of observation is possible. It appears that for signals of short duration the maximum effective time of integration depends on the size of the signal.[3] If this were so in general, the threshold contrast versus disc diameter curves for backgrounds of static and dynamic noise would differ in shape. Comparing threshold contrasts obtained with a background of dynamic noise, derived from X-ray quantum absorptions and displayed on a television monitor, to those obtained with a background of static noise there appears to be no significant difference in shape (Fig. 7.11). In both cases, however, the observations were made with the signal present continuously and the time available for detection was unrestricted. Under these conditions, apparently, the effective integration time for signals of all the sizes investigated is constant. The useful result follows that the spatial and temporal effects of noise are independent.

The spatial sampling aperture

It has been suggested that both an incremental signal, of initial diameter α, and the background noise are sampled by an aperture of an extent related to that of the signal[37] and that there are sampling apertures within the visual system of a range of sizes and shapes: an aperture could be a receptive field or a combination of receptive fields. It is assumed that the neural response evoked by a visual increment (either signal or noise) can be treated as linearly proportional to the intensity of the increment (see p. 243). Since in determining a threshold contrast a sampled signal is always expressed as a ratio to a noise sample, the constant of proportionality can be omitted. As the contrast of a signal is increased from zero the detector connected to the sampling aperture giving the maximum signal-to-noise ratio of responses responds at the lowest contrast. This contrast is the threshold contrast. As the contrast of that particular signal is further increased, however, the decision criteria of other sampling apertures are exceeded. It is at present a matter for speculation whether the responses of these other apertures are suppressed or whether they combine to form a more precise percept of the signal.

In order to achieve the maximum possible signal-to-noise ratio of responses an aperture matched in response profile to the signal profile and modified by the noise spectrum would be required.[90] Detection takes place in the visual cortex, however, after the intensity distribution of the input signal has been distorted by convolution with the PSF, $T(r)$, of the visual system (see Fig. 7.7b), where r is the distance from the stimulus in angular measure. The result of the convolution is represented by its effect on the intensity distribution of the signal in Figure 7.8. A disc-shaped incremental signal of initial diameter α and contrast C displayed on a background of mean luminance I_0 becomes, after the convolution, $I_0 C \Pi(r/\alpha) \star T(r)$, where the function $\Pi(x)$ is defined by:

$$\Pi(x) = 1, |x| < 1/2,$$
$$= 0 \text{ elsewhere.}$$

It is often more convenient to use the Hankel transform of the signal. The transform is $CI_0 M(\omega) \alpha \mathcal{J}_1(\pi \alpha \omega)/2\omega$, where $\mathcal{J}_1(x)$ is the first order Bessel function, $M(\omega)$ is the MTF of the complete visual system and ω is the spatial frequency in reciprocal angular measure. The profile and the transform of the sampling aperture giving a maximum signal-to-noise ratio of responses, however, is determined not only by the signal transform but also by the spectrum of the noise.

In the absence of external noise, it has been suggested that detection is limited by internal noise.[37] It is assumed that the principal source of internal noise is the random absorption of photons in the retina. The noise spectrum has a band-pass characteristic, the low frequency limitation being imposed by lateral inhibition and the high frequency cut-off being determined by the finite size and spacing of the retinal receptors and any further unsharpness introduced by neural processing prior to detection. The high frequency limitation of any signal received, however, is more severe than that of the noise because of the effect of the MTF of the ocular media in addition to any neural unsharpness. Therefore loss of high frequencies in the internal noise spectrum can be neglected. The noise has a power spectral density, $I_0 |L(\omega)|^2$, where $L(\omega)$ is the neural part of the MTF of the visual system. The signal spectrum is $CI_0 M(\omega) \alpha \mathcal{J}_1(\pi \alpha \omega)/2\omega$. Hence, the ideal aperture response profile for maximising the signal-to-noise ratio of responses has a Fourier spectrum proportional to $M(\omega) \alpha \mathcal{J}_1(\pi \alpha \omega)/$

$(2\omega L^2(\omega))$. If the chief source of noise arises external to the visual system (e.g. in the image display system), the noise spectrum is proportional to $|M(\omega)|^2$ and the spectrum of the ideal aperture is proportional to $\alpha \mathcal{J}_1(\pi\alpha\omega)/(2\omega M(\omega))$. It cannot be assumed, however, that the visual system has evolved to provide such an ideal aperture for detection.

It is often assumed for simplicity[37, 79] that the sampling apertures are of uniform response though of a range of diameters. The MTF can be derived from measurements of the contrast sensitivity function, correcting for the effect of noise by multiplying by the frequency (see p. 246). The threshold contrasts can then be calculated for disc-shaped signals of a range of diameters. The response of an aperture of diameter a to a signal of diameter α is

$$S(\alpha, a) = CI_0 \int_0^{a/2} T(r) \star \Pi(r/\alpha) 2\pi r dr \quad (7.1)$$

and to external noise

$$\sigma(a) = \sqrt{[I_0 \int_0^\infty |T(r) \star \Pi(r/a)|^2 2\pi r dr]} \quad (7.2)$$

At threshold, $S_T(\alpha, a) = k\sigma(a)$. This Equation determines the threshold contrast, C_T, of the signal for a given aperture a. It is assumed that the sampling aperture giving a minimum value of C_T is used in detecting the signal. Consequently the minimum value of C_T is the threshold contrast for that signal.

Threshold contrasts have been calculated[18] for disc-shaped signals superimposed on a background of external noise supplied by the magnified image of photographic granularity. Similar calculations have been carried out for experimental conditions in which additional unsharpness is introduced into either the noise or the signals. The value of I_0 is determined by measuring the coefficient of variation of the noise scanned through physical apertures of a range of sizes. The calculated thresholds are compared with those obtained by direct observation of the discs, as illustrated in Figure 7.12. The calculated values are fitted to the observations by adjusting the single parameter k: k values of 2·5, 3·5 and 2 give the best fit for the curves I, II and III, respectively. Agreement between the calculated and observed values of C_T is reasonably satisfactory for discs of diameters greater than 2 mrad. For the smaller discs the agreement is poor, except for the defocused discs where the apparent diameter of a disc is never small. The reason may be that a scanning aperture of uniform response is a poor match to the amplitude distribution of small signals, i.e. when it approaches that of the PSF.

Using a different method to obtain the diameters of the matching apertures, similar values have been obtained[79]. The theoretical predictions were compared with an extensive series of observations of threshold contrasts of discs for backgrounds of uniform luminance from 10^{-2} to 10^3 lx. The agreement obtained was highly satisfactory when k was assigned the value of 2·5. It was necessary, however, also to assume values for quantum efficiency ranging from 0·3 per cent at 10^{-2} lx to 6·1 per cent at 4·5 lx. Unfortunately, values of quantum efficiency obtained otherwise range widely[4] so the goodness of fit of the theoretical values is uncertain to this extent. This source of uncertainty is removed, of course, when external noise, of measured power, limits detectability.

The model offers a qualitative explanation of the shape of the threshold contrast versus diameter curve shown in Figure 7.11. The curve can be divided into three regions, the central one, from approximately 1–10 mrad, being linear and of unity gradient. Signals within this region are only minimally distorted by the spread function of the eye and the relation between the contrast threshold and diameter, α, is that predicted by the Rose-de Vries model. Therefore this region is referred to as the *Rose-de Vries region*. Signals of diameter less than 1 mrad take on the shape of the unsharpness of the eye (Fig. 7.8). Therefore, this region of α is referred to as the *unsharpness region*. The sampling aperture used in detecting these signals is comparable in extent to that of the unsharpness and is constant for all such signals. The intensity of the signal sample is then proportional to α^2 and since the average power of the sampled noise is constant the threshold contrast is proportional to α^{-2}. Signals of diameter greater than 10 mrad are distorted principally by lateral inhibition (Fig. 7.8). With increasing α, the appearance of the signal approximates to an annulus of constant width and the intensity of the signal sample is proportional to α. If the principal source of noise arises distal to the site of the lateral inhibitory mechanism, the noise spectrum is distorted by the mechanism. Sampling the noise with an aperture α is equivalent to sampling white noise with an aperture of annular

254 SCIENTIFIC BASIS OF MEDICAL IMAGING

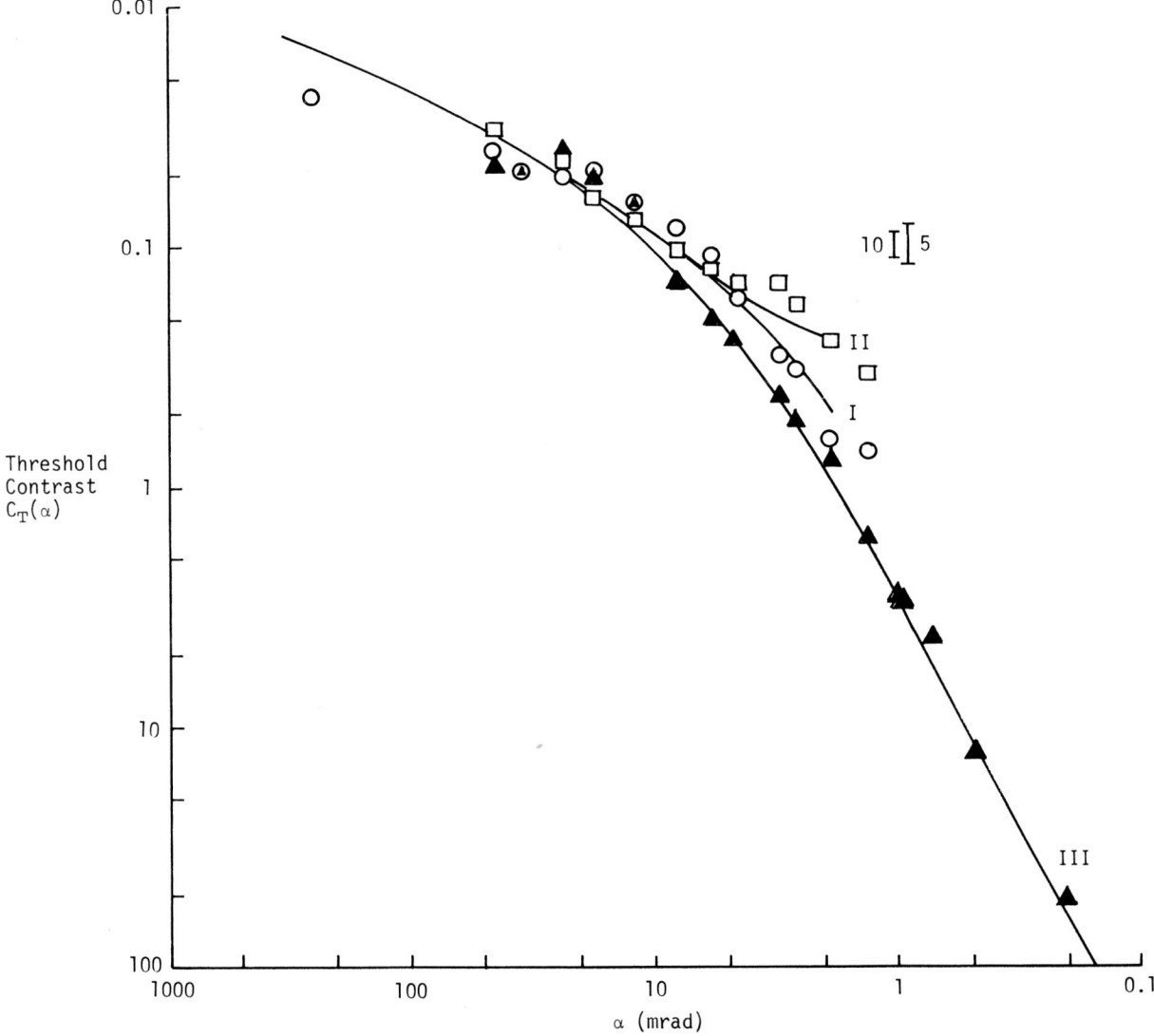

Fig. 7.12 Observed threshold contrasts, $C_T(\alpha)$, for incremental disc-shaped signals of initial diameter α displayed on noise backgrounds of mean luminance 7 cd m^{-2}: both noise and signals focused (○), means of 10 observations; defocused noise and focused signals (□), means of 5 observations; focused noise and defocused signals (▲), means of 5 observations: log scales. The error bars labelled '10' and '5' are 2 × SE of the means of 10 and 5 observations, respectively. The curves I, II and III are theoretical predictions of $C_T(\alpha)$: I, both noise and signals focused; II, defocused noise and focused signals; III, focused noise and defocused signals.

form and of diameter α. Hence the threshold contrast for signals greater than 10 mrad in diameter, where the principal source of noise is external or due to photon absorption in the initial receptors, is proportional to $\sqrt{\alpha}$. It is possible that at high luminances a significant proportion of the noise arises proximal to the lateral inhibitory mechanism (G. A. Hay, personal communication). In this case the noise spectrum is white and the average power of the sampled noise is proportional to α^2. The threshold contrast curve is then asymptotic to a constant value with increasing α.

The detectability of noise

The crucial part played by noise in limiting detectability is sometimes questioned on the grounds that the observer is unaware of the presence of noise under normal viewing conditions. If an additional source of noise is present in the light entering the eye, however, the noise, called *external noise*, can often be detected. The way in which external noise is detected is a matter for speculation at present. The fact that external noise is detectable and internal noise normally is not is a paradox that has not been satisfactorily resolved. Regarded as a signal, for maximum detectability the noise would be scanned by an aperture matched in size to the unsharpness of the noise. The amplitude of the response would only rarely exceed the decision criterion determined by the noise itself, however, if the usual choice of decision criterion was adopted. Detection could occur if the decision criterion was reduced. Although this speculative suggestion can account for the detectability of external noise it also predicts that internal noise should be detectable whereas normally it is not. The dilemma could be resolved by making the further assumption that the decision criterion has a minimum value that is too high to allow the detection of internal noise.

Summary

The visual signals received by the eye are processed by the visual system prior to their arrival at a set of detection units probably sited in the visual cortex. The units sample the incoming processed visual information with sampling apertures of a range of sizes. Both an incoming signal and the background noise are sampled by each unit and the maximum signal-to-noise ratio is attained by the unit whose sampling aperture is matched to the signal but taking account of the spectrum of the noise. Thus the detector of a signal is specific to that signal and detection is limited by noise. This *signal-specific*, *noise-limited* model of detection is referred to subsequently by its initials SSNL.

THE SPATIAL-FREQUENCY-SPECIFIC CHANNEL MODEL

Neurophysiological and psychophysical evidence

Considerable simplification can be achieved by the use of Fourier analysis in investigating the performance of linear imaging systems.[11] The applic-ability of this technique to the visual system has been investigated.[16] The threshold contrast, C_T, of sinusoidal gratings of a range of spatial frequencies has been measured and the MTF of the visual system derived, on the assumption that it is proportional to the contrast sensitivity, C_T^{-1}. Making the further assumption that the threshold contrast is determined by the maximum contrast in the output waveform after attenuation by the MTF, the threshold contrast of a square-wave pattern has been predicted. The predicted values, however, do not agree with those observed: it appears that the higher harmonics are less effective than would have been expected. Therefore it has been suggested that the visual system contains not a single detector following a single spatial frequency filter but a number of channels consisting of independent detectors each preceded by a narrow-band filter tuned to a different frequency. Examples of possible multichannel and single-channel models are illustrated in Figure 7.13. This suggestion has stimulated a considerable amount of research seeking to establish the existence of the channels and their characteristics.

The independence of the channels has been demonstrated.[77] Two superimposed sinusoidal gratings of spatial frequencies differing by more than 25 per cent are detected independently. Adaptation experiments also provide evidence of independence. Prolonged viewing of (adaptation to) a high-contrast grating raises the threshold only for gratings of similar frequencies (within ± 1 octave) and orientations.[7] In Figure 7.14a the contrast sensitivity is shown (as a solid line) prior to adaptation to a spatial frequency of 7·1 cycles deg^{-1}: the circles are the contrast sensitivities after adaptation. In Figure 7.14b is shown the relative threshold elevation following adaptation to the same spatial frequency. Adaptation also causes a shift in the apparent frequency of gratings of neighbouring frequencies away from the frequency of the adapting grating.[8] Further evidence is provided by the frequency-specific effect of external (masking) noise. Figure 7.15a shows the relative threshold elevation for sinusoidal gratings caused by noise of 1 octave bandwidth (of 2·5–5, 5–10 and 10–20 cycles deg^{-1}).[84] The gratings were vertical and the noise consisted of random vertical stripes. In Figure 7.15b the same data are shown for normalised

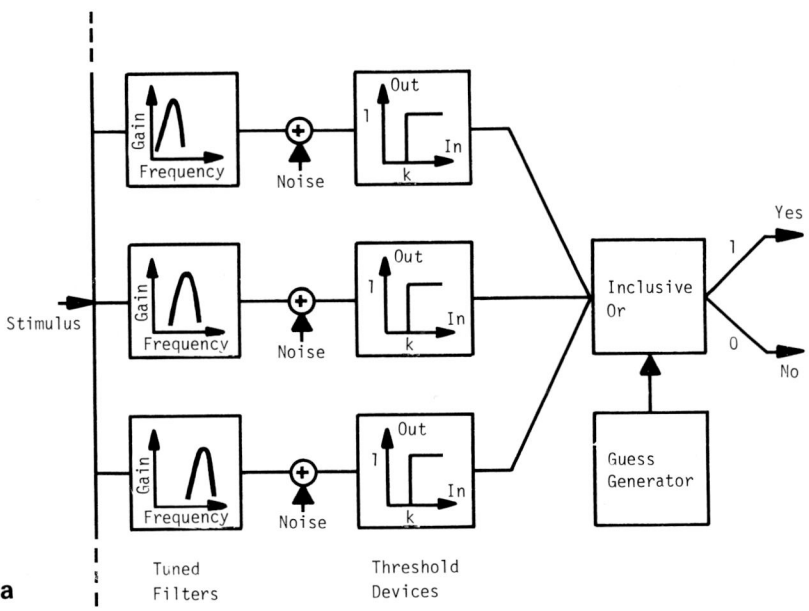

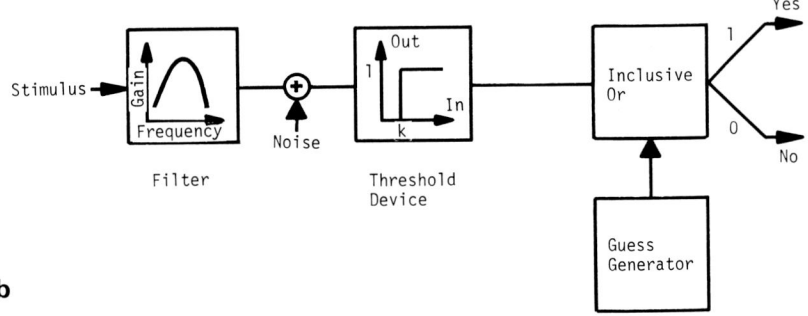

Fig. 7.13 (a) In the multichannel model, the signal passes through a bank of narrow-band filters in parallel. Noise is added and if the sensory threshold, k, is exceeded in one or more threshold devices the signal is detected. A guessing mechanism can also generate a 'yes' response irrespective of the presence or absence of the signal. (b) The single channel model differs from the multichannel model only in that the bank of narrow-band filters is replaced by a single wide-band filter and followed by a single threshold device.[77]

spatial frequencies. Frequencies are expressed as a number of octaves, respectively above or below the upper or lower cut-off frequency of the noise band. Only noise frequencies within ± 1 octave of the frequency of a grating are effective in elevating the threshold contrast of the grating. So far the evidence described has been psychophysical, but a possible neurophysiological basis for the theory has been proposed.[60] It has been shown that in the cat the simple cells of the visual cortex respond to a moving grating by a modulation of their discharge frequency. Any given cell is sensitive to only a narrow band of frequencies (the bandwidth at half maximum is approximately 1 octave) and the centre frequencies for different cells vary from 0·2–2 cycles deg^{-1}. These cells could signal information about the amplitude and phase of any frequency component, and they possess the properties required to act as the independent spatial-frequency-specific channels.

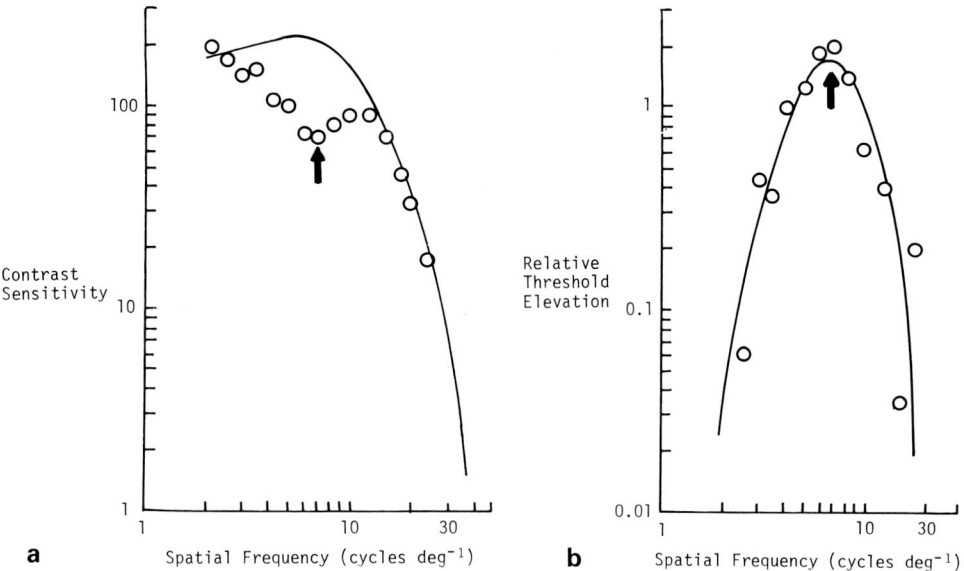

Fig. 7.14 (a) Contrast sensitivities for different spatial frequencies prior to adaptation to a high-contrast grating of 7·1 cycles deg^{-1} (arrowed) are represented by the solid line (log scales): the sensitivities after adaptation are shown as open circles. (b) The relative threshold elevation, i.e. the ratio of the contrast sensitivities before and after adaptation minus 1, is shown as a function of spatial frequency.[7]

The visual system as a Fourier analyser

It has been suggested that the simple cells of the visual cortex are capable of performing a Fourier analysis of the visual image.[60,71,32] It is unlikely, however, that a global two-dimensional transform could be applied to the whole visual image.

The detectability of a beat pattern consisting of three superimposed spatial frequencies can be influenced by the presence of a grating of the same frequency as that of the beat pattern, even though

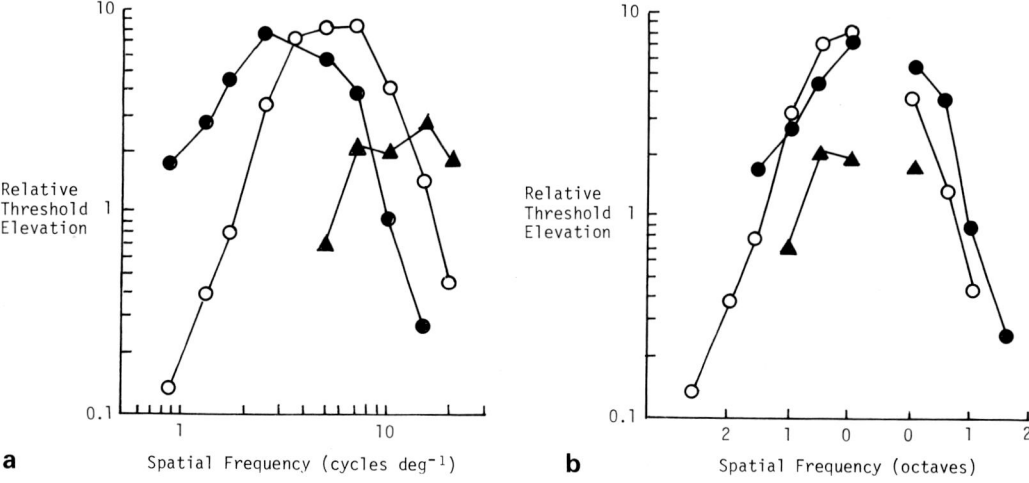

Fig. 7.15 (a) Relative threshold elevation for sinusoidal gratings caused by noise of 1 octave band width: 2·5–5 cycles deg^{-1} (●); 5–10 cycles deg^{-1} (○); 10–20 cycles deg^{-1} (▲): log scales. The average noise contrasts were 0·042, 0·059 and 0·074, respectively. (b) The same relative threshold elevations (log scale) are shown for normalised spatial frequencies. Frequencies are expressed as a number of octaves (linear scale), respectively above or below the upper or lower cut-off frequency of the noise band. Either cut-off frequency is represented as zero.[84]

the beat frequency is 3 octaves below the lowest of the three frequencies that are physically present.[39] Attempts to explain this effect in terms of the non-linearity of the visual system are inconsistent with other evidence. Furthermore, the spatial inhomogeneity of the visual system, demonstrated in humans most directly by the decrease in visual acuity with increasing retinal eccentricity, makes it unlikely that the system is isoplanatic as would be required for a global Fourier analysis. Thus, if any form of Fourier analysis occurs it is likely to be performed piecewise in small homogeneous areas of the retina. Considering the neurophysiological evidence, it has been suggested that, at most, small patches of the image might be analysed into their first three harmonic components.[73] The cells most likely to perform such an analysis are the simple cells of the cortex.

The characteristics of the channels

It has been suggested that channels exist specific to the detection of not only sinusoidal gratings but to edges and bars.[53] Subsequently it has been proposed, however, that the detection of gratings might be explained in terms of the detectability of the individual bars of the grating combined by probability summation.[50] It is then necessary to postulate a disinhibitory mechanism, i.e. an excitatory region outside the inhibitory surround of retinal and ganglion cells.

There is some evidence, however, that appears to contradict the existence of bar-detectors. While adaptation to a sinusoidal grating causes a relative elevation of the threshold contrast of gratings of frequencies only at or near the adapting frequency, the effect of adaptation to bars of specific widths is quite unspecific.[86] Adaptation to bars of either 7·5' or 1·25' elevates the threshold contrast of bars of all widths between 1·25' and 40', approximately to the same degree. This result is more readily explained in terms of frequency-specific rather than width-specific channels. Since any isolated bar has a broad-band spectrum, many frequency-specific channels would be adapted by an isolated bar and their adaptation would to some degree affect the detectability of a bar of any other width.

It has been suggested that the channels possess somewhat different properties.[96,97] Thus at each retinal location there are four kinds of mechanism. All the mechanisms have a centre-surround configuration and are of medium bandwidths but each has a different spatial extent and there are two types of temporal response. The spatial extent of all the mechanisms increases with eccentricity and spatial probability summation across the retina occurs for each type of mechanism. Spatial probability summation is somewhat similar to a discrete form of convolution of the line spread function, LSF, of the mechanism with the spatial pattern. The response is obtained at finely spaced intervals (e.g. 2' intervals) over an 8 degree extent as the LSF of the mechanism is shifted relative to the pattern. Detection can occur at any position and the overall probability of detection is given by probability summation. The model is successful in predicting the spatial modulation transfer function of the visual system from measurements of the LSFs of the mechanisms. The findings appear to be inconsistent with the hypothesis that a Fourier analysis of spatial images is performed. The bandwidths of the detecting mechanisms are too wide (at 1·5–2·5 octaves) to permit any precise spatial frequency analysis. Furthermore, the inhomogeneity of the retina results in a different frequency response at different parts of the retina. Thus the mechanisms should be regarded as size rather than frequency specific.

The response of the channels to non-periodic stimuli

Relatively few attempts have been made to predict or measure the response of the channels to non-periodic stimuli. One such is the experiment previously described[86] in which subjects adapted to bars of selected widths. The subsequent detectability of bars and gratings could be explained if detection occurred when the most sensitive channel (responsive to a spatial frequency of 5 cycles deg^{-1}) reached its threshold. One apparent difficulty,[86,84] is that the perceived appearance of the stimulus does not in general resemble the response profile of the channel.

The experience of seeing can be contrasted with that of hearing where it is quite easy for most people to pick out individual frequencies from a chord. As far as the author knows, however, no one has claimed to recognise the component spatial frequencies of a multi-frequency visual image. There is no reason to assume, of course, that this aspect of vision should resemble that of hearing. It appears, however, that some extension of the model may be necessary to explain how the responses of the channels are combined.

The effect of noise

Proponents of the spatial-frequency-specific channel model generally make no assumption about what determines the threshold level of a channel. There is no suggestion that the level might be related to noise. Alternative single-channel and multichannel models have been proposed[77] in which noise is introduced prior to the site of the threshold decision to represent the uncertainty in the detection process. A guessing mechanism that generates positive responses irrespective of the type of stimulus present is also introduced. Therefore it appears that a high threshold level that is unrelated to the power of the noise in the background has been tacitly assumed.

The well-documented effect of external noise[84] in raising the thresholds of sinusoidal signals is often described as *masking*. Its effect is very similar to that produced by adapting to a high contrast sinusoidal grating. In particular the effect of the noise is found to be frequency specific in that only noise within ± 1 octave of the frequency of the grating causes any elevation of the threshold contrast of that grating. Considerably less attention has been paid to the relation between the power of the noise and the amplitude of the threshold elevation produced. Nevertheless, it has been reported[70,84] that the contrast sensitivity varies linearly with the standard deviation of the noise. One possible interpretation of these results is that noise determines the threshold level of the detector, though as far as the author knows none of the proponents of the spatial-frequency-specific channel model make this assumption.

Summary

Taking into account the available evidence, only some of which has been summarised here, it seems reasonable to conclude that the visual system is organised as a collection of independent channels, each of which has its own filter characteristics and detection mechanism. The precise structure and functioning of the channels has yet to be determined. Although the channels are to some degree selective for spatial frequency, estimates of the bandwidths suggest that they are of the order of ± 1 octave which cannot be considered as highly selective. Probably the most important practical aspect of this model is that it draws attention to the specificity of the interaction between similar spatial frequencies in different signals and in the noise and the signal, a specificity that is also a feature of the previously described signal-specific, noise-dependent model (see p. 247).

SIGNAL DETECTION THEORY

Formulation of the theory

The problem of distinguishing signals from noise arises in many different disciplines, e.g. electronics, acoustics etc., and methods have been developed for achieving this end efficiently. The applicability of these methods to visual detection depends on the assumption that the sensory effect of the signal is indistinguishable from that of the noise except by its amplitude. Thus the amplitude of the signal required for reliable detection depends on the amplitude of the noise.

Other interpretations of the detection process are possible. One, illustrated in Figure 7.16, is that the sensory threshold is a discrete level of sensory excitation, k, much greater than, and independent of, the sensory effect, x, of physiological noise. This interpretation is sometimes called a 'high threshold' theory. The amplitude of the signal required for detection would then be quite independent of the amplitude of the noise. The well-known fact that a signal of constant input contrast is sometimes detected and sometimes not is explained by variability in either the sensory effect of the signal, as shown in Figure 7.16b, or in k. Positive responses when no signal is present are attributed to pure guesswork and can occur also in the presence of a signal that fails to reach the required level. If external noise is present it is sometimes suggested that detectability is reduced by adaptation similar to the effect of a high contrast signal. Although

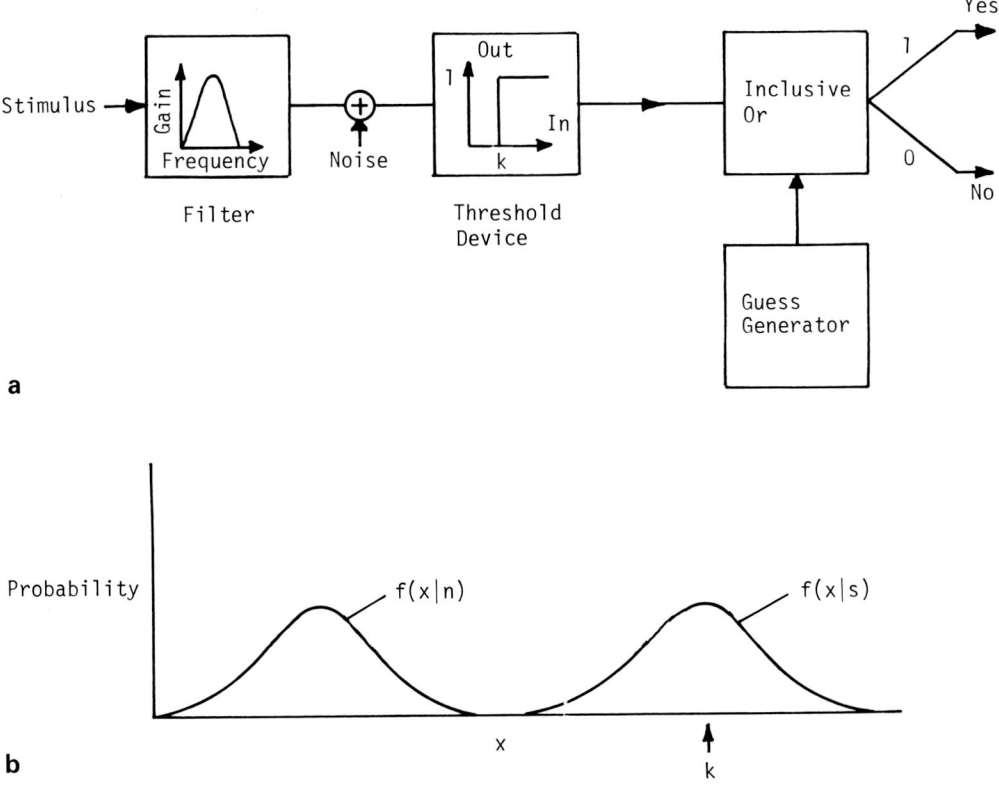

Fig. 7.16 Example of a high-threshold theory of detectability. (a) After filtration noise is added to the signal and if the sensory threshold, k, is exceeded the signal is detected. A guessing mechanism can also generate a 'yes' response irrespective of the presence or absence of the signal. (b) Details of the threshold device showing that the sensory threshold, k, is unlikely to be exceeded by any sensory event, x, generated by noise alone.

this type of theory is consistent with much of the evidence concerning detectability, it offers no very satisfactory explanation of the observer's ability to adjust the true and false positive rates of detection according to the costs of making wrong decisions. This ability is explained very satisfactorily, however, by signal detection theory (SDT).[34]

According to SDT, if a constant signal is presented to an observer the sensory effect produced varies according to a certain probability distribution, $f(x|s)$ (see Fig. 7.10). The probability distribution of the sensory effect due to noise, $f(x|n)$, may or may not be the same as that of the signal but, in general, the mean values of the distributions differ. The observer must decide on the basis of the sensory effect whether or not a signal was present. One possible strategy might be to partition the sensory response axis at a certain level called the 'decision criterion', D. Only if the sensory effect exceeded D would it be accepted as arising from a signal. The choice of D is governed by some decision rule. One such rule is the *Neyman-Pearson objective*. The objective is to keep the probability of false positive detection at an acceptably low value, p, and at the same time to maximise the probability of true positive detection, shown shaded in Figure 7.10. The Neyman-Pearson objective is achieved if D is positioned such that the probability $(x>D|n)$, shown in black in Figure 7.10, is equal to p. The decision criterion can be expressed in units of the standard deviation of the noise, σ, i.e. $D = k\sigma$, where k is determined by the chosen value of p. Clearly, the false positive rate of detection can be reduced by increasing D, but at the same time the true positive rate also decreases. A more satisfactory way of increasing the true positive rate of detection while maintaining the same low false positive rate is to increase the mean separation of the effects of the signal and the noise. If, as is often assumed, the distributions have equal variance, a parameter, d', can be defined as the difference between the means of the distributions divided by their common standard deviation. Increasing d' increases the inherent detectability of the signal by the observer.

A more general decision rule assigns costs to the four possible outcomes, i.e. true and false positive, and true and false negative responses. The mean cost, derived from the probabilities of these outcomes, can be minimised and gives an appropriate value of D. It is of theoretical interest that many decision rules depend on the likelihood ratio, defined as the ratio of the conditional probabilities of an observed event given that the signal was present and given that it was absent. In practice, observers probably do not always adopt a decision criterion that minimises the mean cost.[34] They tend to avoid extreme criteria even when such criteria would be optimal. Certainly, however, observers can easily be persuaded to change their decision criterion in response to rewards and penalties. For example, a high false positive rate of detection, accompanying a high true positive rate of detection, is to be expected and indeed encouraged in a preliminary screening test. If the usual outcome of the positive identification of an abnormality is major surgery, however, the false positive rate of detection is likely to be lower.

The true positive rate of detection of a signal depends on both the mean separation of the sensory effects of the signal and the noise in relation to their standard deviations (d' in the case of equal variances) and the choice of the decision criterion, D. It is one of the strengths of SDT that it can distinguish between these two factors.

ROC curves

The observer can easily be induced to change his decision criterion. From Figure 7.10 it is clear that both the true and false positive rates of detection decrease as D is increased: corresponding values generate a *Receiver Operating Characteristic* (ROC) curve. Although the curve is generated by adopting successively all possible decision criteria its position and shape is criterion-free and depends only on the inherent detectability of the signal by a given observer and with a given noise background.

An ROC curve can be generated by asking the observer to respond 'yes' or 'no' according to his or her judgement of the presence or absence of a signal. Such a yes-no procedure is very time-consuming, however, as at least 100 observations of the signal and the noise are usually considered necessary for each point on the ROC curve.[34] Instead, a rating method can be employed. The observer is required to categorise his or her degree of certainty about the presence of the signal. The categories are sometimes precisely specified, e.g. as the probabilities of the presence of the signal, 0–20 per cent, 20–40 per cent, etc. Alternatively, the categories can be specified by the epithets 'strict, medium strict, medium, medium lax and lax'. The corresponding probabilities of responding to the signal and to the noise within each category are calculated and when plotted generate an ROC curve. It has been shown that the curve so generated does not differ significantly from that generated by the yes-no method. Indeed, if the observer is aware of his degree of certainty in responding to a signal it seems wasteful of information to use only two categories of response, i.e. 'yes' and 'no'. Therefore, there is every reason to use the rating method.

A further psychophysical method of measuring the response to a signal is the forced-choice method. In the simplest form of the method the signal can occur in one of two non-overlapping intervals of time or areas of the display and the subject must choose which interval or area contained the signal. According to SDT, the percentage correct found by this method, like the ROC curve, is independent of the subject's decision criterion. Assuming that the observer chooses the interval in which the amplitude of the response was greatest, the probability that the decision was correct, $P(C)$, is given by,

$$P(C) = \int_{-\infty}^{\infty} f(x = k|s) \int_{-\infty}^{k} f(x|n)dx \, dk \quad (7.3)$$

Clearly the decision criterion must be flexible in this situation and even if the responses in both intervals are low, one interval must be chosen as containing the signal. According to a high threshold theory (p. 259), if the responses are sufficiently low the observer's choice would be pure guesswork. On the basis of SDT, it can be shown[34] that the percentage correct in a forced-choice procedure is equal to the area under the ROC curve generated by a yes-no or rating method. As a measure of detectability, percentage correct is useful in that it is independent of any assumptions about the forms of the distributions of the signal and the noise.

The application of the ROC curve

The classical method for comparing detectabilities of signals is to determine the contrast at which a signal is detected on some fixed percentage (usually 50 per cent) of presentations. In general it is far more time-consuming to generate an ROC curve so the reason for doing so requires justification. Perhaps the chief reason for obtaining an ROC curve is that it can be a criterion-free measure of detectability. Thus it is possible to use ROC curves to compare the detectabilities of signals perhaps generated by two different imaging devices independently of the choice of criterion by the observer. The ROC curve is, of course, also of inherent interest in that it provides information about the detection process.

The question arises, how well an observer can maintain constant, over the extended period necessary for determining ROC curves, the many categories into which his responses must be placed. The classical method requires only one decision criterion to be maintained at a constant level. It has been shown, however, that ROC curves obtained under identical conditions are reproducible,[40] so it appears that the category boundaries can be maintained at constant levels. On the other hand there are considerable differences between the ROC curves obtained from different observers and therefore it is not possible to compare the detectabilities of different signals unless the same observer is employed. The classical method also suffers from this disadvantage.

Any signal that generates an ROC curve wholly above and to the left of another signal is the more detectable.[34] Comparison of ROC curves is qualitative, however, and it is useful to have a quantitative measure of detectability. The measure, d', is often quoted whenever it is applicable, i.e. when the distributions of the signal and the noise are Gaussian and of equal variance, because it has an intuitive interpretation. The percentage correct is perhaps less readily interpreted but is universally applicable.

If it could be established that at least under certain specified conditions the decision criterion was maintained at a constant level, there would be no need to generate a complete ROC curve. Indeed, some evidence is available (see p. 248) that the observer adopts a Neyman-Pearson criterion, with a constant false positive rate, over a wide range of backgrounds and signals. In that case the detectabilities of signals could be compared simply by comparing the contrasts necessary for 50 per cent true positive responses.

In comparing different imaging systems it is possible that some aspect of a system itself causes the observer to change his habitual decision criterion. If this change occurred it could be regarded as an inherent part of the detectability of the signal presented by that system. The comparison of ROC curves, which are criterion-free, could lead to the suppression of this relevant information. In this case, the contrast necessary for 50 per cent detection might be a more relevant comparison. To obtain more complete information, it would be necessary to determine the change in the decision criterion, if it had occurred, by measuring the false positive rates of detection.

To summarise, the ROC curve gives more detailed information about the detectability of a signal than can be derived from the classical method. It offers a criterion-free method of comparing detectabilities. It is more time-consuming, however, and if a constant decision criterion can be assumed or proved to obtain, the threshold contrast can be an adequate measure of detectability.

THE DETECTION AND RECOGNITION OF COMPLEX VISUAL IMAGES

Few attempts have been made to generalise either the noise-limited signal-specific model or the spatial-frequency-specific channel model to the detection and recognition of complex visual images. One theory that attempts to describe the initial processing of such images by the visual system is based on the suggestion that the images received by each eye are filtered through bar- and edge-shaped masks of different sizes and orientations at each point in the image.[62] From the responses to these masks it is possible to identify certain kinds of intensity change (edge, shading edge, line, blob, etc.). Also the position, orientation, contrast, etc. of these changes can be identified. This description of the image is called the 'primal sketch'. The second stage in processing the image is to group together the elements in the primal sketch in such a way as to separate figure from ground. This can be done normally before the shape of the extracted form has been described. Thus downward-flowing information from higher levels in the brain, perhaps relating to a memory of a particular shape, plays little part at this stage. The theory has been extended to account for stereopsis and the representation and recognition of three-dimensional shapes.[63]

APPLICATIONS OF THEORIES OF VISUAL DETECTION

Viewing distance

It would be unusual for a radiologist viewing X-ray images on a television monitor to maintain a fixed distance from the screen. That there is some justification for this flexibility can be shown theoretically and has been confirmed experimentally.

A typical curve relating contrast threshold and diameter for a fixed viewing distance (see Fig. 7.11) can be divided into three regions, depending on the angular diameter subtended at the eye by the signal, as discussed on page 252. Detectability is optimal in the region between about 1 and 10 mrad, i.e. the Rose-de Vries region.[75] The contrast threshold is approximately linearly proportional to the signal diameter, α. The contrast thresholds of signals greater than 10 mrad and less than 1 mrad fall below the line of unity gradient, however, and detectability is less than optimal for these sizes of signal. If the angular unsharpness of the imaging system itself is greater than that of the eye for some viewing distance, the Rose-de Vries region extends from 10 mrad to a diameter only of the order of the system unsharpness. In fact, if the viewing distance is so ill-chosen that the system unsharpness subtends at the eye an angle greater than 10 mrad, no signals are optimally detected.

On the basis of the SSNL model, for images in which the dominant source of noise is external to the eye, it can be shown that the detectability of a signal is constant with variation of viewing distance as long as the angular diameter of the signal falls within the Rose-de Vries region.[17] On the other hand, if at some arbitrarily chosen viewing distance the signal subtends an angle greater than 10 mrad or less than 1 mrad its detectability would be improved if the viewing distance were increased or decreased, respectively, to bring the angular diameter of the signal into the Rose-de Vries region. This theoretical prediction has been confirmed for a range of signal sizes and viewing distances for optically displayed images[17] and for X-ray images displayed on a television monitor (A. R. Cowen, personal communication).

A heuristic explanation for the constancy of detectability within the Rose-de Vries region is illustrated in Figure 7.17. At a viewing distance d_1, a signal subtending an angular diameter α_1 at the eye is imaged on the retina. The size of the retinal image is determined by the angular diameter of the signal. It is assumed that the noise is sampled over the same area as the area of the signal. Since the principal source of noise arises in the object plane, the power of the noise and the signal-to-noise ratio are determined by the area of the object plane, rather than the area of the retina, that is sampled. The area of the object plane remains constant as the viewing distance is decreased to d_2 even though the angular diameter of the signal and its retinal image increase.

For signals subtending angles smaller than 1 mrad at the eye the unsharpness of the eye plays an important role in detectability. The signal takes on the appearance of the unsharpness which, as the viewing distance increases, encompasses a progressively increasing area of the object plane. Therefore, for a given signal, the noise that limits detectability increases progressively and the detectability correspondingly decreases. If, however, the angular unsharpness of the system is greater than that of the eye at some viewing distance the detectability of all small signals is not improved by decreasing the viewing distance. For signals greater than 10 mrad, lateral inhibition reduces detectability to below its optimal value.

If at some initial viewing distance external noise

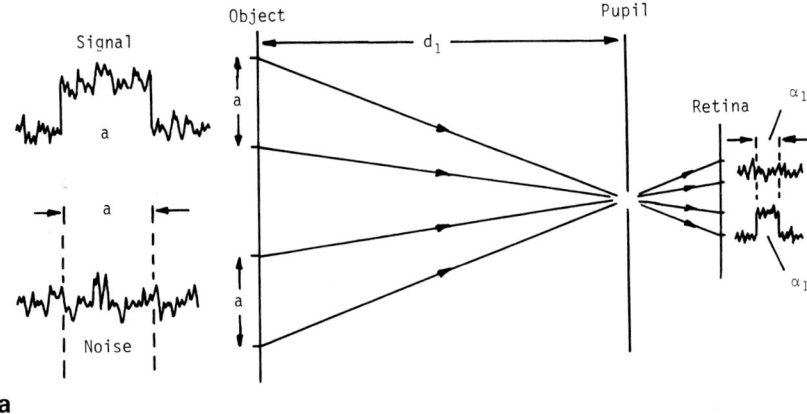

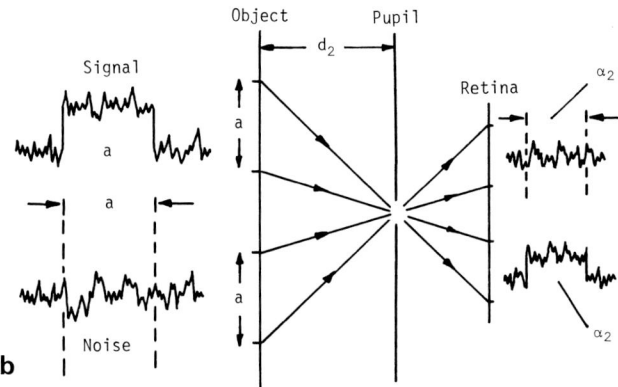

Fig. 7.17 (a) At viewing distance d_1, a disc-shaped signal of diameter a subtends an angle α_1 at the eye. The diameter of the image on the retina is proportional to α_1. Both the signal and the noise are sampled through apertures of diameter α_1 corresponding to apertures of diameter a in the object plane. (b) At viewing distance d_2, the same signal subtends an angle α_2 at the eye. Both the signal and the noise are now sampled through apertures of diameter α_2 which, however, correspond to apertures of diameter a in the object plane.

limits detectability a further consequence of increasing the viewing distance is to reduce the proportion of external noise in the total noise within the image. At greater distances fewer photons enter the pupil of the eye so that internal noise becomes relatively more important and ultimately detectability is reduced (see p. 265). The external noise present in most medical images is of such high power, however, that at any practicable viewing distance external noise is still visible. Therefore, deterioration of detectability at large distances is more likely to be a consequence of moving into the unsharpness region than the loss of photons.

When the dominant source of noise is internal to the visual system the dependence of detectability on viewing distance differs fundamentally from that when external noise dominates. The power of the noise that limits the detectability of a signal of angular diameter α is a function of the area of the retina covered by the signal: the area is determined by α. Theoretically, detectability is expected to be the same for a given value of α whatever the viewing distance. This theoretical prediction has been verified for a range of signal diameters when the viewing distance was increased from 1–2 m.[17] Therefore the changes in detectability with viewing distance can be predicted from the contrast threshold versus diameter curve for a fixed distance.

The above conclusions have been deduced only for isolated, disc-shaped signals. When viewing a medical image, however, the task of detection is likely to be significantly different. The signals to be detected can have a wide range of shapes and it is likely that many signals of different shapes and sizes must be detected simultaneously. The optimum viewing distance must then be a compromise between the ranges of distance that are optimal for the different signals.

There is no experimental evidence known to the author for the way in which an experienced observer chooses the viewing distance to optimise detectability, if indeed the observer does so. The theoretical analysis of the problem presented here gives only general guidelines for the strategy to be adopted. Certainly the observer should be prepared to adjust the viewing distance to suit the characteristics of the signal to be detected. Furthermore, the strategy required for viewing images in which external noise is visible, as in most medical images, differs from that applicable to most conventional images. Whereas reducing the viewing distance to the least distance of distinct vision maximises detectability for conventional images, for noisy images the detectability of some signals can be improved by increasing the viewing distance. In spite of all the theoretical difficulties, however, it is perhaps not over-optimistic to suggest that the experienced observer automatically adjusts the viewing distance to obtain optimal detectability.

Image intensifiers

The introduction of image intensifiers has resulted in a notable improvement in the detectability of X-ray images. There is a limit, however, to the extent of the improvement that can be achieved. One way of identifying the limit has been given on page 29. In this section, the limit is shown to depend on the relative powers of internal and external noise.

The statistics of intensifying systems have been described in detail,[1] but here a very simplified form of intensifier is considered, shown schematically in Figure 7.18a. Unity magnification is assumed. Suppose the image is formed by a mean number, $\bar{N}$, of primary particles falling on an area, A, of the intensifier. The absorption of the primary particle

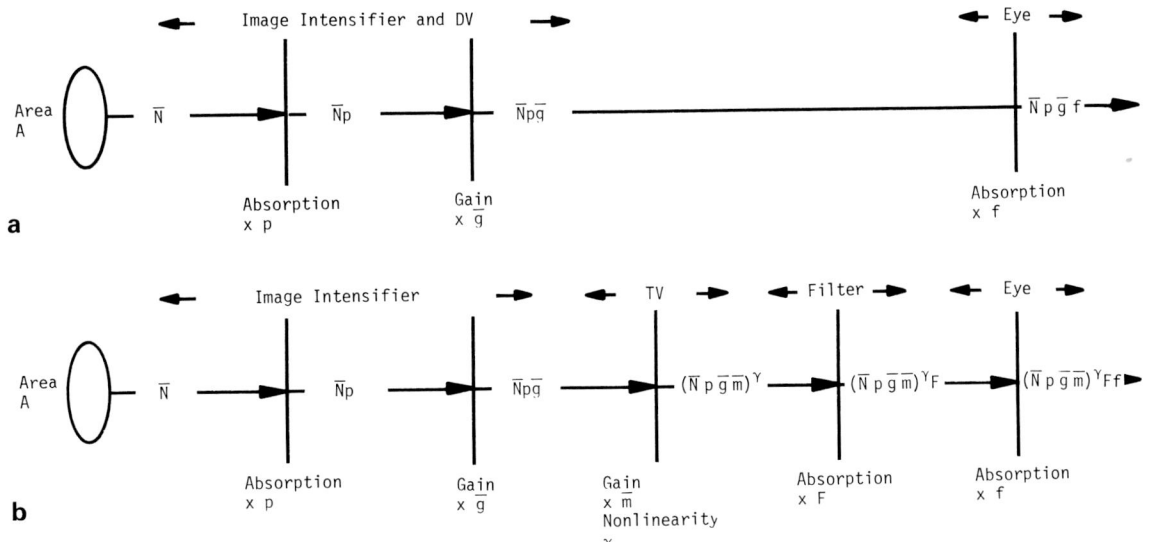

Fig. 7.18 (a) Simplified representation of the conversion processes in an image intensifier with a direct viewer (DV) as the display device. A mean number, $\bar{N}$, of primary particles falls on an area A of the input screen. A fraction p is absorbed and the mean gain per input particle, supplied by the intensifier, is $\bar{g}$. A fraction f of the output particles is absorbed by the eye. (b) A television monitor (TV) is the display device following the image intensifier and the monitor introduces a further mean gain, $\bar{m}$, per input particle and a nonlinearity that takes the form of a power law of exponent γ. A ND filter of absorption F is inserted between the monitor and the eye.

266 SCIENTIFIC BASIS OF MEDICAL IMAGING

is assumed to follow binomial statistics with parameter p so that the mean number of particles absorbed is $\bar{N}p$. A multiplication process is applied to each absorbed particle. It can be described by Poisson statistics with a mean of $\bar{g}$ particles generated per absorbed particle. Thus the mean number of output particles is $\bar{N}p\bar{g}$. Assuming that the output particles are photons and can be detected visually, a mean fraction, f, enters the pupil of the eye and gives rise to a visual sensation. This process follows binomial statistics and because of the small solid angle subtended by the pupil at the least distance of distinct vision, f is small. Finally, the mean number of events, $\bar{n}$, giving rise to a visual sensation, resulting from the initial number, $\bar{N}$, falling on an area A, is given by: $\bar{n} = \bar{N}p\bar{g}f$. The variance of n, $\sigma^2(n)$, is given by:[1]

$$\sigma^2(n) = \bar{N}p\bar{g}f(1 + \bar{g}f) \qquad (7.4)$$

According to the SSNL model, but assuming the effect of unsharpness is negligible, the integrated intensity of a signal of area A and contrast C_T must be equal to $k\sigma(n)$ at threshold (where k is a constant), so that

$$C_T = \sqrt{\frac{1 + \bar{g}f}{\bar{N}p\bar{g}f}} \qquad (7.5)$$

If there were no source of noise other than the absorption of photons the variance of n would be $\bar{n} = \bar{N}p\bar{g}f$. This component of the total variance of n is identified as internal noise and therefore the residual noise, $\bar{N}p(\bar{g}f)^2$ must be the external component.

The effect of increasing the mean gain of the intensifier, $\bar{g}$, can now be explored. Since f is very small, if $g = 1$, i.e. no gain is applied, $\bar{g}f << 1$ and $C_T = k/\sqrt{(\bar{N}p\bar{g}f)}$. This is the value of C_T that would be expected if only internal noise was present. As $\bar{g}$ is increased the mean luminance increases and the value of C_T decreases. However, when $\bar{g}$ reaches a value such that $\bar{g}f \sim 1$, the external noise becomes important. Finally, when $\bar{g}f >> 1$, C_T reaches a constant value, $k/\sqrt{(\bar{N}p)}$, and further increasing $\bar{g}$ results in no improvement in detectability. To summarise, intensification improves detectability initially by increasing the mean luminance level, but as soon as external noise becomes the dominant source of noise no further improvement is possible.

The gain at which $\bar{g}f = 1$ is such that each absorbed primary particle gives rise on average to one detectable event. If the gain is further increased sufficiently to ensure that the probability of detecting a primary particle is close to unity no further improvement in detectability can be expected. Interestingly, it is at about this gain that external noise becomes visible (see p. 29). It may seem paradoxical that to make the external noise visible by increasing the gain in fact improves detectability. It is equally true and perhaps not immediately obvious that eliminating visible noise by decreasing the gain decreases detectability of the signal.

Nonlinearity

Most of the theory of the detectability of images developed elsewhere in this chapter is based on the assumption of linearity. Some imaging devices, however, are well-known to be nonlinear, e.g. television monitors and photographic films. Even though these devices can be treated as approximately linear when the contrasts of the signals being detected are small, as is often the case at threshold, for example in radiology, the non-linearity can have a significant effect.

The effect can be illustrated by comparing the detectability of an intensified image on a direct viewer (DV) and a television monitor (TV) shown schematically in Figure 7.18. The DV is an optical instrument for displaying the output from an image intensifier. The magnification is assumed to be approximately unity in both the DV and the TV images. The TV can be viewed through a neutral density (ND) filter of transmittance such that the mean luminance is equal to that of the DV. The threshold contrast of a signal of area A displayed on a DV has been shown to be:

$$C_T = k\sqrt{\frac{1 + \bar{g}f}{\bar{N}p\bar{g}f}}$$

(Equation 7.5), using the same notation as previously. Therefore the relative contributions of external and internal noise power to the total power are in the ratio $\bar{g}f:1$. The TV both amplifies the input by a factor, m, assumed to obey Poisson statistics, and introduces a nonlinearity that takes the form of a power law with exponent γ of the order of 2·5. The mean number of particles emitted from the area A becomes $(\bar{N}p\bar{g}\bar{m})^\gamma/A^{(\gamma-1)}$ and the variance of the number is given approximately by $(\bar{N}p\bar{g}\bar{m})^{2\gamma}\gamma^2/\bar{N}p \ A^{2(\gamma-1)}$. The integrated intensity of the output signal of input threshold contrast, C_T', is $C_T'\gamma(\bar{N}p\bar{g}\bar{m})^\gamma/A^{(\gamma-1)}$. To restore the mean level to its value at the DV, a ND filter of transmittance, F, is introduced such that $(\bar{N}p\bar{g}\bar{m})^\gamma F/A^{(\gamma-1)} = \bar{N}p\bar{g}$. As for the DV it is assumed that a fraction f of the photons emitted by the area A is absorbed by the eye. The expected value of the threshold contrast, C_T', of the signal displayed on the TV is then given by:

$$C_T' = k \sqrt{\frac{1 + \gamma^2 \bar{g} f}{\gamma^2 \bar{N} p \bar{g} f}} \qquad (7.6)$$

If this expression is compared with that for the threshold contrast, C_T, of the signal displayed on the DV, it is clear that the contribution of external noise to the total power of the noise has increased by γ^2 times. If the gain of the intensifier is such that $\bar{g}f = 1$ then for the DV the contributions of external and internal noise are equal, but for the TV the external noise is the dominant factor. The threshold contrasts are very similar, $C_T' = 0.77 \ C_T$, and yet external noise would probably be visible on the TV whilst almost imperceptible on the DV. When internal noise is the dominant factor in both displays, i.e. $\gamma^2 \bar{g} f << 1$, the threshold contrast of the signal displayed on the TV is expected to be a factor of 2·5 less than if it were displayed on the DV. The TV introduces an additional unsharpness, however, that tends to offset the improvement. When in both displays the image is clearly limited by external noise, i.e. $\bar{g}f >> 1$, then both threshold contrasts should be the same.

Digitisation

Many images, e.g. CT scans and scintiscans, are already digitised before display and it is likely that digitisation will be widely applied to other kinds of image, e.g. X-ray images, in the future (p. 45). One advantage of digitisation is that it enables the image to be processed readily by a computer. Digitisation, however, can itself deteriorate the quality of the image.

In order to represent the image faithfully, it is necessary to consider how many samples should be taken (each sample is sometimes called a *pixel*) and how many *gray levels* are required to display the samples. The number of samples required is obtainable from the sampling theorem.[10] For complete representation of all the information contained in the image, assuming the gray scale is adequate, the sample spacing should be not greater than half the wavelength of the highest spatial frequency occurring in the image. The number of levels of gray required to display the image is also related to the size of the detail to be detected. The number depends also on the type of image. The lowest threshold contrasts recorded occur in the detection of large area signals displayed in CT scans and are of the order of 0·1 per cent.[48] Such contrasts cannot be seen with the unaided eye[5] presumably because they fall below the internal noise level of the visual system. After amplification, however, they can be detected.[48] To represent such contrasts, a gray scale of at least 2000 levels is required. In most medical images, however, the external noise present is of greater power and the minimum detectable contrast is likely to be greater than 1 per cent. The noise consists of either random fluctuations of luminance or irrelevant anatomical detail. Experience shows that often 64 gray levels are adequate.[33]

The Mach effect

The visual system accentuates sharp increments in luminance. The effect produced, first described by Mach,[58] is shown in Figure 7.19. The perceived

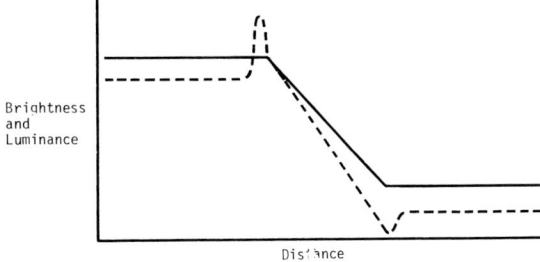

Fig. 7.19 The objective luminance distribution across a step in luminance is represented by the solid line. The corresponding subjective brightness distribution is shown by the dashed line.[27]

brightness (shown as a dashed line) of a step in luminance does not correspond exactly to the objective luminance (shown as a solid line). The MTF of the visual system is characterised by a low frequency attenuation approximately proportional to the square of the spatial frequency (see p. 246). The square law dependence is equivalent to spatial double differentiation and results in enhancement of the transition in luminance at an edge. It is important that a diagnostician working with images should be aware of the phenomenon as the dark and light bands of the Mach effect might be interpreted as real anatomical structures.[54, 22]

It is possible that the Mach effect also enhances the detectability of small differences in contrast between adjacent areas. If the boundary between the areas is made diffuse, the difference in luminance becomes less detectable.[80] It is not clear, however, whether edges are detected by specialised edge detectors or whether the areas of different luminance separated by an edge are detected.

A phenomenon related to the Mach effect is the poor detectability of low frequency stimuli. In the spatial domain the contrast of a large area of uniform luminance is suppressed. It is tempting to speculate that the visual system has evolved so that those areas of the image carrying the most information are enhanced.

IMAGE PROCESSING

The objective

It is often the case that a feature of interest in a medical image cannot be seen as clearly as the observer would wish. If the contrast of the feature is low it can easily be obscured by other anatomical details or by random background noise. It is usually not possible to improve detectability either by increasing the signal-to-noise ratio, because of the need to restrict the dose of radiation delivered to the patient, or by physically removing the unwanted anatomical details. Consequently, there is considerable interest in methods of processing the image to improve the detectability of the feature. Processing can be carried out most easily by digital computer. Indeed, processing has been applied almost exclusively to those images in which computers play a part, e.g. computed tomography and radioisotope scanning. These methods may become applicable to conventional X-ray images when digital radiography (p. 45) becomes more widely used.

Two types of processing can be distinguished; one is image enhancement and the other is restoration. The former comprises methods that, it is hoped, increase the capacity of the human observer to detect a feature of interest. The latter seeks to restore the image to as nearly as possible a faithful copy of the original object. For example, all imaging devices introduce some degree of unsharpness; restoration can be used to counteract its effects.

It should be emphasised that the aim of processing a medical image is to enhance the detectability of a feature of interest. It may not be necessary to improve the fidelity of the whole image nor to maximise the aesthetic appeal of the image unless the latter effect at the same time improves detectability. The general appearance of an image is not a reliable guide to the detectability of any particular feature of the image although it is often used as such. Consequently, the success of any method of processing should be measured by quantitative psychophysical assessment of the improvement in detectability. Whether the recognition of a feature can be improved by further processing once it is clearly detectable must be the subject of further study.

Image enhancement

Histogram modification operating on the gray scale of the image

The probability distribution of the gray levels in an image contains part of the information content of the image. In a digitised image the levels are discrete and the probability distribution is a histogram. The modification is equivalent to a transformation (in general nonlinear) of the intensities. Often it is advantageous to use a transform that leads to a histogram of uniform density: this transformation is called histogram equalisation. In Figure 7.20, the gray levels, r, in the original image, having a probability distribution, $p(r)$, are transformed to new gray levels, s, by the transformation $s = T(r)$. The transformation has been chosen so that the probability distribution of s is uniform. The transform is most likely to be useful if the original image contains only a limited dynamic range. A more general transformation can be used

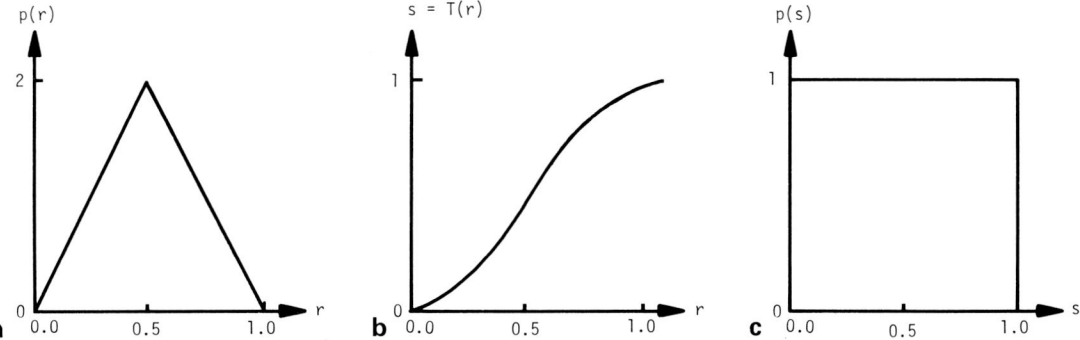

Fig. 7.20 (a) The probability density, $p(r)$, of gray levels, r, in the original image. (b) The transformation, $T(r)$ to new gray levels, s. (c) The probability density, $p(s)$, of s is uniform.

to produce any desired probability distribution in the final image.

Image smoothing

Image smoothing is intended to reduce spurious fluctuations of luminance, i.e. noise, in the image. Smoothing can be carried out in either the spatial or the spatial frequency domains.

In the spatial domain, smoothing can be achieved by neighbourhood averaging. The spatial extent of a neighbourhood is defined and the intensity at each point in the image is replaced by the intensity averaged over the neighbourhood of the point. Sometimes a weighted average is used. Clearly, the greater the extent of the neighbourhood, the smoother the resulting image. Smoothing introduces unsharpness, however, and can result in deterioration instead of enhancement of image quality. In practical images the signal-to-noise ratio can vary across the image. A variable amount of smoothing can be used to achieve, for example, a constant signal-to-noise ratio over each area of the image.[89] If the shape of the signal is known, optimal detectability can be achieved by filtering the image with a matched filter[90] which is equivalent to introducing optimal smoothing. Unfortunately, the signal is rarely known in advance. If the signal is small, however, the shape of its image approximates the PSF of the imaging system and so should the matching filter.

In the spatial frequency domain, smoothing is equivalent to the reduction of the high-frequency content of the image. Therefore, smoothing can be achieved by filtering the image with a low-pass filter. A so-called 'ideal' filter, illustrated in Figure 7.21a, is one whose transfer function, $H(\omega)$, satisfies the relation:

$H(\omega) = 1$, if $0 \leq \omega \leq \omega_0$, where ω_0 is a constant and ω is spatial frequency,

$= 0$, elsewhere.

Multiplying by such a filter is equivalent, in the spatial domain, to convoluting with a PSF (Fig. 7.21b), $h(r) = \omega_0 \mathcal{J}_1(\pi\omega_0 r)/2r$, where $\mathcal{J}_1(x)$ is the first order Bessel function.[10] Convolution is equivalent to a kind of weighted neighbourhood averaging and the diameter of the neighbourhood is of the order of $1/\omega_0$. The PSF corresponding to any ideal filter, however, is characterised by a central core surrounded by successive rings of progressively decreasing intensity. These rings can often be seen in the filtered image and can be confused with the true image. The rings arise because of the sharp edge of the ideal filter. Other low-pass filters have been designed to circumvent this problem. One such filter is the *Butterworth* low-pass filter. High frequencies are severely attenuated by this filter, but since there is no sharp discontinuity in the frequency response, no spurious rings are introduced into the image. Another filter with similar properties is called the *exponential* filter. The *convexity* or *concavity operator*[28] sometimes used in radioisotope scanning also introduces smoothing. Over an organ such as the liver, the distribution of activity along a line is expected to be a convex function, but a tumour, which is usually an area of low activity called a 'cold spot', appears as a concavity, as illustrated in Figure 7.22. To detect the

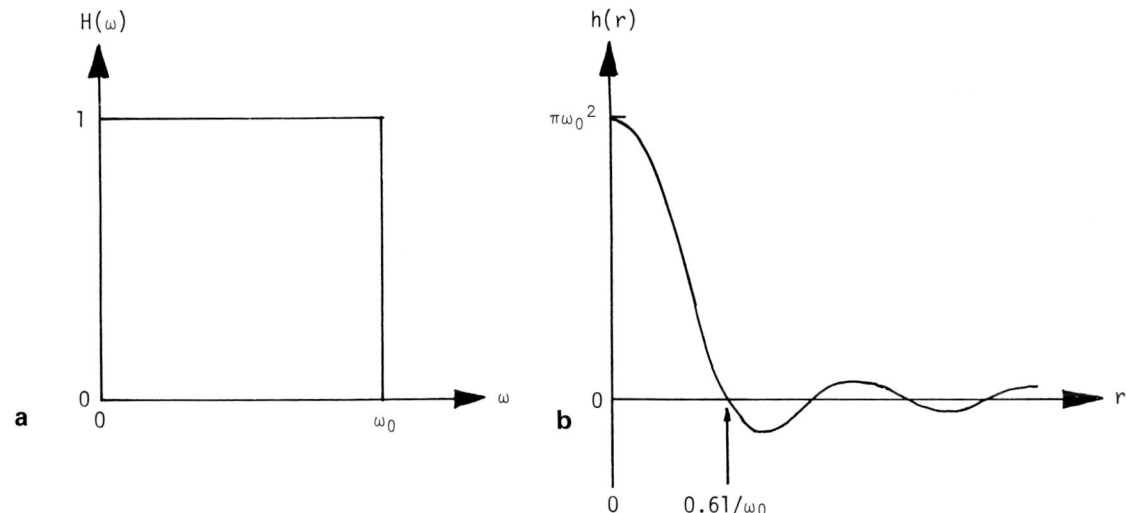

Fig. 7.21 (a) The response, $H(\omega)$, of an 'ideal' filter as a function of the radial spatial frequency, ω, with cut-off frequency ω_0. (b) The point spread function, $h(r)$, corresponding to the 'ideal' filter shown in (a).

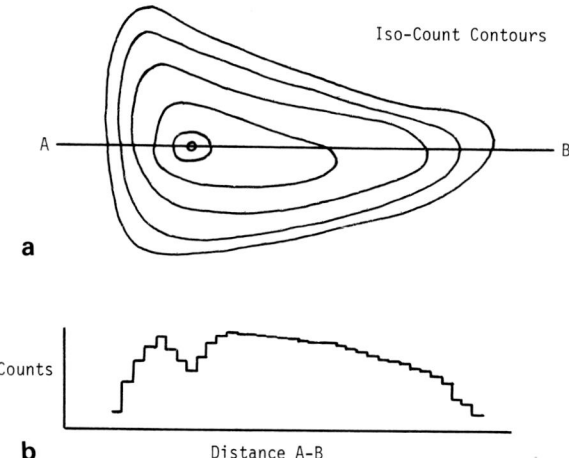

Fig. 7.22 (a) Scan of a liver phantom showing isocount contours at fixed percentages of the maximum count density (hypothetical data). (b) Integrating counts over segments of constant length along the line AB indicates the presence of a 'cold spot' as a concavity in the count distribution.[78]

concavity, the image is first integrated along consecutive lengths, the choice of the length being determined by the width of the collimator spread function. Then if the activity within a length is significantly less than the average of the activities in two neighbouring lengths for at least one direction the presence of a concavity is recorded. Only concavities are displayed and it is claimed that the presence of cold spots is revealed more clearly than in the original image.

It is sometimes possible to reduce the relative contribution of noise to an image by summing many representations of the same object. This procedure is followed in the computer-of-average-transients and to some extent in CT scanners. The noisy image, $g(x,y)$, is given at each point (x,y) by: $g(x,y) = f(x,y) + n(x,y)$, where $f(x,y)$ is the true image and $n(x,y)$ is the noise contribution. After N presentations, the true signal contribution is $Nf(x,y)$, but the standard deviation of the noise contribution has increased by only $\sqrt{N}$, so that the signal-to-noise ratio has improved by $\sqrt{N}$. If the image is produced by a certain dose of radiation and the principal source of noise is quantum fluctuation the above procedure is entirely equivalent to increasing the dose N-fold.

Image sharpening

Image sharpening has the opposite effect to image smoothing. It enhances edges and if noise is present in the image, the noise is also enhanced.

One way of enhancing sharp transitions of luminance is by replacing the luminance at each point of the image by the absolute value of its gradient. In such an image, edges are clearly revealed but all areas of uniform luminance are presented as dark areas. This technique is useful when the area of a lesion is required, e.g. for making quantitative estimates of the uptake of a radioisotope. Many variations on this technique are practised. One example is to replace the image by its gradient only when the value of the gradient lies above a certain threshold. Otherwise the image luminance itself is retained. In this example significant edges are enhanced while information about gradual changes in luminance is retained.

As in smoothing, it is possible to filter the image in the frequency domain to achieve the desired sharpening effect. To achieve sharpening a high-pass filter is required. The response of an 'ideal' filter is given by:

$H(\omega) = 0$, if $0 \leq \omega \leq \omega_0$, where ω is spatial frequency and ω_0 is constant,

= 1, elsewhere.

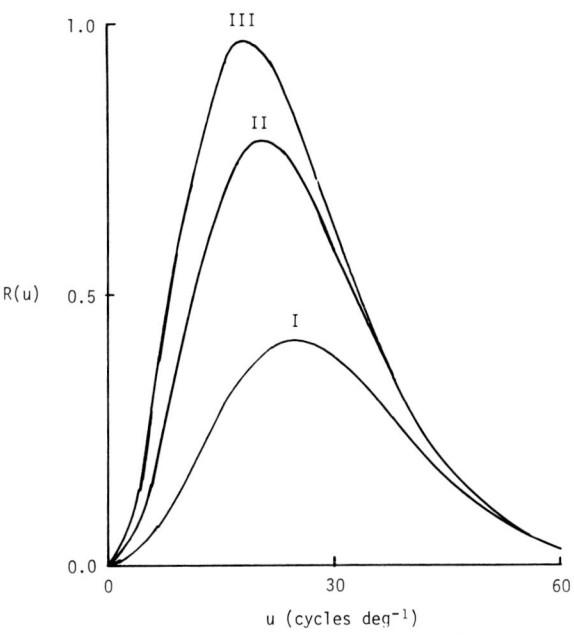

Fig. 7.23 Examples of unsharp masking or Canterbury filters: the relative filter responses, $R(u)$, are: I, $[M(u)-M^2(u)]$; II, $[M(u)-M^4(u)]$ and III, $[M(u)-M^6(u)]$; where $M(u)$ is the response of a smoothing filter.

Such a filter introduces spurious rings into the filtered image and hence either a Butterworth or exponential high-pass filter is preferable. After high-pass filtering there is inevitably a loss of low frequency information. This information can be retained by using a filter response consisting of a constant plus a high-pass response. Further improvement can sometimes be obtained by carrying out histogram equalisation of the filtered image.

Two filters commonly used in nuclear medicine are the *Canterbury*[20] and *Metz*[64] filters. These introduce both sharpening and smoothing. They have the additional merit that processing is rapid. The N-fold multiplication of a low-pass smoothing filter, $M(u)$, with itself provides a set of N low-pass filters, $[M(u)]^N$. Subtracting each filter, $[M(u)]^N$, from the original filter, $M(u)$, yields a set of band-pass or Canterbury filters as illustrated in Figure 7.23.

A filter with a similar characteristic is the '*optimum filter*'.[87] This filter is designed to achieve better resolving power than a matched filter. If the signal-to-noise ratio is low, a matched filter, which introduces smoothing, is required for optimal detectability. If the signal-to-noise ratio is higher, however, the degree of smoothing can be reduced while still retaining acceptable detectability so that the sharpness of the image can be enhanced. A constraint is applied to keep the enhancement of the noise within acceptable limits.

The use of colour

An image consisting of gray levels can be converted into a '*pseudo colour*' image by associating different gray levels with different colours. The use of colour could be advantageous because the number of colours that can be distinguished at a constant luminance is greater than the number of gray levels. About 20 000 chromaticities can be detected,[57] whereas the number of gray levels is probably about 100 (see p. 267).

One way of associating gray levels and colour is to divide the gray scale into regions and to associate each one with a different colour. This representation is sometimes referred to as a *geographical* display. One such display is illustrated in Figure 7.24. Areas of the image corresponding to one of the intervals in the gray scale are represented by the corresponding colour.

A more sophisticated method is to perform three different transformations on the gray level image. Each one is associated with a primary colour, red, green or blue. The three colour transforms are then added resulting in a different colour associated with each gray level present in the image. The trans-

272 SCIENTIFIC BASIS OF MEDICAL IMAGING

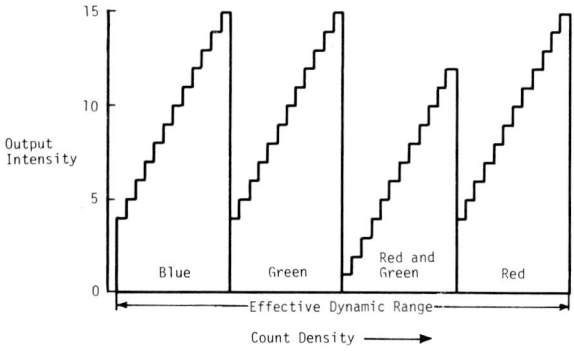

Fig. 7.24 Geographical display. Each count density is represented by one of 15 intensity levels of either blue, green, red-plus-green, or red: red-plus-green appears as yellow.[44]

forms can be chosen so that as the gray scale luminance increases there is a transition from red, through orange and yellow, to white: this transformation is known as a '*heated-object spectrum*', an example of which is shown in Figure 7.25, and has been used in scintigraphy[44] and ultrasound.[65]

occurs in the X-radiography of blood vessels. Two X-ray images are formed, one prior to the injection of radiopaque medium, one following. After subtraction of the first image from the second, most of the structure noise in the background is removed revealing the vessels more clearly (see p. 42).

Image restoration

Image restoration differs from image enhancement in that it seeks to reconstruct an image that has been degraded in some known way. Degradation can occur as part of the image forming process, for example, the collimator used in scintiscanning introduces unsharpness. The process of degradation can be represented as a convolution with a known PSF, $h(x,y)$. Then if the original image is represented by $f(x,y)$, the resulting image, $g(x,y)$, is given by

$$g(x,y) = h(x,y) \star f(x,y) + n_2(x,y) \qquad (7.7)$$

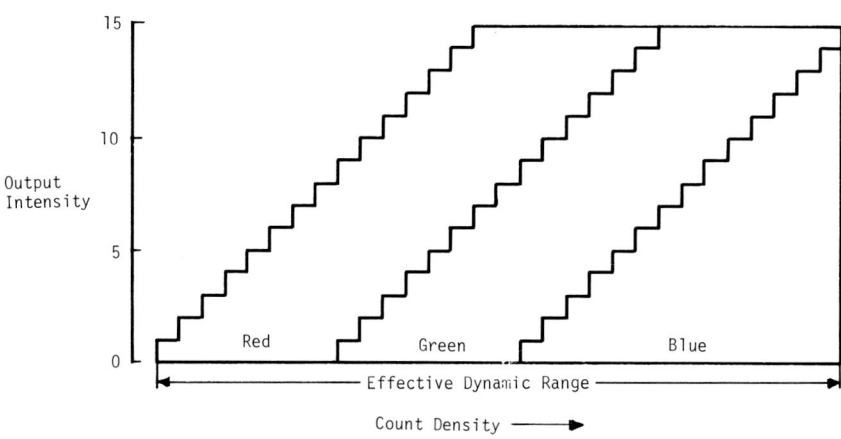

Fig. 7.25 'Heated-object spectrum' display. Each count density is represented by a different colour resulting from a unique combination of red, green and blue intensities.[44]

A similar, three colour, transform can be carried out in the frequency domain where, for example, high frequencies predominate in the red transform, medium frequencies in the green, and low frequencies in the blue.

Subtraction

One undeniably successful form of processing that is applicable to some medical images is subtraction of unwanted detail in the image. A typical example

where $n_2(x,y)$ is a random noise added to the image after the convolution. The original image, $f(x,y)$, sometimes comprises a signal, $f_1(x,y)$, plus a noise component, $n_1(x,y)$. In the spatial frequency domain convolution is replaced by multiplication so that

$$G(u,v) = H(u,v)F(u,v) + N_2(u,v), \qquad (7.8)$$

where $G(u,v)$, $H(u,v)$, $F(u,v)$ and $N_2(u,v)$ are the Fourier transforms of $g(x,y)$, $h(x,y)$, $f(x,y)$ and $n_2(x,y)$ respectively.

Inverse filtering

One method of restoration suggests itself immediately as a result of Equation 7.8. An estimate of $F(u,v)$, $\hat{F}(u,v)$, can be obtained from

$$\hat{F}(u,v) = \frac{G(u,v)}{H(u,v)} + \frac{N_2(u,v)}{H(u,v)} \qquad (7.9)$$

In the absence of the noise, $N_2(u,v)$, the estimate $\hat{F}(u,v)$, would be identical to $F(u,v)$, provided $H(u,v) \neq 0$, and inverse Fourier transformation would yield the original image, $f(x,y)$. When noise is present, serious discrepancies can arise between the estimate, $\hat{F}(u,v)$, and the original signal, $F(u,v)$. If the filter function, $H(u,v)$, is small for some u and v, the noise term can make a very large contribution to the restored image. The contribution of the original noise term, $N_1(u,v)$, however, should be the same after restoration as before degradation.

The Wiener filter

A general method for obtaining an estimate, $\hat{f}(x,y)$, of a signal $f(x,y)$, from data corrupted by noise is one that minimises the quantity $E\{[f(x,y) - \hat{f}(x,y)]^2\}$, where E denotes the expectation value. The method is useful in the restoration of degraded images since the constraint applied controls, on average, the amplification of noise. The estimate, $\hat{F}(u,v)$, is given by:

$$\hat{F}(u,v) = \frac{1}{H(u,v)} \cdot \left\{ \frac{|H(u,v)|^2}{|H(u,v)|^2 + [S_{n1}(u,v)|H(u,v)|^2 + S_{n2}(u,v)]/S_f(u,v)} \right\} \cdot G(u,v) \qquad (7.10)$$

where $S_{n1}(u,v)$, $S_{n2}(u,v)$ and $S_f(u,v)$ are the power spectra of the two sources of noise and the signal, respectively. The expression within the square brackets is the so-called '*Wiener filter*'. It is interesting to note that if the noise contribution is negligible, the required filter is simply the inverse filter. If, on the other hand, the noise contribution is large, the filter is a matched filter. In order to carry out the restoration strictly according to Equation 7.10, knowledge of the power spectra is required and is usually not available. A useful degree of restoration can sometimes be achieved, however, by assuming that $[S_{n1}(u,v)|H(u,v)|^2 + S_{n2}(u,v)]/S_f(u,v)$ is equal to some constant value.

Other similar constraints can be applied to obtain the estimate, $\hat{f}(x,y)$. One such constraint[69] ensures that the estimate, $\hat{f}(x,y)$, is not subject to large fluctuations, tacitly assuming that the true signal is a smoothly varying function. Whereas the Wiener filter controls only on average the amplification of noise, this alternative constraint is effective for any given image.[33] The constraint can be applied by minimising some function of the second derivative of $\hat{f}(x,y)$. The procedure is generally applicable because no prior knowledge of the original signal is required, and only an estimate of the mean and variance of the noise is necessary.

Interactive restoration

The above methods of restoration are applicable when the process of degradation is known. Even without such prior knowledge, however, it is sometimes possible to recognise from the appearance of the degraded image that a particular form of degradation has occurred and to counteract it. An example of such a degradation is a sinusoidal interference pattern. The pattern appears in the Fourier transform of the degraded image as one or more pairs of frequency impulses. A small region of the frequency plane containing the interference frequencies can sometimes be filtered out with consequent improvement in the image. Of course, it may not always be clear which frequency components are interference and which belong to the true image.

The efficacy of image processing

Practical tests of processing

Many different forms of image processing have been tried particularly in scintigraphy and CT scanning where computers are used in presenting the image. Those forms of processing commonly applied to scintigraphic images have been compared and the efficacy of each type of display has been assessed by measuring the detectability of computer-simulated lesions superimposed on either brain or normal liver images.[42,43] Two quantitative methods of measuring the improvement in detectability were used: localisation receiver operating characteristic curves[82] and a points system scoring true and false positives.[42] The results indicate that no one method of processing is consistently better than all others, although the Canterbury[20] and optimum[87] filters as well as the convexity operator[78] are often successful in improving detectability. The type of display, particularly the size of the matrix used, as well as the degree of experience of a particular observer appear to be important. Although there are some favourable reports following the clinical evaluation of some types of processing they are few in number compared with the general availability of facilities for processing. It has been speculated that there is perhaps under-reporting of trials in which processing procedures are not shown to be successful.[89] Thus the clinical efficacy of image processing should be regarded as unproven at present.

Although in the comparative study just mentioned[43] smoothing was not a noticeably successful form of processing, other studies have reached different conclusions. Thus an increase in detectability after smoothing a scintigraphic image consisting of a small hot-spot in a uniform field has been shown,[40] although the analysis of the results has been questioned. A 'noise-cheating' algorithm equivalent to smoothing has been described which was judged subjectively to improve the quality of digitised, defocused, photographic images.[99] A subjective improvement in CT images after smoothing has also been shown.[48]

There are fewer examples of the use of image sharpening than of smoothing in medical images. The Canterbury filter[20] is a band-pass filter used in scintigraphic images and has been shown[43] to be relatively successful. A method of electronic enhancement of details for use in X-ray television systems has been described.[29] The image is defocused and subtracted from the original image so that low frequencies are removed. The resulting image is then added to the original yielding a final image in which high frequencies are enhanced. It is claimed that the detection of small details is improved although the danger of introducing artifacts by this process has been pointed out.

Image restoration is often attempted in scintigraphy. Although Wiener filters have been used, it has been pointed out that the conventional Wiener filter is inappropriate in that its use assumes no cross-correlation between the signal and the noise.[13] Clearly, in scintigraphic images there is such a correlation. An alternative approach is to deconvolute the image, seeking the smoothest solution.[69] Efficient methods of implementing this constraint have been developed.[9] The method has been used clinically in angiography[9] and it is claimed that lesions are rendered more apparent.

In CT scanning the reconstructed image is routinely subjected to some form of restoration. Most methods of reconstruction use back projection which results in an image each point of which is blurred by a function, $f(r)$, proportional to $1/r$, where r is the distance from the image point.[88] The reconstruction algorithm usually contains a component that corrects for the blurring function, $f(r)$, in addition to other forms of processing. The effect of the algorithm can be described in terms of its MTF, $M_{alg}(f)$, where f is the spatial frequency. Neglecting non-algorithmic blurring, it has been shown[94] that the noise power spectrum is proportional to $|M_{alg}(f)|^2 \times f$. The effect of the algorithm on the noise power spectrum is reminiscent of that of lateral inhibition on a visual signal (see p. 246). Whereas lateral inhibition affects the visual signal as well as any source of noise arising distal to the site of the inhibitory mechanism, however, the spectrum of the signal in a reconstructed CT image is multiplied only by $M_{alg}(f)$ and not by f. Therefore there is an apparent enhancement of the signal-to-noise ratio of low frequency signals proportional to $f^{-1/2}$ in a reconstructed CT image.

Different forms of colour display of scintigraphic images have been compared with gray-scale displays[44] using the same type of computer-simulated lesions as in the assessment of other forms of processing.[42] The gray-scale displays consisted of only 16 levels of gray: in one, black-on-white, white corresponded to the lowest count-density, and in the other, white-on-black, the intensity scale was reversed. These displays were compared with two types of colour display, a geographical display, using 50 levels, and a heated-object spectrum display, using 30 levels. The latter display has been used also in ultrasound imaging.[65] The heated-object spectrum display proved to be the best for brain images, while for liver images no significant differences emerged. These comparisons, however, do not provide a clear-cut comparison of the use of colour and gray level displays. In both colour displays a greater number of levels were used. Furthermore, in the heated-object spectrum display, the luminance differences were greatest in the orange thus aiding detectability in brain images which lie mainly in the region of orange.

Theoretical considerations

The physiology of the visual system is such as to suggest that the image received is processed prior to detection (see p. 246). The MTF of the visual system is equivalent to a band-pass filter. The attenuation of low frequencies results in the enhancement of edges (p. 267) and the high frequency limitation introduces some degree of smoothing. In order to enhance detectability, any processing of the visual scene must be either more effective than or must complement that of the visual system. Furthermore, the detection mechanism itself is relevant in determining whether any particular kind of processing is effective. Unfortunately, the proposed models of the visual detection mechanism are of limited scope. Nevertheless, certain predictions can be made about the efficacy of some kinds of processing.

According to the SSNL model the effect of smoothing on the detectability of isolated signals is expected to be at best ineffective and possibly detrimental. The effect of smoothing on a signal is to remove or diminish high frequency components. Only those frequencies in the spectrum of the noise that form part of the signal spectrum interfere with the detectability of the signal. It is immaterial whether high frequency components, not present in the signal, are present in the noise as they are prior to smoothing, or not, after smoothing. Thus, smoothing the noise to the same degree as the signal cannot be expected to enhance the detectability of the signal. Indeed the signal-to-noise ratio decreases for small signals leading to a decrease in detectability. A similar conclusion has been drawn on the basis of the Rose model.[93,47] Some of the experimental results of smoothing, however, suggest that detectability can be enhanced.[40,48,94] A possible explanation is that smoothing can be effective when the noise is overwhelming and the ability of the visual system to carry out smoothing is limited.[48] In some measurements of detectability using optically projected images and a noise background of power sufficient to increase the threshold contrast to five times the value for a uniform background, however, smoothing by defocusing decreased detectability, as shown in Figure 7.26.

There are theoretical reasons for expecting histogram modification to be successful under certain conditions. If any external noise present in the image is of low power, detection of small contrasts is limited by the internal noise of the visual system. If the contrast of the image is increased by histogram modification a previously undetectable signal can be amplified above the decision criterion set by internal noise and rendered detectable. If external noise is the limiting factor in the detectability of the original image, however, no such improvement can be expected as the noise is amplified to the same extent as the signal.

Image restoration can be expected to be effective if the noise present in the image is of low power. If significant noise is present, provided it arises before the degradation of the image, restoration might improve detectability. If the noise arises after the degradation, however, the noise contribution can be amplified by the restoration and artifacts appear in the image.

A colour display could in theory be more effective than a gray-level display if the number of potentially distinguishable levels in the image was in excess of 100 (see p. 267). The number depends on the power of the noise inherent in the image and, for example, in CT scans can approach 2000[48] although in most other medical images the number rarely exceeds 100. Because of the internal noise present in the visual system, the human observer cannot distinguish more than about 100 gray levels whereas it is claimed[57] that about 20 000 chromaticities are distinguishable. Colour representation, however, could affect detectability or pattern recognition in other ways that are as yet uninvestigated.

ASSESSMENT OF IMAGE QUALITY

The choice of methods of assessment

In medical images probably the most important criterion of image quality is detectability (see p. 237). Methods of assessing image quality fall into two broad categories, viz. objective and sub-

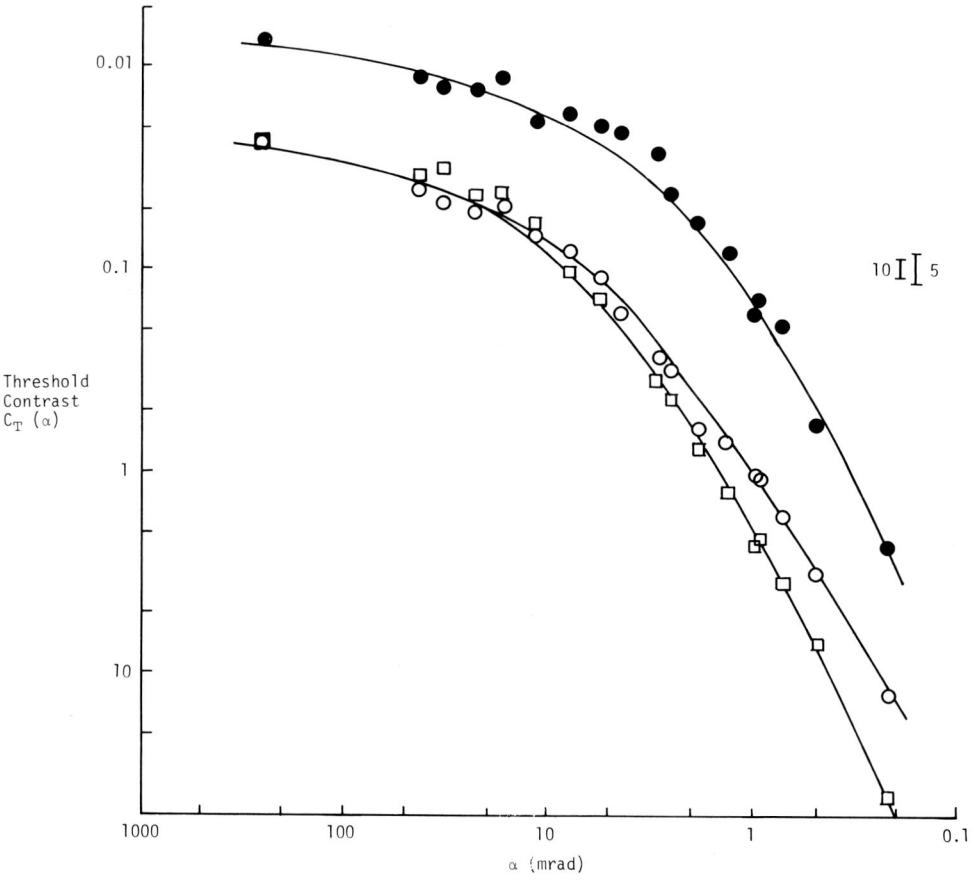

Fig. 7.26 Threshold contrasts, $C_T(\alpha)$, for incremental disc-shaped signals of initial diameter α mrad displayed on noise and uniform, i.e. zero power noise, backgrounds of mean luminance 7 cd m^{-2}: full power focused noise and focused signals (○); defocused noise and signals (□); and zero power noise and focused signals (●); log scales. Points labelled '○' and '●' are means of 10 observations: points labelled '□' are means of 5 observations. The error bars labelled '10' and '5' are 2 × SE of the means of 10 and 5 observations, respectively.

jective. A subjective method is one in which a human observer judges the quality of an image on the basis of its appearance. The judgement can be quantitative, e.g. measurement of an ROC curve, or qualitative, e.g. based on purely aesthetic considerations. An objective method involves the measurement of some characteristic of the image that is believed to affect its detectability.

If observers are asked to give a qualitative, subjective assessment of image quality they are free to choose any criterion and that criterion may not be detectability. Often a picture in which noise is clearly visible is regarded as inferior to one in which noise does not appear. This judgement can well be fallacious. For example, if the gain of an X-ray image intensifier is insufficient to render each X-ray quantum clearly visible, detectability is not optimal (see p. 265). Nevertheless, the picture has less visible noise than one in which the gain is sufficient for optimal detectability. It is important that diagnosticians working with medical images should realise that visible noise is not an insuperable barrier to detectability, although it is possible that some experience is needed to achieve maximum performance. In qualitative judgements of image quality, sharpness appears to be a frequently used criterion. Nevertheless, it can be inappropriate to a particular detection task, for example the detection of a large low contrast lesion.

Quantitative subjective methods of assessment

can give direct answers to questions of image quality, based on a criterion of detectability, but can be criticised on the grounds that the answers can vary from observer to observer. For example, ROC curves can be shown to be reasonably reproducible for a given observer and image but there is considerably more variation between observers.[40]

Although objective measurements could be more reproducible they give only indirect information about image quality. A comprehensive and reliable theory of visual detection would be required before objective measurements alone could be used to assess the quality of an image. Such a theory is not available at present. Some information about image quality, however, can be inferred from certain objective measurements. For example, it is true in general that a sharp image is of high quality and a noisy image is not. Nevertheless, quantitative subjective measurements, averaged over several observers, are at present probably the most reliable means of assessment.

The conditions under which image quality is to be assessed can have a crucial influence on the choice of the most suitable method. There is a need for a simple method of assessment to monitor the quality of imaging devices in routine use. Elaborate laboratory methods are clearly inappropriate as well as impractical. Quantitative subjective assessment, even by a single observer, is probably all that is required.

There have been many attempts to summarise the quality of an image in a single figure of merit. Limiting resolution is often quoted as such; its inadequacies are discussed on page 36. It seems rather unlikely that any such figure can be found.

The most relevant measure of any improvement in image quality produced by processing is increased detectability. It is particularly important, however, to measure not only the rate of true detectability but also the false positive rate. Determination of an ROC curve, of course, necessitates measuring both. Restoration of noisy images can create artifacts and it would be possible to find an increase not only in the true positive rate of detection but also in the false positive rate. Such an outcome would not be regarded as satisfactory. Unfortunately, the detectability of a particular lesion in a complex medical image probably depends on the location of the lesion in relation to surrounding anatomical structures. It is possible that the dectectability of the lesion is not improved if processing enhances the surrounding structures to the same degree as the lesion. Thus although it may be possible to draw some general conclusions about the efficacy of processing from the detectability of particular signals it is also necessary to verify whether these conclusions apply in any particular class of medical image.[89]

Phantoms and test objects for subjective assessment

Perhaps the best subjective test of an imaging system would be measurement of the detectability of a typical lesion in a typical patient. The practical difficulties of such a measurement, however, are insurmountable. Therefore attempts have been made to simulate the lesion and the patient in a phantom. The phantom can be either a physical construction, for example the Burger phantom,[14] or, where computers are used in presenting the image, it can be created mathematically.[42]

Such phantoms cannot be guaranteed to represent all the characteristics of the lesion and the patient that are important for detectability, however, since these characteristics may not be known. Therefore it is perhaps reasonable to simplify the design of the phantom making it easier to construct. There is a further gain in that the detectability of a simple shape can be easier to correlate with theories of visual detection. Geometrically-shaped phantoms called test objects have been used to test X-ray systems (p. 36), CT scanners,[19] and scintigraphic imaging devices.[67]

Disc-shaped test objects of a range of diameters and contrasts can be used to measure the threshold contrast. Figure 1.32 shows the 'Leeds' test object as it would appear on a perfect fluorescent screen. If the range of diameters is sufficient, information can be obtained about the power of the noise in the system and the sharpness of the system. The performance of the system measured by such test objects is probably an adequate representation of its performance in relation to most isolated lesions, e.g. small calcifications. Test objects of different shapes, e.g. metal wires simulating blood vessels, could be used to test whether the performance of the system depended on the shape of the test object. Other commonly used test objects are gratings consisting of parallel strips of high contrast material. A set of gratings with different spacings between the strips could be used to measure the contrast sensitivity curve of an imaging system giving information about the noise inherent in the image and the sharpness of the image. Grating patterns in which the spacing increases progressively across the pattern, however, are more commonly found and are used to measure only limiting resolution.

Acknowledgements

I am particularly grateful to my colleagues G. A. Hay and A. R. Cowen for reading the manuscript and for many helpful discussions of the material in this chapter. My thanks are also due to Mrs P. Smith and Miss M. Frost for their help in producing the typescript.

I acknowledge with thanks permission to reproduce copyright material as follows: B. B. Boycott and the Editor of the *Proceedings of the Royal Society of London* for Figure 7.2, K. H. Ruddock and the Editor of *Reports on Progress in Physics* for Figures 7.3 and 7.4, and D. H. Hubel and the Editor of the *Journal of Physiology* for Figure 7.5.

REFERENCES

1. Albrecht, C. (1965) Noise sources in image intensifying devices. In *Diagnostic Radiological Instrumentation: Modular Transfer Function*, ed. Moseley, R. D. Jr & Rust, J. H., pp. 291–311. Springfield: Thomas.
2. Barlow, H. B. (1958) Intrinsic noise of cones. In *Nat. Phys. Lab. Symposium (No. 15) on Visual Problems of Colour*, pp. 617–30. London: HMSO.
3. Barlow, H. B. (1958) Temporal and spatial summation in human vision at different background intensities. *J. Physiol. (Lond.)*, **141**, 337–50.
4. Barlow, H. B. (1977) Retinal and central factors in human vision limited by noise. In *Vertebrate Photoreception*, pp. 337–58. London: Academic Press.
5. Blackwell, H. R. (1946) Contrast thresholds of the human eye. *J. opt. Soc. Am.*, **36**, 624–43.
6. Blackwell, H. R. (1963) Neural theories of simple visual discriminations. *J. opt. Soc. Am.*, **53**, 129–60.
7. Blakemore, C. & Campbell, F. W. (1969) On the existence of neurones in the human visual system selectively sensitive to the orientation and size of retinal images. *J. Physiol. (Lond.)*, **203**, 237–60.
8. Blakemore, C., Nachmias, J. & Sutton, P. (1970) The perceived spatial shift: evidence for frequency-selective neurones in the human brain. *J. Physiol. (Lond.)*, **210**, 727–50.
9. Boardman, A. K. (1979) Constrained optimisation and its application to scintigraphy. *Physics Med. Biol.*, **24**, 363–71.
10. Bracewell, R. (1965) *The Fourier Transform and its Applications*. New York: McGraw-Hill.
11. Brown, E. B. (1965) *Modern Optics*, pp. 479–521. New York: Reinhold.
12. Brown, P. H. & Wald, G. (1964) Visual pigments in single rods and cones of the human retina. *Science*, **144**, 45–52.
13. Budinger, T. F. (1973) Clinical and research quantitative nuclear medicine system. In *Medical Radioisotope Scintigraphy*, vol. I, pp. 501–55. Vienna: IAEA.
14. Burger, G. C. E. (1950) Phantom tests with X rays. *Philips techn. Rev.*, **11**, 291–8.
15. Campbell, F. W. & Gubisch, R. W. (1966) Optical quality of the human eye. *J. Physiol. (Lond.)*, **186**, 558–78.
16. Campbell, F. W. & Robson, J. G. (1968) Application of Fourier analysis to the visibility of gratings. *J. Physiol. (Lond.)*, **197**, 551–66.
17. Chesters, M. S. (1973) *The Influence of Visual Noise on Visual Detection Thresholds*. University of Leeds: Ph.D. thesis.
18. Chesters, M. S. (to be published). The theory of the visual detection of images. In *Proceedings of the HPA Conference on Physical Aspects of Medical Imaging*.
19. Cohen, G. & DiBianca, F. A. (1979) The use of contrast-detail-dose evaluation of image quality in a computed tomographic scanner. *J. comput. assist. Tomogr.*, **3**, 189–95.
20. Corfield, J. R. (1976) Development of a fast enhancement filter for routine use. In *Proc. 13th Internationale Jahrestagung der Gesellschaft für Nuclearmedizin, E.V.*, Copenhagen, 1975.
21. Crozier, W. J. (1935) On the variability of critical illumination for flicker fusion and intensity discrimination. *J. gen. Physiol.*, **19**, 503–22.
22. Daffner, R. H. (1980) Visual illusions in computed tomography: phenomena related to Mach effect. *Am. J. Roentg.*, **134**, 261–4.
23. De Vries, H. (1943) The quantum character of light and its bearing upon threshold of vision, the differential sensitivity and visual acuity of the eye. *Physica*, **10**, 553–64.
24. Dowling, J. E. & Boycott, B. B. (1966) Organization of the primate retina: electron microscopy. *Proc. R. Soc. Lond. (Biol)*, **166**, 80–111.
25. Enroth-Cugell, C. & Robson, J. G. (1966) The contrast sensitivity of retinal ganglion cells of the cat. *J. Physiol. (Lond.)*, **187**, 517–52.
26. Fechner, G. T. (1860) *Elemente der Psychophysik*. Leipzig.
27. Fiorentini, A. & Radici, T. (1957) Binocular measurements of brightness on a field representing a luminance gradient. *Atti. Fond. Giorgio Ronchi*, **12**, 453–61.
28. Fiorentini, A., Sireteanu, R. & Spinelli, D. (1976) Lines and gratings: different interocular after-effects. *Vision Res.*, **16**, 1303–9.
29. Fuchs, W. A., Messerschmid, U., Herren, U. & Steck, W. (1972) Electronic detail enhancement in Roentgen

television. *Invest. Radiol.*, **7**, 140–6.
30. Georgeson, M. A. & Sullivan, G. D. (1975) Contrast constancy: deblurring in human vision by spatial frequency channels. *J. Physiol. (Lond.)*, **252**, 627–56.
31. Ginsburg, A. P., Casson, M. W. & Nelson, M. A. (1980) Suprathreshold processing of complex visual stimuli: evidence for linearity in contrast perception. *Science*, **208**, 619–21.
32. Glezer, V. D., Invanoff, V. A. & Tscherbach, T. A. (1973) Investigation of complex and hypercomplex receptive fields of visual cortex of the cat as spatial frequency filters. *Vision Res.*, **13**, 1875–904.
33. Gonzalez, R. C. & Wintz, P. A. (1977) *Digital Image Processing*. Massachusetts: Addison-Wesley.
34. Green, D. M. & Swets, J. A. (1966) *Signal Detection Theory and Psychophysics*. New York: Wiley.
35. Hartline, H. K. (1940) The receptive fields of optic nerve fibers. *Am. J. Physiol.*, **130**, 690–9.
36. Hay, G. A. (1966) New aspects of visual perception thresholds. *Nature*, **211**, 1380–1.
37. Hay, G. A. & Chesters, M. S. (1977) A model of visual threshold detection. *J. theor. Biol.*, **67**, 221–40.
38. Hecht, S., Schlaer, S. & Pirenne, M. H. (1942) Energy, quanta and vision. *J. gen. Physiol.*, **25**, 819–40.
39. Henning, G. B., Hertz, B. G. & Broadbent, D. E. (1975) Some experiments bearing on the hypothesis that the visual system analyses spatial patterns in independent bands of spatial frequency. *Vision Res.*, **15**, 887–97.
40. Herath, K. B. & Sharp, P. F. (1976) Effects of 'matched filter' smoothing as measured by receiver operating characteristic curve. *Phys. Med. Biol.*, **21**, 442–6.
41. Holway, A. H. (1937) On the precision of photometric observations. *J. opt. Soc. Am.*, **27**, 120–3.
42. Houston, A. S. & Macleod, M. A. (1979) An intercomparison of computer assisted image processing and display methods in liver scintigraphy. *Phys. Med. Biol.*, **24**, 559–70.
43. Houston, A. S., Sharp, P. F., Tofts, P. S. & Diffey, B. L. (1979) A multicentre comparison of computer assisted image processing and display methods in scintigraphy. *Phys. Med. Biol.*, **24**, 547–58.
44. Houston, A. S. (1980) A comparison of four standard scintigraphic TV displays: concise communication. *J. nucl. Med.*, **21**, 512–7.
45. Howell, E. R. & Hess, R. F. (1978) The functional area for summation to threshold for sinusoidal gratings. *Vision Res.*, **18**, 369–74.
46. Hubel, D. H. & Wiesel, T. N. (1968) Receptive fields and functional architecture of monkey striate cortex. *J. Physiol. (Lond.)*, **195**, 215–43.
47. Joseph, P. M. (1978) Image noise and smoothing in computed tomography (CT) scanners. *Opt. Eng.*, **17**, 396–9.
48. Joseph, P. M., Hilal, S. K., Schultz, R. A. & Kelcz, F. (1980) Clinical and experimental investigation of a smoothed CT reconstruction algorithm. *Radiology*, **134**, 507–16.
49. King-Smith, P. E. (1973) The optical density of erythrolabe determined by retinal densitometry using the self-screening method. *J. Physiol. (Lond.)*, **230**, 535–49.
50. King-Smith, P. E. & Kulikowski, J. J. (1975) The detection of gratings by independent activation of line detectors. *J. Physiol. (Lond.)*, **247**, 237–71.
51. Kuffler, S. W. (1953) Discharge patterns and functional organization of mammalian retina. *J. Neurophysiol.*, **16**, 37–68.
52. Kuffler, S. W., Fitzhugh, R. & Barlow, H. B. (1957) Maintained activity in the cat's retina in light and darkness. *J. gen. Physiol.*, **40**, 683–702.
53. Kulikowski, J. J. & King-Smith, P. E. (1973) Spatial arrangement of line, edge and grating detectors revealed by subthreshold summation. *Vision Res.*, **13**, 1479–86.
54. Lane, E. J., Proto, A. V. & Phillips, T. W. (1976) Mach bands and density perception. *Radiology*, **121**, 9–17.
55. Linfoot, E. H. (1966) *Fourier Methods in Optical Image Evaluation*. London: Focal Press.
56. Longhurst, R. S. (1967) *Geometrical and Physical Optics*, p. 386. London: Longman.
57. MacAdam, D. L. (1942) Visual sensitivities to color differences in daylight. *J. opt. Soc. Am.*, **32**, 247–74.
58. Mach, E. (1865) Über die Wirkung der räumlichen Vertheilung des Lichtreizes auf die Netzhaut, I. *Sber. math.-nat. Classe Kaiselichen Akad. Wiss.*, **52**, 303–22.
59. Maffei, L. & Fiorentini, A. (1972) Processes of synthesis in visual perception. *Nature*, **240**, 479–81.
60. Maffei, L. & Fiorentini, A. (1973) The visual cortex as a spatial frequency analyser. *Vision Res.*, **13**, 1255–67.
61. Marg, E. (1973) Recording from single cells in the human visual cortex. In *Handb. Sens. Physiol.*, vol VII/3B, pp. 441–50. New York: Springer-Verlag.
62. Marr, D. (1976) Early processing of visual information. *Phil. Trans. R. Soc. Lond. (Biol.)*, **275**, 483–524.
63. Marr, D. & Poggio, T. (1979) A computational theory of human stereovision. *Proc. R. Soc. Lond. (Biol.)*, **204**, 301–28.
64. Metz, C. E. (1970) *A mathematical investigation of radio-isotope scan image processing*. Ph.D. Thesis. University Microfilms, Ann Arbor.
65. Milan, J. & Taylor, K. J. W. (1975) The application of the temperature scale to ultrasonic imaging. *J. clin. Ultrasound*, **3**, 171–3.
66. Morgan, R. H. (1965) Threshold visual perception and its relationship to photon fluctuation and sine wave response. *Am. J. Roentg.* **93**, 982–97.
67. Murray, K. J., Elliott, A. T. & Wadsworth, J. (1979) A new phantom for the assessment of nuclear medicine imaging equipment. *Phys. Med. Biol.*, **24**, 188–92.
68. O'Brian, B. (1951) Vision and resolution in the central retina. *J. opt. Soc. Am.*, **41**, 882–94.
69. Phillips, D. L. (1962) A technique for the numerical solution of certain integral equations of the first kind. *J. ass. Comput. Mach.*, **9**, 84–97.
70. Pollehn, H. & Roehrig, H. (1970) Effect of noise on the modulation transfer function of the visual channel. *J. opt. Soc. Am.*, **60**, 842–8.
71. Pollen, D. A. & Taylor, J. H. (1974) The striate cortex and the spatial analysis of visual space. In *The Neurosciences, Third Study Program*, pp. 239–47. Cambridge: MIT Press.
72. Polyak, S. L. (1941) *The Retina*. Chicago: Chicago University Press.
73. Robson, J. G. (1975) Receptive fields: neural representation of the spatial and intensive attributes of the visual image. In *Handbook of Perception*, ed. Carterette, E. C. & Friedman, M. P., vol. V, pp. 81–116. New York: Academic Press.
74. Rose, A. (1942) The relative sensitivities of television pickup tubes, photographic film, and the human eye. *Proc. I.R.E.*, **30**, 293–300.
75. Rose, A. (1948) The sensitivity performance of the

human eye on an absolute scale. *J. opt. Soc. Am.*, **38**, 196–208.
76. Ruddock, K. H. (1977) The organization of human vision for pattern detection and recognition. *Rep. Prog. Phys.*, **40**, 603–63.
77. Sachs, M. B., Nachmias, J. & Robson, J. G. (1971) Spatial-frequency channels in human vision. *J. opt. Soc. Am.*, **61**, 1176–86.
78. St. Clair Neill, G. D. & Hutchinson, F. (1971) Computer detection and display of focal lesions on scintiscans. *Br. J. Radiol.*, **44**, 962–9.
79. Schnitzler, A. D. (1973) Image-detector model and parameters of the human visual system. *J. opt. Soc. Am.*, **63**, 1357–68.
80. Shapley, R. M. & Tolhurst, D. J. (1973) Edge detectors in human vision. *J. Physiol. (Lond.)*, **229**, 165–83.
81. Snyder, A. W. & Miller, W. H. (1977) Photoreceptor diameter and spacing for highest resolving power. *J. opt. Soc. Am.*, **67**, 696–8.
82. Starr, S. J., Metz, C. E., Lusted, L. B. & Goodenough, D. J. (1975) Visual detection and localization of radiographic images. *Radiology*, **116**, 533–8.
83. Stevens, S. S. (1960) The psychophysics of sensory function. *Am. Scient.*, **48**, 226–53.
84. Stromeyer, C. F. III & Julesz, B. (1972) Spatial-frequency masking in vision: critical bands and spread of masking. *J. opt. Soc. Am.*, **62**, 1221–32.
85. Sturm, R. E. & Morgan, R. H. (1949) Screen intensification systems and their limitations. *Am. J. Roentg.* **62**, 617–34.
86. Sullivan, G. D., Georgeson, M. A. & Oatley, K. (1972) Channels for spatial frequency selection and the detection of single bars by the human visual system. *Vision Res.*, **12**, 383–94.
87. Tanaka, E. & Iinuma, T. A. (1970) Approaches to optimal data processing in radioisotope imaging. *Phys. Med. Biol.*, **15**, 683–94.
88. Tanaka, E. & Iinuma, T. A. (1975) Correction functions for optimizing the reconstructed image in transverse section scan. *Phys. Med. Biol.*, **20**, 789–98.
89. Todd-Pokropek, A. (1980) Image processing in nuclear medicine. *I.E.E.E. Trans. nucl. Sci.*, **NS-27**, 1080–94.
90. Turin, G. L. (1960) An introduction to matched filters. *I.R.E. Trans. inform. Theory*, **IT-6**, 311–29.
91. Van Meeteren, A. & Vos, J. J. (1972) Resolution and contrast sensitivity at low luminances. *Vision Res.*, **12**, 825–33.
92. Van Meeteren, A. (1974) Calculations on the optical modulation transfer function of the human eye for white light. *Optica Acta*, **21**, 395–412.
93. Wagner, R. F. (1977) Toward a unified view of radiological imaging systems. Part II: Noisy images. *Med. Phys.*, **4**, 279–96.
94. Wagner, R. F., Brown, D. G. & Pastel, M. S. (1979) Application of information theory to the assessment of computed tomography. *Med. Phys.*, **6**, 83–94.
95. Werblin, F. S. & Dowling, J. E. (1969) Organization of the retina of the mudpuppy, *Necturus maculosus*. II. Intracellular recording. *J. Neurophysiol.*, **32**, 339–55.
96. Wilson, H. R. & Giese, S. C. (1977) Threshold visibility of frequency gradient patterns. *Vision Res.*, **17**, 1177–90.
97. Wilson, H. R. & Bergen, J. R. (1979) A four mechanism model for threshold spatial vision. *Vision Res.*, **19**, 19–32.
98. Zwass, F. & Alpen, M. (1976) The density of human rhodopsin in the rods. *Vision Res.*, **16**, 121–7.
99. Zweig, H., Silvestri, A., Hu, P. & Barrett, E. (1976) Experiments in digital restoration of defocussed grainy photographs by noise cheating and Fourier techniques. *Proc. S.P.I.E.*, **74**, 10–6.

Index

Absorption unsharpness, 13
Absorption,
    ultrasonic, 145
Acoustic microscopy 171–4
Air-gap effect, 15
Aliasing, 79–80
Anatomy, visual system, 237–41
Angiography, 47
Angiology, 178–9, 187–9
Angular frequency, 143
Annihilation photon tomography, 106
Antirheumatic drug therapy, 205–6
Aperture transfer function, 76
Aperture,
    spatial sampling, 252–4
    temporal sampling, 250–2
Artifact
    partial detection, 81–2
    ring, 81
    streak, 80–1
    ultrasonic multiple reflexion, 154
    X-ray CT, 78–82
A-scope, ultrasonic, 151
Attenuation,
    X-ray, 4–6, 56
    ultrasonic, 144–7
Atomic nuclei, 212–3
Automatic control,
    brightness, 32
    density, 32
    time gain, 151–2

Back projection reconstruction, 55, 58–9
Beam hardening, 80
Biological effects,
    NMR imaging, 233
    ultrasound, 176–7
Bi-plane serial changer, 47
Biopolar cells, 237
Black body, 195
Blurring, X-ray image, 11–3
Body scanning, X-ray CT, 87
Bolometer, 195
Bone studies, X-ray CT, 88–9
Boundary, behaviour of wave at, 139–41
Brain physiology, 237–44

Brain,
    radionuclide imaging, 111–6
    radionuclide perfusion study, 111–6
Breast thermography, 202–4
Bremsstrahlung, 3
B-scope, ultrasonic, 154

Canterbury filter, 271
Cardiac studies,
    X-ray CT, 90
    radionuclide, 117–21
    ultrasonic, 179–81, 189–91
C-d diagram, 38
Central nervous system, radionuclide imaging, 111–6
Cerebral spinal fluid dynamics, 116
Characteristic
    impedance, 140–1
    radiation, 3
Channel
    characteristic, 258
    response, 258–9
    model, spatial frequency specific, 255–9
Chemical shift, 219
Cholesteric liquid crystal, 194
Cine-fluorography, 35
Clinical applications,
    nuclear magnetic resonance imaging 232–3
    radionuclide imaging, 111–33
    thermographic imaging, 202–8
    traditional X-ray imaging, 46–52
    ultrasonic imaging, 178–90
    X-ray CT, 86–9
Colour, 271–2
Compton scattered radiation, 5
Computed tomography,
    emission radionuclide, 106–7
    ultrasonic, 171–2
    X-ray, 54–92
Concavity operator, 269
Cones, 237
Continuous wave Doppler systems, 163–4
Contrast
    detail diagram, 38
    media, 48
    scale, 75

Contrast,
    effect of scattered radiation on primary, 8–10
    factors affecting primary, 8
    objective, 21
    X-ray, 6–10
Convexity operator, 269
Cost-effectiveness, X-ray CT, 90–1
Crozier's law, 250
CT number, 67, 69, 82–3
Cupping effect, 80
Cyclotron, 96

Deadtime, 98
Decay process, radioactive, 95
Decibel notation, 144–5
Deep vein thrombosis, 207
Detection of complex visual images, 262–3
Detection, signal-specific noise-limited models, 244–55
Detector,
    semi-conductor, 110
    thermal, 195–6
    X-ray CT, 65–6
Diamagnetism, 213
Diffraction, NMR, 219
Digital radiography, 45–6
Digitisation of images, 267
Directionally sensitive Doppler systems, 164–7
Display, X-ray CT, 68–73
Doppler
    diagnostic methods, 162–70
    effect, ultrasonic, 143–4
    imaging, two-dimensional, 168–70
    signal analysis, 167–8
Dose, radiation,
    traditional X-ray, 27
    X-ray CT, 83–5
Duplex scanning, 170
Dynamic range, 66, 152

Echoplanar NMR, 223
Effective focal spot, 3
Elasticity, 138
Electronic real-time B-scanning, 157–61
Endocrinology, 129–30, 180
Evaluation of images, 237–80

Extra-focal radiation, 16
Eye physiology, 237–44

Fan beam, 63–4
Ferromagnetism, 213
Field
  size, 98
  uniformity, 98
Film
  badge, 24
  non-screen, emulsion design, 23–5
Filtered back projection, 62
Filtering, image, 69–71
Fluorescent screen
  characteristics, 19
  quantum limit, 18–19
Fluorography, 35, 46–7
Fluoroscopy, 19, 28–9, 46–7
Focused nuclear resonance, 224
Focusing, ultrasonic, 150
FONAR, 224
Foreign body localisation, 48
Fourier
  techniques, 15–16
  zeugmatography, 223–4
Fovea centralis, 238
Fraunhofer zone, 149
Free induction decay, 215
Fresnel zone, 149
Frequency
  -of-seeing curve, 243
  spectrum analyser, 167–8
Frequency, angular, 143
Full-width-half-maximum, 97
Future trends,
  NMR imaging, 233–4
  radionuclide imaging, 133
  thermographic imaging, 208–10
  ultrasonic imaging, 190–2
  X-ray CT, 89–91

Gamma camera, 101–6
Ganglion cells, 237
Gastric mucosal imaging, 131–2
Gastroenterology, 180–3
Genitourinary imaging, 127–9
Geometrical unsharpness, 11
Gray scale, 155, 267
Gynaecology, 184–5

H & D curve, 22
Haematological system, 124
Half-value layer, 4
Harmonisation, 43, 61
Hazard, possibility of in
  NMR imaging, 233
  ultrasonic imaging, 177–8
Head scanning, X-ray CT, 86–7
Heated-object spectrum, 272
High-kV radiography, 7–8
Histogram equalisation, 268
Holography, ultrasonic, 174–5
Hounsfield number, 82
Huygen's principle, 149

Image
  assessment methods, 275–7
  detection, 36–46
  distortion, 99
  enhancement, 43–4, 268–73
  evaluation, 237–80
  intensifier, 29–31, 265–6
    viewing and recording output, 31–2
    X-ray, 35–6
  latent photographic, 20
  linearity, 99
  perception, 36–46, 237–80
  processing, 268–75
    efficiency, 273–5
  quality,
    assessment, 275–8
    X-ray CT, 74–8
  restoration, 272
    iterative, 273
  sharpening, 270–1
  smoothing, 43, 269–70
  storage devices, 33–4, 155–6
  subtraction, 44, 272
  X-ray transducer, new types, 44–6
Imaging time, NMR, 229–31
Inflammation imaging, 130–1
Infrared thermography, 195
Intensity, ultrasonic, 144–5
Interference, ultrasonic wave, 141–3
Inverse
  filtering, 273
  square law, 4
Ionisation chamber, xenon, 66
Ionography, 44

Lacrimal duct imaging, 133
Large-field-of-view gamma camera, 102
Larmor theorem, 213
Lateral resolution, ultrasonic, 153
Leeds test object, 37
Line
  scan, NMR, 223
  spread function, 15
Linear
  array, ultrasonic, 157–61
  energy transfer, 95
Liquid crystal thermography, 194–5
Liver imaging, 124–7
Loss, ultrasonic, in biological materials, 147

M-mode, 154–5
Mach effect, 41, 44, 267–8
Macroradiography, 11, 14–5, 48
Magnetic moment, 213
Magnets for NMR, 225
Metz filter, 271
Microscopy, acoustic, 171–4
Microwave thermography, 209–10
Minification, 29
Modulation transfer function, 15–6, 76, 98, 246–7

Movement
  artifacts, 81
  unsharpness, 12
Multiple sensitive point, 222
Multiwire proportional chambers, 44–5

Neurology, 183–4
Noise
  detectability, 254–5
  equivalent
    power, 197
    temperature difference, 197
  masking, 259
Noise,
  effective, 246
  signal-specific effect of, 247–8
  visual, 243
  X-ray
    CT picture, 74
    transducer, 28
Nonlinearity, visual detection 266–7
Nuclear
  induction signal, 214
  magnetic resonance
    classical view, 213–5
    continuous wave spectroscopy, 220
    diffraction, 220
    Fourier zeugmatography, 223–4
    frequency, operating, 224–5
    high-resolution spectroscopy, 218–9
    images, 226–8
    imaging, 212–38
    imaging, future prospects, 233–4
    imaging methods, 219–24
    imaging systems, 224–6
    liquids and solids, in, 217–8
    magnets, 225
    performance of imaging systems, 226–33
    principles, 212–9
    pulsed spectroscopy, 220
    quantum view, 215–6
    resolution and imaging time, 229–31
    selective irradiation, 223
    simple apparatus, 215–6
    spectrometry and image display, 225–6
    spin-warp method, 231
    steady-state free precession, 220
    tissue discrimination, 229
  magnetic resonance,
    comparison of imaging methods, 231–2
    possibility of hazard, 233
    potential clinical applications, 232–5
  magneton, 213
  relaxation, time, 215–7
Nyquist frequency, 77

Objective contrast, 21
Obstetrics, 184–5
Oncology, 185–7

Ophthalmology, 186
Orthographic transmission imaging, 170–1

Paramagnetism, 213
Partial detection artifact, 81–2
Pattern recognition, 42–4
Perception of images, 237–80
Period, wave, 139
Phantoms, 36, 277–8
Phase angle, 142–3
Phased array, 160
Photoelectric absorption, 5
Photographic emulsion, 19–21
  characteristic curve, 21–4
Photomultiplier, 65, 101, 105
Photon
  detector, thermal 195–6
  tomography, annihilation, 106
Physiology, eye and brain, 237–44
Piezoelectricity, 146–9
Plane waves, ultrasonic, 141–3
Point spread function, 15, 61, 246–7
Positron tomography, 95, 106
Power, ultrasonic, 144–5
Precession, nuclear, 213
Precision, X-ray CT, 74–5
Profile, X-ray attenuation, 57
Projection, NMR reconstruction, 219–21
Proton, 212–3
Pseudo colour, 271
Pulmonary imaging, 116–7
Pulsed Doppler systems, 164
Pyroelectric detector, 196

Quality control, X-ray CT, 85
Quality, X-ray beam, 4
Quantum efficiency, 19

ROC curve, 244, 261–4
Radiographic contrast, 21
Radiography, 46–7
  as an imaging system, 25–7
  non-screen, 24
  sensitivity, 28
  serial, 47
  stereoscopic, 47–8
  unusual kV, 47
Radioisotope scanning, 93
Radiological distortion and magnification, 10–1
Radionuclide
  emission computed tomography, 106–7
  imaging, 93–137
    collimator, 97
    sensitivity, 98
    systems, 99–111
    instrumentation, 97–111
Radiopharmaceuticals, 93–6
Radiotherapy treatment planning, X-ray CT, 87–8
Rare earth screens, 27

Raynaud's disease, 206
Real-time ultrasonic scanners, 156–61, 191
Receiver operating characteristic (ROC) curve, 244, 261–4
Receptive field, 241–3
Recognition of complex visual images, 262–3
Rectilinear scanner, 99–101
Reconstruction,
  algebraic technique (ART), 60
  analogue methods, 64
  convolution, 61–3
  fan beam, 64
  iterative
    techniques, 59–61
    least squares technique (ILST), 60
  principles, 56–63
  simultaneous iterative technique (SIRT), 60
  X-ray CT analogue, 73–4
Recording, X-ray CT images, 68–73
References,
  nuclear magnetic resonance imaging, 234–6
  perception and evaluation of images, 278–80
  radionuclide imaging, 134–7
  thermographic imaging, 210–1
  traditional X-ray imaging, 52–3
  ultrasonic imaging, 192–3
  X-ray CT, 91–2
Reflexion of ultrasound, 140–1
Refraction of ultrasound, 139
Relaxation
  process, ultrasonic, 145–6
  time, nuclear, 215–7
  time, visual, 251
Renal imaging, 127–9
Resolution,
  energy, 98
  nuclear magnetic resonance, 229–31
  radionuclide imaging, 97
  ultrasonic
    Doppler, 167
    pulse-echo, 152–54
  X-ray
    CT, 75–8
    limiting, 36
Retina, 238–41
Ring artifact, 81
Rods, 237
Rose-de Vries model, 246
Rotating frame zeugmatography, 224

Salivary gland imaging, 131
Scan
  converter, 158
  speed, X-ray CT, 84
Scanning instruments, X-ray CT, 63–74
Scanogram, 67
Scattering, ultrasonic, 141–3
Scintillation
  camera, 97

Scintillation (cont'd.)
  detector, 93
Screen unsharpness, 13
Screening, 19, 28–9
  constant, 218
Scrotal thermography, 204–5
Secondary
  electron, 5
  radiation grid, 10
Sensitometric curve, 22
Serial changer, 47
Shift frequency, Doppler ultrasonic, 144
Signal detection theory, 248
  visual, 259–62
Single
  photon tomography, 106
  sensitive point, 222
Skeletal studies, 121–4
Skin lesions, 206
Small-field-of-view gamma camera, 102
Sodium iodide scintillator, 65, 93
Sound spectogram, 168
Spatial sampling aperture, 252–4
Specular reflexion, 140
Speed, ultrasonic, 138–9
Spin
  mapping, 221–2, 231
  -warp NMR, 231
Spleen imaging, 124–7
Spot film, 31
Static B-scanner, ultrasonic, 156
Steered array, ultrasonic, 160
Stomach motility, 132
Storage time, brain, 6
Streak artifacts, 80–1
Swept gain, 151–2

Television
  monitors, 34–5
  system, X-ray, 32–3
Temperature reference aperture, 198
Temporal sampling aperture, 250–2
Test objects, 36–8, 277–8
Theories of visual detection, application of, 263–8
Thermal
  detector performance, 197
  display systems, 198–200
  imaging systems, 197–8
Thermographic
  imaging, 194–211
  index, 205
Thermography,
  infrared, 195
  liquid crystal, 194–5
  microwave, 209–10
  physical and physiological factors, 200–8
Threshold
  contrast, 38, 245
  detection, 36, 43
Thrombus detection, 133
Time
  gain control, 151–2

Time (cont'd.)
  interval
    difference imaging, 46
    histogram, 168
  -position recording, 154–5
Tissue
  characterisation, ultrasonic, 175–6
  discrimination, NMR, 229
Tomography,
  annihilation photon and positron, 106
  computed
    emission, 106–7
    X-ray, 54–92
  positron emission, 95
  reconstruction, 53
  single photon, 106
  traditional X-ray, 48
  transverse axial, 54
  X-ray, 11–3
Traditional X-ray imaging, 1–53
Transducer,
  ultrasonic diagnostic, 146–9
  X-ray, 18–36
Translate-rotate scanning, 63
Transverse relaxation time, 215
Trauma, 208
Tumour imaging, 130–1
Two-dimensional B-scan, 155–62

Ultrasound detection and generation, 146–9
Ultrasound, fundamental physics, 138–44
Ultrasonic
  A-scope, 151
  B-scope, 154
  beam focusing, 150
  computed tomography, 171–2
  diagnosis, possible hazards of, 176–9
  distance measurements, 161
  Doppler
    diagnostic methods, 162–70
    imaging, 168–70
    resolution, 167
    signal analysis, 167–8
  duplex scanner, 170
  field, 149–51
    steady state, 149–50
    transient, 150–1
  high-resolution real-time scanning, 191
  holography, 174–5
  imaging, 138–93

Ultrasonic (cont'd.)
  intraoperative scanning, 192
  M-mode, 154–5
  orthographic transmission imaging, 170–1
  M-mode, 154–5
  orthographic transmission imaging, 170–1
  portable real-time scanning, 191
  pulse, 148–9
  time-position recording, 154–5
  tissue characterisation, 175–6
  transmission methods, 170–5
  two-dimensional
    arrays, 191–2
    B-scan, 155–62
  ultrafast scanning, 191
Ultrasonics,
  biological effects, 176–7
  future prospects, 190–2
Unsharpness,
  addition and effects, 13–5
  X-ray image, 11–3
Urology, 186–7

Vascular disorders, 206–8
Video-tape recorders, 33–4
Vidicon, pyroelectric, 209–10
Viewing
  box, 21
  distance, 263–5
Visual
  detection, 36
  effects in radiology, 41–2
  noise, 243
  pattern recognition, 36
  perception, 36
  system
    anatomy, 237–41
    Fourier analyser, as a, 257–8
    linearity, 243–4
    modification of object by, 246–7
    threshold detection model, 39–41

Water-bath B-scanner, 156
Wavelength, 138–9, 195
Waves, ultrasonic, 138–9
Weber's law, 243
Wiener filter, 273
Window, X-ray CT, 69–70

X-ray
  attenuation, typical in clinical situation, 6
  CT, system performance, 74–85
  coning, 9
  contrast, 6–10
    formation mechanisms, 6–7
    medium, 8
  detectors for CT, 65–6
  filter, 3
  fluorography and cine-fluorography, 35
  image
    formation and detection, 1–2
    intensifiers, 29–31
    sharpness, 10
    unsharpness, 11–3
    transducers, fluorescent screens, 18–9
    transducers, fluoroscopy and image intensifiers, 28–36
    radiography, 20–8
  images, clinical examples, 48–52
  imaging, shapes and fine structure: Fourier techniques, 10–8
  information in continuous and intermittent exposures, 6
  intensifying screen, 20
  interaction with matter, 4–6
  primary contrast calculation, 7–8
  production, 2–4
  quantum limit, 18
  sources, 64–5
  television systems, 32–4
  tomography, 11–3
  transducer characteristics, 27–8
  tube spectra, 3–4
  tubes, 2–3
  tube intensity distributions, 16–8
X-ray,
  characteristic radiation, 3
  factors affecting primary contrast in practice, 8
  general relationships in clinical practice, 6
  history, 1
  interactive mechanisms, 4–6
  linear attenuation coefficient, 4
  nature, 1
  quality of beam, 4
Xeroradiography, 44

Zero crossing counter, 167
Zeugmatography, 212, 219

NO LONGER THE PROPERTY
OF THE
UNIVERSITY OF R.I. LIBRARY